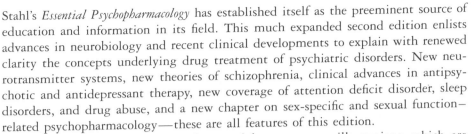

Stahl's *Essential Psychopharmacology* has established itself as the preeminent source of education and information in its field. This much expanded second edition enlists advances in neurobiology and recent clinical developments to explain with renewed clarity the concepts underlying drug treatment of psychiatric disorders. New neurotransmitter systems, new theories of schizophrenia, clinical advances in antipsychotic and antidepressant therapy, new coverage of attention deficit disorder, sleep disorders, and drug abuse, and a new chapter on sex-specific and sexual function—related psychopharmacology—these are all features of this edition.

The fully revised text is complemented by many new illustrations, which are instructive and entertaining as before and enhanced to reflect new knowledge and topics covered for the first time. The illustrations and their captions may be used independently of the main text for a rapid introduction to the field or for review. CME self-assessment tests are also included.

Even more, this will be the essential text for students, scientists, psychiatrists, and other mental health professionals, enabling them to master the complexities of psychopharmacology and plan sound treatment approaches based on current knowledge.

**Stephen M. Stahl** is Adjunct Professor of Psychiatry at the University of California, San Diego. He received his undergraduate and medical degrees from Northwestern University in Chicago and his Ph.D. degree in pharmacology and physiology from the University of Chicago and has trained in three specialties, internal medicine, neurology, and psychiatry. As a faculty member at Stanford University, the University of California at Los Angeles, the Institute of Psychiatry in London, and currently at the University of California at San Diego, Dr. Stahl has conducted numerous research projects awarded by the National Institute of Mental Health, the Veterans Administration, and the pharmaceutical industry. The author of more than 200 articles and chapters, Dr. Stahl is an internationally recognized clinician, researcher, and teacher. Lectures and courses based on *Essential Psychopharmacology* have taken him to dozens of countries to speak to tens of thousands of physicians, mental health professionals, and students at all levels.

# ESSENTIAL
# PSYCHOPHARMACOLOGY

## Neuroscientific Basis and Practical Applications
### Second Edition

## STEPHEN M. STAHL, M.D., Ph.D.

Adjunct Professor of Psychiatry
University of California, San Diego

*With illustrations by*
Nancy Muntner

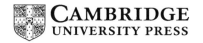

**CAMBRIDGE**
**UNIVERSITY PRESS**

PUBLISHED BY THE PRESS SYNDICATE OF THE UNIVERSITY OF CAMBRIDGE
The Pitt Building, Trumpington Street, Cambridge, United Kingdom

CAMBRIDGE UNIVERSITY PRESS
The Edinburgh Building, Cambridge CB2 2RU, UK
40 West 20th Street, New York, NY 10011-4211, USA
477 Williamstown Road, Port Melbourne, VIC 3207, Australia
Ruiz de Alarcón 13, 28014 Madrid, Spain
Dock House, The Waterfront, Cape Town 8001, South Africa

http://www.cambridge.org

Every effort has been made in preparing this book to provide accurate and up-
to-date information, which is in accord with accepted standards and practice at
the time of publication. Nevertheless, the authors, editors, and publisher can
make no warranties that the information contained herein is totally free from
error, not least because clinical standards are constantly changing through
research and regulation. The authors, editors, and publisher therefore
disclaim all liability for direct or consequential damages resulting from the
use of material contained in this book. Readers are strongly advised to pay
careful attention to information provided by the manufacturer of any drugs
or equipment that they plan to use.

First published 2000
Reprinted 2000, 2001, 2002 (twice)

Printed in the United States of America

Typeset in Garamond

*A catalog record for this book is available from the British Library*

*Library of Congress Cataloging-in-Publication Data*

Stahl, S. M.
    Essential psychopharmacology : neuroscientific basis and practical application / Stephen M. Stahl ;
with illustrations by Nancy Muntner.—2nd ed.
        p. ; cm.
    Includes bibliographical references and index.
    ISBN 0-521-64154-3 (hardback)—ISBN 0-521-64615-4 (pbk.)
    1. Mental illness—Chemotherapy.   2. Psychopharmacology.   I. Title.
    [DNLM:   1. Mental Disorders—drug therapy.   2. Central Nervous System—drug effects.
3. Psychotropic Drugs—pharmacology. WM 402 S78105e 2000]
    RC483 .S67 2000
    616.89′18—dc21
                                                                                                99-089281

ISBN 0 521 64154 3 hardback          ISBN 0 521 79560 5 hardback plus CD-ROM (teacher's set)
ISBN 0 521 64615 4 paperback         ISBN 0 521 78788 2 teacher's CD-ROM

# Reviews of *Essential Psychopharmacology, First Edition*

In memory of Daniel X. Freedman, mentor, colleague, and scientific father.

To Cindy, my wife, best friend, and tireless supporter.

To Jennifer and Victoria, my daughters, for their patience and understanding of the demands of authorship.

# PREFACE TO THE SECOND EDITION

Much has changed in psychopharmacology since the publication of the first edition of *Essential Psychopharmacology* four years ago. This second edition attempts to reflect the advances in neuroscience, in the understanding of psychiatric disorders, and in the dozens of new medications for psychiatric disorders that have dramatically advanced the field of psychopharmacology in this brief period of time. Thus, two chapters have been added, 11 of the 12 earlier chapters have been extensively revised, and the length of the written text has been increased by about 50%. What has not changed is the didactic style of the first edition, which continues in this edition and is largely based on updated lectures, slides, and articles of the author. Thus, new materials are presented, with an emphasis on color pictures, which have more than doubled in this edition to over 500 in total.

Also newly included in this edition are materials at the end of each chapter for readers interested in using the text materials to receive continuing medical education credits. Since the lessons in these chapters are used widely by the author for lecturing to medical practitioners, they have been accredited by the University of California, San Diego as enduring materials for up to 54 category I continuing medical education credit hours according to the guidelines of the Accreditation Council of Continuing Medical Education (ACCME) of the American Medical Association. Tests are included at the end of each chapter, and instructions for submitting them and the required fees are all explained at the end of the textbook for those readers who are interested.

In general, this text attempts to present the fundamentals of psychopharmacology in simplified and readily readable form. Thus, this material should prepare the reader to consult more sophisticated textbooks as well as the professional literature. The organization of the information here also applies principles of programmed learning for the reader, namely repetition and interaction, which have been shown to enhance retention.

Therefore, it is suggested that novices first approach this text by going through it from beginning to end, reviewing only the color graphics and the legends for these graphics. Virtually everything covered in the text is also covered in the graphics and icons. Once having gone through all the color graphics in these chapters, it is recommended that the reader then go back to the beginning of the book and read the entire text, reviewing the graphics at the same time. Finally, after the text has been read, the entire book can be rapidly reviewed merely by referring to the various color graphics.

This approach to using the materials will create a certain amount of programmed learning by incorporating the elements of repetition as well as interaction with visual learning through graphics. Hopefully, the visual concepts learned via graphics will reinforce abstract concepts learned from the written text, especially for those of you who are primarily "visual learners" (i.e., those who retain information better from visualizing concepts than from reading about them).

For those who are already familiar with psychopharmacology, this book should provide easy reading from beginning to end. Going back and forth between the text and the graphics should provide interaction. Following review of the complete text, it should be simple to review the entire book by going through the graphics once again.

The text is purposely written at a conceptual level rather than a pragmatic level and includes ideas that are simplifications and rules, while sacrificing precision and discussion of exceptions to rules. Thus, this is not a text intended for the sophisticated subspecialist in psychopharmacology.

One other limitation of the book is that it is not extensively referenced to original papers but rather to textbooks and reviews, including several of the author's.

For those interested in the specific updates made in the second edition, the first section on basic science has expanded coverage of gene expression and transcription factors; of developmental neurobiology, neuronal selection, synaptogenesis, and growth factors; of the complex genetics of psychiatric disorders; and of new concepts of neurodegeneration such as apoptosis, with dozens of new color graphics.

The second section on clinical science has been increased by two chapters to accommodate the increase in the numbers of drugs and advances in knowledge about psychiatric disorders. Three new neurotransmitter systems are introduced and illustrated: substance P and the neurokinin family; nitric oxide; and the endocannabinoids such as anandamide (the "brain's own marijuana"). Also amplified is coverage of the classical neurotransmitter systems, especially intercommunications now illustrated between serotonin and dopamine and between norepinephrine/noradrenaline and serotonin. Also included are numerous new illustrations of noradrenergic and cholinergic pathways.

In the clinical syndrome chapters, there is now coverage of several new topics, including bipolar disorders, attention deficit disorder, erectile dysfunction, the role of estrogen in mood and cognitive disorders across the female life cycle, disorders in children and adolescents (in part), and pharmacokinetics of psychopharmacologic drugs. Some sections have been revised, including those on sleep disorders, and schizophrenia and psychotic disorders. In the clinical therapeutics chapters, the explosion of new therapeutics is reflected by the inclusion of over 30 new icons for drugs that appear for the first time in the second edition, including new antidepressants, mood stabilizers, atypical antipsychotics, acetylcholinesterase inhibitors, phosphodiesterase inhibitors, sedative hypnotics, and several others.

I would be remiss if I did not thank my editors at Cambridge University Press for their most helpful suggestions and exhortations to get this edition in on time.

Best wishes for your first step on your journey into this fascinating field of psychopharmacology.

STEPHEN M. STAHL, M.D., Ph.D.

# CONTENTS

# CHAPTER 1

# PRINCIPLES OF CHEMICAL NEUROTRANSMISSION

Modern psychopharmacology is largely the story of chemical neurotransmission. To understand the actions of drugs on the brain, to grasp the impact of diseases on the central nervous system (CNS), and to interpret the behavioral consequences of psychiatric medicines, one must be fluent in the language and principles of chemical neurotransmission. The importance of this fact cannot be overstated for the student of psychopharmacology. What follows in this chapter will form the foundation for the entire book and the roadmap for one's journey through one of the most exciting topics in science today, namely the neuroscience of how drugs act on the CNS.

## The Synapse

The best understood chemical neurotransmission occurs at synapses, specialized sites that connect two neurons. Neurons are organized so that they can both send synaptic

1

information to other neurons and receive synaptic information from other neurons. Figure 1–1 is an artist's concept of how a neuron is organized in order to *send* synaptic information. This is accomplished by a long *axon* branching into terminal fibers ready to make synaptic contact with other neurons. Figure 1–2, by contrast, shows how a neuron is organized to *receive* synaptic information on its dendrites, cell body, and axon. The synapse itself is enlarged conceptually in Figure 1–3, showing its specialized structure, which enables chemical neurotransmission to occur.

## Three Dimensions of Neurotransmission

Chemical neurotransmission can be described in three dimensions: space, time and function.

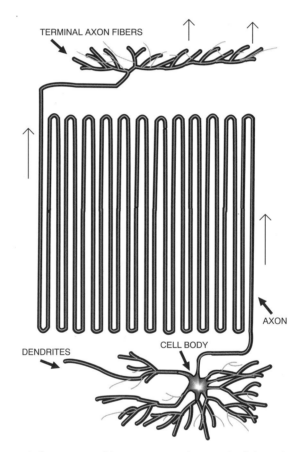

TERMINAL AXON FIBERS

AXON

DENDRITES

CELL BODY

FIGURE 1–1. This is an artist's concept of how a neuron is organized in order to **send** synaptic information. It does this via a long **axon**, which sends its information into numerous branches called **terminal axon fibers**. Each of these axon terminals can potentially make presynaptic contacts with other neurons. Also shown is the **cell body**, which is the command center of the nerve, contains the nucleus of the cell, and processes both incoming and outgoing information. The **dendrites** are organized largely to capture information from other neurons (see also Fig. 1–2).

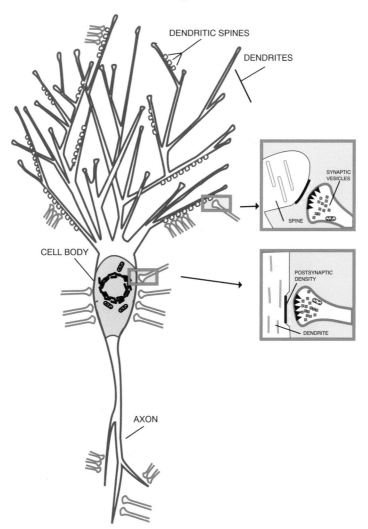

FIGURE 1−2. This figure shows how a neuron is organized to **receive** synaptic information. Presynaptic input from other neurons can be received postsynaptically at many sites, but especially on **dendrites**, often at specialized structures called **dendritic spines**. Other postsynaptic neuronal sites for receiving presynaptic input from other neurons include the **cell body** and **axon terminal**.

## Space: *The Anatomically Addressed Nervous System*

Classically, the central nervous system has been envisioned as a series of "hard-wired" synaptic connections between neurons, not unlike millions of telephone wires within thousands upon thousands of cables (Fig. 1−4). This idea has been referred to as the "anatomically addressed" nervous system. The anatomically addressed brain is thus a complex wiring diagram, ferrying electrical impulses to wherever the "wire" is plugged in (i.e., at a synapse). There are an estimated 100 billion neurons, which make over 100 trillion synapses, in a single human brain.

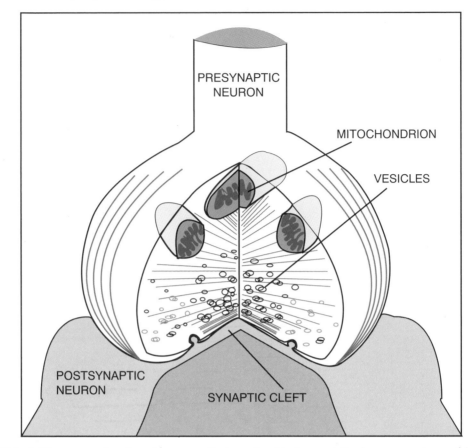

FIGURE 1–3. The synapse is enlarged conceptually here showing its specialized structures that enable chemical neurotransmission to occur. Specifically, a **presynaptic neuron** sends its **axon terminal** to form a synapse with a **postsynaptic neuron**. Energy for this process is provided by mitochondria in the presynaptic neuron. Chemical neurotransmitter is stored in small vesicles ready for release on firing of the presynaptic neuron. The **synaptic cleft** is the connection between the presynaptic neuron and the postsynaptic neuron. Receptors are present on both sides of this cleft and are key elements of chemical neurotransmission.

Neurons send electrical impulses from one part of the cell to another part of the same cell via their axons, but these electrical impulses do not jump directly to other neurons. Neurons communicate by one neuron hurling a chemical messenger, or neurotransmitter, at the receptors of a second neuron. This happens frequently, but not exclusively, at the sites of synaptic connections between them (Fig. 1–3). Communication *between* neurons is therefore chemical, not electrical. That is, an electrical impulse in the first neuron is converted to a chemical signal at the synapse between it and a second neuron, in a process known as chemical neurotransmission. This occurs predominantly in one direction, from the presynaptic axon terminal, to any of a variety of sites on a second postsynaptic neuron. However, it is increasingly apparent that the postsynaptic neuron can also "talk back" to the presynaptic neuron with chemical messengers of its own, perhaps such as the neurotransmitter nitric oxide. The frequency and extent of such cross-communication may determine how

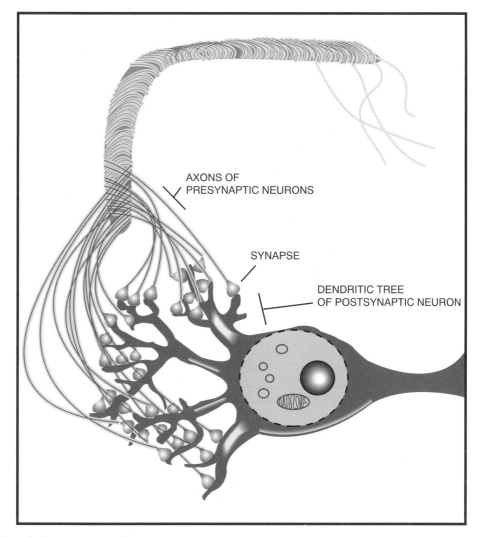

FIGURE 1–4. The **anatomically addressed nervous system** is the concept that the brain is a series of hard-wired connections between neurons, not unlike millions of telephone wires within thousands and thousands of cables. Shown in the figure is a cable of axons from many different neurons, all arriving to form synaptic connections with the dendritic tree of the postsynaptic neuron.

well that synapse functions. Thus, mental "exercise" may provoke progressive structural changes at a synapse, which increase the ease of neurotransmission there (Fig. 1–3).

### Space: The Chemically Addressed Nervous System

More recently, neurotransmission without a synapse has been described, which is called *volume neurotransmission* or nonsynaptic diffusion neurotransmission. Chemical messengers sent by one neuron to another can spill over to sites distant to the synapse by diffusion. Thus, neurotransmission can occur at any compatible receptor within the diffusion radius of the neurotransmitter, not unlike modern communication with cellular telephones, which function within the transmitting radius of a given cell (Fig. 1–5). This concept is called the *chemically addressed* nervous system, where neurotransmission occurs in chemical "puffs." The brain is thus not only a collection of wires but also a sophisticated "chemical soup." The chemically addressed nervous system is particularly important in understanding the actions of drugs that act at various neurotransmitter receptors, since such drugs will act wherever there are relevant receptors and not just where such receptors are innervated with synapses by the anatomically addressed nervous system.

## Time: Fast-Onset versus Slow-Onset Signals

Some neurotransmitter signals are very fast in onset, starting within milliseconds of receptors being occupied by neurotransmitter. Two of the best examples of fast-onset signals are those caused by the neurotransmitters glutamate and gamma-aminobutyric acid (GABA). Glutamate is a neurotransmitter that universally stimulates almost any neuron, whereas GABA is a messenger that universally inhibits almost any neuron (Fig. 1–6). Both of these neurotransmitters can cause fast onset of chemical signaling by rapidly changing the flux of ions, thus altering within milliseconds the excitability of the neuron.

On the other hand, signals from other neurotransmitters can take longer to develop, ranging from many milliseconds to even several full seconds of time. Sometimes these neurotransmitters with slower onset are called neuromodulators, since slow-onset ionic signals may last long enough to carry over and modulate a subsequent neurotransmission by another neurotransmitter (Fig. 1–6). Thus, a slow-onset but long-acting neuromodulating signal can set the tone of a neuron and influence it not only by a primary action of its own, but also by a modifying action on the neurotransmission of a second chemical message sent before the first signal is gone. Examples of slow-onset, long-acting neurotransmitters are the monoamines norepinephrine and serotonin, as well as various neuropeptides. Although their signals can take seconds to develop, the biochemical cascades that they trigger can last for days.

## Function: Presynaptic Events

The third dimension of chemical neurotransmission is function, namely that cascade of molecular and cellular events set into action by the *chemical signaling* process. First come the presynaptic and then the postsynaptic events. An electrical impulse in the first, or presynaptic, neuron is converted into a chemical signal at the synapse by a process known as *excitation-secretion coupling*.

Once an electrical impulse invades the presynaptic axon terminal, it causes the release of chemical neurotransmitter stored there (Fig. 1–3). Electrical impulses open ion channels, such as *voltage-gated calcium channels* and *voltage-gated sodium channels*, by changing the ionic charge across neuronal membranes. As calcium flows into the presynaptic nerve, it anchors the synaptic vesicles to the inner membrane of the nerve terminal so that they can spill their chemical contents into the synapse. The way is paved for chemical communication by previous synthesis and storage of neurotransmitter in the first neuron's presynaptic axon terminal.

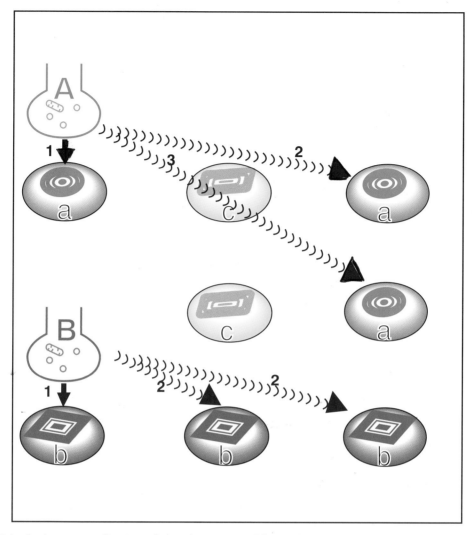

FIGURE 1–5. A conceptualization of the **chemically addressed nervous system** is shown. Two anatomically addressed synapses (neurons A and B) are shown communicating (*arrow 1*) with their corresponding postsynaptic receptors (*a* and *b*). However, there are also receptors for neurotransmitter *a*, neurotransmitter *b*, and neurotransmitter *c*, which are distant from the synaptic connections of the anatomically addressed nervous system. If neurotransmitter A can diffuse away from its synapse before it is destroyed, it will be able to interact with other receptor a sites distant from its own synapse (*arrow 2*). If neurotransmitter A encounters a different receptor not capable of recognizing it (receptor *c*), it will not interact with that receptor even if it diffuses there (*arrow 3*). Thus, a chemical messenger sent by one neuron to another can spill over by diffusion to sites distant from its own synapse. Neurotransmission can occur at a compatible receptor within the diffusion radius of the matched neurotransmitter. This is analogous to modern communication with cellular telephones, which function within the transmitting radius of a given cell. This concept is called the **chemically addressed** nervous system, in which neurotransmission occurs in chemical "puffs." The brain is thus not only a collection of wires (Fig. 1–2 and the anatomically addressed nervous system), but also a sophisticated "chemical soup" (Fig. 1–3 and the chemically addressed nervous system).

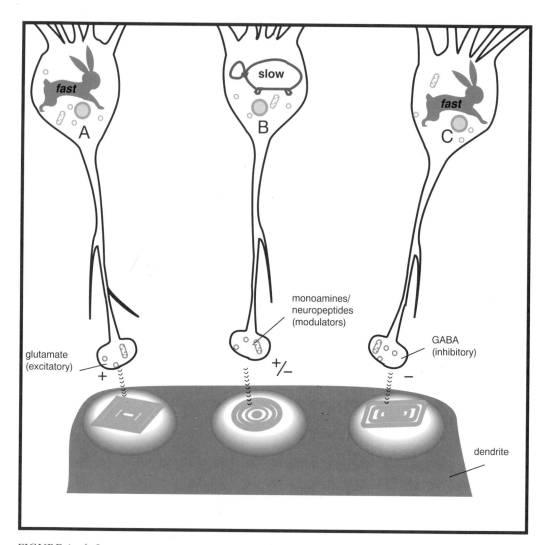

FIGURE 1–6. Some neurotransmitter signals are **fast** in onset (rabbit/hare neurons A and C) whereas other transmitter signals are **slow** in onset (tortoise neuron B). The neurotransmitter **glutamate** (neuron A) is fast in onset and **excitatory** (+), whereas the neurotransmitter **GABA** (neuron C) is fast on onset and **inhibitory** (−). In contrast to the fast glutamate and GABA signals, neurotransmission following those neurotransmitters known as **monoamines** or **neuropeptides** tends to be slow in onset (neuron B) and either excitatory (+) or inhibitory (−). Fast in this context is a few milliseconds, whereas slow signals are many milliseconds or even several full seconds of time. Slower-onset neurotransmitters may nevertheless be long-acting. They are sometimes called **neuromodulators**, since they may modulate a different signal from another neurotransmitter. In this figure, three neurons (A, B, and C) are all transmitting to a postsynaptic dendrite on the same neuron. If the slow signal from B is still present when a fast signal from A or C arrives, the B signal will modulate the A or C signal. Thus, a long-acting neuromodulating signal of neuron B can set the tone of the postsynaptic neuron, not only by a primary action of its own but also by modifying the action of neurons A and C.

When presynaptic neurons use monoamine neurotransmitters, they manufacture not only the monoamine neurotransmitters themselves but also the *enzymes* for mono-amine synthesis (Fig. 1–7), the *receptors* for monoamine reuptake and regulation (Fig. 1–8) and the *synaptic vesicles* loaded with monoamine neurotransmitter. They do this on receiving instructions from the "command center" or headquarters, namely the cell nucleus containing the neuron's deoxy-ribonucleic acid (DNA). These activities occur in the cell body of the neuron, but then monoamine presynaptic neurons send all of these items to the presynaptic nerve terminals, which act as "field offices" for that neuron throughout the brain (Figs. 1–1 to 1–3, 1–7, 1–8). Neurotransmitter is thus packaged and stored in the presynaptic neuron in vesicles, like a loaded gun ready to fire.

Since the enzyme machinery to manufacture more monoamines is present in axon terminals (Fig. 1–7), additional monoamine neurotransmitters can be synthesized there. Since a reuptake pump, which can recapture released monoamines, is present on the presynaptic neuron (Fig. 1–8), monoamines used in one neurotransmission can be captured for reuse in a subsequent neurotransmission. This is in contrast to the way in which neuropeptides function in neurotransmission (Fig. 1–9).

In the case of neuropeptides, presynaptic neurotransmission synthesis occurs only in the *cell body* because the complex machinery for neuropeptide synthesis is *not* transported into the axon terminal. Synthesis of a specific neuropeptide begins with the *pre-propeptide gene* in the cell nucleus (Fig. 1–9). This gene is transcribed into primary ribonucleic acid (RNA), which can be rearranged, or "edited," to create different versions of RNA, known as alternative splice variants, such as pre-propeptide RNA.

Next, this RNA is translated into a pre-propeptide, which enters the endoplasmic reticulum (Fig. 1–9). This is the "precursor of a precursor," sometimes also called the "grandparent" of the neuropeptide neurotransmitter. This pre-propeptide grand-parent neuropeptide has a peptide "tail," called a signal peptide, which allows the pre-propeptide to enter the endoplasmic reticulum, where the tail is clipped off by an enzyme called a signal peptidase with formation of the propeptide, or "parent" of the neuropeptide. The propeptide is the direct precursor of the neuropeptide neurotransmitter itself.

This parental propeptide then leaves the endoplasmic reticulum and enters synaptic vesicles, where it is finally converted into the neuropeptide itself by a converting enzyme located there. Since only the synaptic vesicles loaded with neuro-peptide neurotransmitters and not the synthetic enzyme machinery to make more neuropeptides, are transported down to the axon terminals, no local synthesis of more neuropeptide neurotransmitter can occur in the axon terminal.

Furthermore, there does not appear to be any significant reuptake pump for neu-ropeptides, so once they are released, they are not recaptured for subsequent reuse (Fig. 1–9). The action of peptides is terminated by catabolic peptidases, which cut the peptide neurotransmitter into inactive metabolites.

## *Function: Postsynaptic Events*

Once neurotransmitter has been fired from the presynaptic neuron, it shoots across the synapse, where it seeks out and hits target sites on receptors of the postsynaptic neuron that are very selective for that neurotransmitter. (This will be discussed in

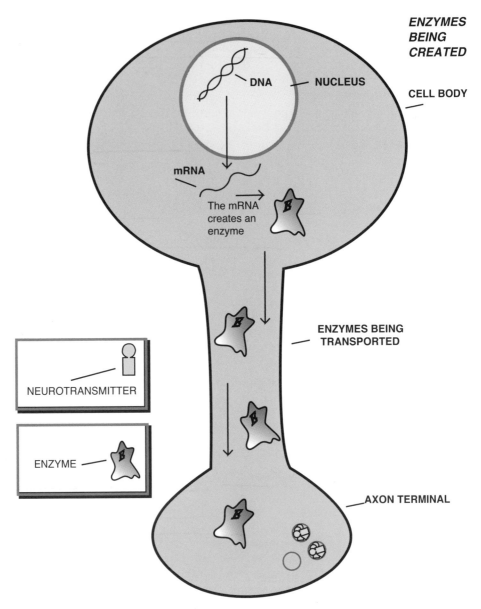

FIGURE 1–7. Shown here is the axonal transport of monoamine-synthesizing enzymes in a monoaminergic neuron. Enzymes are protein molecules, which are **created** (synthesized) in the **cell body**,
starting in the cell **nucleus**. Once synthesized, enzymes may be **transported** down the axon to the
**axon terminal** to perform functions necessary for neurotransmission, such as making or destroying
neurotransmitter molecules. **DNA** in the cell nucleus is the "command center," where orders to carry
out the synthesis of enzyme proteins are executed. DNA is a template for **mRNA** synthesis, which
in turn is a template for protein synthesis in order to form the enzyme by classical molecular rules.

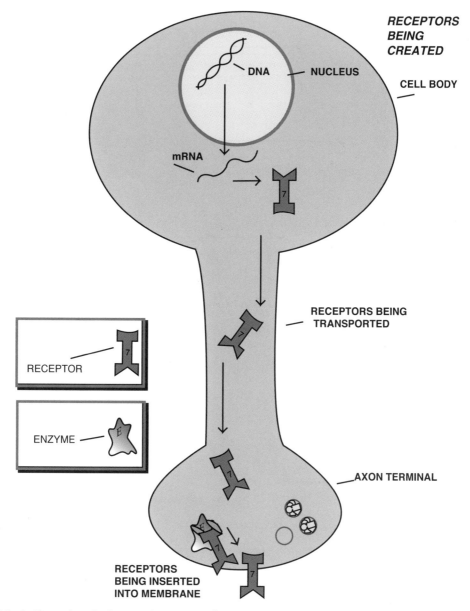

FIGURE 1–8. Shown here is the axonal transport of a presynaptic receptor in a monoaminergic neuron. In analogy with the process shown in Figure 1–7, receptors are also protein molecules created (synthesized) in the cell body of the neuron. Receptors can also be transported to various parts of the neuron, including the axon terminal, where they can be inserted into neuronal membranes to perform various functions during neurotransmission, such as capturing and reacting to neurotransmitters released from incoming signals sent by neighboring neurons.

11

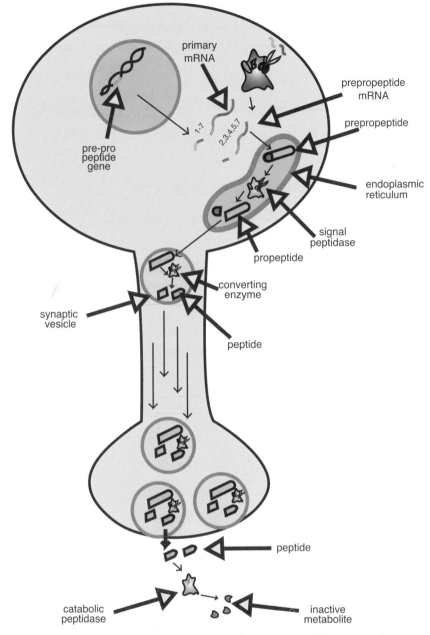

FIGURE 1–9. Neurotransmitter synthesis in a neuropeptidergic neuron. Neurotransmitter synthesis occurs only in the **cell body** because the complex machinery for neuropeptide synthesis is not transported into the axon terminal. Synthesis of a specific neuropeptide begins with the transcription of the pre-propeptide gene in the cell nucleus into primary RNA, which can be rearranged or "edited" to create different versions of RNA, known as alternative splice variants or **pre-propeptide** RNA. Next, RNA is translated into a **pre-propeptide**, which enters the endoplasmic reticulum, where its peptide tail is clipped off by an enzyme called a signal peptidase to form the propeptide, the direct precursor of the neuropeptide neurotransmitter. Finally, the propeptide enters synaptic vesicles, where it is converted into the **neuropeptide** itself. Synaptic vesicles loaded with neuropeptide neurotransmitters are transported down to the axon terminals, where there is no reuptake pump for neuropeptides. The action of peptides is terminated by catabolic peptidases, which cut the peptide neurotransmitter into inactive metabolites.

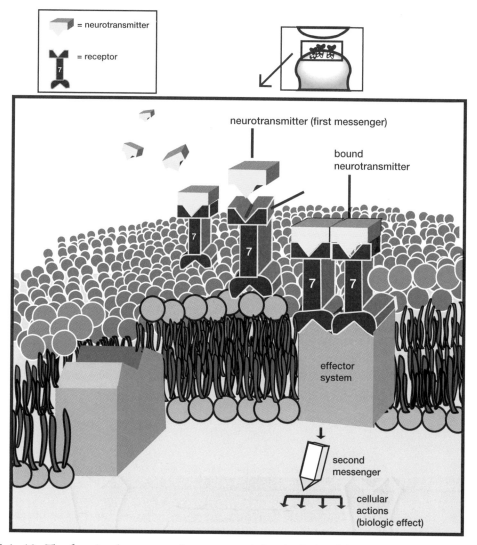

FIGURE 1–10. The functional outcome of neurotransmission is depicted here in the postsynaptic neuron. **Neurotransmitter** released from the presynaptic neuron is considered the **first messenger**. It binds to its **receptor** and the **bound neurotransmitter** causes an **effector system** to manufacture a **second messenger**. That second messenger is inside the cell of the postsynaptic neuron. It is this second messenger that then goes on to create **cellular actions** and **biological effects**. Examples of this are the neuron beginning to synthesize a chemical product changing its firing rate. Thus, information in the presynaptic neuron is conveyed to the postsynaptic neuron by a chain of events. This is how the brain is envisioned to do its work—thinking, remembering, controlling movement, etc. —through the synthesis of brain chemicals and the firing of brain neurons.

much greater detail in the section below on molecular neurobiology and in Chapters 2, 3, and 4). Receptor occupancy by neurotransmitter binding to highly specific sites begins the postsynaptic events of chemical neurotransmission (Fig. 1–10). This process is very similar to the binding of substrates by enzymes at their active sites. The neurotransmitter acts as a key fitting the receptor lock quite selectively.

Classically, it has been held that this neurotransmitter-receptor complex initiates a process that reconverts the chemical message back into an electrical impulse in the second nerve. This is certainly true for rapid-onset neurotransmitters and can explain the initial actions of some slow-onset neurotransmitters as well. However, it is now known that the postsynaptic neuron has a vast repertoire of responses beyond just whether it changes its membrane polarization to make it more or less likely to "fire." Indeed, many important biochemical processes are triggered in the postsynaptic neuron by neurotransmitters occupying their receptors. Some of these begin within milliseconds, whereas others can take days to develop (Figs. 1–11 to 1–13).

Thus, chemical neurotransmission in the postsynaptic neuron begins with receptor occupancy by the neurotransmitter, the *first messenger*. This leads to numerous intracellular events, starting with additional messengers within the cell (Fig. 1–10). The *second messenger* is an intracellular chemical, which is created by the first messenger neurotransmitter occupying the receptor outside of the cell, in the synaptic connection between the first and the second neuron. The best examples of second messengers are cyclic adenosine monophosphate (cAMP) and phosphatidyl inositol. Some receptors are linked to one type of second messenger and others to different second messengers.

The second messenger intracellular signal eventually tells the second neuron to change its ionic fluxes, to propagate or disrupt neuronal electrical impulses, to phosphorylate intracellular proteins, and to perform many, many other actions. It does this by a biochemical cascade, which eventually reaches the cell nucleus and results in genes being turned on or turned off (Fig. 1–11). Once gene expression is so triggered, a second biochemical cascade based on the direct consequences of which specific genes have been turned on or off is initiated (Fig. 1–12). Many of these events are still mysteries to neuroscientists. These events of postsynaptic neurotransmission are akin to a molecular "pony express" system, with the chemical information encoded within a neurotransmitter-receptor complex being passed along from molecular rider to molecular rider until the message is delivered to the appropriate DNA mailbox in the postsynaptic neuron's genome (Fig. 1–11).

Thus, the function of chemical neurotransmission is not so much to have a presynaptic neurotransmitter communicate with its postsynaptic receptors as to have a *presynaptic genome converse with a postsynaptic genome*: DNA to DNA; presynaptic command center to postsynaptic command center.

In summary, the message of chemical neurotransmission is transferred via three sequential molecular pony express routes: (1) a presynaptic neurotransmitter synthesis route from the presynaptic genome to the synthesis and packaging of neurotransmitter and supporting enzymes and receptors (Figs. 1–7, 1–8, and 1–9); (2) a postsynaptic route from receptor occupancy through second messengers (Fig. 1–10) all the way to the genome, which turns on postsynaptic genes (Fig. 1–11); and (3) another postsynaptic route, starting from the newly expressed postsynaptic genes transferring information as a molecular cascade of biochemical consequences throughout the postsynaptic neuron (Fig. 1–12).

It should now be clear that neurotransmission does not end when a neurotransmitter binds to a receptor or even when ion flows have been altered or second messengers have been created. Events such as these all start and end within milliseconds to seconds following release of presynaptic neurotransmitter (Fig. 1–13). The ultimate goal of neurotransmission is to alter the biochemical activities of the

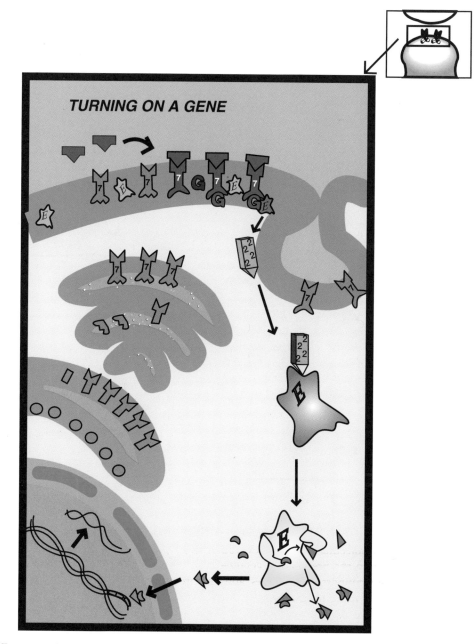

FIGURE 1–11. Shown here is a neurotransmitter setting off a cascade that results in turning on a gene. The neurotransmitter binds to its receptor at the top, creating a second messenger. The second messenger activates an intracellular enzyme, which results in the creation of transcription factors (*red arrowheads*) that cause gene activation (red DNA segment).

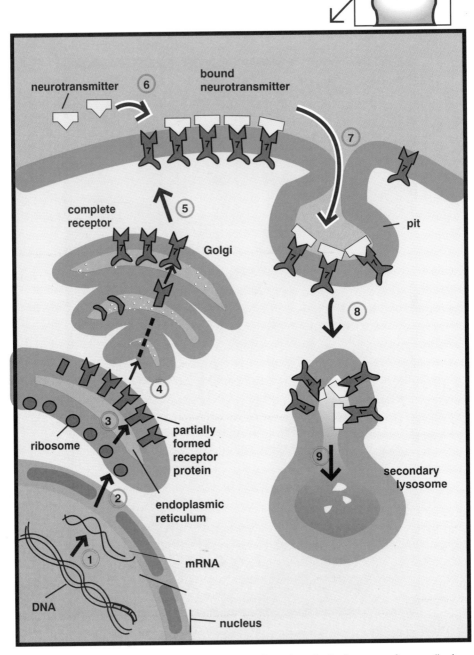

FIGURE 1–12. As in Figures 1–7 to 1–9, DNA in the cell nucleus is the "command center," where orders to carry out the synthesis of receptor proteins are executed. DNA is a template for **mRNA** synthesis, which in turn is a template for protein synthesis in order to form the receptor by classical molecular rules. Shown in this figure is the molecular neurobiology of receptor synthesis. The process begins in the cell nucleus, when a gene (red DNA segment) is transcribed into messenger RNA

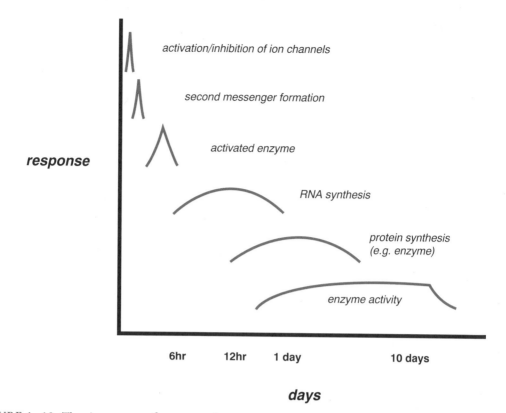

response

activation/inhibition of ion channels

second messenger formation

activated enzyme

RNA synthesis

protein synthesis
(e.g. enzyme)

enzyme activity

6hr    12hr    1 day              10 days

days

FIGURE 1–13. The time course of postsynaptic responses to presynaptic neurotransmitter are shown here. At the top, the most immediate actions are on **ion channels** or **second messenger formation**. Next comes **activation of intracellular enzymes**, leading to transcription of genes into **RNA synthesis**. This leads naturally to translation of RNA into **proteins**. Proteins have functions, which include such actions as **enzyme activity**. By the time enzyme activity has begun, it is already hours after the initial neurotransmission event. Once so activated, the functional changes in enzyme activity can last for many days. Thus, the ultimate effects of neurotransmission are not only delayed but long-lasting.

(*arrow 1*). Messenger RNA then travels to the endoplasmic reticulum (*arrow 2*), where ribosomes cause the messenger RNA to be translated into partially formed receptor protein (*arrow 3*). The next step is for partially formed receptor protein to be transformed into complete receptor molecules in the golgi apparatus (*arrow 4*). Completely formed receptor molecules are proteins and these are transported to the cell membrane (*arrow 5*) where they can interact with neurotransmitters (*arrow 6*). Neurotransmitters can bind to the receptor, as shown in Figure 1–10. In addition to causing second messenger systems to be triggered, as shown in Figure 1–10, the bound neurotransmitter may also reversibly cause the membrane to form a *pit* (*arrow 7*). This process takes the bound receptor out of circulation when the neuron wants to decrease the number of receptors available. This can be reversed or it can progress into **lysosomes** (*arrow 8*), where receptors are destroyed (*arrow 9*). This helps to remove old receptors so that they can be replaced by new receptors coming from DNA in the cell nucleus.

postsynaptic target neuron in a profound and enduring manner. Since the post-synaptic DNA has to wait until molecular pony express messengers make their way from the postsynaptic receptors, often located on dendrites, to the postsynaptic neuron's nucleus (Fig. 1–11), it can take a while for neurotransmission to begin influencing the postsynaptic target neurons' biochemical processes (Fig. 1–13). The time it takes from receptor occupancy by neurotransmitter to gene expression is usually hours. Furthermore, since the last messenger triggered by neurotransmission, called a transcription factor, only initiates the very beginning of gene action (Fig. 1–11), it takes even longer for the gene activation to be fully implemented via the series of biochemical events it triggers (Figs. 1–12 and 1–13). These biochemical events can begin many hours to days after the neurotransmission occurred and can last days or weeks once they are put in motion (Fig. 1–13).

Thus, a brief puff of chemical neurotransmission from a presynaptic neuron can trigger a profound postsynaptic reaction, which takes hours to days to develop and can last days to weeks or even longer. Every conceivable component of this entire process of chemical neurotransmission is a candidate for modification by drugs. Most psychotropic drugs act on the processes that control chemical neurotransmission at the level of the neurotransmitters themselves or of their enzymes and especially their receptors. Future psychotropic drugs will undoubtedly act directly on the biochemical cascades, particularly on those elements that control the expression of pre- and postsynaptic genes. Also, mental and neurological illnesses are known or suspected to affect these same aspects of chemical neurotransmission.

## Multiple Neurotransmitters

The known or suspected neurotransmitters in the brain already number several dozen (Table 1–1). Based on theoretical considerations of the amount of genetic material in neurons, there may be several hundred to several thousand unique brain chemicals. Originally, about half a dozen "classical" neurotransmitters were known. In recent years, an ever increasing number of neurotransmitters are being discovered. The classical neurotransmitters are relatively low molecular weight amines or amino acids. Now we know that strings of amino acids called *peptides* can also have neurotransmitter actions, and many of the newly discovered neurotransmitters are peptides, which are specifically called *neuropeptides* (Fig. 1–9).

### God's Pharmacopoeia

Some naturally occurring neurotransmitters may be similar to drugs we use. For example, it is well known that the brain makes its own morphine (i.e., beta endorphin), and its own marijuana (i.e., anandamide). The brain may even make its own antidepressants, it own anxiolytics, and its own hallucinogens. Drugs often mimic the brain's natural neurotransmitters. Often, drugs are discovered prior to the natural neurotransmitter. Thus, we knew about morphine before the discovery of beta-endorphin; marijuana before the discovery of cannabinoid receptors and anandamide; the benzodiazepines diazepam (Valium) and alprazolam (Xanax) before the discovery of benzodiazepine receptors; and the antidepressants amitriptyline (Elavil) and fluoxetine (Prozac) before the discovery of the serotonin transporter site. This un-

Table 1–1. *Neurotransmitters in brain*

*Amines*
- Serotonin (5HT)
- Dopamine (DA)
- Norepinephrine (NE)
- Epinephrine (E)
- Acetylcholine (Ach)
- Tyramine
- Octopamine
- Phenylethylamine
- Tryptamine
- Melatonin
- Histamine

*Pituitary Peptides*
- Corticotropin (ACTH)
- Growth hormone (GH)
- Lipotropin
- Alpha-melanocyte–stimulating hormone (alpha-MSH)
- Oxytocin
- Vasoporessin
- Thyroid-stimulating hormone (TSH)
- Prolactin

*Circulating Hormones*
- Angiotensin
- Calcitonin
- Glucagon
- Insulin
- Leptin
- Atrial natriuretic factor
- Estrogens
- Androgens
- Progestins
- Thyroid hormones

*Hypothalamic-Releasing Hormones*
- Corticotropin-releasing factor (CRH)
- Gonadotropin-releasing hormone (GnRH)
- Somatostatin
- Thyrotropin-releasing hormone (TRH)

*Amino Acids*
- Gamma-aminobutyric acid (GABA)
- Glycine
- Glutamic acid (glutamate)
- Aspartic acid (aspartate)
- Gamma-hydroxybutyrate

*Gut Hormones*
- Cholecystokinin (CCK)
- Gastrin
- Motilin
- Pancreatic polypeptide
- Secretin
- Vasoactive intestinal peptide (VIP)

*Opioid Peptides*
- Dynorphin
- Beta-endorphin
- Met-enkephalin
- Leu-enkephalin
- Kyotorphin

*Miscellaneous Peptides*
- Bombesin
- Bradykinin
- Carnosine
- Neuropeptide Y
- Neurotensin
- Delta sleep factor
- Galanin
- Oxerin

*Gases*
- Nitric oxide (NO)
- Carbon monoxide (CO)

*Lipid Neurotransmitter*
- Anandamide

*Neurokinins/Tachykinins*
- Substance P
- Neurokinin A
- Neurokinin B

derscores the point made above that the great majority of drugs that act in the CNS act on the process of neurotransmission. Indeed, this apparently occurs at times in a manner that often replicates or mimics the actions of the brain itself when the brain uses its own chemicals.

## Co-transmitters

Each neuron was originally thought to use one neurotransmitter only and to use it at all of its synapses. Today, we now know, however, that many neurons have more than one neurotransmitter (Table 1–2). Thus, the concept of co-transmission has arisen. This often involves a monoamine coupled with a neuropeptide. Under some conditions, the monoamine is released alone; under other conditions, both are released, adding to the repertoire of options for chemical neurotransmission by neurons that contain both neurotransmitters.

Incredibly, the neuron thus uses a certain "polypharmacy" of its own. The rationale behind the use and action of many drugs, however, grew up in the era of thinking about one neuron using only one neurotransmitter, so that the more selective a drug, perhaps the better it could modify neurotransmission. This may be true only to a point. That is, the physiological function of many neurons is now known to be that of communicating by using more than one neurotransmitter.

To replace or influence abnormal neurotransmission, it may therefore be necessary to use multiple drug actions. If the neuron itself uses polypharmacy, perhaps occasionally so should the psychopharmacologist. Today we still lack a rationale for specific multiple drug uses based on the principle of co-transmission, and so much polypharmacy is empirical or even irrational. As understanding of co-transmission increases, the scientific basis for multiple drug actions may well become established for clinical applications. In fact, this may explain why drugs with multiple mechanisms or multiple drugs in combination are the therapeutic rule rather than the exception in psychopharmacology practice. The trick is to be able to do this rationally.

Table 1–2. *Co-transmitter pairs*

| Amine/Amino Acid | Peptide |
| --- | --- |
| Dopamine | Enkephalin |
| Dopamine | Cholecystokinin |
| Norepinephrine | Somatostatin |
| Norepinephrine | Enkephalin |
| Norepinephrine | Neurotensin |
| Epinephrine | Enkephalin |
| Serotonin | Substance P |
| Serotonin | Thyrotropin-releasing hormone |
| Serotonin | Enkephalin |
| Acetylcholine | Vasoactive intestinal peptide |
| Acetylcholine | Enkephalin |
| Acetylcholine | Neurotensin |
| Acetylcholine | Luteinizing-hormone-releasing hormone |
| Acetylcholine | Somatostatin |
| Gamma aminobutyric acid (GABA) | Somatostatin |
| Gamma aminobutyric acid (GABA) | Motilin |

## Molecular Neurobiology

As mentioned earlier, the purpose of chemical neurotransmission is to alter the function of postsynaptic target neurons. To understand the long-term consequences of chemical neurotransmission on the postsynaptic neuron (e.g., Fig. 1–13), it is necessary to understand the molecular mechanisms by which neurotransmission regulates gene expression. It is estimated that the human genome contains approximately 80,000 to 100,000 genes located within 3 million base pairs of DNA on 23 chromosomes. Incredibly, however, genes only occupy about 3% of all this DNA. The other 97% of DNA is not well understood, but it is obviously there for some reason. We may need to await the completion of the *Human Genome Project*, which hopes to sequence the entire 3 million base pairs within a few years, before the function of all this DNA is clarified. Once the DNA is sequenced, it will be easier to figure out what it does.

The general function of the various gene elements within the brain's DNA is well known; namely, they contain all the information necessary to synthesize the proteins that build the structures that mediate the specialized functions of neurons. Thus, if chemical neurotransmission ultimately activates the appropriate genes, all sorts of changes can occur in the postsynaptic cell. Such changes include making, strengthening, or destroying synapses; urging axons to sprout; and synthesizing various proteins, enzymes, and receptors that regulate neurotransmission in the target cell.

How does chemical neurotransmission regulate gene expression? We have already discussed how chemical neurotransmission converts receptor occupancy by a neurotransmitter into the creation of a second messenger (Fig. 1–10), followed by activation of enzymes, which in turn form transcription factors that turn on genes (Fig. 1–11). Most genes have two regions, a *coding* region and a *regulatory* region (Fig. 1–14). The coding region is the direct template for making its corresponding RNA. This DNA can be transcribed into its RNA with the help of an enzyme called *RNA polymerase*. However, RNA polymerase must be activated, or it will not function.

Luckily, the regulatory region of the gene can make this happen. It has an *enhancer element* and a *promoter element* (Fig. 1–14), which can initiate gene expression with the help of transcription factors. Transcription factors themselves can be activated when they are phosphorylated, which allows them to bind to the regulatory region of the gene (Fig. 1–15). This in turn activates RNA polymerase, and off we go with the coding part of the gene *transcribing* itself into its mRNA (Fig. 1–16). Once transcribed, of course, the RNA goes on to *translate* itself into the corresponding protein (Fig. 1–16).

If such changes in genetic expression lead to changes in connections and in the functions that these connections perform, it is easy to understand how genes can *modify behavior.* The details of nerve functioning, and thus the behavior derived from this nerve functioning, are controlled by genes and the products they produce. Since mental processes and the behavior they cause come from the connections between neurons in the brain, genes therefore exert significant control over behavior. But can behavior modify genes? Learning as well as experiences from the environment can indeed alter which genes are expressed and thus can give rise to changes in neuronal connections. In this way, human experiences, education, and even psychotherapy may change the expression of genes that alter the distribution and "strength" of specific synaptic connections. This, in turn, may produce long-term changes in behavior.

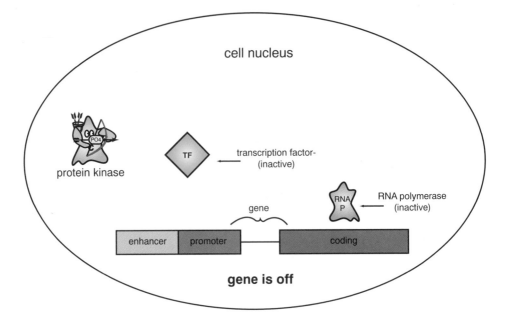

FIGURE 1–14. Activation of a gene, part 1. Here the **gene is "off."** The elements of gene activation include the enzyme **protein kinase**, a **transcription factor**, the enzyme **RNA polymerase**, and the gene itself. This gene is off because the transcription factor has not yet been activated. The gene contains both a **regulatory region** and a **coding region**. The regulatory region has both an **enhancer element** and a **promoter element**, which can initiate gene expression when they interact with activated transcription factors. The coding region is directly transcribed into its corresponding RNA once the gene is activated.

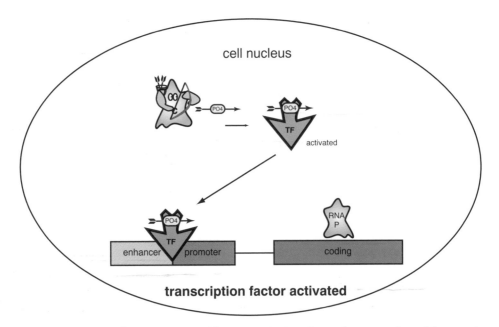

FIGURE 1–15. Activation of a gene, part 2. The **transcription factor** is now **activated** because it has been phosphorylated by protein kinase allowing it to bind to the regulatory region of the gene.

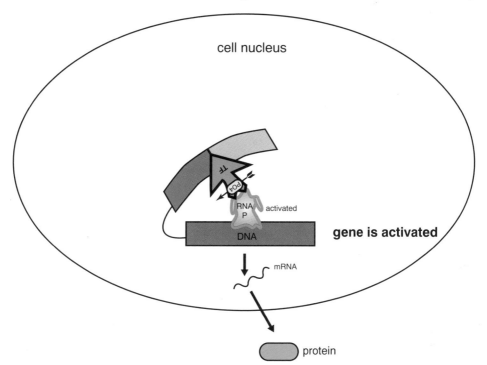

FIGURE 1–16. Activation of a gene, part 3. The **gene** itself is now **activated** because the transcription factor has bound to the regulatory region of the gene, activating in turn the enzyme RNA polymerase. Thus, the gene is transcribed into mRNA, which in turn is translated into its corresponding protein. This protein is thus the product of activation of this particular gene.

caused by the original experience and mediated by the genetic changes triggered by that original experience. Thus, genes modify behavior and behavior modifies genes.

Enzymes (Fig. 1–7) and receptors (Fig. 1–8) are specific examples of proteins encoded within the neuron's genes and synthesized when the appropriate gene is turned on (see also Fig. 1–12). A complete understanding of receptor function involves knowing the exact structure of the receptor protein, based on its amino acid sequence. This can be derived from cloning the receptor by standard molecular techniques. Subtle differences in receptor structure can be the key to explaining distinctions between receptors in various species (e.g., humans versus experimental animals), in certain diseases (i.e., "sick" versus healthy receptors), and in pharmacological subtypes of receptors (i.e., receptors that bind the same neurotransmitters but do so quite differently and with vastly different pharmacologic properties). This will be amplified in Chapter 2.

Molecular neurobiology techniques thus help to clarify receptor functioning in neurotransmission by giving scientists the structure of the receptor. Knowledge of receptor structure also assists in refining receptors as targets for chemists trying to develop new drugs. Knowing the structure of receptors especially allows comparisons of receptor families of similar structure and may ultimately lead to describing changes in receptor structure caused by inherited disease and by drug administration.

Although receptors are usually discovered after neurotransmitters and drugs are found to bind to them, sometimes it happens the other way around. That is, if the gene for a receptor with no known ligand is characterized, it is known as an "orphan receptor," waiting to be adopted by a ligand to be discovered in the future.

The conceptual point to grasp here is that the genome (i.e., DNA) is responsible for the production of receptors, and the production of receptors can be modulated by physiological adaptations, by drugs, and by diseases.

## Neurodevelopment and Neuronal Plasticity

Understanding of human brain development is advancing at a rapid pace. Most neurons are formed by the end of the second trimester of prenatal life (Fig. 1–17). Neuronal migration starts within weeks of conception and is largely complete by birth. Thus, human brain development is more dynamic before birth than during adulthood, and brain volume is 95% of its adult size by age 5. On the other hand, several processes affecting brain structure persist throughout life. Myelination of axon fibers and branching, or arborization, of neurons into their tree-like structures continue at least throughout adolescence. Synaptogenesis seemingly occurs throughout a lifetime.

Thus, both the neuron and its synapses are quite "plastic," changeable, and malleable. Surprising recent reports suggest that some neurons can divide after birth, even in mature mammalian brains and possibly even in human brains. Equally shocking, however, is the discovery that periodically throughout the life cycle and under certain conditions neurons kill themselves in a type of molecular hari-kari called *apoptosis*. In fact, up to 90% of the neurons that the brain makes during fetal development commit apoptotic suicide before birth. Since the mature human brain contains approximately 100 billion neurons, perhaps nearly 1 trillion are initially formed and hundreds of billions apoptotically destroyed between conception and birth.

How do neurons kill themselves? Apoptosis is programmed into the genome of various cells including neurons, and when activated, causes the cell to self-destruct. This is not the messy affair associated with cellular poisoning or suffocation known as necrosis (Fig. 1–18). Necrotic cell death is characterized by a severe and sudden injury associated with an inflammatory response. By contrast, apoptosis is more subtle, akin to fading away. Apoptotic cells shrink, whereas necrotic cells explode (Fig. 1–18). The original scientists who discovered apoptosis coined that term to rhyme with necrosis, and also to mean literally a "falling off," as the petals fall off a flower or the leaves fall from a tree. The machinery of cell death is a set of genes that stand ever ready to self-destruct if activated.

Why should a neuron "slit its own throat" and commit cellular suicide? For one thing, if a neuron or its DNA is damaged by a virus or a toxin, apoptosis destroys and silently removes these sick genes, which may serve to protect surrounding healthy neurons. More importantly, apoptosis appears to be a natural part of development of the immature CNS. One of the many wonders of the brain is the built-in redundancy of neurons early in development. These neurons compete vigorously to migrate, innervate target neurons, and drink trophic factors necessary to fuel this process. Apparently, there is survival of the fittest, because 50 to 90% of many types of neurons normally die at this time of brain maturation. Apoptosis is a natural mechanism to eliminate the unwanted neurons without making as big a molecular mess as necrosis would.

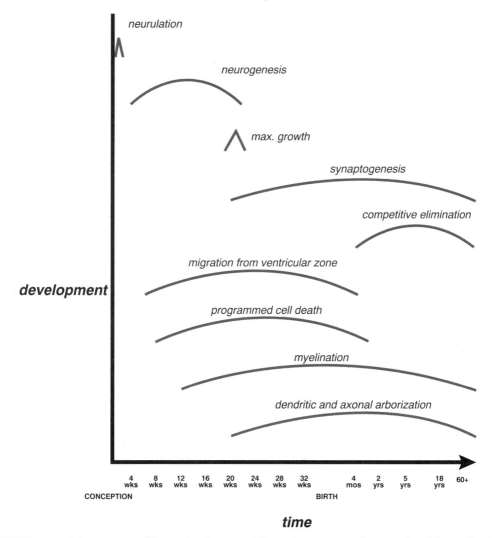

FIGURE 1–17. Time course of brain development. The earliest events of neuronal and brain development in humans are shown at the top, with subsequent and longer-lasting events shown in the lower panels. **Maximum growth** of new neurons is complete before birth, as are the processes of **neuronal migration** and **programmed cell death**. After birth, **synaptogenesis, myelination,** and **dendritic and axonal arborization** occur throughout the individual's lifetime. **Competitive elimination** of synapses, not neurons, is at its peak around pubescence.

Dozens of neurotrophic factors regulate the survival of neurons in the central and peripheral nervous systems (Table 1–3). A veritable alphabet soup of neurotrophic factors contributes to the brain broth of chemicals that bathe and nourish nerve cells. Some are related to nerve growth factor (NGF), others to glial cell line–derived neurotrophic factor (GDNF) and still others to various other neurotrophic factors (Table 1–3). Some neurotrophic factors can trigger neurons to commit cellular suicide by making them fall on their apoptotic swords. The brain seems to choose which nerves live or die partially by whether a neurotrophic factor nourishes them

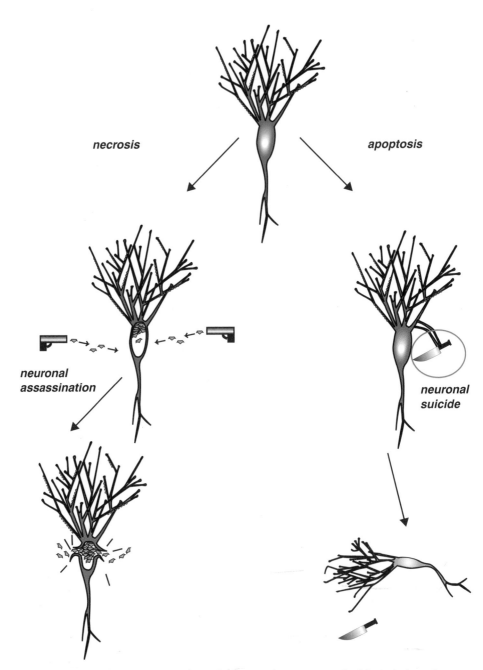

FIGURE 1–18. Neuronal death can occur by either **necrosis** or **apoptosis**. Necrosis is analogous to neuronal assassination, in which neurons explode and cause an inflammatory reaction after being destroyed by poisons, suffocation, or toxins such as glutamate. On the other hand, apoptosis is akin to neuronal suicide and results when the genetic machinery is activated to cause the neuron to literally "fade away" without causing the molecular mess of necrosis.

Table 1–3. *Neurotrophin factors: An alphabet soup of brain tonics*

| | |
|---|---|
| NGF | Nerve growth factor |
| P75 | Proaptotic receptors |
| TrkA | Antiaptotic receptors |
| GDNF | Glial cell line–derived neurotrophic factors including neurturin, c-REF, and R-alpha |
| BDNF | Brain-derived neurotrophic factor |
| NT-3, 4 and 5 | Neurotrophins 3, 4, and 5 |
| CNTF | Ciliary neurotrophic factr |
| ILGF I and II | Insulin-like growth factors |
| FGF | Fibroblast growth factor (comes in both acidic and basic forms) |
| EGF | Epidermal growth factor |

Table 1–4. *Recognition molecules*

PSA-NCAM, polysialic acid–neuronal cell adhesion molecule
NCAM, neuronal cell adhesion molecules (such as H-CAM, G-CAM, VCAM-1)
APP, amyloid precursor protein
Integrin
N-Cadherin
Laminin
Tenscin
Proteoglycans
Heparin-binding growth-associated molecule
Glial hyaluronate–binding protein
Clusterin

or chokes them to death. That is, certain molecules (such as NGF) can interact at proapoptotic "grim reaper" receptors to trigger apoptotic neuronal demise. However, if NGF decides to act on a neuroprotective "bodyguard" receptor, the neuron prospers.

Not only must the correct neurons be selected, but they must migrate to the right parts of the brain. While the brain is still under construction in utero, whole neurons wander. Later, only their axons can move. Neurons are initially produced in the center of the developing brain. Consider that 100 billion human neurons, selected from nearly 1 trillion, must migrate to the right places in order to function properly. What could possibly direct all this neuronal traffic? It turns out that an amazing form of chemical communication calls the neurons forth to the right places and in the right sequences. At speeds up to 60 millionths of a meter per hour, they travel to their proper destination, set up shop, and then send out their axons to connect with other neurons.

These neurons know where to go because of a series of remarkable chemical signals, different from neurotransmitters, called *adhesion molecules* (Table 1–4). First, glial cells form a cellular matrix. Neurons can trace glial fibers like a trail through the brain to their destinations. Later, neurons can follow the axons of other neurons

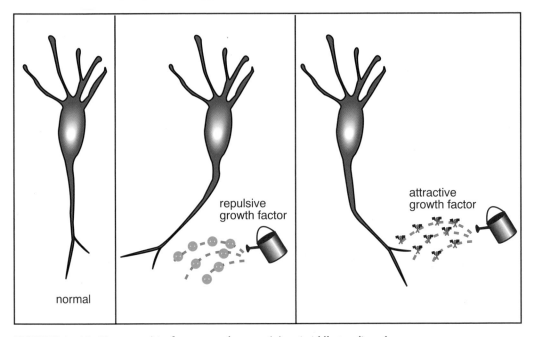

FIGURE 1–19. Neurotrophic factors can be **repulsive** (*middle panel*) and cause axons to grow away from such molecules. Neurotrophic factors can also be **attractant** and encourage axonal growth toward such molecules. Neurotrophic factors thus direct axonal traffic in the brain and help determine which axons synapse with which postsynaptic targets.

already in place and trace along the trail already blazed by the first neuron. Adhesion molecules are coated on neuronal surfaces of the migrating neuron, and complementary molecules on the surface of glia allow the migrating neuron to stick there. This forms a kind of molecular Velcro, which anchors the neuron temporarily and directs its walk along the route paved by the appropriate cell surfaces. Settlement of the brain by migrating neurons is complete by birth, but axons of neurons can grow for a lifetime on activation.

Once neurons settle down in their homesteads, their task is to form synapses. How do their axons know where to go? Neurotrophins not only regulate which neuron lives or dies, but also whether an axon sprouts and which target it innervates. During development in the immature brain, neurotrophins can cause axons to cruise all over the brain, following long and complex pathways to reach their correct targets. Neurotrophins can induce neurons to sprout axons by having them form an axonal growth cone. Once the growth cone is formed, neurotrophins as well as other factors make various recognition molecules for the sprouting axon, presumably by having neurons and glia secrete these molecules into the chemical stew of the brain's extracellular space.

These recognition molecules can either repel or attract growing axons, sending directions for axonal travel like a semaphore signaling a navy ship (Fig. 1–19). Indeed, some of these molecules are called semaphorins to reflect this function. Once the axon growth tip reaches port, it is told to collapse by semaphorin molecules called collapsins, allowing the axon to dock into its appropriate postsynaptic slip

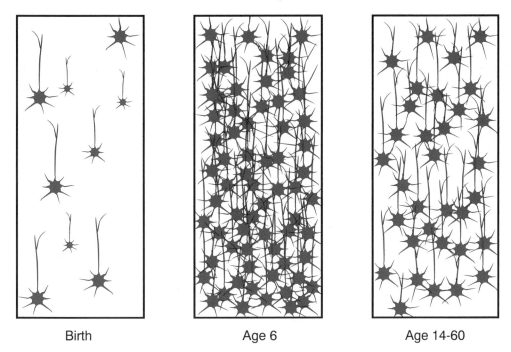

| Birth | Age 6 | Age 14-60 |

FIGURE 1–20. Synapses are **formed** at a furious rate between birth and age 6. However, there is **competitive elimination** and **restructuring** of synapses, a phenomenon that peaks during pubescence and adolescence, leaving about half to two-thirds of the synapses present in childhood to survive into adulthood.

and not sail past it. Other recognition molecules direct axons away by emitting repulsive axon guidance signals (RAGS) (Fig. 1–19).

As brain development progresses, the travel of axonal growth cones is greatly impeded but not completely lost. The fact that axonal growth is retained in the mature brain suggests that neurons continue to alter their targets of communication, perhaps by repairing, regenerating, and reconstructing synapses as demanded by the evolving duties of a neuron. A large number of recognition molecules supervise this. Some of these include not only semaphorins and collapsins but also molecules such as netrins, neuronal cellular adhesion molecules (NCAMS), integrins, cadherins, and cytokines (Table 1–4).

Interestingly, more synapses are present in the brain by age 6 than at any other time in the life cycle (Fig. 1–20). During the next 5 to 10 years and into adolescence, the brain then systematically removes half of all synaptic connections present at age 6. This leaves about 100 trillion synapses and up to 10,000 individual synapses for some neurons. Excitotoxicity may mediate the pruning of synaptic connections (as will be discussed in much greater detail in Chapter 4). Hopefully, neurodevelopmental experiences and genetic programming lead the brain to select wisely which connections to keep and which to destroy. If this is done appropriately, the individual prospers during this maturational task and advances gracefully into adulthood. Bad selections theoretically could lead to neurodevelopmental disorders such as schizophrenia or even attention deficit hyperactivity disorder.

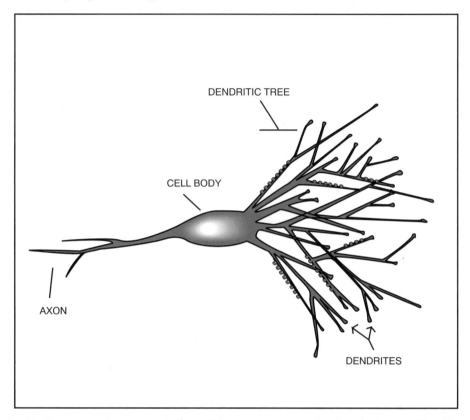

FIGURE 1–21. The neuron is composed of a **cell body**, an **axon** and a **dendritic tree** (literally, a tree of branching dendrites). The dendritic tree is in constant flux and revises its synaptic connections throughout life.

That growth of new synapses and the pruning of old synapses then proceeds throughout a lifetime, but at a much slower pace and over shorter distances than earlier in development. Thus, the axons and dendrites of each neuron are constantly changing, establishing new connections, and removing old connections, in a manner reminiscent of the branches of a tree (Fig. 1–21). Indeed, the *arborization* of neuronal terminals and the *dendritic tree* are terms implying this constant branching (Fig. 1–22) and pruning (Fig. 1–23) process, which proceeds throughout the lifetime of that neuron. After the dramatic reductions in neurons before birth and in synapses during late childhood and early adolescence are complete, activity calms down considerably in the mature brain, where maintenance and remodeling of synapses continue to modest extents and over more limited distances.

Although the continuous structural remodeling of synapses in the mature brain, directed by recognition molecules, cannot approximate the pronounced long-range growth of early brain development, this restriction could be beneficial, in part because it allows structural plasticity while restricting unwanted axonal growth. This would stabilize brain function in the adult and could furthermore prevent chaotic rewiring of the brain by limiting both axonal growth away from appropriate targets and ingrowth from inappropriate neurons. On the other hand, the price of such

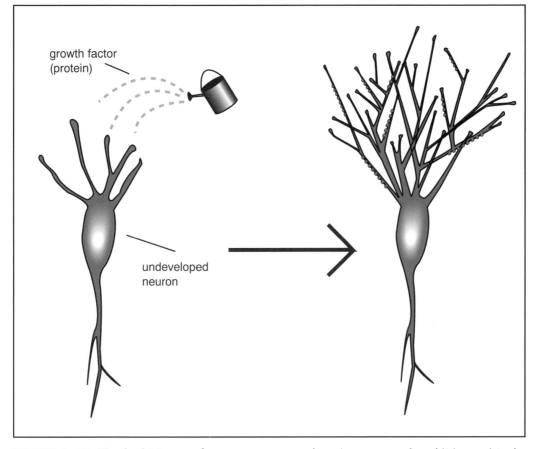

FIGURE 1–22. The dendritic tree of a neuron can sprout branches, grow, and establish a multitude of new synaptic connections throughout its life. The process of making dendritic connections on an **undeveloped neuron** may be controlled by various **growth factors**, which act to promote the branching process and thus the formation of synapses on the dendritic tree.

growth specificity becomes apparent when a long-distance neuron in the adult brain or spinal cord dies, thus making it difficult to reestablish original synaptic connections, even if axonal growth is turned on.

As previously discussed, neurons and their supportive and neighboring glia elaborate a rich array of neurotrophic factors, which promote synaptic connections (Fig. 1–22) or eliminate them (Fig. 1–23). The potential for releasing growth factors is preserved forever, which contributes to the possibility of constant synaptic revision throughout the lifetime of that neuron. Such potential changes in synaptogenesis may provide the substrate for learning, emotional maturity, and the development of cognitive and motor skills throughout a lifetime. However, it is not clear how the brain dispenses its neurotrophic factors endogenously during normal adult physiological functioning. Presumably, demand to use neurons is met by keeping them fit and ready to function, a task accomplished by salting the brain broth with neurotrophic factors that keep the neurons healthy. Perhaps thinking and learning provoke the release of neurotrophic factors. Maybe "use it or lose it" applies to adult neurons,

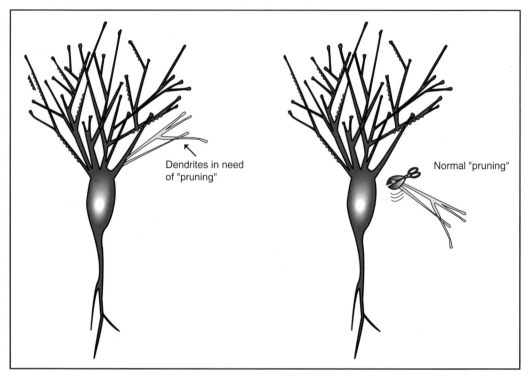

FIGURE 1–23. The dendritic tree of a neuron not only sprouts branches, grows, and establishes a multitude of new synaptic connections throughout its life, as shown in Figure 1–22, but it can also remove, alter, trim, or destroy such connections when necessary. The process of dismantling synapses and dendrites may be controlled by removal of growth factors or by a naturally occurring destructive process sometimes called *excitotoxicity*. Thus, there is a **normal "pruning"** process for removing **dendrites in need of pruning**.

with neurons being preserved and new connections being formed if the brain stays active. It is even possible that the brain could lose its "strength" in the absence of mental exercise. Perhaps inactivity leads to pruning of unused, "rusty" synapses, even triggering apoptotic demise of entire inactive neurons. On the other hand, mental stimulation might prevent this, and psychotherapy may even induce neurotrophic factors to preserve critical cells and innervate new therapeutic targets to alter emotions and behaviors. Only future research will clarify how to use drugs and psychotherapy to balance the seasonings in the tender stew of the brain.

## Summary

The reader should now appreciate that chemical neurotransmission is the foundation of psychopharmacology. It has three dimensions, namely, space, time, and function. The *spatial* dimension is both that of "hard wiring" as the anatomically addressed nervous system and that of a "chemical soup" as the chemically addressed nervous system. The *time* dimension reveals that neurotransmission can be fast (milliseconds) or slow (up to several seconds) in onset, depending on the neurotransmitter or neuromodulator, of which there are dozens. Neurotransmission can also cause actions that are short-acting (milliseconds) or very long acting (days to weeks or longer). The *functional* dimension of chemical neurotransmission is the process whereby an electrical impulse in one neuron is converted into a chemical message at the synaptic connection between two neurons and then into a chemical message that can alter gene expression in the second neuron.

This chapter has also emphasized a few additional points: Chemical neurotransmission sometimes occurs with more than one neurotransmitter in a single neuron. Naturally occurring neurotransmitters are often mimicked by drugs (for example, marijuana and morphine). Molecular neurobiology and its techniques demonstrate that the genetic materials of a neuron are responsible for the production of neuronal proteins in general and neurotransmitter receptors in particular. This can be modulated by physiological adaptations, by drugs, and by diseases. Finally, the neuron is dynamically modifying its synaptic connections throughout its life, in response to learning, life experiences, genetic programming, drugs, and diseases.

# CHAPTER 2

# RECEPTORS AND ENZYMES AS THE TARGETS OF DRUG ACTION

In Chapter 1 we discussed how modern psychopharmacology is essentially the study of chemical neurotransmission. In this chapter we will become more specific and discuss how virtually all central nervous system (CNS) drugs act in one of two very specific ways on chemical neurotransmission: first and most prominently as stimulators (agonists) or blockers (antagonists) of neurotransmitter receptors; or second, and less commonly, as inhibitors of regulatory enzymes.

Given the far-reaching importance of receptors and enzymes in our current thinking about how drugs work in the brain, this chapter will explore the properties of these very interesting targets of CNS drug action. We will first explore the organization of single receptors and how they form binding sites for neurotransmitters and drugs. We will then describe how receptors work as members of a synaptic neurotransmission team, including ions, ion channels, transport carriers, second messenger systems, transcription factors, genes, and gene products. Finally, we will

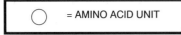

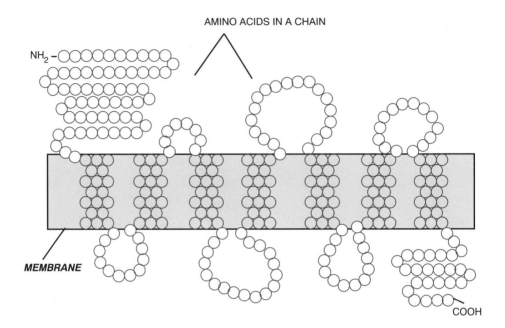

FIGURE 2–1. This figure is a schematic diagram of a receptor, showing that it is a protein arranged essentially as a long **chain of amino acids**. The chain winds in and out of the cell several times, creating three regions of the receptor: first, the extracellular portions are those parts of the chain entirely **outside** the neuron; second, the intracellular portions are those bits of the chain entirely **inside** the neuron; and third, the transmembrane portion, which comprises the regions of the receptor that reside within the **membrane** of the neuron.

discuss how enzymes and receptors are sites of drug actions and how such drug actions in turn modify chemical neurotransmission.

## The Organization of a Single Receptor: Three Parts of a Receptor

Receptors are long chains of amino acids and therefore a type of protein (Fig. 2–1). Receptors reside partially within neuronal membranes (Figs. 2–1 and 2–2). In fact, neurotransmitter receptors can be thought of as containing three portions: an extracellular portion, a transmembrane portion and an intracellular portion (Fig. 2–2). The chain of amino acids constituting the receptor is not arranged in a straight line as might be implied by oversimplified representations in diagrams such as Figures

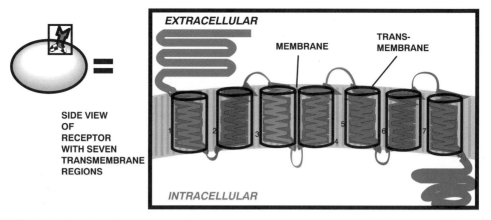

FIGURE 2–2. A side view of a receptor with seven **transmembrane regions** is shown here. This is a common structure of many receptors for neurotransmitters and hormones. That is, the string of amino acids goes in and out of the cell several times to create three portions of the receptor: first, that part that is outside of the cell (called the extracellular portion); second, the part that is inside the receptor that is inside the cell (called the intracellular portion; and finally, the part that traverses the membrane several times (called the **transmembrane** portion). Throughout this text, this receptor will be represented in a simplified schematic manner with the icon shown in the small box.

2–1 and 2–2, but rather in an alpha helical manner, as a spiral around a central core (Figs. 2–3 and 2–4). The binding site for the neurotransmitter is inside the central core for many receptors (i.e., inside the helix of Figs. 2–3 and 2–4).

The *extracellular binding portion* of a receptor is the part of the receptor that is located outside the cell. It was originally believed that this portion of the receptor contained the selective binding site for its neurotransmitter. However, as mentioned above, it is now known that the selective binding site for a neurotransmitter is often located within the second portion of the receptor, its transmembrane regions (Figs. 2–3 and 2–4).

Some drugs may compete with the neurotransmitter for its own binding site, attempting to mimic the neurotransmitter that normally binds there or to block that neurotransmitter. As we will discuss in more detail in Chapter 3 under the topic of allosteric modulation, drugs may also act at totally separate and unique binding sites at other locations on the receptor to change the actions of the neurotransmitter on its receptor. The locations of such binding sites are still under intense investigation, but these sites may also be located in the transmembrane regions, yet separate from the neurotransmitter's binding site. This recognition site for the neurotransmitter receptor is quite unique from one receptor to the next and indeed may be one of the major distinguishing characteristics of one receptor versus another. Some receptors even have binding sites for two distinct neurotransmitters, in which case they are called *co-transmitters*.

The *transmembrane regions* (Figs. 2–2 and 2–3) probably also serve in part a structural purpose, holding the receptor in place or allowing a certain movement of the receptor relative to the membrane itself. Transmembrane regions of one neurotransmitter receptor can be quite similar to those of other neurotransmitter receptors,

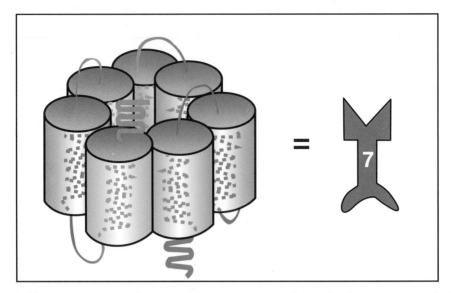

FIGURE 2–3. The seven **transmembrane** regions are not arranged in a line but rather in a circle. In the middle of this circle is a **central core**, where neurotransmitters find their **binding sites**. This figure depicts each transmembrane region as a spiral, since each is actually an alpha-helix. Also shown is how these spirals are arranged so that the seven of them form a circle. In the middle of the circle is the binding site for the neurotransmitter. Since there are seven transmembrane regions (left), the icon representing this will have the number 7 on it (right).

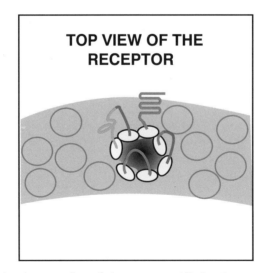

FIGURE 2–4. This figure shows a top view of the receptor. All that is seen are the **extracellular portions** of the receptors sticking out of the membrane. These extracellular regions of the receptor connect the various transmembrane regions to each other. In the center of the bits of receptor is the **central core**, where the neurotransmitter for that receptor binds.

forming large families of receptors (sometimes called superfamilies), which are structurally similar but which use different neurotransmitters.

One example of this is the super-family of receptors organized with seven transmembrane regions (Fig. 2–3). This is a structure common to many neurotransmitter receptors that use second-messenger systems and are "slow" in responding (e.g., serotonin-2A receptors and beta-2 adrenergic receptors). A description of the seven-transmembrane region superfamily of receptors will be amplified below in our discussion of receptors linked to second-messenger systems.

A second important example of the organization of a receptor structure that is shared by many different neurotransmitter receptors is that of four transmembrane regions common to many other neurotransmitter receptors that interact with ion channels (Fig. 2–5). In this case, multiple copies of each four-transmembrane region receptor are clustered around a central ion channel (Fig. 2–6). A description of the four-transmembrane region superfamily of receptors will be amplified below in our discussion of receptors interacting with ion channels.

There is even a third prominent example of how a receptor can be organized, namely, the 12-transmembrane region transporter systems (Fig. 2–7). A description of such transporters will be given in greater detail in the section on monoamine reuptake, which follows later in this chapter.

The third part of a neurotransmitter receptor is *intracellular* (Figs. 2–2 and 2–3). These intracellular section of the receptor, sometimes termed cytoplasmic loops, can interact with other transmembrane proteins or with intracellular proteins in order to trigger second-messenger systems (as shown in Figs. 1–10 and 1–11). The great majority of neurotransmitter and hormone receptors interact with second-messenger systems to modify the transition of molecular information from the neurotransmitter first-messenger to the second-messenger system and on to the genetic machinery (i.e., DNA) of the cell nucleus.

## Synaptic Teamwork

Much importance and emphasis is given to the selective interaction of neurotransmitter with its unique binding site on its *receptor* because this is how information is encoded and decoded, both by neurotransmitters and by drugs mimicking neurotransmitters. Indeed, the majority of psychopharmacologic agents are thought to act at such sites on various receptors. However, this is far from a complete description of chemical neurotransmission or of all the sites at which drugs can potentially modulate neurotransmission.

Chemical neurotransmission can be described more completely as a *team* of molecular players. The neurotransmitter may be the captain of the team, but it is only one key player. Other molecular players on the synaptic transmission team include the specific ions (Fig. 2–8), that interact with the ion channels (e.g., Fig. 2–6), various enzymes (Fig 2–9), transport carriers (Fig. 2–10), active transport pumps (Fig. 2–11), second messengers (Fig. 2–12), receptors (Fig. 2–13), transcription factors (Fig. 2–14), genes (Fig. 2–15), and gene products (Fig. 2–16).

In addition to the role of these players in chemical neurotransmission, each molecule is a known or potential site of drug interactions. Each is also a theoretical site of malfunction that could possibly contribute to a nervous or mental disorder, as

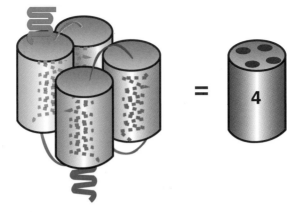

FIGURE 2–5. A type of structure that is shared by many receptors linked to an **ion channel** is that of **four transmembrane regions**. This will be represented by the icon on the right, and labeled with a 4. It is not the whole receptor but just a subunit of the receptor as shown in Figure 2–6.

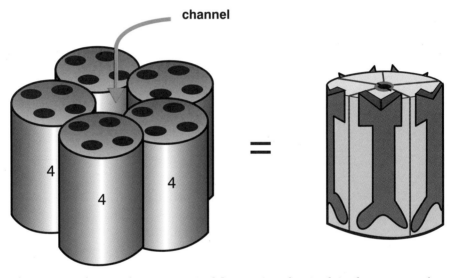

FIGURE 2–6. **Ion channels** are often composed of **five copies** of each of the four-transmembrane-region receptor subunits shown in Figure 2–5. In the **center** of these five copies is the ion channel itself. We will use the icon on the right to represent receptor–ion channel complexes comprising five copies of the four-transmembrane-region subunits.

will be discussed in general terms in Chapter 4 and in specific relationship to various psychiatric disorders throughout the rest of the book.

The molecular players beyond the second messenger are particularly important in gene regulation. They include both active and inactive forms of protein kinase, an enzyme that phosphorylates various intracellular proteins, and protein dephosphatase enzymes, which reverse this (Fig. 2–9). Also included are transcription factors, which

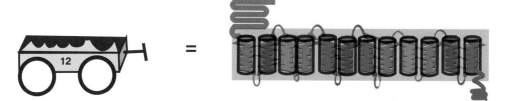

FIGURE 2–7. Another prominent example of how a receptor can be organized is provided by the **12-transmembrane-region** proteins that comprise the binding sites for various **neurotransmitter transporter systems**. The icon on the left will be used to represent this type of receptor.

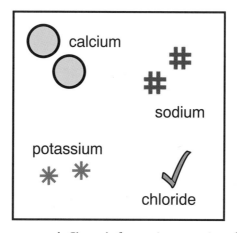

FIGURE 2–8. Various **ions** are represented. Channels for one ion are unique from channels for other ions. The ions include **sodium, potassium, chloride,** and **calcium**.

activate genes (Fig. 2–14) by allowing RNA polymerase to spring into action, transcribing DNA into RNA (Figs. 1–16 and 2–9).

Immediate early genes (early response genes) with exotic names such as cJun and cFos are some of the very first that can be transcribed directly following neurotransmitter action at postsynaptic receptors (Fig. 2–15). In fact, the gene products of "early genes," such as the Fos gene product from the cFos gene and the Jun gene product from the cJun gene, can themselves form transcription factors with equally exotic names, such as leucine zipper (Fig. 2–14). Later-onset genes (Fig. 2–15) are turned on by these products of early-onset genes to perpetuate the cascade begun way back with the neurotransmitter. These late-onset genes are the ultimate regulators of the postsynaptic neuron, as their gene products include all the important proteins that target neurons make, including enzymes, receptors, transcription factors, growth factors, structural proteins, and many more (Fig. 2–16).

The spatial arrangement of these different molecules relative to one another facilitates their mutual interactions. These various elements of chemical neurotransmission, represented as icons in Figures 2–5 through 2–16, can be arranged to cooperate on teams to accomplish various aspects of chemical neurotransmission, as will be shown in several of the figures that follow.

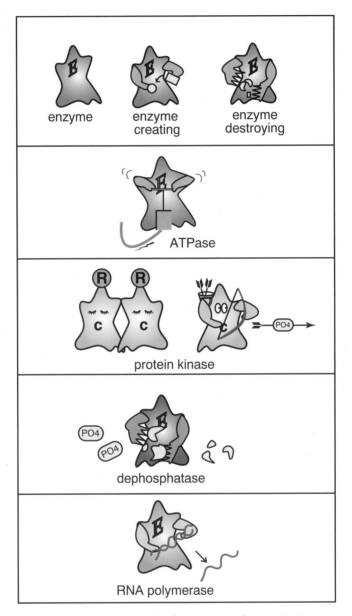

FIGURE 2–9. **Enzymes** are very important to the functioning of the cell. Some enzymes **create** molecules (i.e., build them up) and some enzymes **destroy** molecules (i.e., tear them apart). One enzyme responsible for using energy is **ATPase**. Three important classes of enzymes that regulate gene expression include both active and inactive forms of protein kinases, various **dephosphatases**, which can reverse the actions of protein kinases, and finally, **RNA polymerase** enzymes, which catalyze the transcription of DNA into RNA.

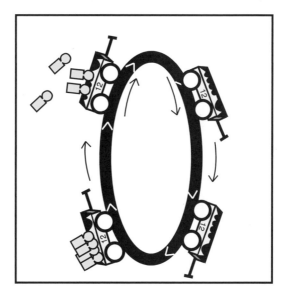

FIGURE 2–10. A **transport carrier** is used to shuttle molecules into cells that otherwise would not be able to get into the cell through the membrane.

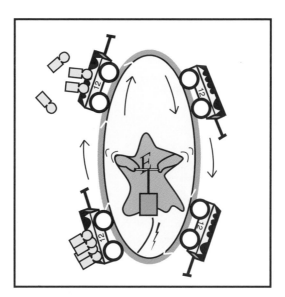

FIGURE 2–11. If a transport carrier is coupled with an energy-providing enzyme such as **ATPase**, it is called an **active transport pump**.

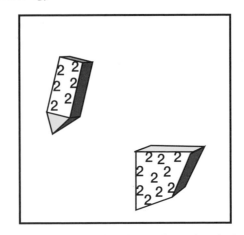

FIGURE 2–12. **Second messengers** are intracellular chemicals produced when some neurotransmitters bind to their receptors. Such receptors are capable of converting the binding information of their neurotransmitter into the synthesis of these second messengers.

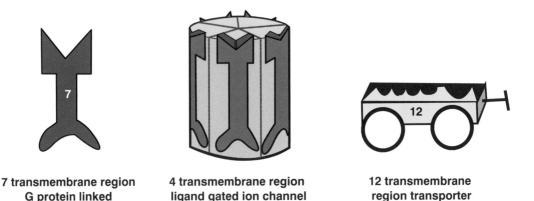

| 7 transmembrane region<br>G protein linked | 4 transmembrane region<br>ligand gated ion channel | 12 transmembrane<br>region transporter |

FIGURE 2–13. Icons for **various receptors** are shown here, including the seven-transmembrane region G-protein-linked second messenger system (left), the ligand-gated ion channel comprising five subunits with four transmembrane regions (middle), and the 12-transmembrane region transporter (right).

## Ion Channels

Some transmembrane proteins form channels, lining the neuronal membrane to enable ions to traverse the membrane (Figs. 2–6, 2–17, and 2–18). Channels exist for many ions, including, for example, sodium, potassium, chloride, and calcium (Fig. 2–8). Ion channels in the CNS can be modulated in such a way that the channel may be open or permeable at times (Fig. 2–17) and closed or impermeable at other times (Fig. 2–18). There are two principal ways to regulate the opening and closing of ion channels, with electricity or with a molecular gatekeeper (Fig. 2–19). Those that use electricity are called *voltage-gated*; those that use a neurotransmitter ligand binding to a receptor near the ion channel are called *ligand-gated* (Fig. 2–19).

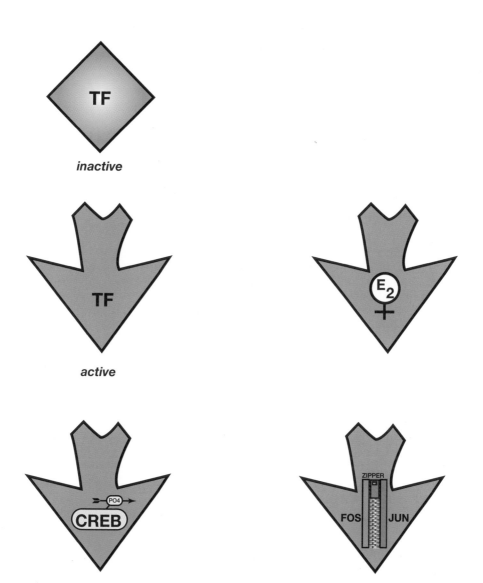

FIGURE 2–14. Multiple **transcription factors** are represented here, including active and inactive forms, estradiol (E2), cyclic AMP response binding element (CREB), and the leucine zipper formed by Fos and Jun.

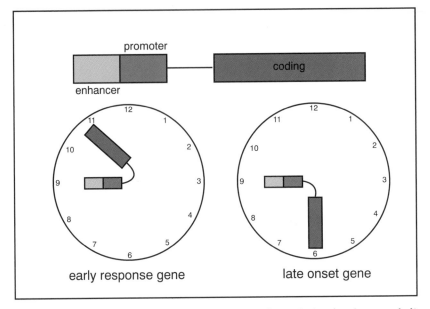

FIGURE 2–15. Many different genes are important to neuronal regulation by drugs and diseases. The prototypical gene is a sequence of DNA that has a regulatory region comprising an enhancer and a promoter, plus a coding region, which is directly transcribed into RNA. Some genes are quickly activated and are known as **early-response genes** or immediate early genes. Others take longer to be activated, and are **late-onset genes**.

## Transport Carriers and Active Transport Pumps

Membranes normally serve to keep the internal milieu of the cell constant by acting as a barrier against the intrusion of outside molecules and the leakage of internal molecules. However, selective permeability of the membrane is required to allow uptake as well as discharge of specific molecules to respond to the needs of cellular functioning. This has already been mentioned with regard to ions but also applies to a number of other specific molecules. For example, glucose is transported into the cell in order to provide energy for neurotransmission. Neurotransmitters are also transported into neurons as a recapture mechanism following their release and use during neurotransmission. This is done in order for neurotransmitter to be repackaged and reused in a subsequent neurotransmission.

In order to accomplish selective shuttling of certain molecules across an otherwise impermeable membrane, other molecules known as *transport carriers* work to bind that molecule needing a trip inside the cell (Figs. 2–11 and 2–20 through 2–22). The transport carrier is thus itself a type of receptor. In order for some transport carriers to concentrate the shuttling molecules within the cell, they require energy.

One example of molecular transport requiring energy is the reuptake of neurotransmitter into its presynaptic neuron, as already mentioned above. In this case, the energy comes from linkage to an enzyme known as sodium-potassium ATPase (Fig. 2–9). An *active transport pump* is the term for this type of organization of two neurotransmitters, namely a transport carrier and an energy-providing system, which function as a team to accomplish transport of a molecule into the cell (Fig. 2–11).

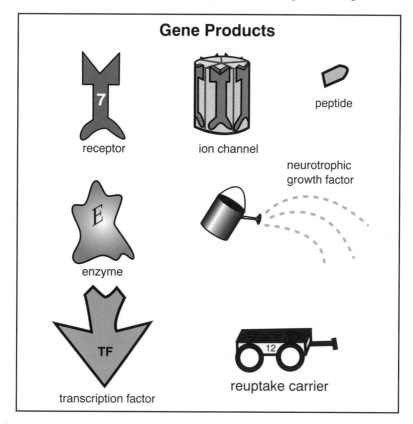

**FIGURE 2–16. Gene products** are various proteins with a wide spectrum of functions, including receptors, ion channels, peptide neurotransmitters, enzymes, neurotrophic factors, transcription factors, reuptake carriers, and many, many more.

### *Neurotransmitter Synaptic Reuptake—an Example of Molecular Transport Using an Active Transport Pump*

In the case of the active transport pump for presynaptic transport of neurotransmitter, the job is to sweep synaptic neurotransmitter molecules out of the synapse and back into the presynaptic neuron. The reuptake pump comprises a carrier for neurotransmitter (Fig. 2–20). However, in the absence of sodium it cannot bind that neurotransmitter very well (see carrier with no sodium binding, no neurotransmitter binding, and "flat tires" in Figure 2–20). However, in the presence of sodium the carrier does bind to neurotransmitter molecules (see Figure 2–21 with sodium in the tires, which are now pumped up, and the carrier now binding neurotransmitter as well). This reuptake pump can also be inhibited so that neurotransmitter molecules can no longer bind to the reuptake carrier (Figure 2–22 shows sodium gone, neurotransmitter gone, and an inhibitor in place causing the tires to go flat again). Many antidepressants act by targeting one or another of the reuptake pumps for monoamine neurotransmitters, especially the serotonin transporter, the norepinephrine transporter, and the dopamine transporter.

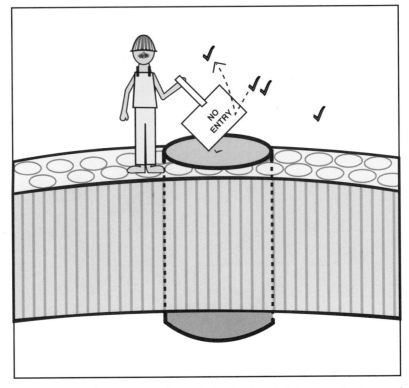

FIGURE 2–17. This schematic shows an **ion channel** that is **closed**. It has a molecular **gatekeeper**, shown here keeping the channel closed so that ions cannot get into the cell.

This reuptake pump takes an active part in the neurotransmission process, which begins with the firing of the presynaptic neuron and release of neurotransmitter (Fig. 2–23). The neurotransmitter diffuses across the synapse, binds its neurotransmitter receptors selectively, and triggers all the subsequent events that translate that chemical message into another neuronal impulse in the postsynaptic neuron, activate postsynaptic genes, and regulate various cellular functions in the target neuron. The neurotransmitter then diffuses off its receptor and can be destroyed by enzymes or transported back into the presynaptic neuron.

When neurotransmitter successfully diffuses back to the presynaptic neuron, a transport carrier, which has been waiting there for it (Fig. 2–23), binds it in the presence of sodium (Fig. 2–23) and, with the help of its teammate energy-providing enzyme system sodium-potassium ATPase, shuttles the neurotransmitter back into the neuron for repackaging and reuse, while simultaneously exchanging sodium for potassium with the neuron. Several molecules therefore cooperate to make this reuptake complex function so as to transport neurotransmitter back into the neuron. The most important of these are the transport carrier (Figs. 2–20, 2–21, and 2–23) and the enzyme sodium-potassium ATPase (Figs. 2–9 and 2–23). Also involved is sodium, which increases the affinity of the transporter for its neurotransmitter (Figs.

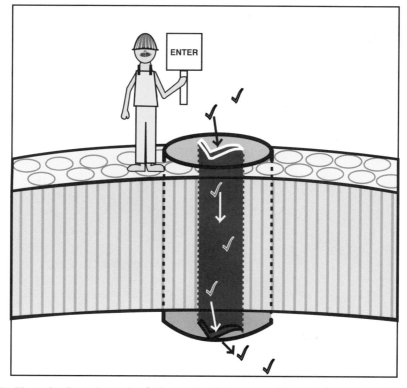

FIGURE 2–18. Here the **ion channel** of Figure 2–17 is **open**. The **gatekeeper** has acted, on instruction from some neurotransmitter, to open the channel and allow ions to travel into the cell.

2–21 and 2–23). As will be discussed in detail in Chapter 6, inhibiting this transport of one or another of the monoamine neurotransmitters is the mechanism of action of most antidepressant drugs (Figs. 2–22 and 2–24).

Reuptake of synaptic neurotransmitter is thus another example of how molecules cooperate with each other as players on a team in order to accomplish a complex but elegant dimension of chemical neurotransmission.

## Second-Messenger Systems

A neurotransmitter receptor can also cooperate with a team of specialized molecules comprising what is known as a second-messenger system (Figs. 2–25 through 2–28). The *first* messenger is considered to be the neurotransmitter itself (Fig. 2–25). It transfers its message to a second messenger, which is intracellular (see Fig. 1–10 and 2–25 through 2–28). It does this via two receptors, which cooperate with each other. These two receptors are the neurotransmitter receptor itself and another receptor associated with the inner membrane of the cell, known as a *G protein*. Once these two receptors have interacted (Figs. 2–26 and 2–27), this permits yet another interaction, namely that of the two receptors with an enzyme (Figs. 2–27 and 2–

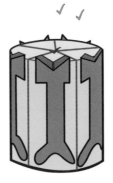

**ligand gated**

✓ = chloride

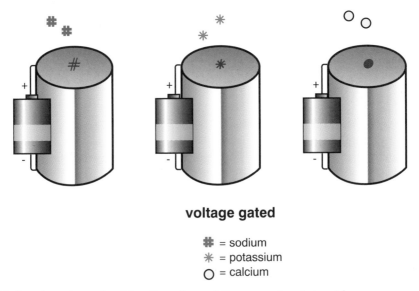

**voltage gated**

⌗ = sodium
✳ = potassium
○ = calcium

FIGURE 2–19. Ion channels can be either **ligand-gated** (i.e., opened and closed by neurotransmitter ligands) or **voltage-gated** (i.e., opened or closed by the voltage charge across the channel). Many different ions have their own channels, including sodium, potassium, and calcium.

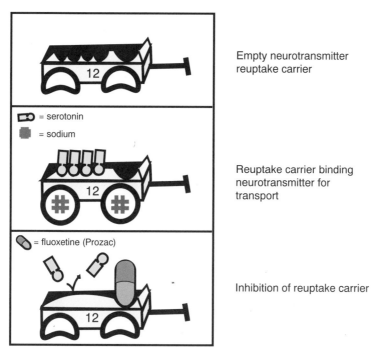

Empty neurotransmitter reuptake carrier

= serotonin

= sodium

Reuptake carrier binding neurotransmitter for transport

= fluoxetine (Prozac)

Inhibition of reuptake carrier

FIGURE 2–20. The **transport carrier** for neurotransmitter reuptake is like a box car with reserved seats for molecules for neurotransmitter. Here the transport carrier is **empty**. Its tires are flat, and it is unable to transport neurotransmitter.

FIGURE 2–21. The neurotransmitter reuptake **transporter** can bind neurotransmitter molecules at specific binding sites. Here the neurotransmitter is bound to transporter sites, ready for a trip inside the neuron. It is now binding the neurotransmitter serotonin (SHT) because it has found **sodium** ions, which have increased its affinity for serotonin, resulting in the tires being pumped up and full of air, ready for transport.

FIGURE 2–22. If an **inhibitor** of the **transport carrier** binds to its own binding site, it **prevents** neurotransmitter molecules from being able to bind to their sites. This figure shows an antidepressant, **fluoxetine (Prozac)**, binding to the serotonin transporter. When this drug binds to the serotonin transporter, it essentially bumps serotonin neurotransmitter molecules out of their seats on the transport carrier. This causes **inhibition** or **blockade** of neurotransmitter transport into the neuron. Sodium binding is also decreased, and the tires go flat, so that transport is halted.

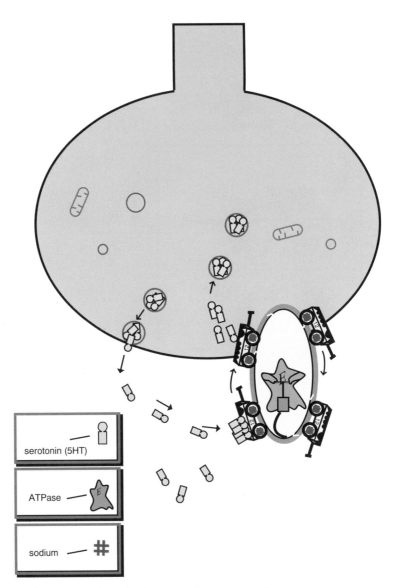

FIGURE 2–23. This figure shows how the box cars of neurotransmitter transporters are arranged on a track to act as a **neurotransmitter shuttle system**. Once the neurotransmitter molecules are released by the neuron, they can be snatched by the transport carrier, given a seat on the shuttle, and driven into the cell on the track created by the **transport carrier** using energy provided by **ATPase**. Once inside the cell, the neurotransmitter gets out of its seat on the shuttle and is stored again in synaptic vesicles so that it can be reused in a subsequent neurotransmission.

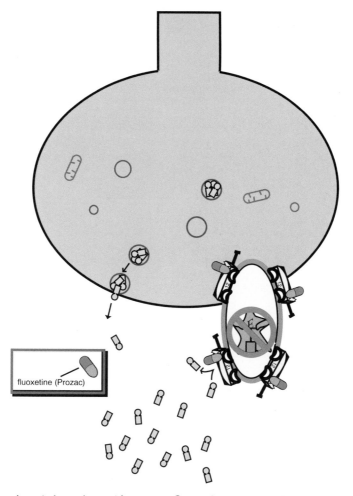

FIGURE 2–24. Shown here is how the antidepressant **fluoxetine (Prozac)** disrupts neurotransmitter from shuttling into the neuron. In this case, binding of the transport carrier by fluoxetine prevents serotonin neurotransmitter molecules from taking a seat on the shuttle. Thus, there is no ride for the serotonin into the neuron. This means that the neurotransmitter serotonin remains in the synapse until it diffuses away or is destroyed by enzymes.

28). The enzyme manufactures a second messenger in response to its interactions with the dual cooperating receptors (Fig. 2–28) but cannot do this by interaction with either of the receptors separately.

A second-messenger system thus includes several elements (Figs. 2–25 through 2–28): (1) the first messenger (neurotransmitter); (2) the neurotransmitter's receptor; (3) a second receptor called a G protein, which interacts with the neurotransmitter receptor; (4) an enzyme triggered into action by the interacting pair of receptors; (5) and a second-messenger molecule manufactured by this enzyme. The two best known examples of second messengers are cyclic adenosine monophosphate (cAMP) and phosphatidyl inositol (PI). The systems that produce these second messengers are also sometimes known as the cAMP second messenger system and the PI second

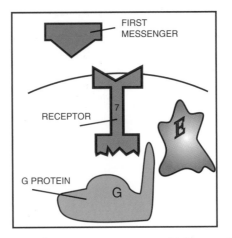

FIGURE 2–25. Shown here is a **second messenger system**, which comprises four elements. The first element is the neurotransmitter itself, sometimes also referred to as the **first messenger**. The second element is the neurotransmitter **receptor**. The third element is a connecting protein called a **G protein**. The fourth element of the second messenger system is an **enzyme**, which can synthesize a second messenger.

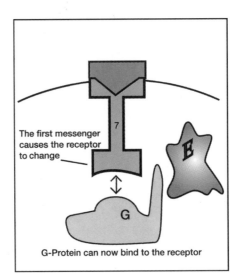

FIGURE 2–26. In this figure the neurotransmitter has docked into its receptor. The first messenger does its job by **transforming** the receptor, indicated here by turning the same color as the neurotransmitter, in order to make it **capable of binding to the G** protein. This requires a **conformational change** of the neurotransmitter receptor, shown here as a change in the shape of its bottom.

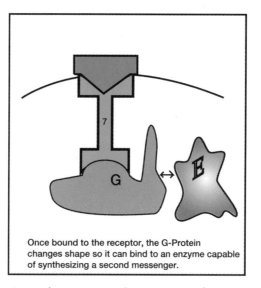

Once bound to the receptor, the G-Protein changes shape so it can bind to an enzyme capable of synthesizing a second messenger.

FIGURE 2–27. The next stage in producing a second messenger is for the transformed neurotransmitter receptor to **bind to the G protein**, depicted here by the G protein turning the same color as the neurotransmitter and its receptor. Binding of the binary neurotransmitter receptor complex to the G protein causes yet another **conformational change**, this time in the G protein, represented here as a change in the shape of the right-hand side of the G protein. This prepares the G protein to bind to the enzyme capable of synthesizing the second messenger.

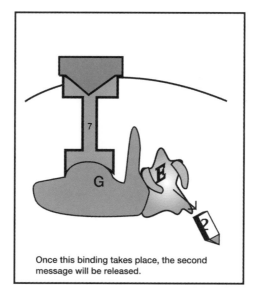

Once this binding takes place, the second message will be released.

FIGURE 2–28. The final step in formation of the second messenger is for the ternary complex neurotransmitter–receptor–G protein to bind to a **messenger-synthesizing enzyme**, depicted here by the enzyme turning the same color as the ternary complex. Once the enzyme binds to this ternary complex, it becomes activated and capable of **synthesizing the second messenger**. Thus, it is the cooperation of all four elements, wrapped together as a quaternary complex, which leads to the production of the second messenger. Information from the first messenger thus passes to the second messenger through use of receptor–G protein–enzyme intermediaries.

messenger system, respectively. Although the actions of a stimulatory G protein are shown here, other types of G proteins are inhibitory and slow down or prevent coupling of the receptor with the enzyme that makes the second messenger.

Thus, the transfer of first messenger to second messenger is accomplished by means of a molecular cascade: neurotransmitter to neurotransmitter receptor (Fig. 2–25); neurotransmitter receptor to G protein (Fig. 2–26); binary complex of two receptors to enzyme (Fig. 2–27); and enzyme to second-messenger molecule (Fig. 2–28).

## Ion Regulation

As if this were not complex enough, the cascade put into motion by the first messenger and continued by the second messenger in fact does not stop here. The exact molecular events of this continuing cascade are the subject of intense current investigation and are just beginning to be unraveled. The cascade continues as second messengers change various cellular activities. Usually, the next step is for the second messenger to activate enzymes (Fig. 2–29) that are capable of altering virtually any function within the cell. One of the most important functions triggered by enzymes activated by second messengers is to change the membrane's permeability to ions such as calcium (Fig. 2–30). Altering fluxes of ions in the neuron is one of the key ways to modify the excitability of the neuron that the second messenger is trying to influence. This happens fairly soon after neurotransmission has occurred. Other events take longer to develop and last longer once they have been started.

## Gene Regulation

Second messengers frequently activate enzymes and cause them to phosphorylate proteins and other enzymes inside the cell (Figs. 2–31 through 2–35). This can alter the synthesis of various molecules in the cell that are subject to regulation by the second messenger. Specifically, in order to modify the functioning of a neuron, these molecules must alter the genes that control the synthesis of the proteins that implement all the functions the postsynaptic cell can perform. Eventually the message is passed along via messenger after messenger (Figs. 2–31 through 2–33) until the information reaches the cell nucleus and the DNA (genes) in it (Fig. 2–34). Once the message has been received at this site, virtually any biochemical change is possible, since the DNA is the command center of the cell and has the power to change any and all biochemical events of which the cell is capable.

Thus, genes do not directly regulate cellular functioning. Rather, they directly regulate the proteins that bring about cellular functioning. Thus, changes in function have to wait until the changes in protein synthesis occur and the events that they cause start to take place.

Let us now trace the events that the common second messenger cAMP can trigger. Once cAMP is formed (Fig. 2–31), it can interact with a family of important regulatory enzymes called protein kinases. Once cAMP binds to the inactive or "sleeping" version of one of these enzymes, the enzyme "wakes up" and becomes activated protein kinase (Fig. 2–32). Protein kinase's job is to activate transcription factors by phosphorylating them (Fig. 2–33). It does this by traveling straight to the cell nucleus and finding a "sleeping" transcription factor, to which it attaches a

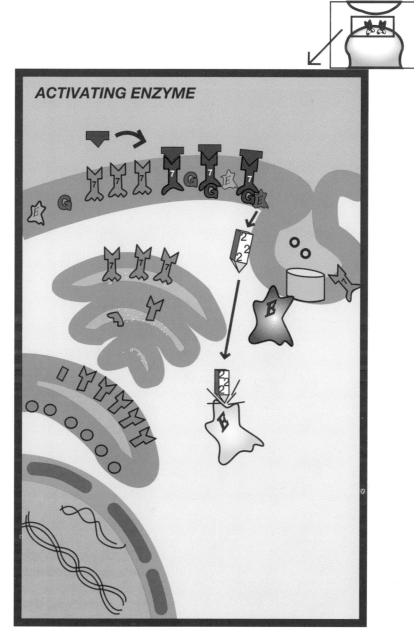

FIGURE 2–29. Once the second messenger has been synthesized, it can continue the information transfer by further molecular conversations. Shown here is second messenger synthesis, depicted as blue neurotransmitter binding extracellularly and cascading the transfer of blue information through receptor, G protein, and enzyme to produce a second messenger, indicated in Figures 2–25 through 2–28. However, this figure goes past second messenger synthesis to depict the second messenger **activating** an intracellular **enzyme**. Note that the ion channel is closed in this figure and that no information is being directed at the cell's DNA here.

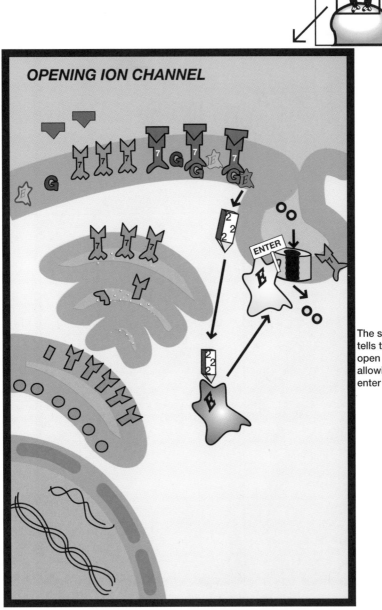

**OPENING ION CHANNEL**

The second messenger tells the enzyme to open an ion channel, allowing Calcium to enter the cell.

FIGURE 2–30. One of the consequences of activation of an intracellular enzyme by a second messenger is that some activated enzymes can instruct **ion channels to open**. This may be mediated by a complicated molecular cascade, set in motion by a second messenger activating an intracellular enzyme, which itself creates still further molecular instructions to an ionic gatekeeper to **open the ion channel**.

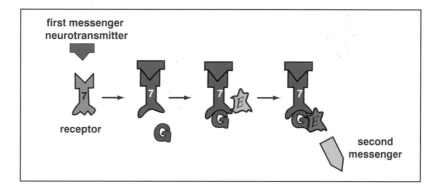

FIGURE 2–31. Gene regulation by neurotransmitters, part 1. Neurotransmitters begin the process of **activating genes** by producing a **second messenger**, as previously shown in Figures 2–25 through 2–28.

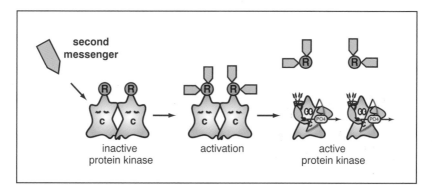

FIGURE 2–32. Gene regulation by neurotransmitters, part 2. Here a second messenger is activating an intracellular enzyme, **protein kinase**. This enzyme is inactive when it is paired with another copy of the enzyme plus two regulatory units (R). In this case, two copies of the second messenger interact with the regulatory units, dissociating them from the copies of protein kinase. This activates protein kinase, readying this enzyme to **phosphorylate** other proteins (PO₄).

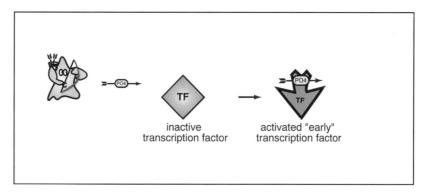

FIGURE 2–33. Gene regulation by neurotransmitters, part 3. Once activated, protein kinase phosphorylates a **transcription factor** (TF). Attaching phosphate (PO₄) to this transcription factor activates it so it can bind to the regulatory region of a gene.

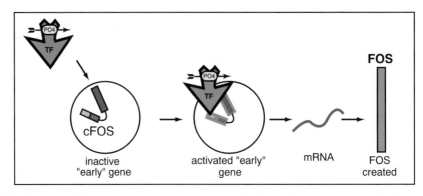

FIGURE 2–34. Gene regulation by neurotransmitters, part 4. The activated transcription factor now binds to the regulatory region of the gene and activates it. The gene shown here is called cFos. **Activation of a gene** means that it is transcribed into RNA and then the RNA is translated into the protein for which it codes. In this example, the protein is Fos from the gene cFos.

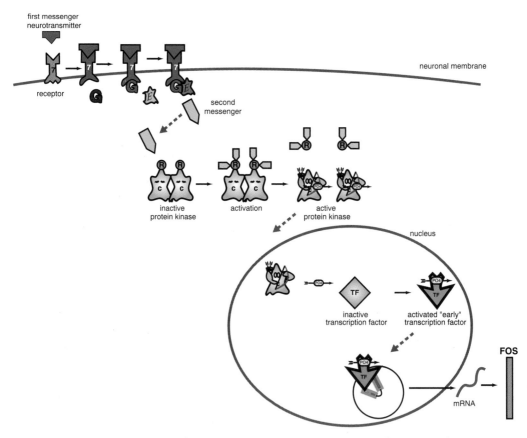

FIGURE 2–35. Gene regulation by neurotransmitters, part 5. Here all four parts of Figures 2–31 through 2–34 are put together into a **continuous cascade** from first-messenger neurotransmitter to gene activation and production of the gene product, Fos protein.

60

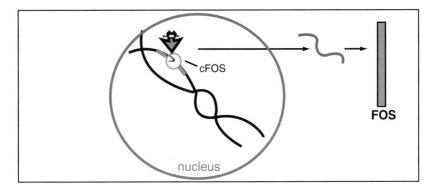

FIGURE 2–36. How early genes activate late genes, part 1. Here, a transcription factor is **activating the immediate early gene** cFos and producing the protein product Fos, as described in detail in Figures 2–31 through 2–35.

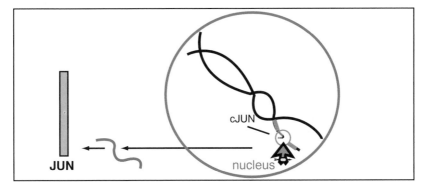

FIGURE 2–37. How early genes activate late genes, part 2. While the cFos gene is being activated in Figure 2–38, another immediate early gene is being simultaneously activated. This **second gene** is called cJun and it is producing its protein product Jun.

phosphate group; by so doing the protein kinase is able to "wake up" that transcription factor (Fig. 2–33). Once a transcription factor is activated, it will bind to genes.

Some genes are known as immediate early genes (Fig. 2–34). They have weird names such as cJun and cFos (Figs. 2–34 through 2–40) and belong to a family called leucine zippers (Fig. 2–38). These genes function as rapid responders to the neurotransmitter's input, like the first troops sent into combat once war has been declared. Such rapid deployment forces of immediate early genes are the first to respond to the neurotransmission signal by making the proteins they encode. In this example, these are Jun and Fos proteins coming from cJun and cFos genes (Figs. 2–36 and 2–37). These are nuclear proteins, that is, they live and work in the nucleus. They get started within 15 minutes of receiving a neurotransmission, but only last for a half hour to an hour (Fig. 2–41).

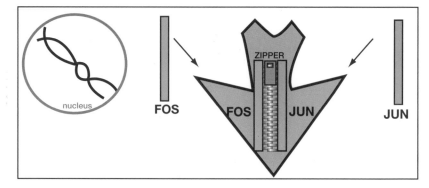

FIGURE 2–38. How early genes activate late genes, part 3. Once Fos and Jun proteins are synthesized, they can collaborate as partners and produce a Fos-Jun combination protein, which now acts as a **transcription factor for late genes**. Sometimes the Fos-Jun transcription factor is called a **leucine zipper**.

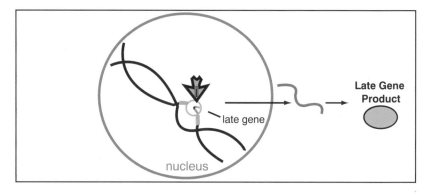

FIGURE 2–39. How early genes activate late genes, part 4. The leucine zipper transcription factor formed by the products of the activated early genes cFos and cJun now returns to the genome and finds another gene. Since this gene is being activated later than the others, it is called a **late gene**. Thus, **early genes activate late genes** when the products of early genes are themselves transcription factors. The product of the late gene can be any protein the neuron needs, such as an enzymes, transport, or growth factor, as shown in Figure 2–16.

When Jun and Fos team up, they form a leucine zipper type of transcription factor (Fig. 2–38), which in turn activates many kinds of later onset genes (Figs. 2–39 through 2–42). Thus, Fos and Jun serve to wake up the much larger army of inactive genes. Which individual soldier genes are so drafted to active gene duty depends on a number of factors, not the least of which is which neurotransmitter is sending the message, how frequently it is sending the message, and whether it is working in concert with or in opposition to other neurotransmitters addressing other parts of the same neuron at the same time.

When Fos and Jun operate as partners to form a leucine zipper type of transcription factor, this can lead to the activation of genes to make anything you can think of, from enzymes to receptors to structural proteins (see Fig. 2–42).

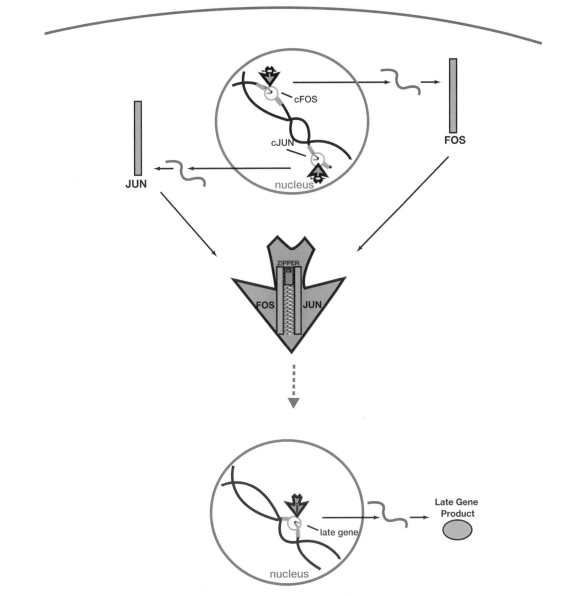

FIGURE 2–40. How early genes activate late genes, part 5. This figure shows the process of activating a late gene, incorporating the elements illustrated in Figures 2–36 through 2–39. At the top, immediate early genes cFos and cJun are expressed, and their protein products Fos and Jun are formed. Next, a transcription factor, namely a leucine zipper, is created by the cooperation of Fos and Jun together. Finally, this transcription factor goes on to activate a late gene, resulting in the expression of its own gene product.

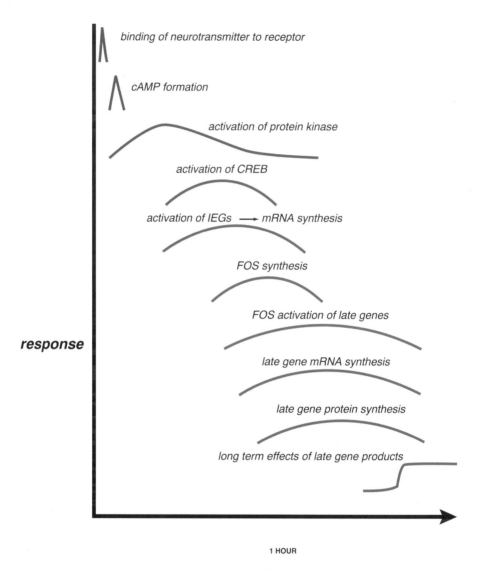

FIGURE 2–41. The **time course** of neurotransmitter-induced **activation of late genes** is shown here. This encompasses the activities illustrated in Figures 2–31 through 2–40. A similar time course was outlined in less detail in Figure 1–13. Here, the earliest events start at the top, and the later events cascade down through the graph. Neurotransmitter binding to receptor is immediate, and many important events occur within the first hour. Immediate early genes are probably activated within 15 minutes and late genes within the first hour. However, it is only many hours to days after activation of the late genes that the profound physiological actions are seen, such as regulation of enzymes and receptors and synaptogenesis.

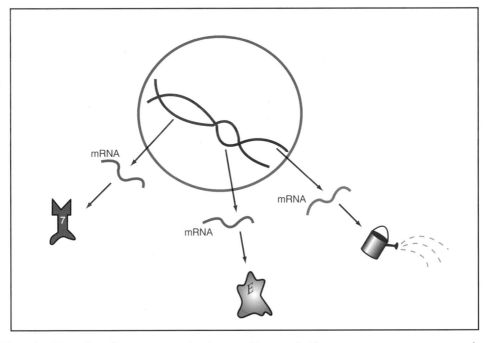

FIGURE 2–42. Examples of **late gene activation** are illustrated. Thus, a receptor, an enzyme, and a neurotrophic growth factor are all being expressed owing to activation of their respective genes. Such gene products go on to modify neuronal function for many hours or days.

## Receptors as Sites of Drug Action

One common example of a neurotransmitter-induced change is the regulation of the number of the neurotransmitter's own receptors. By asking for more copies or fewer copies of its receptors, the neurotransmitter enables the neurotransmission process to come full circle from receptor to gene and back to receptor again (Figs. 2–43 and 2–44). Drugs acting at a receptor can also affect the number of these neurotransmitter receptors by similarly decreasing the rate of receptor synthesis. When the rate of a neurotransmitter receptor's synthesis is decreased, it is sometimes called down regulation or desensitization (see Figs. 2–43 and 2–45). This process takes days. Changes in the rates of receptor synthesis can powerfully modify chemical neurotransmission at the synapse. That is, a decreased rate of receptor synthesis results in less receptor being made and less being transported down the axon to the terminal for insertion into the membrane (see Figs. 1–8, 2–43, and 2–45). This would theoretically diminish the sensitivity of neurotransmission. A neurotransmitter or drug can also cause a faster form of desensitization by activating an enzyme that phosphorylates the receptor, making the receptor immediately insensitive to its neurotransmitter.

When the rate of a neurotransmitter receptor's synthesis is increased, it is sometimes called up regulation (Figs. 2–44 and 2–45). In fact, receptors may be synthesized in excess under some conditions, especially if these receptors are blocked by a drug for a long period of time (Figs. 2–44 and 2–45). Too much receptor

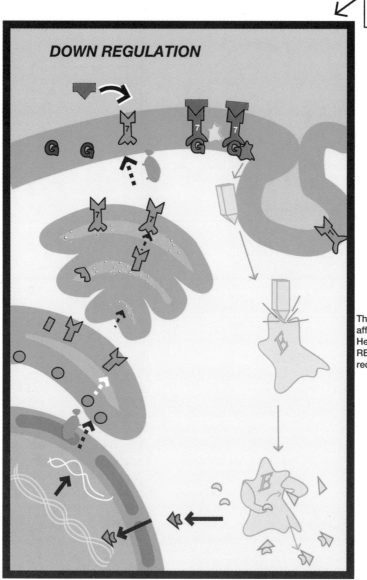

**DOWN REGULATION**

The new chemical affects the cell's DNA. Here, it causes DOWN-REGULATION of receptors.

FIGURE 2–43. The production of chemical instructions by intracellular enzymes can include orders for the cell's DNA. Shown here is the blue neurotransmitter cascade leading to second messenger formation, followed by second messenger activation of an intracellular enzyme, which in turn has triggered yet another intracellular enzyme to produce red molecules. These red molecules contain instructions for the cell's DNA, which order it to **slow down** the synthesis of the neurotransmitter receptor. Thus, fewer blue neurotransmitter receptors are being formed, as represented by the tortoise on the arrows of neurotransmitter receptor synthesis. Such slowing of neurotransmitter receptor synthesis is called **down regulation**.

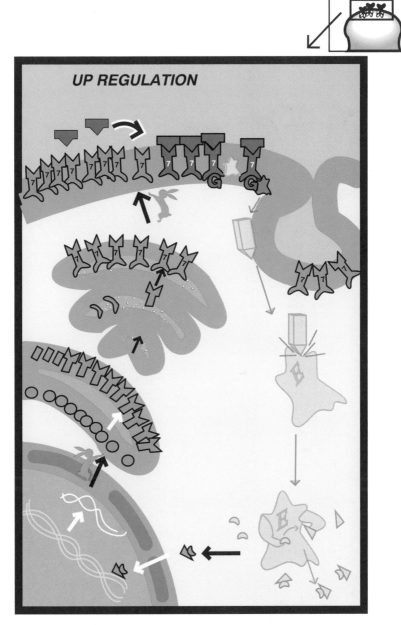

FIGURE 2–44. The production of chemical instructions by intracellular enzymes can also include orders for the cell's DNA to speed up the synthesis of neurotransmitter receptors. Thus, the blue neurotransmitter cascade leads to second messenger formation, which is followed by second messenger activation of an intracellular enzyme, which in turn has triggered yet another intracellular enzyme to produce red molecules. In contrast to the molecules of Figure 2–43, the red molecules depicted here contain instructions for the cell's DNA, which order it to **speed up** the synthesis of the neurotransmitter receptor. Thus, a greater number of blue neurotransmitter receptors are being formed, as represented by the hare on the arrows of neurotransmitter receptor synthesis. Such an increase in neurotransmitter receptor synthesis is called **up regulation**.

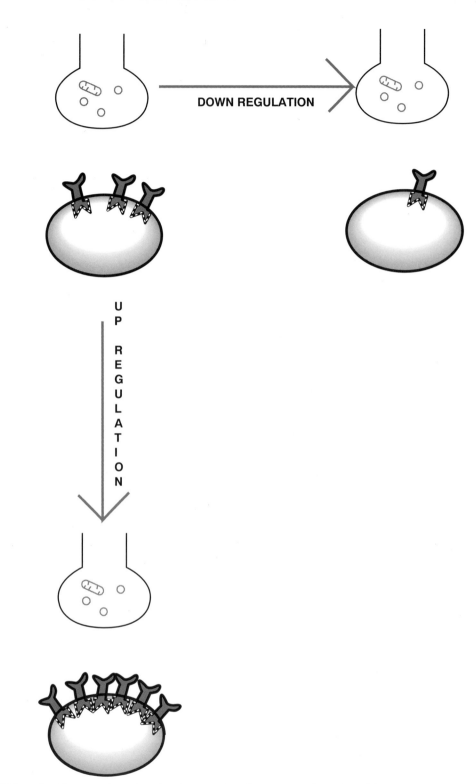

FIGURE 2–45. The complicated molecular cascades of Figures 2–43 and 2–44 are shown here with simplified icons. Thus, when **fewer** neurotransmitter receptors are formed, the process is called **down regulation**. When **more** neurotransmitter molecules are formed, it is called **up regulation**.

After a substrate binds to an enzyme, it is turned into a product which is then released from the enzyme.

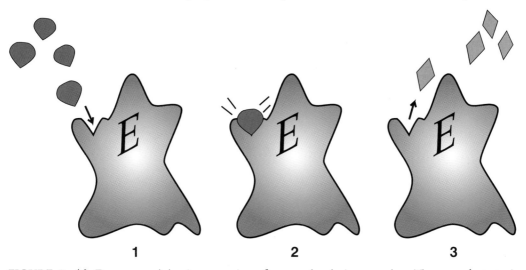

**1**                    **2**                    **3**

FIGURE 2–46. **Enzyme activity** is conversion of one molecule into another. Thus, a **substrate** is said to be turned into a **product** by enzymatic modification of the substrate molecule. The enzyme has an active site at which the substrate can bind specifically (1). The substrate then finds the active site of the enzyme, and binds to it (2), so that a molecular transformation can occur, changing the substrate into the product (3).

synthesis may not only increase the sensitivity of neurotransmission but may also produce a disease. Exactly this is suspected to be the case for the condition known as tardive dyskinesia (see Chapter 11, antipsychotics), which is apparently caused when drugs that block dopamine receptors cause abnormal changes in the number or sensitivity of dopamine receptors.

Neurotransmitter-induced molecular cascades into the cell nucleus of course lead not only to changes in the synthesis of the neurotransmitter's own receptors, but also to changes in the synthesis of many other important postsynaptic proteins, including enzymes and receptors for other neurotransmitters.

In summary, second-messenger systems (Figs. 2–25 through 2–28) have a general theme of using neurotransmitter first messengers occupying their receptors in order to precipitate a cascade of molecular events, carried out by a team of molecular players that interact with one another cooperatively, handing over the message from one molecule to another. This accomplishes the transfer of information sent via a transmitting neuron's neurotransmitter outside of the receiving neuron (Fig. 2–25) to inside that receiving neuron (Figs. 2–26 through 2–28), with many potential effects on intracellular processes (Figs. 2–29 through 2–45).

Once the extracellular first messenger from the transmitting neuron has handed over a message to an intracellular second messenger of the receiving neuron, the message then penetrates deep inside the recipient cell in a complex molecular cascade, which reaches enzymes, receptors, ion channels, and ultimately DNA, in order to transmit the information of how the neurotransmitter from the transmitting

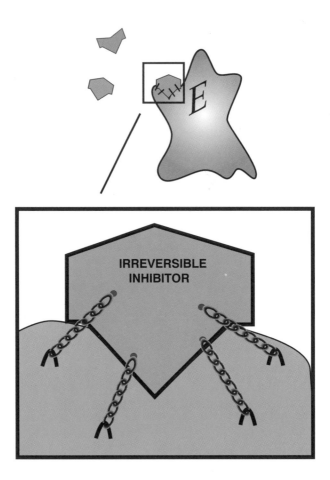

The "suicide inhibitor." This enzyme inhibitor binds
irreversibly to the enzyme protein, permanently
inhibiting the enzyme.

FIGURE 2–47. Some drugs are **inhibitors of enzymes**. Shown here is an **irreversible inhibitor** of an enzyme, depicted as binding to the enzyme with chains. The binding is locked so permanently that such irreversible enzyme inhibition is sometimes called the work of a "suicide inhibitor," since the enzyme essentially commits suicide by binding to the irreversible inhibitor. Enzyme activity cannot be restored unless another molecule of enzyme is synthesized by the cell's DNA. The enzyme molecule that has bound the irreversible inhibitor is permanently incapable of further enzymatic activity and therefore is essentially "dead."

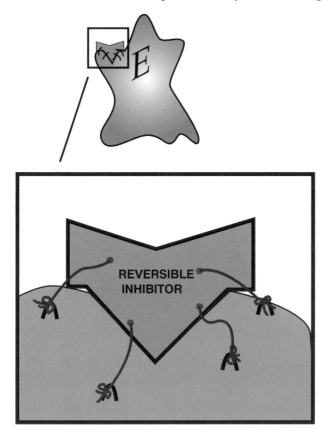

The reversible inhibitor. This inhibitor can come off of the
enzyme protein and thus can be reversed.

FIGURE 2–48. Other drugs are **reversible enzyme inhibitors**, depicted as binding to the enzyme
with a string. It is possible for the inhibitor to be chased off the enzyme under the right circumstances,
in which case the inhibition is reversed and the enzyme becomes fully functional again.

neuron will alter cellular function in the receiving neuron (Figs. 2–35 and 2–40
through 2–42). At each point along the way, there is a potential site of action for
psychotropic drugs or for contributions to psychiatric and neurological diseases.

Finally, altering the rates of synthesis of enzymes that can either create or destroy
neurotransmitters can also affect the amount of chemical neurotransmitter available
for neurotransmission and thereby alter the chemical neurotransmission process itself.

## Enzymes as Sites of Drug Action

Enzymes are involved in multiple aspects of chemical neurotransmission, as discussed
earlier in this chapter. Every enzyme is the theoretical target for a drug acting as
an enzyme inhibitor. However, in practice only a minority of currently known drugs
are enzyme inhibitors.

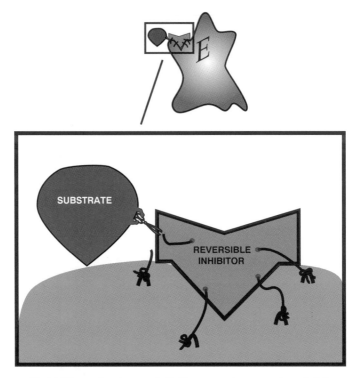

The inhibitor can then be moved off of the enzyme by a competing substrate.

FIGURE 2–49. This **reversible enzyme inhibitor** is being challenged by the **substrate** for this same enzyme. In the case of a reversible inhibitor, the molecular properties of the substrate are such that it can get rid of the reversible inhibitor, which is depicted as scissors cutting the string that binds the reversible inhibitor to the enzyme.

The enzymes most important in the neurotransmission process are those that make and destroy the neurotransmitters. Thus, precursors are transported into the neuron with the aid of an enzyme-assisted transport pump and converted into neurotransmitters by a series of neurotransmitter-synthesizing enzymes (Figs. 1–7 through 1–9). Once synthesis of the neurotransmitter is complete, it is stored in vesicles, where it stays until released by a nerve impulse. In the vesicle, the neurotransmitter is also protected from enzymes capable of breaking it down. Once released, however, the neurotransmitter is free not only to diffuse to its receptors for synaptic actions but also to diffuse to enzymes capable of destroying the neurotransmitter or to the reuptake pump already discussed above and represented in Figures 2–20 through 2–24.

Enzyme activity is thus the conversion of one molecule into another, namely a substrate into a product. The substrates for each enzyme are very unique and selective, as are the products. The inhibitors of an enzyme are also very unique and selective for one enzyme as compared with another. Enzymes doing their normal work bind their substrates prior to converting them into products (Fig 2–46). How-

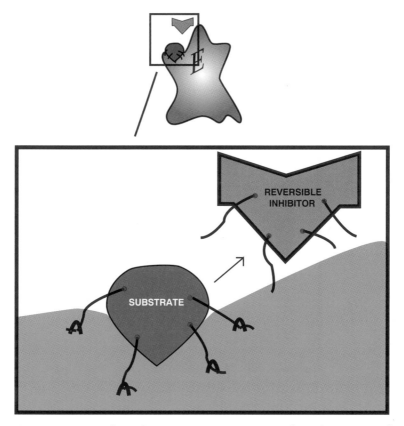

FIGURE 2–50. The consequence of a **substrate competing successfully** for reversal of enzyme inhibition is that the substrate essentially **displaces** the inhibitor and **shoves it off**. Because the substrate has this capability, the inhibition is said to be **reversible**.

ever, in the presence of an enzyme inhibitor, the enzyme can also bind to the inhibitor, which prevents the binding of substrate and the making of products (Figs. 2–47 through 2–51). The binding of inhibitors can be either reversible (Figs. 2–48 through 2–50) or irreversible (Figs. 2–47 and 2–51).

In the case of reversible enzyme inhibitors, an enzyme's substrate is able to compete with that reversible inhibitor for binding to the enzyme (Fig. 2–49) and literally to shove it off the enzyme (Fig. 2–50). Whether the substrate or the inhibitor "wins" or predominates depends on which one has the greater affinity for the enzyme and/or is present in the greater concentration.

However, when an irreversible inhibitor binds to the enzyme, it cannot be displaced by the substrate and thus binds irreversibly (Fig. 2–51). The irreversible type of enzyme inhibitor is sometimes called a "suicide inhibitor" because it covalently and irreversibly binds to the enzyme protein, permanently inhibiting it and therefore essentially "killing" the enzyme by making it nonfunctional forever (Fig. 2–51). Enzyme activity in this case is only restored when new enzyme molecules are synthesized.

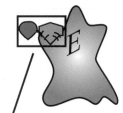

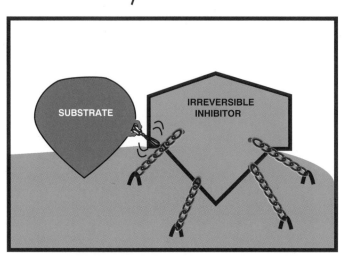

The suicide inhibitor cannot be moved off of the enzyme by a competing substrate.

FIGURE 2–51. The consequence of a **substrate competing unsuccessfully** for reversal of enzyme inhibition is that the substrate is **unable to displace** the inhibitor. This is depicted as scissors unsuccessfully attempting to cut the chains of the inhibitor. In this case, the inhibition is **irreversible**.

These concepts can be applied potentially to any enzyme system. Given the rapid clarification of increasing numbers of enzymes, we should expect to see an ever-growing number of enzyme inhibitors entering psychopharmacology in future years.

## Summary: How Drugs Modify Chemical Neurotransmission

This chapter has discussed the role of receptors and enzymes in the fascinating and dynamic processes of chemical neurotransmission. The importance of understanding of fundamentals of how receptors and enzymes affect neurotransmission cannot be underestimated. Much of contemporary neuropharmacology is predicated on the premise that most of the drugs and many of the diseases that affect the CNS do so at the level of the synapse, as well as on the process of chemical neurotransmission.

The chapter has specifically reviewed how receptors and enzymes are the targets of drug actions in psychopharmacology. We have explored the components of individual receptors and discussed how receptors function as members of a synaptic neurotransmission team, which has the neurotransmitter as captain and receptors as major team players interacting with other players on the team including ions, ion channels, transport carriers, active transport pumps, second-messenger systems, and enzymes. The reader should also have an appreciation for the elegant if complex molecular cascade precipitated by a neurotransmitter, with molecule-by-molecule transfer of the transmitted message inside the neuron receiving that message eventually altering the biochemical machinery of that cell in order to carry out the message sent to it.

# CHAPTER 3

# Special Properties of Receptors

The study of receptor psychopharmacology involves understanding not only that receptors are the targets for most of the known drugs but also that they have some very special properties. This chapter will build on the discussion of the general properties of receptors introduced in Chapter 2 and will introduce the reader to some of the special properties of receptors that help explain how they participate in key drug interactions. Specifically, we will discuss three important psychopharmacological principles of receptors: first, that they are organized into multiple subtypes; second, that their interactions with drugs can define not only agonists and antagonists but also partial agonists and inverse agonists; and finally, that allosteric modulation is an important theme of receptor modulation by drugs.

## Multiple Receptor Subtypes

### Definition and Description

There are at least two ways to categorize receptors. One is based on describing all the receptors that share a common neurotransmitter. This is sometimes called pharmacological subtyping. The other organizational scheme for receptors is to classify them according to their common structural features and molecular interactions, a classification sometimes called receptor superfamilies.

Additional classification schemes will not be discussed here in any detail but include those with related gene and/or chromosome localizations and those with the same effector systems. (e.g., stimulatory or inhibitory G proteins or sodium, potassium, chloride, or calcium channels). These features of different receptors will be discussed as specific neurotransmitter receptors are mentioned throughout the rest of the book.

### Pharmacological Subtyping

To increase the options for brain communication, each neurotransmitter can act on more than one neurotransmitter receptor. That is, there is not a single acetylcholine receptor, nor a single serotonin receptor, nor a single norepinephrine receptor. In fact, multiple subtypes have been discovered for virtually every known neurotransmitter receptor.

It is as though the neurotransmitter keys in the brain can open many receptor locks. Thus, the neurotransmitter is the master key. Whereas some drugs act like duplicates of master keys, others can be made more selective and act at only one of the receptors, like a submaster key for a single lock (Fig. 3–1).

This makes for clever engineering of the communications that occur via the brain's neurotransmitters and receptors. Because the system of chemical neurotransmission uses *multiple* neurotransmitters, each working through *multiple* receptors, chemical signaling provides the features of both selectivity and amplification. That is, while there is *selectivity* of a receptor family for a single neurotransmitter, there is nevertheless *amplification* of receptor communication due to the presence of a great variety of neurotransmitter receptors for the same neurotransmitter. Thus, each neurotransmitter has not only the property of selectivity when compared with other neurotransmitters but also a redundancy of receptor subtypes sharing the same neurotransmitter. Receptor subtypes allow a single neurotransmitter to perform quite different functions, depending not only on which particular subtype it is binding but also on where in the brain's topography any receptor subtype is localized.

### Receptor Superfamilies

There are two major superfamilies of receptors. The first is the superfamily of which all members have seven transmembrane regions, all use a G protein, and all use a second-messenger system (represented as an icon in Fig. 3–2). This was extensively discussed in the text and figures of Chapter 2. Individual member receptors within this class may, however, use various different neurotransmitters and still be a member of this same superfamily. What makes one member of the family use one neuro-

## Drugs for six neurotransmitter
## receptor subtypes

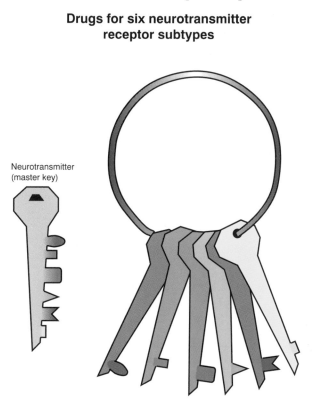

Neurotransmitter
(master key)

FIGURE 3–1. Neurotransmitters have multiple **receptor subtypes** with which to interact. It is as though the neurotransmitter is the master key capable of unlocking each of the multiple receptor subtype locks. Drugs can be made that mimic the neurotransmitter. The most selective drugs are capable of mimicking the natural neurotransmitter's action at just one of the receptor locks. This figure shows a neurotransmitter capable of interacting with six different receptor subtypes (i.e., the master key). Also shown are six different drugs on a key chain. Each of these drugs is selective for a different single subtype of the neurotransmitter receptors.

transmitter and another member of this same family use another neurotransmitter is probably the molecular makeup of that portion of the transmembrane region that binds the neurotransmitter (see Figs. 2–3, 2–5, and 2–6). The molecular configuration of the neurotransmitter binding site differs from one receptor to the next in the same family. This is how different neurotransmitters can be used in the same receptor superfamily. The differences in binding sites between receptors in the same superfamily are generally based on substitution of different amino acids at a few critical places in the receptor's amino acid chain (Fig. 2–1). Precise substitution of amino acids in just a few key places can thus transform a receptor with binding characteristics for one neurotransmitter into a receptor with vast changes in its binding characteristics so that it now recognizes and binds an entirely different neurotransmitter. This has been previously discussed in Chapter 2 and represented in earlier figures, including Figures 2–1 to 2–3.

A second superfamily of receptors shares a common molecular makeup in which every member has four transmembrane regions, with five copies of each receptor configured around an ion channel (represented as icons in Figs. 3–3 and 3–4; see

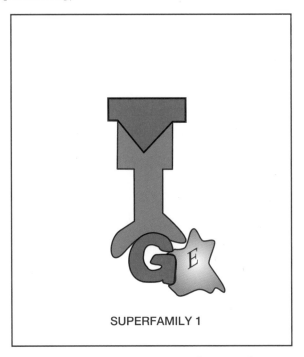

SUPERFAMILY 1

FIGURE 3–2. Represented here is one of the two major **superfamilies of neurotransmitter recep-tors**. This superfamily is called the **G protein–linked receptor superfamily**. Each member of this family has a receptor containing **seven transmembrane regions** (shown in Figs. 2–1 and 2–2) but given here as a simple receptor icon. Each receptor in this family is linked to a **G protein** and also uses a **second-messenger system** triggered by a cooperating **enzyme**. A more detailed breakdown and explanation of this superfamily with a series of icons was given in Figures 2–25 through 2–22.

also Figs. 2–5 and 2–6). The ion channel may differ from one receptor to another in this superfamily, and the neurotransmitter may also differ from one family member to another. However, all are arranged in a similar molecular form, concentrically around the ion channel.

Another common feature of this superfamily is that not only are there multiple copies of each receptor but many different types of receptor are present. Thus, the ion channel is surrounded by *multiple* copies of *many* different receptors (Fig. 3–3). This allows the critical passage of ions into the cell via the ion channel to be regulated by multiple neurotransmitters and drugs rather than just a single neuro-transmitter. It seems that regulating an ion channel is too important a job to be left up to a single neurotransmitter. Thus, the brain has arranged for many different gatekeepers to watch over the passage of ions into the neuron. Sometimes the various gatekeepers that have a say in the regulation of the channel compete with each other to neutralize each other. Sometimes they cooperate to boost each other's actions. There may even be two neurotransmitters that can be active at such receptors; these are known then as co-transmitters.

The ion channel itself is essentially a column of columns. By binding to the binding sites in the receptor columns, the neurotransmitter causes the opening and closing of the ion channel column in the center of all the columns (i.e., within the

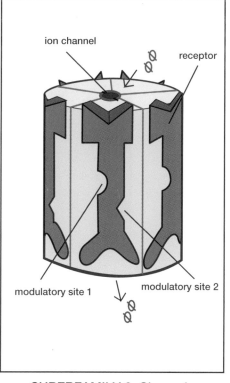

**SUPERFAMILY 2; Channel
in resting state**

FIGURE 3–3. The second major superfamily of neurotransmitter receptors is represented here. This superfamily is called the **ligand-gated ion channel receptors**. This receptor has five copies of subunits each of which have four transmembrane regions. (See also Figs. 2–5 and 2–6.) Since multiple copies of each such receptor are arranged as columns in a circle they can serve as **molecular gatekeepers** for an **ion channel**. The ion channel is located in the middle of the circle of receptors. On each receptor, there is not only the **receptor binding site** but also various different **modulatory sites** for additional neurotransmitters and drugs. In this figure, the ion channel is partially open.

column of columns) (Fig 3–3). This arrangement is best documented for the nicotinic acetylcholine receptor, and for the gamma-aminobutyric acid (GABA)–benzodiazepine receptor, but is hypothesized to be a general theme for several types of ligand-gated ion channels, including glycine receptors. However, this may not be the exact structural configuration for ion channels that use glutamate as the gatekeeping ligand.

As mentioned in Chapter 1 and represented pictorially in Figure 1–6 depicting slow and fast neurotransmission, the members of the superfamily with seven transmembrane regions linked to second-messenger systems have slower-onset modulatory signals, eventually amplified into gene activation minutes to hours later. However, the members of the superfamily with four transmembrane region ion channels have faster onset in that they immediately change the ionic condition of the neuron and thus facilitate excitatory or inhibitory neurotransmission.

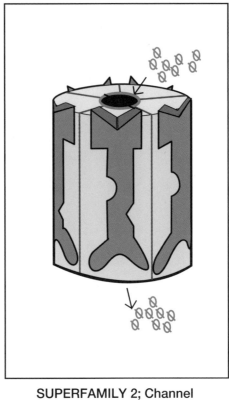

**SUPERFAMILY 2; Channel
open**

FIGURE 3–4. Another version of the ligand-gated ion channel receptor superfamily is shown here with the **ion channel opened** to a greater extent than in Figure 3–3. The **opening and closing of the ion channel** is controlled by the various ligands that can bind to the different binding sites on the receptors in this family. That is why this superfamily is called **ligand-gated**.

## Agonists and Antagonists

Naturally occurring neurotransmitters stimulate receptors. These are called agonists. By contrast, the portfolio of options for drugs is far greater than just stimulation of receptors. In fact, a whole spectrum of possibilities exists, sometimes called the agonist spectrum (Fig. 3–5). Some drugs do stimulate receptors just as do the natural neurotransmitters and are therefore agonists. Other drugs actually block the actions of a natural neurotransmitter at its receptor and are called antagonists. True antagonists only exert their actions in the presence of agonist; they have no intrinsic activity of their own in the absence of agonist. Still other drugs do the opposite of what agonists do and are called inverse agonists. Thus, drugs acting at a receptor exist in a *spectrum* from full agonist to antagonist to inverse agonist (Fig. 3–5).

Examples of the actions of agonists can be taken from each of the two major molecular superfamilies. For the family of seven-transmembrane-region receptors linked to G proteins and enzymic second-messenger systems, the agonist would turn on the synthesis of second messenger to the greatest extent possible (i.e., the action

# THE AGONIST SPECTRUM

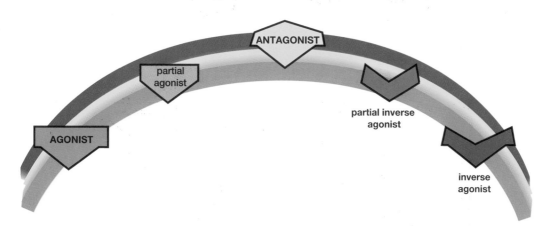

FIGURE 3–5. Shown here is the agonist spectrum. This spectrum reaches from agonists through antagonists to inverse agonists. Naturally occurring neurotransmitters are agonists. It is a common misconception that antagonists are the opposite of agonists because they block the actions of agonists. However, inverse agonists are really the opposite of agonists. Antagonists can block anything in the agonist spectrum, including inverse agonists. If an agonist is not as strong as the full agonist, it is called a **partial agonist**. Similarly, if an inverse agonist is partial and not as strong as a full inverse agonist, it is called a **partial inverse agonist**. Examples of the psychopharmacological actions of an agonist would be to **reduce** anxiety or to reduce pain. An inverse agonist, by analogy, would cause anxiety or pain. A partial agonist would **weakly reduce** anxiety or pain, and a partial inverse agonist would **weakly cause** anxiety or pain. An **antagonist** would block the full and partial agonists from reducing any anxiety or pain and would also block the full and partial inverse agonists from causing any anxiety or pain. However, an antagonist would neither reduce nor cause pain in itself.

of a *full* agonist). The full agonist is generally represented by the naturally occurring neurotransmitter itself, although some drugs can also act in as full a manner as the natural neurotransmitter. Often the term agonist is therefore imprecise, and the better term is full agonist.

For the family of four-transmembrane-region receptors, with multiple copies of each arranged as individual columns forming an ion channel in the center, a full agonist acts by multiple molecules of the agonist each finding the transmembrane binding site for the agonist within the receptor columns surrounding the ion channel. This in turn opens the ion channel column more completely; thus, the full agonist action (Fig. 3–6). At baseline the ion channel is only partially open, and a full agonist therefore opens it much more (Fig. 3–6).

## Antagonists

Antagonists block the actions of everything in the agonist spectrum (Fig. 3–5). By themselves, antagonists have no intrinsic activity and therefore are sometimes referred to as "silent" (Fig. 3–7). However, in the presence of an agonist, an antagonist will block the actions of that agonist (Fig. 3–8).

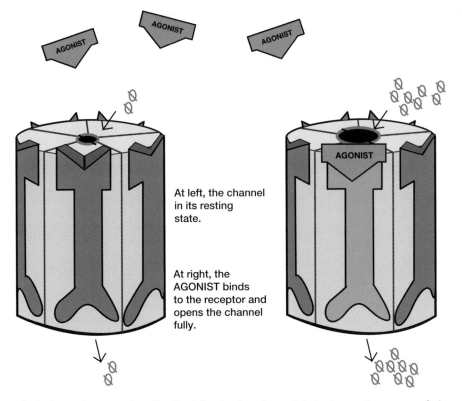

At left, the channel in its resting state.

At right, the AGONIST binds to the receptor and opens the channel fully.

FIGURE 3–6. Actions of an agonist. On the left, the ion channel is in its resting state, a balance between being opened and closed. On the right, the agonist occupies its binding site on the ligand-gated ion channel receptor and as gatekeeper, opens the ion channel. This is represented as the red agonist turning the receptor red and opening the ion channel as the agonist docks into its binding site.

## Inverse Agonists

Inverse agonists do the *opposite* of agonists. An example of their action can also be taken from receptors linked to an ion channel. By contrast to agonists and antagonists, an *inverse agonist* neither opens the ion channel as does an agonist (Fig. 3–6) nor blocks the agonist from opening the channel as does an antagonist (Fig. 3–8); rather, it binds the neurotransmitter receptor in such a fashion as to provoke an action opposite to that of the agonist, namely, causing the receptor to *close* the ion channel (Fig. 3–9).

It might seem at first look that there is no difference between an inverse agonist and an antagonist. There is, however, a very important distinction between them. Whereas an antagonist blocks an agonist (Fig. 3–8), it has no particular action in the absence of the agonist, when it is thus silent (Fig. 3–7). An inverse agonist has an action *opposite* to that of an agonist (Fig. 3–9). Furthermore, an antagonist will actually block the action of an inverse agonist (Fig. 3–10), just as it will block the action of a full agonist (Fig. 3–7).

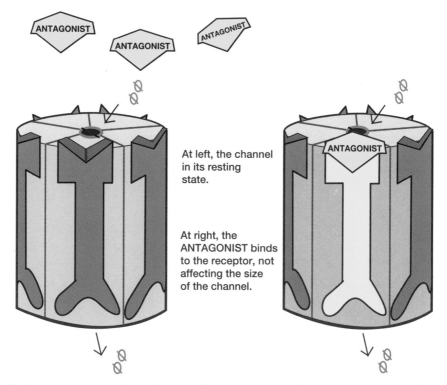

FIGURE 3–7. Antagonist acting alone. On the left, the **ion channel** is in its resting state, a balance between being open and closed. On the right, the **antagonist** occupies the binding site normally occupied by the agonist on the ligand-gated ion channel receptor. However, there is **no consequence** to this, and the **ion channel neither opens further nor closes**. This is represented as the yellow antagonist turning the receptor yellow and neither opening nor closing the ion channel as the antagonist docks into the binding site.

## Partial Agonists

To add even more options to the actions of drugs at neurotransmitter receptors and to influence neurotransmission in even more ways, there is a class of agents known as *partial agonists*. A partial agonist exerts an effect similar to but weaker than that of the full agonist. Thus, in the example of the neurotransmitter system controlling an ion channel, a partial agonist would open the ion channel to a certain extent (Fig. 3–11) but only partially as compared with the full agonist (Fig. 3–6). Partial agonists are also blocked by antagonists (Fig. 3–12). It is even possible for the inverse agonists to be partial (Fig. 3–13). In this case, the partial inverse agonist closes the ion channel to a lesser extent (Fig. 3–13) than a full inverse agonist (Fig. 3–9).

This means that there is a spectrum of degree to which a receptor can be stimulated (Fig. 3–14). At one end of the spectrum, there is the full agonist, which elicits the same degree of physiologic receptor-mediated response as the natural neurotransmitter agonist itself. At the other end of the spectrum is a full inverse agonist, which in concept does the opposite of the agonist. In the middle is the

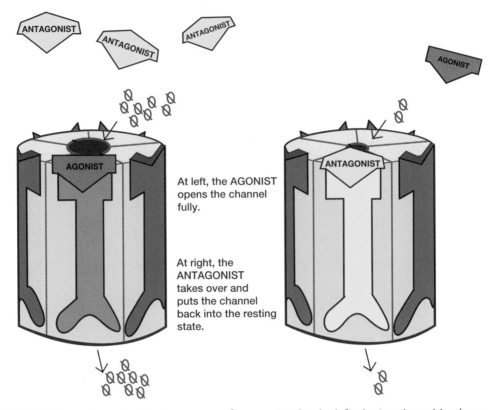

FIGURE 3–8. Antagonist acting in the presence of an agonist. On the left, the ion channel has been opened by the agonist occupying its binding site on the ligand-gated ion channel receptor and as gatekeeper, **opening the ion channel**, just as in Figure 3–6. This is represented as the red agonist turning the receptor red and opening the ion channel as it docks into its binding site, as in Figure 3–6. On the right, the yellow **antagonist prevails** and shoves the red agonist off the binding site, **reversing the agonist's actions**. Since the agonist had opened the ion channel, the antagonist reverses this by partially closing the ion channel to restore the resting state. Thus, the ion channel has been caused to return to its status before the agonist acted.

antagonist, which blocks the effects of all participants in the spectrum but has no properties of its own in changing the ion channel.

The spectrum thus goes from full agonist to partial agonist to antagonist to partial inverse agonist to full inverse agonist (Fig. 3–14). Although this concept of agonists, antagonists, and partial agonists is well developed for several neurotransmitter systems, there are relatively few examples of inverse agonists.

### Light and Dark as an Analogy for Partial Agonists

It was originally considered that a neurotransmitter could act at the receptor as does a light switch, to turn it on or off. We now know that the synapse and its receptors can function rather more like a rheostat. That is, a full agonist will turn the lights all the way on (Fig. 3–15), but a partial agonist will only turn the light on partially (Fig. 3–16). If neither full agonist nor partial agonist is present, the room is dark (Fig. 3–17).

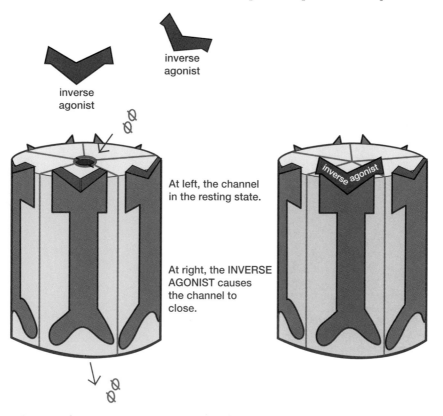

At left, the channel in the resting state.

At right, the INVERSE AGONIST causes the channel to close.

FIGURE 3–9. Actions of an inverse agonist. On the left, the **ion channel** is in its resting state, a balance between being opened and closed. On the right, the **inverse agonist** occupies the binding site on the ligand-gated ion channel receptor as gatekeeper, **closes the ion channel**. This is the **opposite** of what the agonist does (cf. Fig. 3–6). Inverse agonist is represented as the light blue inverse agonist turning the receptor light blue and closing the ion channel as the inverse agonist docks into its binding site.

Each partial agonist has its own set point engineered into the molecule, so that it cannot make lights brighter with a higher dose. No matter how much partial agonist is given, only a certain degree of brightness will result. A series of partial agonists will differ one from the other in degree of partiality, so that theoretically all degrees of brightness can be covered within the range from "off" to "on," but each partial agonist is associated with its own unique degree of brightness.

What is so interesting about partial agonists is that they can appear as net agonists or as net antagonists, depending on the amount of naturally occurring full agonist neurotransmitter that is present. Take, for example, the case of neurotransmitters controlling an ion channel. When no full agonist neurotransmitter is present, a partial agonist will be a net agonist, that is, it will *open* the channel from its resting state (Fig. 3–18). However, when a full agonist neurotransmitter agonist is present, the same partial agonist will become a net antagonist, it will *close* the channel from its full agonist state (Fig. 3–18). Thus, a partial agonist can simultaneously *boost* deficient neurotransmitter activity yet *block* excessive neurotransmitter activity (Fig. 3–18).

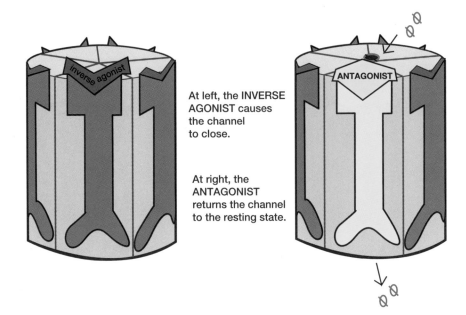

At left, the INVERSE AGONIST causes the channel to close.

At right, the ANTAGONIST returns the channel to the resting state.

FIGURE 3–10. Antagonist acting in the presence of an inverse agonist. On the left, the **ion channel** has been closed by the inverse agonist occupying the binding site on the ligand-gated ion channel receptor and as gatekeeper, **closing the ion channel**, just as shown in Figure 3–9. This is represented as the light blue inverse agonist turning the receptor light blue and closing the ion channel as it docks into its binding site, as in Figure 3–9. On the right, the yellow antagonist prevails and shoves the light blue inverse agonist off the binding site, **reversing the inverse agonist's actions**. Since the inverse agonist had previously closed the ion channel, the antagonist reverses this closing by opening the ion channel to restore the resting state. This causes the ion channel to return to its status before the agonist acted. In this way, the antagonist's effect on an inverse agonist's actions is similar to that on an agonist's actions, namely, it **returns the ion channel to its resting state** (cf. Fig. 3–8). However, in the case of an inverse agonist, the antagonist opens the channel, whereas in the case of an agonist, the same antagonist **closes** the channel (cf. Figs. 3–8 and 3–10). Thus, an antagonist can **reverse either an agonist or an inverse agonist** despite the fact that it does nothing on its own (Fig. 3–7).

Returning to the light switch analogy, a room will be dark when agonist is missing and the light switch is off (Fig. 3–17). A room will be brightly lighted when it is full of natural full agonist and the light switch is fully on (Fig. 3–15). Adding partial agonist to the dark room where there is no natural full agonist neurotransmitter will turn the lights up, but only as far as the partial agonist works on the rheostat (Figure 3–16). Relative to the dark room as a starting point, a partial agonist acts therefore as a net agonist. On the other hand, adding a partial agonist to the fully lighted room will have the effect of turning the lights down to a level of lower brightness on the rheostat (Fig. 3–16). This is a net antagonistic effect relative to the fully lighted room. Thus, after adding partial agonist to the dark room and to the brightly lighted room, both rooms will be equally lighted.

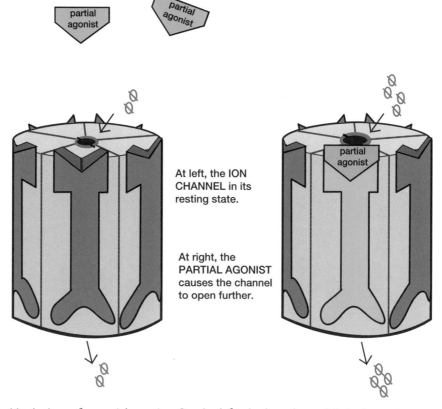

At left, the ION
CHANNEL in its
resting state.

At right, the
PARTIAL AGONIST
causes the channel
to open further.

FIGURE 3–11. Actions of a partial agonist. On the left, the **ion channel** is in its resting state, a balance between being opened and closed. On the right, the **partial agonist** occupies its binding site on the ligand-gated ion channel receptor and as gatekeeper, **partially opens the ion channel**. This is represented as the orange agonist turning the receptor orange and partially, but not fully, opening the ion channel as the partial agonist docks into its binding site. The ion channel is thus more open than it was in the resting state once a partial agonist acts, but less open than after a full agonist acts (cf. Figure 3–6).

The degree of brightness is that obtained with the lights partially turned on as dictated by the properties of the partial agonist. However, in the dark room, the partial agonist has acted as a net agonist, whereas in the brightly lighted room, it has acted as a net antagonist.

An agonist and an antagonist in the same molecule provide quite a new dimension to therapeutics. This concept has led to proposals that partial agonists could treat not only states that are theoretically deficient in full agonist but also states that theoretically have an excess of full agonist. An agent such as a partial agonist may even be able to treat simultaneously states that are mixtures of both excessive and deficient neurotransmitter activity.

## Allosteric Modulation

By now, it should be clear that a neurotransmitter and its receptor act as members on a team of specialized molecules, all working together in numerous ways to carry

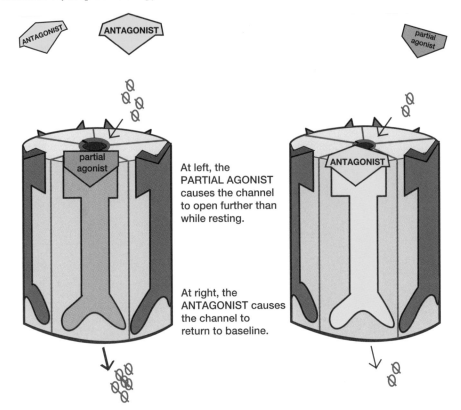

FIGURE 3–12. Antagonist acting in the presence of a partial agonist. On the left, the **ion channel** has been opened by the partial agonist occupying its binding site on the ligand-gated ion channel receptor and as gatekeeper, partially opening the ion channel, just as in Figure 3–11. This is represented as the orange agonist turning the receptor orange and partially opening the ion channel as the partial agonist docks into its binding site, as in Figure 3–11. On the right, the yellow antagonist prevails and shoves the orange partial agonist off the binding site, reversing the partial agonist's actions. Since the partial agonist had partially opened the ion channel, the antagonist reverses this partial opening by restoring the resting state of the ion channel that existed prior to the partial agonist's actions.

out the specialized functions necessary for the chemical neurotransmission of neuronal information. Another specific example of molecular interactions during chemical neurotransmission is the configuration of two or more neurotransmitter receptor sites such that one can boost or blunt the activities of the other. In some instances, the two interacting receptor binding sites may be located on the same receptor molecule; in other cases, the binding sites may be on neighboring receptors of different classes.

When two different receptor sites utilizing different neurotransmitters are arranged so as to influence a single receptor, there is generally considered to be a primary neurotransmitter receptor site, which influences its receptor in the usual manner (i.e., it turns on a second messenger or alters an ion channel). In this example, furthermore, there is a second receptor site, which can influence the receptor generally only when the primary neurotransmitter is binding at the primary receptor

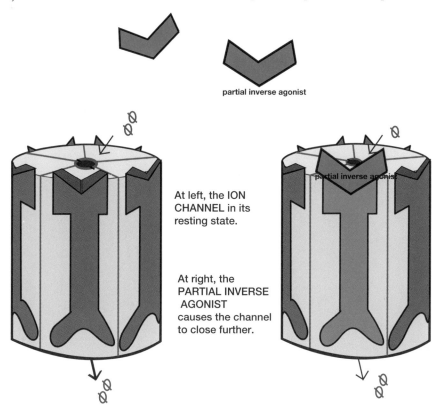

At left, the ION CHANNEL in its resting state.

At right, the PARTIAL INVERSE AGONIST causes the channel to close further.

FIGURE 3–13. Actions of a partial inverse agonist. On the left, the **ion channel** is in its resting state, a balance between being opened and closed. On the right, the **partial inverse agonist** occupies its binding site on the ligand-gated ion channel receptor and as gatekeeper, **partially closes** the ion channel. This is represented as the green inverse agonist turning the receptor green and partially closing the ion channel as the partial inverse agonist docks into its binding site.

site. Thus, a second neurotransmitter interacting at the secondary site only acts *indirectly* and through an interaction with the receptor when the primary neurotransmitter is simultaneously binding at its primary (and different) receptor site. Since the binding of the secondary neurotransmitter to its secondary receptor site is influencing the receptor by a mechanism other than direct binding to the primary receptor site, it is said to be modulating that receptor *allosterically* (literally, at an "other site"). The other site is the second receptor binding site, which utilizes a second neurotransmitter, yet influences the same receptor as does the primary neurotransmitter at its primary receptor binding site, but only when the primary neurotransmitter is present at that primary binding site. As mentioned earlier, this allosteric modulation can either amplify or block the actions of the primary neurotransmitter at the primary receptor binding site.

This allosteric cooperation among synaptic transmission teammates, in which one player interacts with a second player in order to modify or control it, is another example of a common recurring theme in chemical neurotransmission: A cascade of molecular interactions is triggered by the neurotransmitter–receptor binding site events.

# THE AGONIST SPECTRUM

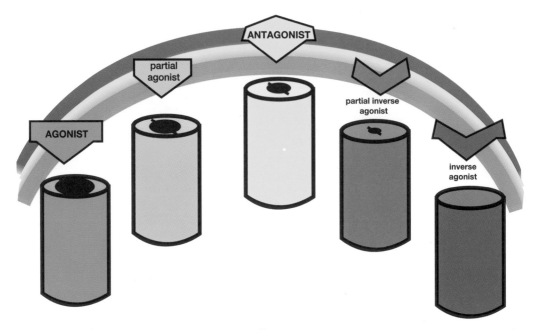

FIGURE 3–14. The agonist spectrum and its effects on the ion channel. Shown again is the **agonist spectrum**, this time with the corresponding effects of each agent on the ion channel. This spectrum ranges from **agonists**, which fully open the ion channel, through **antagonists**, which retain the resting state between open and closed, to **inverse agonists**, which close the ion channel. Between the extremes are **partial agonists**, which partially open the ion channel, and partial inverse agonists, which partially close the ion channel. Antagonists can block anything in the agonist spectrum, returning the ion channel to the resting state in each instance.

## Positive Allosteric Interactions

An example of positive allosteric modulation is shown by the influence of modulatory sites on the gatekeepers at ligand-gated ion channels. In this case, the primary neurotransmitter is the gatekeeper, which opens the ion channel as discussed previously. To explain allosteric modulation, we will introduce a second receptor binding site, which can interact with the gatekeeper and its receptor. Thus, following occupancy of the gatekeeper receptor by the primary gatekeeper, that receptor in turn interacts with an ion channel to open it a bit, as previously discussed for agonist actions (Fig. 3–19).

Near the gatekeeper's receptor site is not only the ion channel but also another neurotransmitter receptor binding site, namely, a receptor capable of allosterically modulating the gatekeeper's receptor (Fig. 3–19). Allosteric modulatory sites do not directly influence the ion channel. They do so indirectly by influencing the gatekeeper receptor, which in turn influences the ion channel. Thus, the allosteric modulatory site acts literally at another site to influence the ion channel. Since the meaning of allosteric is other site, one can easily understand why this term is applied

**FULL AGONIST --** light is at its brightest

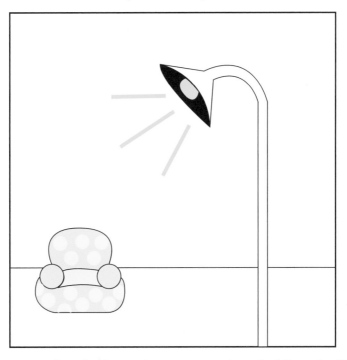

FIGURE 3–15. Light as an analogy for the agonist spectrum: actions of a full agonist. Light will be **brightest** after a full agonist turns the light switch **fully on.** When a **partial agonist** is added to the fully lighted (i.e. full agonist) room, it will "dim" the lights; thus, the partial agonist in this case acts as a **net antagonist.**

to such modulatory receptor sites and their neurotransmitters. The allosteric modulatory site thus has a knock-on effect on the conductance of ions through the ion channel.

The mechanism of allosteric modulation is such that when an allosteric modulator binds to its own receptor site, which is a neighbor of the gatekeeper receptor binding site, nothing happens if the gatekeeper is not also binding to its own gatekeeper receptor. On the other hand, when the gatekeeper is binding to its receptor site, the simultaneous binding of the allosteric modulator to its binding site causes a large amplification in the gatekeeper's ability to increase the conductance of ion through the channel (Fig. 3–19).

Why is this necessary? It turns out that most gatekeepers can increase ionic conductance through ion channels only to a certain extent by themselves. Allosteric modulators cannot alter ionic conductance at all when working by themselves. However, allosteric modulation is a formula to maximize ionic conductance beyond that which the gatekeeper alone can accomplish. Thus, the gatekeeper can increase ionic conductance through an ion channel much more dramatically when an allosteric modulator is helping than it can when it is working alone.

Evident in this discussion of allosteric modulation of one receptor binding site by another receptor binding site is the possibility of *numerous* allosteric sites for a

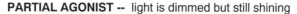

**PARTIAL AGONIST --** light is dimmed but still shining

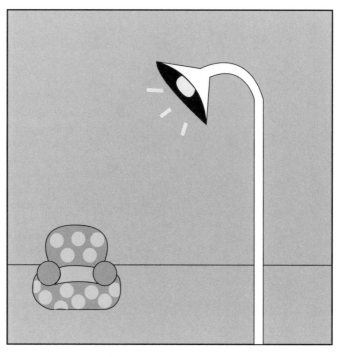

FIGURE 3–16. Light as an analogy for the agonist spectrum: actions of a partial agonist. By itself, a partial agonist turns the light neither fully on or fully off. Rather, a **partial agonist** acts like a rheostat, or dimming switch, which turns on the light but only **partially**.

single receptor. As will be developed in greater detail in subsequent chapters, it is hypothesized that the anxiolytic, hypnotic, anticonvulsant, and muscle relaxant properties of numerous drugs, including the benzodiazepines, barbiturates, and anticonvulsants, are all mediated by allosteric interactions at molecular sites around the GABA receptor and the chloride channel. It is possible that a variety of allosteric sites, analogous to the benzodiazepine sites, modulate GABA-induced increases at chloride channels by a wide variety of drugs, even including alcohol.

## Negative Allosteric Interactions

An example of negative allosteric modulation is the case of the antidepressants, which act as neurotransmitter reuptake blockers for the neurotransmitters norepinephrine and serotonin. This has already been discussed in Chapter 2. When the neurotransmitters norepinephrine and serotonin bind to their own selective receptor sites, they are normally transported back into the presynaptic neuron, as shown in Figure 2–23. Thus the empty reuptake carrier (Fig. 2–20) binds to the neurotransmitter (Fig. 2–21) to begin the transport process (Fig. 2–23). However, when certain antidepressants bind to an allosteric site close to the neurotransmitter transporter (represented as an icon in Figs. 2–22 and 2–24), this causes the neurotransmitter to no longer be able to bind there, thereby blocking synaptic re-

**NO AGONIST --** light is off

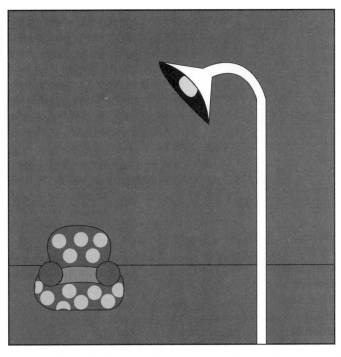

FIGURE 3–17. Light as an analogy for the agonist spectrum: actions when no agonist is present. When **no agonist** is present, the situation is analogous to the light switch being off. Adding the **partial agonist** when the lights are off has the effect of turning the lights partially on, to the level preset in the partial agonist rheostat. Thus, in the **absence of a full agonist**, adding a partial agonist will turn up the lights. In this case, the **partial agonist acts as a net agonist**.

uptake transport of the neurotransmitter. Therefore, norepinephrine and serotonin cannot be shuttled back into the presynaptic neuron.

An antidepressant drug, which blocks norepinephrine and serotonin reuptake, can be said to modulate in a *negative allosteric* manner the presynaptic neurotransmitter transporter and thereby block neurotransmitter reuptake (Figs. 2–22 and 2–24). As developed in detail in later chapters, this action may have therapeutic implications for a number of disorders, including depression, panic disorder, and obsessive-compulsive disorder.

It should now be clear from these numerous examples that when neurotransmitter receptor binding sites are arranged as neighbors, they can interact with each other allosterically to promote or control some aspect of neurotransmission. This theme is amplified over and over again throughout psychopharmacology, with varying receptors, transmitters, ion channels, and allosteric modifying receptors and their transmitters. The exact architecture of specific sites is being discovered at a fast pace. It has only been well worked out for a few specific neurotransmitters, for example the benzodiazepine complex, nicotinic cholinergic receptors, and glutamate receptors. However, the most important thing to remember is the concept, not necessarily the details of allosteric modulation.

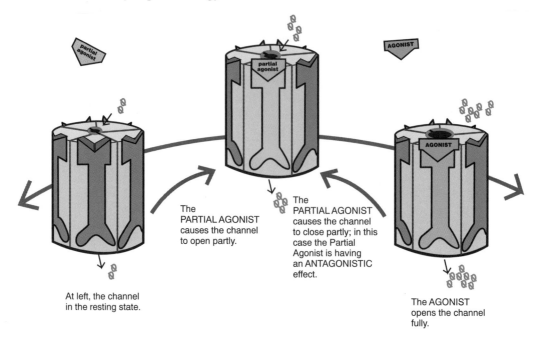

FIGURE 3–18. Partial agonist acting either as net agonist or as net antagonist. When full agonist is absent, a partial agonist partially opens the ion channel, since it increases the opening relative to the resting state. In this instance, the **partial agonist** is acting as a **net agonist**, just as in Figure 3–11. However, in the **presence of full agonist**, a partial agonist partially closes the ion channel, since it decreases the opening relative to the open state of the ion channel. In this instance, the **partial agonist** is acting as a **net antagonist**.

In summary, allosteric modulation is a specific concept in which neurotransmitters and their receptors may cooperate with each other to work much more powerfully and through a much greater range of action than they can by themselves. This may be mediated in many instances by the guarding of ion channels. Drugs can act at a myriad of sites, to influence this process. So can diseases. There are at a minimum ion channel sites, neurotransmitter sites, and allosteric sites as targets of drug (and disease) action. Data are developing so quickly, that the details are changing constantly. However, as a general principle, understanding this architecture of receptor-mediated chemical neurotransmission should provide the reader with the basis to understand a vast array of drug actions, and how such actions modify and impact chemical neurotransmission.

## Co-transmission versus Allosteric Modulation

Why isn't allosteric modulation just called "co-transmission?" That is, two chemicals are influencing neurotransmission together. Indeed, some systems do incorporate co-transmitters, such as both glutamate and glycine at some glutamate receptor sub-types. In the case of co-transmitters, each can work somewhat independently of the other, and although their effects can be additive if they are working simultaneously, it is not necessary for both to be present for either one to have an effect. However, in the case of allosteric modulation, there is only one neurotransmitter, whereas the

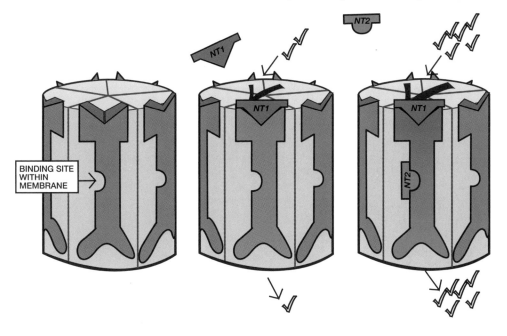

When a neurotransmitter binds to receptors making up an ion channel,
the channel opens. However, when BOTH the neurotransmitter and
a second chemical are bound to the receptor, the channel opens further
allowing more ions into the cell.

FIGURE 3–19. Allosteric modulation of the ligand-gated ion channel receptor. On the left, the receptor is shown not only with its agonist binding site for neurotransmitter 1 (NT1), but also with a **second binding site** within the membrane for neurotransmitter 2 (NT2). The ion channel is shown on the left to be **closed** in the absence of binding of their NT1 or NT2. When neurotransmitter full agonist (**NT1**) binds to its binding site, it of course **opens the ion channel**, as shown in the middle of the figure also in Figure 3–6. This is represented in the middle of the figure as purple NT1 binding to its agonist site, turning the receptor purple, and opening the ion channel to the greatest extent possible by the full agonist. If allosteric modulator (**NT2**) binds to the second binding site in the **absence** of neurotransmitter binding to its own binding site, it has **no particular effect**. However, if neurotransmitter (**NT1**) is already binding to its binding site, addition of allosteric modulator (**NT2**) binding to the second membrane site has the effect of dramatically opening the ion channel even further than a full agonist can on its own, as shown on the right. This is graphically represented as purple NT1 binding to the receptor and turning it partially purple; as green NT2 binding to the receptor and turning it partially green; and as the ion channel opening to an extent much greater than can be achieved by the action of a full agonist alone.

other has been called an allosteric modulator, *not* a co-transmitter. The difference is that the neurotransmitter can work in the absence of the allosteric modulator, but the allosteric modulator cannot work in the absence of the neurotransmitter. Thus, these chemicals are not independent of each other and are not considered to be co-transmitters.

## Summary

This chapter has introduced the reader to three special properties of receptors. The first of these is the classification of receptors by their subtypes and by their molecular configurations. Several receptor subtypes can bind the exact same neurotransmitter. Also, families of receptors can share common molecular characteristics even if they do not share the same neurotransmitter. Specifically, individual receptors within superfamilies of receptors can all be arranged in similar configurations with second messengers or with ion channels. The second of the special properties of receptors discussed here is the action of receptors with neurotransmitters and drugs that bind to them to produce a spectrum of output ranging from full agonists to partial agonists to antagonists to partial inverse agonists to full inverse agonists. Finally, the reader has been introduced to the concept of allosteric modulation of one receptor by another. This provides for regulation of neurotransmission through either the boosting or blocking one receptor's action by another. The allosterically modulating receptor was shown to act *indirectly* either as a referee or as a coach but not by participating directly in the action game of neurotransmission.

# CHAPTER 4

# CHEMICAL NEUROTRANSMISSION AS THE MEDIATOR OF DISEASE ACTIONS

## Receptors and Enzymes as Mediators of Disease Action in the Central Nervous System

The reader should now know that enzymes make things and receptors make things happen, especially by activating genes. We have already discussed in Chapter 2 that the most powerful way known to change the functioning of a neuron with a *drug* is to interact at one of its key receptors or to inhibit one of its important enzymes. However, this is only one perspective in psychopharmacology, namely, that enzymes and receptors are the sites of *drug* action. A second and equally important perspective in psychopharmacology will be developed in this chapter. That perspective is that enzymes and receptors in their various neuronal pathways and circuits can also be the mediators of *disease* actions.

99

If receptors and enzymes are so important for explaining the actions of *drugs* on chemical neurotransmission, it should not be surprising that alterations of these same enzymes and receptors could disrupt brain function. That is, if the normal flow of chemical neurotransmission leads to the healthy growth, development, and implementation of normal brain functions, abnormal neurotransmission could therefore lead to behavioral or motor abnormalities expressed by patients who suffer from psychiatric and neurological disorders. Obviously, different aspects of neurotransmission would hypothetically be disrupted in different brain disorders. Given the vast complexity of chemical neurotransmission, there are certainly a lot of possibilities for sites of abnormally acting receptors and/or enzymes. Since these receptors and enzymes live in different neuronal pathways, when something happens to damage, misdirect, or remove a pathway, the resultant aberrant neurotransmission could be quite disruptive to normal brain functioning.

Psychopharmacology is a science dedicated in part to discovering where molecular lesions exist in the nervous system in order to determine what is wrong with chemical neurotransmission. Knowledge of the molecular problem that leads to abnormal neurotransmission can generate a rationale for developing a drug therapy to correct it, thereby removing the psychiatric and neurological symptoms of the brain disorder. This concept has proved to be quite complex to apply to specific brain disorders. The general nature of investigating the molecular basis of psychiatric disorders will first be discussed in a broad and general manner in this chapter. Later, once the reader is familiar with the general concepts outlined here, these scientific strategies will be applied in the subsequent chapters to many specific psychiatric and neurological disorders.

In particular, this chapter will discuss how diseases of the central nervous system (CNS) are approached by three disciplines: neuroscience, biological psychiatry, and psychopharmacology. We will then show how these three approaches can be applied to learning how modifications in chemical neurotransmission might lead to various brain disorders. Specific concepts that will be explained are the molecular neurobiology and genetics of psychiatric disorders, neuronal plasticity, and excitotoxicity. Also, the reader will learn how CNS disorders may be linked either to no neurotransmission, too much neurotransmission, an imbalance among neurotransmitters, or the wrong rate of neurotransmission.

## Diseases in the Central Nervous System: A Tale of Three Disciplines

### Neurobiology

Neurobiology is the study of brain and neuronal functioning, usually emphasizing normal brain functioning in experimental animals rather than in humans (Table 4–1). Obviously, one must first understand normal brain functioning and normal chemical neurotransmission in order to have any chance of detecting, let alone understanding, neurobiological abnormalities that cause psychiatric and neurological disorders. For example, neurobiological investigations have led to the clarification of certain principles of chemical neurotransmission, to the enumeration of specific neurotransmitters, to the discovery of multiple receptor subtypes for each neurotransmitter, to the understanding of the enzymes that synthesize and metabolize the neurotransmitters, and to the unfolding discoveries of how genetic information con-

Table 4–1. *Neurobiology*

*Limited definition*
    The study of brain and neuronal functioning

*Approach*
    Studies using experimental animals
    Use of drugs to probe neurobiological and molecular regulatory mechanisms

*Findings relevant to psychopharmacology*
    Discovery of neurotransmitters and their enzymes and receptors
    Principles of neurotransmission
    Genetic and molecular regulation of neuronal functioning
    Neurobiological regulation of animal behaviors

trols this whole process. The discipline of neurobiology uses drugs as tools to interact selectively with enzymes and receptors—and with the DNA and RNA systems that control the synthesis of enzymes and receptors—in order to elucidate their functions in the normal brain. Many of the lessons derived from this approach have already been discussed in the preceding chapters.

## Biological Psychiatry

Biological psychiatry, on the other hand, is oriented toward discovering the abnormalities in brain biology associated with the causes or consequences of mental disorders (Table 4–2). Making such discoveries is proving to be very difficult. However, the importance of pursuing the causes of mental disorders is underscored by how frequent these illnesses are in our society and how limited current treatments for them can be. That is, as many as one in five persons may experience a mental illness during their lifetimes, and about 4% of the population has a chronic and severe mental disorder. Furthermore, currently available treatments in psychopharmacology are not strictly "curative" but are merely palliative, reducing symptoms without necessarily offering sustained relief. Better treatments of the future now depend on discovering the causes of mental illness. This is the central goal of biological psychiatry.

This discipline uses the results of neurobiological investigations of normal brain functioning as a basis for the search for the substrate of abnormal brain functioning in psychiatric disorders. Scientists have long suspected that abnormalities in brain enzymes or receptors are major contributors to the causes of mental illness and have been searching for an enzyme or receptor deficiency that could be identified as the cause of specific psychiatric disorders. Some of the earliest tools of biological psychiatry were less elegant than those of basic neurobiology, since practical and ethical considerations limit the manner in which patients and their CNS can be studied, compared with the techniques available for use in laboratories with experimental animals. Such tools available for use in humans include studies of enzymes, receptors, and genes in postmortem brain tissues and in peripheral tissues that can be ethically

Table 4–2. *Biological psychiatry*

*Limited definition*

The study of abnormalities in brain neurobiology associated with the causes or consequences of mental illnesses

*Approach*

Studies using patients with psychiatric disorders

Taking direction from psychopharmacological studies indicating that drugs with known mechanisms of action on receptors or enzymes predictably alter symptoms in a specific psychiatric disorder

Search for abnormalities in receptors, enzymes, neurotransmitters, genes, or gene products that correlate with the diagnosis of a particular mental illness

Biochemical measurements using blood, urine, cerebrospinal fluid, peripheral tissues such as platelets or lymphocytes, postmortem brain tissues, or plasma hormones after provoking hormone secretion by drugs

Measurements of structural abnormalities using CT or MRI brain scans

Measurements of functional or physiological abnormalities using PET, EEG, evoked potentials, or magnetoencephalography

*Findings relevant to psychopharmacology*

Few strong biological findings demonstrating lesions in specific psychiatric disorders

Example: discovery of changes in serotonin receptors and metabolites in depression, schizophrenia, and suicidal behavior

Search for the genetic basis of specific neurological and psychiatric illnesses

---

sampled in living patients, such as blood platelets or lymphocytes, whose enzymes, receptors, and genes are similar or identical to those in brain. Metabolites of neurotransmitters can be studied in cerebrospinal fluid, plasma, and urine. Metabolic rates and cerebral blood flow reflecting neuronal firing patterns, as well as the number and function of several neurotransmitter receptors, can be visualized in living patients by use of positron emission tomography (PET) scans. Receptors for neurotransmitters can also be studied indirectly by using selective drug probes, which cause hormones to be released into the blood that can be measured and therefore serve as a reflection of brain receptor stimulation. Structural brain abnormalities can be detected by computed tomography (CT) and magnetic resonance imaging (MRI). The latter modality can also detect functional changes in brain activity with a technique called functional MRI. Abnormalities in brain electrical activity can be measured with electroencephalography (EEG), evoked potentials, or magnetoencephalography.

Unfortunately, little progress has been made yet in defining the biological causes of mental illnesses by using these approaches. No single reproducible abnormality in any neurotransmitter or in any of its enzymes or receptors has been shown to cause any common psychiatric disorder. Indeed, it is no longer considered likely that one will be found, given the complexity of psychiatric diagnosis and the profound interaction of environmental factors with genetics in psychiatric disorders. More recently, biological psychiatry has shifted from a strategy of pursuing a single unique biochemical lesion as the cause of each psychiatric disorder to the discovery and enumeration of risk factors that do not *cause* illness by themselves but *contribute to the risk* of a psychiatric disorder. This approach is sometimes called *complex genetics* because it is indeed complicated, as we shall see below.

The potential usefulness of this approach is underscored by findings from genetic studies of mental illnesses. Despite strong evidence from twin studies that genetic susceptibility exists for both bipolar disorder and schizophrenia, no specific gene has been unambiguously identified for the usual forms of any common mental disorder. Thus, it is already clear that the cause of major psychiatric disorders is *not* going to be a single abnormality in a major genetic locus of DNA, as already proved for Huntington's disease, sickle cell anemia, and cystic fibrosis. Rather, the genetics of major psychiatric disorders are likely to be at best contributors in multiple complex ways to these illnesses, just as is currently suspected for coronary artery disease, diabetes, and hypertension.

Methods to approach the complex genetics of mental illnesses are just evolving and include such techniques as *linkage, linkage disequilibrium,* and *association studies* to name a few. Rather than looking for a single major abnormality in DNA as the cause of mental disorders, the idea behind these methods is to identify multiple genes that each make a small contribution to the overall vulnerability to mental illness, perhaps only when other critical genetic vulnerabilities and critical environmental inputs are also present. If this approach does not prove to explain the causes of psychiatric disorders as defined in the Diagnostic and Statistical Manual of Mental Disorders, 4th edition (DSM-IV), as appears likely, it may unravel the causes of simpler symptom complexes or even variations in personality.

Thus, biological psychiatry no longer deems it likely that any single abnormality in DNA in a psychiatric disorder leads to abnormalities in the synthesis of gene products that are sufficient on their own to cause mental illness. Rather, a whole list of abnormally acting genes and their corresponding gene products, triggered by both inherited and acquired risk factors, are hypothesized to act together or in just the right sequence to cause clusters of symptoms that appear in different psychiatric disorders. No wonder they call this field complex genetics!

Once the complete list of genes and environmental factors that comprise all the vulnerabilities to a psychiatric illness is determined, it will be necessary to understanding how all the corresponding gene products participate in the neuronal functioning and especially the chemical neurotransmission that mediate the mental illness. The long-term hope, of course, is that by knowing this, a logical biochemical rationale can be found for reversing these abnormalities with drug therapies. The question of how this could lead to a rational drug therapy to halt, reverse, or compensate for these multiple simultaneous biochemical events leaves us in a complete quandary at present.

It might be possible to pursue treatments based on this knowledge if the abnormal gene products proved to be enzymes or receptors that could be stimulated or blocked by drugs. However, it is not likely to be this simple, as multiple simultaneous drugs acting to compensate for each genetic abnormality that contributes to the disease vulnerability might prove to be necessary. At any rate, the biological psychiatry hunt is on, but treatments based on this approach certainly do not appear to be right around the corner.

Table 4–3. *Psychopharmacology*

| |
|---|
| *Limited definition* |
|     The use of drugs to treat symptoms of mental illness |
|     The science of drug discovery, targeting enzymes and receptors |
| *Approach* |
|     Studies in patients with psychiatric disorders |
|     Serendipitous clinical observations |
|     In clinical investigations, the use of drugs with known mechanisms of action to provoke biological or behavioral responses that would provide clues where abnormalities in brain functioning may exist in specific psychiatric disorders |
|     In drug discovery, theory-driven targeting of enzymes and receptors hypothesized to regulate symptoms in a psychiatric disorder |
| *Psychopharmacological results* |
|     In clinical investigations, the first observation is often a serendipitous discovery of clinical efficacy, after which the biochemical mechanism of action is discovered |
|     In drug discovery, specific enzymes or receptors are first targeted for drug action. The earliest experiments use chemistry to synthesize drugs; experimental animals to test the biochemical, behavioral, and toxic actions of the drugs; and human subjects, both normal volunteers and patients, to test the safety and efficacy of the drugs |
|     Discovery and use of antidepressants, anxiolytics, antipsychotics, and cognitive enhancers as well as drugs of abuse |

## Psychopharmacology

As mentioned previously, the discipline of psychopharmacology is oriented not only toward discovering new drugs and understanding the actions of drugs on the CNS, but also toward understanding diseases of the CNS by altering them through the use of drugs whose actions are known (Table 4–3). That is, if a drug with a well understood mechanism of action on a receptor or enzyme causes reproducible effects on the symptoms of a patient with a brain disorder, it is likely that those symptoms are also linked to the same receptor that the drug is targeting. Using drugs as tools in this manner can help map which receptors and enzymes are linked to which psychiatric or neurological disorder.

Since drug actions are much better known than disease actions at the present time, the use of drug tools in this manner has so far proved to be the more productive approach to understanding diseases as compared with the biological psychiatry approach of looking for abnormal receptors, enzymes, or genes. Indeed, much of what is known, hypothesized, or theorized about the neurochemical abnormalities of brain disorders is derived from the approach of using drugs as tools.

Therefore, in general, contemporary knowledge of CNS disorders, as will be discussed for specific entities in subsequent chapters, is in fact largely predicated on knowing how drugs act on disease symptoms, and then inferring pathophysiology by knowing how the drugs act. Thus, pathophysiology is inferred rather than proved, since we do not yet know the primary enzyme, receptor, or genetic deficiency in any given psychiatric or neurological disorder.

The discipline of psychopharmacology has therefore been useful, not only in generating empirically successful treatments for CNS disorders, but also in generating the leading theories and hypotheses about psychiatric disorders. These theories, in fact, direct the biological psychiatry researcher where to look for proof of disease abnormalities. Thus, psychopharmacology is bidirectional in the sense that certain drugs, namely, those that have a known neurochemical mechanism of action and that are also effective in treating brain disorders, help to generate hypotheses about the causes of those brain disorders. The other direction of psychopharmacology is that in the case of a brain disorder with a known or suspected pathophysiology, drugs can be rationally designed to act on a specific receptor or enzyme to correct the known or suspected pathophysiology and thereby treat the disorder.

It would be advantageous for new drug development to proceed from knowledge of pathophysiology to the invention of new therapeutics, but this must await the elucidation of such pathophysiologies, which, as emphasized here, are yet largely unknown. Virtually all effective psychopharmacological drugs that have been discovered to date were found by serendipity (good luck) or by empiricism, that is, by probing disease mechanisms with a drug of known action but no prior proof that such actions would necessarily be therapeutic. Hopefully, a rational route from pathophysiology to drug development will become increasingly available as the molecular causes of such disorders are elucidated in coming years.

A new approach to selecting specific drugs for individual patients called *pharmacogenetics* is dawning in psychopharmacology. Although in its infancy, pharmacogenetics attempts to match the likelihood of a positive or negative clinical response to a given drug with the specific genetic makeup of the patient. The idea is that knowing the critical genetic information about a patient, not just the psychiatric diagnosis, could lead to a more rational decision as to which drug to prescribe for that patient.

Currently, there is no rational way to predict which antidepressant is more likely than another to work in any depressed patient or which antipsychotic would be best for a given schizophrenic patient. Such selections often are made by trial and error. Perhaps certain genetic characteristics will predict the likelihood of a better therapeutic response or better tolerability of one drug over another. To date, no such genetic factors are yet known that can assist the prescriber in selecting psychotropic drugs for individual patients.

## How Synaptic Neurotransmission Mediates Emotional Disorders

Despite a frustrating lack of knowledge of specific pathophysiological mechanisms for various psychiatric disorders, a good deal of progress has been made in our thinking about mechanisms whereby synaptic neurotransmission can mediate disease processes. Discussed below are several general concepts relating to how psychiatric disorders are thought to be associated with modifications in synaptic neurotransmission.

### *Molecular Neurobiology and Psychiatric Disorders*

A modern formulation of psychiatric disorders involves the integration of at least four key elements: (1) genetic vulnerability to the expression of a disease; (2) life event stressors that come that individual's way (divorce, financial problems, etc.); (3) the individual's personality, coping skills, and social support available from others;

and (4) other environmental influences on the individual and his or her genome, including viruses, toxins, and various diseases.

*Genetic Vulnerability.* Geneticists no longer talk about inheriting a mental illness; they talk about inheriting vulnerability to a mental illness. Such vulnerability theoretically arises from a set of abnormally functioning genes, and some of this abnormal functioning is inherited. Since genes control all functions of the neuron, all psychiatric disorders at some level are genetic. However, that does not necessarily mean that all abnormal functions of genes are inherited. Some of the problems of gene function can arise from the person's experiences, from stressors arising in the environment, and from chemicals and toxins outside the brain. Vulnerability factors for psychiatric disorders are as yet poorly understood, multiple in number, and very complicated. Nevertheless, a few important principles of genetic vulnerability have been established.

For instance, if the rate of illness is greater among monozygotic (single-egg) twins than among dizygotic (two-egg) twins, then heredity is an important factor. At least two important examples of this, bipolar illness and schizophrenia, are well documented in psychiatry. The monozygotic twin of a schizophrenic has a 50% chance of having schizophrenia, whereas a dizygotic twin has only about a 15% chance. Similarly, the monozygotic twin of a person with bipolar illness has up to an 80% chance of being bipolar, whereas a dizygotic twin has only about an 8 to 10% chance. Despite this proof of genetic vulnerability, no specific gene has been established for these illnesses because it is now believed that there is no single genetic abnormality within the affected subject's DNA that by itself causes these or any other common psychiatric disorders.

Rather, the current thinking is that multiple sites in DNA within the genome must interact to produce most of the causation of a psychiatric illness. Such genes may act independently, additively, or even synergistically; they may also act at different critical times during brain development. There may be both positive and negative modifier genes, which if present also influence the likelihood that the illness will occur. Thus, unlike Mendelian disorders such as Huntington's disease, in which single genes contribute large effects (e.g., Fig. 4–1), in psychiatric disorders we are looking for many different genes, each of which contributes only a small effect or even no effect unless its effects coincide with the expression of other critical genes (Fig. 4–2). To make things even more complicated, different genes may be abnormal in different families with the same psychiatric illness. This situation is called heterogeneity.

The biochemical expression of vulnerability to a psychiatric disorder occurs when many different genes make many important proteins in the wrong amounts, at the wrong places, or at the wrong times. This in turn causes abnormal structures and functions of neurons. Even when all this happens in a manner to create the maximum amount of risk, there still may not be a psychiatric disorder unless nongenetic factors, especially from the environment, interact in just the right way to convert latent vulnerability into manifest disease. In such a case, only a conspiracy of several genetic and environmental risks produces an emotional disorder. Detection of a single conspirator without rounding up all the coconspirators is inadequate to explain the genetic basis of the disease.

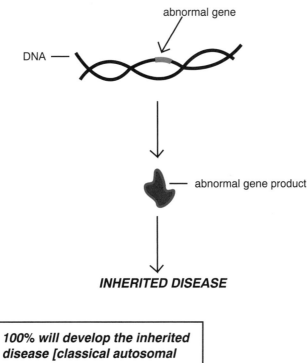

abnormal gene

DNA

abnormal gene product

**INHERITED DISEASE**

**100% will develop the inherited disease [classical autosomal dominant pattern]**

FIGURE 4–1. This figure depicts the **classical view of an inherited disease**. In this case, the abnormal gene expresses some sort of abnormal gene product. The consequences of making this deficient gene product is that cellular functioning is compromised, resulting in the inherited disease.

*Life Events and the Two-Hit Hypothesis of Psychiatric Disorders.* One theory that tries to explain this combination of genetic vulnerabilities and environmental factors as the basis of many psychiatric disorders is the "two-hit" hypothesis. That is, in order to manifest an overt psychiatric disorder, one must not only sustain the first hit, namely all the critical genetic vulnerabilities, but one must also sustain a second hit of some type from the environment (Figs. 4–2 through 4–5). Thus, psychiatric disorders are increased in incidence in first-degree relatives of patients with a wide variety of psychiatric disorders but not to an extent that allows one to predict which specific individuals will or will not eventually develop a specific psychiatric disorder.

This supports the concept that one does not inherit the mental disorder per se; one inherits vulnerability factors for the mental disorder (the genetic first hits) (Figs. 4–2 through 4–5). The chance of actually manifesting a psychiatric illness apparently depends not only on whether one inherited all the necessary vulnerability factors but also on numerous other factors (i.e., second hits from nongenetic environmental sources) (Fig. 4–4).

Some mental disorders, such as schizophrenia or bipolar illness, may have a higher chance of being expressed in vulnerable individuals as compared with disorders such as depression, anxiety, or obsessive-compulsive disorder, which may more frequently lie dormant in the vulnerable individual (Fig. 4–5). Thus, genetic endowment gives

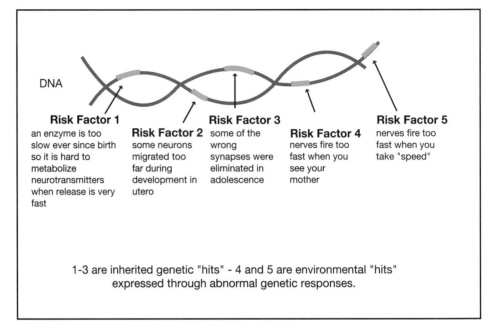

FIGURE 4–2. Depicted here is the hypothesis of **complex genetics of psychiatric disorders**. Here, three risk factors are inherited and two risk factors come from the environment. In this case, these five factors combine to produce a hypothetical case of schizophrenia in a young adult. Thus, this individual inherited not only an aberrant enzyme (**genetic risk factor 1**) but also neurons with abnormal neuronal migration in utero (**genetic risk factor 2**), plus synapses that were incorrectly eliminated in adolescence (**genetic risk factor 3**). Compounding these inherited abnormalities in the biological functioning of the brain, there are neurodevelopmental problems due to bad parenting (**environmental risk factor 4**) and neuronal toxicities from ingesting drugs of abuse (**environmental risk factor 5**). When they are put all together in the right sequence, the result is schizophrenia.

an individual a certain degree of risk for a psychiatric disorder, and certain disorders may have more of a propensity to become manifest than other disorders, but genetic vulnerability alone is not enough to express overt psychiatric illness.

*Childhood Development, Personality, Coping Skills, and Social Support as Factors in Psychiatric Illnesses.* Several environmental interactions are hypothesized to affect the expression of information present in the genome and therefore may dictate whether a disorder remains only a latent possibility or breaks down into overt psychiatric pathology (Fig. 4–4). These include *early life experiences*, which cause a person to develop learned patterns of coping that together constitute his or her personality, or in some cases, personality disorder (Figs. 4–3 and 4–4). Also, there are *adult life experiences*, which an individual encounters from social interaction with the environment, including events commonly called stressful, such as divorce, death of a loved one, financial difficulties, and medical problems (Fig. 4–4).

Personality traits (Fig. 4–3) may themselves be genetically influenced (e.g., impulsivity, shyness) or environmentally determined by early childhood developmental

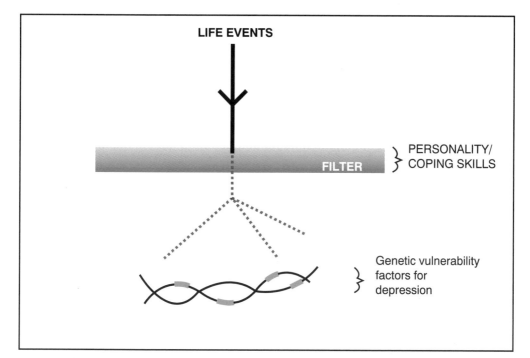

**LIFE EVENTS**

FILTER

⟩ PERSONALITY/
⟩ COPING SKILLS

⟩ Genetic vulnerability
⟩ factors for
⟩ depression

FIGURE 4–3. This figure demonstrates how **life events** from the environment test the postulated vulnerability genes for a psychiatric illness (in this case, several postulated genes capable of triggering depression if expressed in the critical manner). Life events, sometimes called stressors, challenge the organism, and this manifests itself as a biological demand on the individual's genome. Such stressors are modified by the individual and processed so that the nature of the biological demand may be similarly modified. That is, persons who have developed an **adaptive personality** with good **coping skills** and **social support** may be able to mitigate, blunt, or lessen the biological demand on their genetic code for latent depression. On the other hand, those who have developed an abnormal personality with poor coping skills may actually worsen, accelerate, or even recruit potentially damaging psychosocial stressors to play on the genome. Thus, personality and coping skills are either a **filter** or a **magnifying glass** through which psychosocial stressors pass on their journey to test and challenge the genome where a potential psychiatric disorder may or may not be waiting for a chance to be expressed.

experiences. Personality traits generate coping skills, which can either blunt or exacerbate the impact of adult life events on that individual's genome (Fig. 4–3). The ability of an individual to buffer stressors or even to grow and prosper when exposed to them versus breaking down into a mental disorder may be the product of which life events occur and how much coping skill and social support exist prior to being layered onto a genome. Also, that genome may be robust or vulnerable, and the particular vulnerability may explain why some people develop depression, others obsessive-compulsive disorder, and still others no disorder at all despite similar life experiences and similar personalities.

   The nature of genetic risk may thus be quite different for different psychiatric disorders. Given comparable genetic material and comparable personalities and coping skills, it may be the severity of psychosocial stressors from the environment that determines how often a vulnerable individual develops a mental illness. According

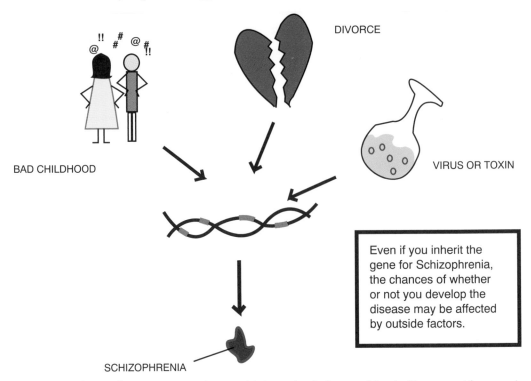

BAD CHILDHOOD

DIVORCE

VIRUS OR TOXIN

Even if you inherit the gene for Schizophrenia, the chances of whether or not you develop the disease may be affected by outside factors.

SCHIZOPHRENIA

FIGURE 4–4. This figure represents the **two-hit hypothesis for psychiatric illnesses** with a genetic component. In this hypothesis, inheriting a set of abnormal genetic risks (the **first hit** shown as the **red genes** on the black strands of DNA) is not sufficient for manifestation of a psychiatric disorder. One must also sustain just the right **second hit** from the **environment**, postulated to be life events such as a bad childhood or divorce or insults from the environment such as a virus or a toxin. Thus, those with just one hit do not develop the disorder, even though they have the identical genetic makeup as those who do develop the psychiatric disorder. What distinguishes those who ultimately develop an illness from those who do not is whether the individual at risk and vulnerable for the illness (i.e., having the red genes of vulnerability to a specific psychiatric disorder) also is exposed to just the right second hit (shown as inputs to the gene) necessary to **trigger the abnormal genes** into making their abnormal gene products and thereby causing the disease in that individual.

to this model, the more biologically determined disorders, with the more vulnerable genomes, would require only minor stressors for a person develop that mental illness to develop (e.g., schizophrenia in Fig. 4–5). On the other hand, a less vulnerable disorder such as depression might theoretically require moderate stressors to become manifest (Fig. 4–5). Finally, some stressors could be so severe (e.g., rape, combat, witnessing atrocities) that even a normal robust genome might break down to cause a mental disorder (e.g., posttraumatic stress disorder [PTSD] in Fig. 4–5).

*Other Environmental Influences on Individuals and Their Genomes.* Finally, the environment provides numerous potential biochemical influences on the genome, such as exposure to viruses, toxins, or diseases (Fig. 4–4). These, too, could contribute to the probability that genetic vulnerabilities for a psychiatric illness will become manifest.

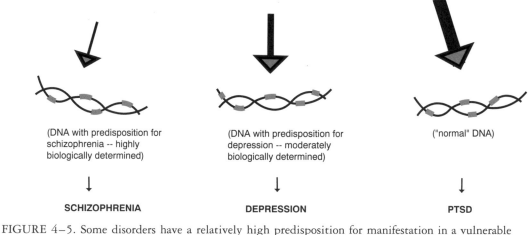

FIGURE 4–5. Some disorders have a relatively high predisposition for manifestation in a vulnerable individual, whereas others have a relatively low predisposition, as shown in Figure 4–2. Thus, it may take only relatively **minor or usual stressors** for the set of schizophrenia vulnerability genes of a vulnerable individual to be activated into producing a disease (left panel). On the other hand, since fewer individuals with the postulated genetic potential for depression or bipolar disorder may actually manifest this disorder, it may take at least **moderate or more unusual stressors** for the vulnerable individual to have his or her set of bipolar disorder vulnerability genes activated into producing a disease (middle panel). Finally, even those with apparently normal DNA, with no known predisposition to any given psychiatric disorder, may decompensate under **major and overwhelming stressors** (such as rape or combat or natural disasters) to produce a breakdown of cellular functioning through the breakdown of normal DNA to produce yet other psychiatric disorders (right panel). This latter mechanism is one hypothesis for the development of posttraumatic stress disorder (PTSD), for example.

## Neuronal Plasticity and Psychiatric Disorders

*Neurodevelopmental Disorders.* Neurons and their synapses must develop properly and then be adequately maintained or else a disorder in the functioning of the brain could result. First, the correct neurons must be selected in utero (Fig. 4–6), and then they must migrate to their predesignated locations (Fig. 4–7) for the brain to function properly. Epilepsy and mental retardation are disorders that in part may result from neurons getting lost and migrating to the wrong places during fetal development (Fig. 4–7). Abnormal neuronal migration may even contribute to the causes of schizophrenia and dyslexia.

Failure of neuronal migration could be caused by genes giving the wrong directions. Bad instructions could be inherited and thus be preprogrammed, or they could be acquired in utero, after the mother takes cocaine and alcohol or her uterus sustains radiation for some reason. One mechanism whereby the wrong genetic information or toxins such as drugs or radiation could cause abnormal neuronal selections would be for them to cause a "grim reaper" growth factor to be inappropriately turned on instead of a "bodyguard" growth factor (Fig. 4–6). This could cause the wrong cell to turn on its apoptotic suicide system (see Fig. 1–18). What may be left are puny cells with bad molecular "Velcro" (e.g., cadherins), which therefore cannot crawl along glia/fibers to get where they need to go. Thus, a neuronal migration disorder is begun by improper selection of neurons in the first place.

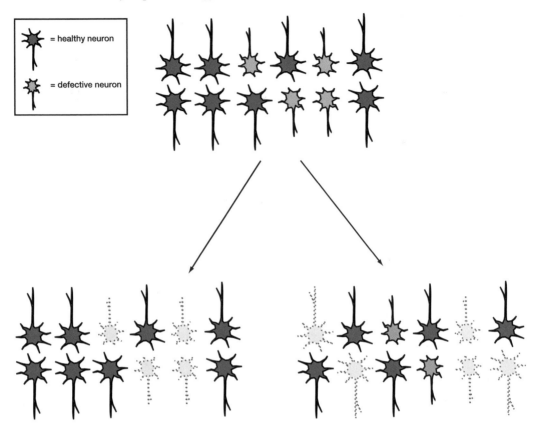

Good neuronal selection                    Bad neuronal selection

FIGURE 4–6. Neurons are formed in excess prenatally (top panel of neurons). Some are healthy and others may be defective. Normal neurodevelopment **chooses the good neurons** (left), but in a developmental disorders, some **defective neurons may be chosen** and thus cause a neurological or psychiatric disorder later in life when that neuron is called on to perform its duties (right panel).

Other neurodevelopmental problems could result from abnormal synaptogenesis. As discussed in Chapter 1, synapses are dynamic and constantly changing, being laid down, maintained, and in some cases removed. Many things influence this process of adding, maintaining, and removing synapses. If the neuron receives the wrong semaphore signal (from neurotrophic semaphorin molecules), it may sail its axonal growth tip into the wrong postsynaptic targets (cf. Figs. 4–8 and 4–9). Since the synapse is the substrate of chemical neurotransmission, information transfer in the brain is vitally dependent on axons innervating the correct targets.

Once innervation is complete, information transfer in the brain continues to be dependent on how the synapse is maintained, including the processes of branching, pruning, growing, or dying of neuronal axons and dendrites (see Chapter 1 and Figs. 1–21 through 1–23, as well as Fig. 4–10). If the process of synaptogenesis is interrupted early in development, the brain may not reach its full potential, as occurs in mental retardation, autism, and as is now hypothesized for schizophrenia (Fig.

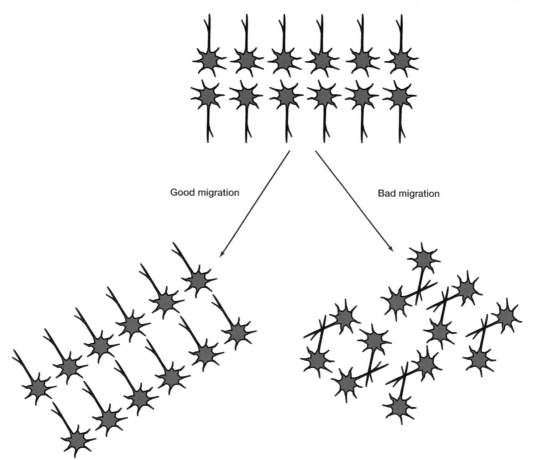

FIGURE 4–7. Neurons are formed in central growth plates (top panel) and then migrate out into the growing brain. If this is done properly (left panel), the neurons are **properly aligned** to grow, develop, form synapses, and generally function as expected. However, if there is **abnormal migration of neurons** (right panel), the neurons are not in the correct places, and do not receive the appropriate inputs from incoming axons, and therefore do not function properly. This may result in a neurological or psychiatric disorder.

4–10). The *wrong neuronal wiring* of the anatomically addressed nervous system could thus be quite problematic for proper brain functioning.

Drug treatments themselves may not only modify neurotransmission acutely but also could potentially interact with neuronal plasticity. Harnessing the neurochemistry of the brain's plasticity is an important goal of new drug development. For example, certain growth factors may provoke the neuron to sprout new axonal or dendritic branches and to establish new synaptic connections (see Chapter 1 and Fig. 1–22, as well as Fig. 4–10). If applied early enough in the course of a neurodevelopmental disorder, such treatments might be able to compensate for problems in cell selection, cell migration, or synapse formation. On the other hand, these problems are so anatomically discrete that it is hard to envision how one could program a drug for delivery only at the critical time during neurodevelopment and just at the critical places.

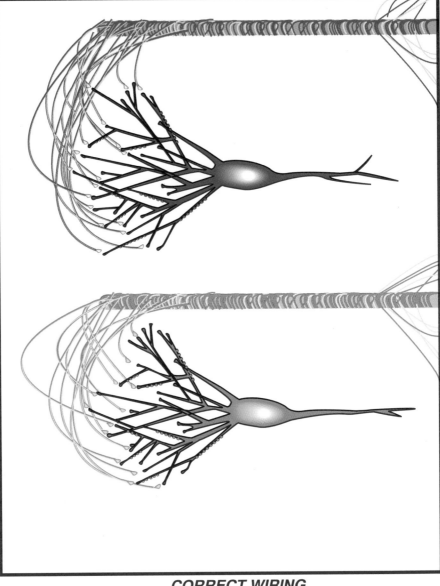

## CORRECT WIRING

FIGURE 4–8. This figure represents the **correct wiring** of two neurons. During development, the incoming blue axons from all different parts of the brain are appropriately directed to their **appropriate target dendrites** on the blue neuron. Similarly, the incoming red axons from various regions of the brain are appropriately paired with their correct dendrites on the red neuron.

*Neurodegenerative Disorders and Neurotrophic Growth Factors.* Not only can psychiatric illness result if synapses are malformed early in life, but brain disorders can also occur if normal healthy synapses are inappropriately interrupted late in life. Thus, the brain may regress from the potential it had realized and result in various types of dementia (Fig. 4–10). A milder form of this may occur in "normal aging," if it

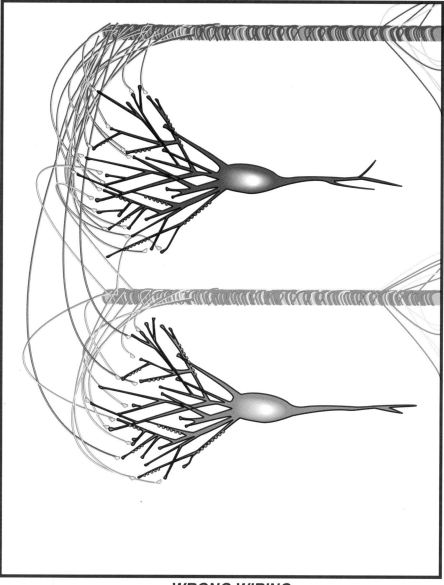

## *WRONG WIRING*

FIGURE 4–9. This figure represents simplistically a possible disease mechanism in neurodevelop-mental disorders. In this case, the neurons do not fail to develop connections; the neurons also do not die or degenerate. What happens here is that the **synapse formation is misdirected**, resulting in the **wrong wiring**. This could lead to abnormal information transfer, confusing neuronal communi-cations, and the inability of neurons to function, which are postulated to occur in schizophrenia, mental retardation, and other neurodevelopmental disorders. This state of chaos is represented here as a tangle of axons, where red axons inappropriately innervate blue dendrites and blue axons inappro-priately pair up with red dendrites. This is in contrast to the organized state represented in Figure 4–8.

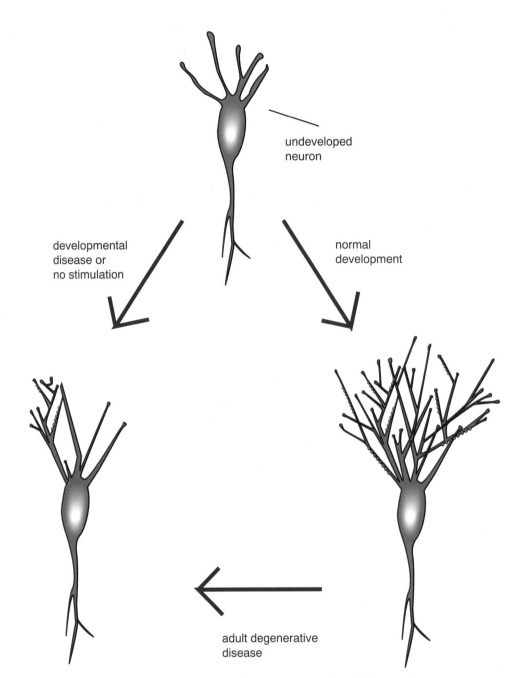

FIGURE 4–10. An **undeveloped neuron** may fail to develop during childhood either because of a **developmental disease** of some sort or because of the lack of appropriate neuronal or environmental stimulation for proper development (*left arrow*). In other cases, the undeveloped neuron does develop normally (*right arrow*), only to lose these gains when an **adult-onset degenerative disease** strikes it (*bottom arrow*).

116

can be considered normal to stop exercising the brain as one gets older. Just as neglect and abuse of other tissues contribute to breakdown of peripheral organ systems as they age, so could the lack of mental exercise lead to "rusty" and irritable synapses in the brain. Fortunately, challenging the brain throughout a lifetime by honing acquired skills and developing new ones may prevent this type of age-associated brain impairment.

Frank brain failure, however, can occur when neurons die and synapses are ruined. Two of the principal final common pathways for neuronal and synaptic destruction are necrosis and apoptosis, as discussed in Chapter 1 (see also Fig. 1–18). In neurological disorders, necrotic inflammatory demise of neurons can be triggered if they are poisoned by toxins and infections or hammered by physical trauma, or if their oxygen is choked off during a stroke, for example. More subtle loss of neurons occurs when apoptosis is activated inappropriately after the brain has developed, as may occur in Alzheimer's dementia, frontotemporal dementia, Lewy body dementia, and perhaps schizophrenia. Even if apoptosis can explain *how* neurons die in these illnesses, it is still a major mystery *why* they do this. Although neurological illnesses such as Alzheimer's disease and Parkinson's disease are classically considered to be the illnesses typified by neurodegeneration, there are now hints that a subtle form of neurodegeneration may be operative in the progressive course of schizophrenia and in the development of treatment resistance in depression, panic, and other psychiatric illnesses. Neurodegenerative phenomena may also play a role in the apparent "kindling" phenomena of various affective disorders, such as the development of rapid cycling in bipolar disorder, and in the increased risk of recurrence of depression during a shift in reproductive hormones in women who have had an affective episode associated with a previous shift in reproductive hormones.

Exploitation of normal neuronal plasticity to develop new drugs to halt degenerative diseases of the nervous system is only beginning to be investigated. Drugs are not yet available that can reliably turn on and direct the plasticity process. Theoretically, it should become possible to salvage degenerating neurons, to establish new synapses, and to reestablish preexisting synapses. Such possible modifications of degenerative nerve diseases are being pursued in several different ways.

First, the search is on for abnormal genes or abnormal gene products that might be mediating the breakdown of neurons. Once these are identified, it should theoretically be possible to stop the production or block the action of unwanted gene products. It should also be possible to turn on the production or provide a substitute for desirable but absent gene products.

Second, attempts are being made to make neurotrophic factors "get on your nerves" to rescue degenerating neurons and halt the progression of neurodegenerative disorders (Figs. 4–11 through 4–13). This might be particularly effective if acquired deficiencies in neurotrophic factors were causing previously healthy neurons to degenerate. Hypothetically, the ideal cocktail of molecules could help nourish back to health all sorts of ailing neurons (Figs. 4–12 and 4–13). Applying knowledge of the actions of neurotrophic factors and recognition molecules that help guide sprouting axons might some day increase the odds that dysfunctional neurons in the mature nervous system can be salvaged or even that desirable synaptic connections can be facilitated.

It might in theory be possible to have growth factors get on your nerves by direct delivery of the growth factor if a delivery method could ever be devised. There are

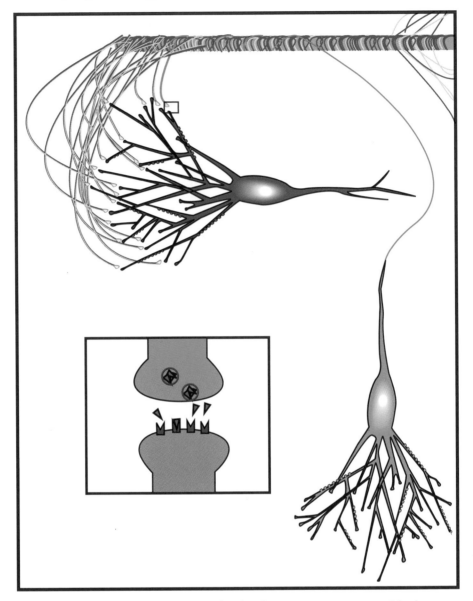

FIGURE 4–11. Shown here is **normal communication** between two neurons, with the synapse between the red and the blue neuron magnified. Normal neurotransmission from the red to the blue neuron is being mediated here by neurotransmitter binding to postsynaptic receptors by the usual mechanism of synaptic neurotransmission.

numerous problems in using neurotrophic factors as therapeutic agents. Such a large number of neurons are responsive to them that systemic administration may well activate all kinds of axonal sprouts that are not desired. Perhaps high doses or chronic use could stimulate unwanted cell division of neurons or even increase the risk of cancer. Thus, local administration to the desired site of action or site-selective actions

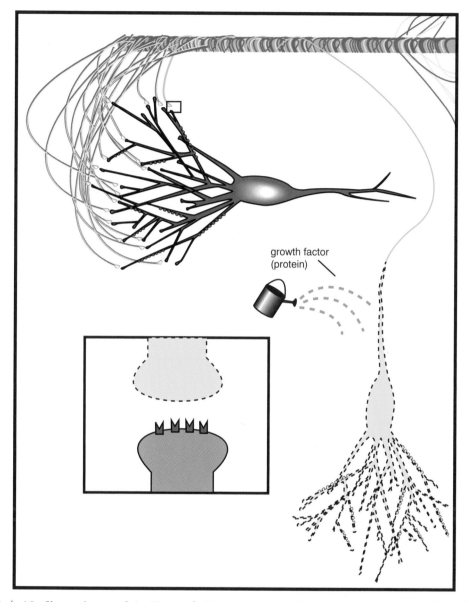

FIGURE 4–12. Shown here and in Figure 4–13 is a conceptually more complex mechanism of compensation for the loss of a **degenerating neuron**. The ailing but not yet degenerated red neuron indicated here is no longer functioning to allow normal neurotransmission with the blue neuron (*see box*) and is about to die. Also indicated is the application of a **growth factor** to the degenerating neuron. This could be conceived as either a natural reparative mechanism that the dying neuron could activate (see Fig. 1–22 and Table 1–3) or a drug that could mimic this.

of systemically administered neurotrophic factors may be required if treatment is going to be safe.

To complicate the potential utility of growth factors for neurodegenerative disorders is that fact that many growth factors are large protein or peptide molecules,

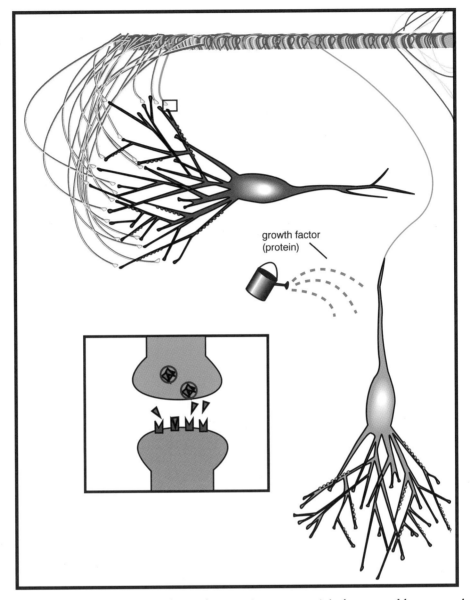

FIGURE 4–13. This figure demonstrates how a degenerating neuron might be **rescued by a growth factor**. In this case, the dying neuron of Figure 4–12 is salvaged by a growth factor, which restores the function of neurotransmission to reactivate normal communications between the red neuron and the blue neuron (*see box*).

which are unable to survive intact when administered orally and unable to cross the blood-brain barrier when administered intravenously. This has led to several different approaches to delivering neurotrophic factors to their desired targets in the CNS.

First, the protein itself can be infused directly into the cerebrospinal fluid or implanted in a biodegradable, slow-release preparation. Second, the active protein can travel across the blood-brain barrier by hiding inside a "Trojan horse" molecule

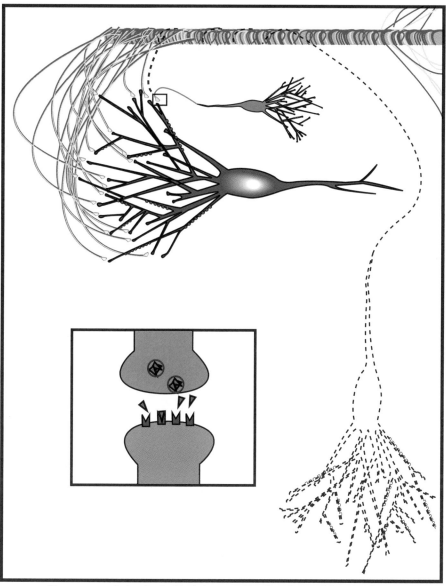

New neuron is implanted to take over the functions of the dead neuron

FIGURE 4–14. **Transplantation of a new neuron** by neurosurgical techniques is another potential mechanism for replacing the function of a degenerated neuron. In this case, the turquoise transplanted neuron makes the same neurotransmitter as the formerly red neuron made (see Fig. 4–11) prior to degenerating here. Synaptic neurotransmission is restored when the transplanted neuron takes over the lost function of the degenerated neuron (*see box*). This has already been performed for patients with Parkinson's disease, in which transplanted fetal substantia nigra neurons can successfully improve functional neurotransmission of degenerated substantia nigra neurons in some patients.

that is normally translocated across this blood-brain barrier. Third, low molecular weight chemicals might be able to get into the brain and pharmacologically induce the formation of a trophic factor. This action, in fact, has been suggested for cholinesterase inhibitors, which not only increase acetylcholine levels but subsequently increase nerve growth factor. Finally, a high-tech idea is to transfer genes that produce the trophic factor directly into the brain by grafting cells that normally make it, by genetically engineering cells to make it, or by delivering the gene in a carrier virus. All of these possibilities are under active investigation.

A third long-term therapeutic approach to neurodegenerative disorders is transplantation of neurons. Neuronal transplantation is being investigated as a way to substitute new neurons for degenerated neurons (Fig. 4–14). This is not a Frankenstein-style transplant of an entire brain but rather a selective introduction of specific and highly specialized nerves, which produce specialized chemicals and neurotransmitters capable of compensating for and replacing the functions of the degenerated and destroyed neurons that caused disease in the first place. Transplantation of neurons into human brain is already occurring in Parkinson's disease, where dopamine-producing neurons have been successfully transplanted into the brains of patients with this condition. Experimental use of cholinergic neurons holds promise for the treatment of experimental models of Alzheimer's disease.

## From Excitement to Brain Burn: Too Much Excitatory Neurotransmission Could Be Hazardous to Your Health

If Benjamin Franklin said "nothing in excess, including moderation" he may have anticipated contemporary thinking about excitatory neurotransmission. Excitatory neurotransmission with glutamate ranges from talking to neurons (Fig. 4–15), to screaming at them (Fig. 4–16), to strangling their dendrites, and even to assassinating them (Fig. 4–17).

Glutamate normally opens an ion channel so that the nerve can drink calcium (Figs. 4–15 and 4–18). Sipping calcium is exciting to a neuron and a normal reaction when glutamate is speaking pleasantly. However, when glutamate screams at a neuron, the neuron reacts by drinking more calcium (Figs. 4–16 and 4–19). Imbibing too much calcium may lead in part to excitatory symptoms such as panic, seizures, mania, or psychosis (Figs. 4–19 and 4–20). Too much calcium eventually will anger intracellular enzymes, which then generate nasty chemicals called free radicals. A small commune of free radicals can crash the chemical party in the postsynaptic dendrite and strangle it (Fig. 4–21). A mob of free radicals can kill the whole neuron, perhaps by triggering apoptosis (Fig. 4–22; see also Fig. 1–18).

Why would the neuron allow this to happen? It is possible that the brain needs this excitotoxic mechanism so that glutamate can act as a gardener in the brain, pruning worn out branches from dendritic trees so that healthy new sprouts may prosper (Fig. 1–23). However, this also equips the neuron with a powerful weapon, which can potentially be misused to cause various neurodegenerative conditions due literally to pruning neurons to death (Fig. 4–22). Such an excitotoxic mechanism could be activated if the genetic program controlling it is turned on or potentially by ingestion of toxins or toxic drugs of abuse. That is, when glutamate decides to act as an abusive bully for whatever reason, neurons may seize, panic, become manic, or become psychotic (Fig. 4–20). Furthermore, such symptoms of calcium intoxi-

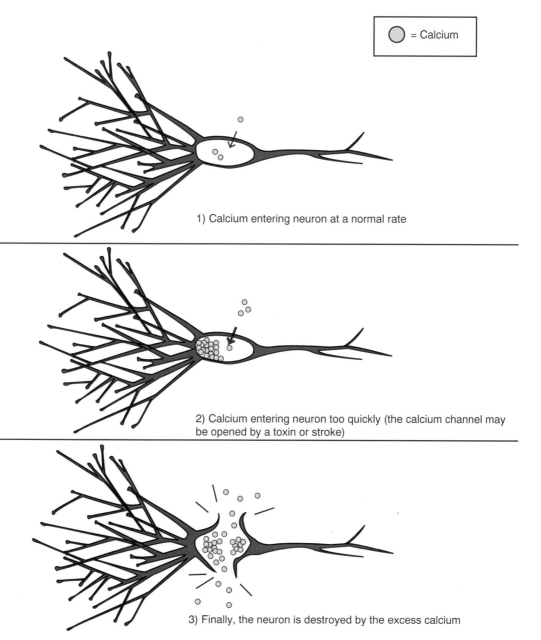

= Calcium

1) Calcium entering neuron at a normal rate

2) Calcium entering neuron too quickly (the calcium channel may be opened by a toxin or stroke)

3) Finally, the neuron is destroyed by the excess calcium

FIGURE 4–15. The **calcium** ion is a key regulator of **neuronal excitability** and is constantly entering and leaving neurons through ion channels of various sorts that are conducting the normal business functions of the neuron. When this occurs at a **normal rate**, it modifies neuronal excitability but is not damaging to the neuron (but see Figs. 4–16 and 4–17).

FIGURE 4–16. **Calcium** may also rush into cells **too quickly** if its ion channels are opened too much, as is postulated to occur as a result of certain toxins, by stroke, or by neurodegenerative conditions (see Fig. 4–17).

FIGURE 4–17. If **too much calcium** gets into the neuron and overwhelms any sinks and buffers there, it can **destroy the neuron** and cause it to degenerate and die. This mechanism of excessive excitation is called **excitotoxicity** and is a major current hypothesis of the cause of various psychiatric and neurological disorders. This idea postulates that for such diseases, neurons are literally *"excited to death."*

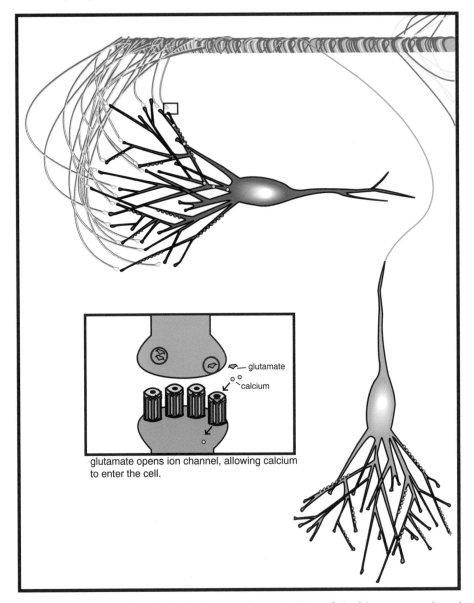

glutamate

calcium

glutamate opens ion channel, allowing calcium
to enter the cell.

FIGURE 4–18. Shown here are details of calcium entering a dendrite of the blue neuron when the
red neuron excites it with glutamate during normal excitatory neurotransmission. This was shown in
a more simplistic model in Figure 4–15. Glutamate released from the red neuron travels across the
synapse, docks into its agonist slot on its receptor, and as ionic gatekeeper, opens the calcium channel
to allow calcium to enter the postsynaptic dendrite of the blue neuron to mediate **normal excitatory
neurotransmission** (*see box*).

cation may be followed by an unfortunate glutamate hangover in the form of destroyed dendrites, which can never be excited again (Fig. 4–21).

Other illnesses such as Alzheimer's disease, Parkinson's disease, amytrophic lateral
sclerosis (Lou Gehrig's disease), and even schizophrenia may hire glutamate as a

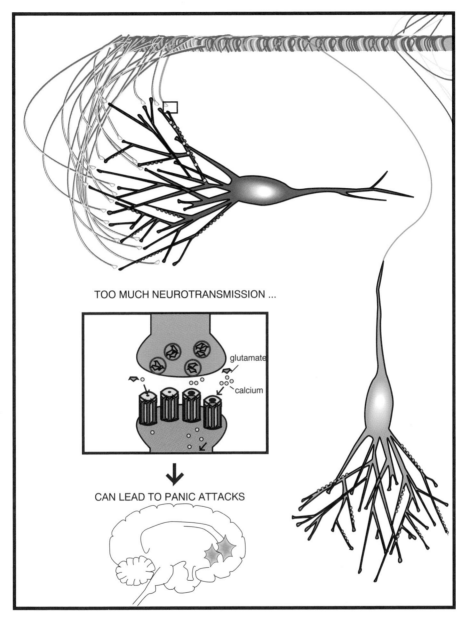

TOO MUCH NEUROTRANSMISSION ...

glutamate

calcium

CAN LEAD TO PANIC ATTACKS

FIGURE 4–19. Shown here is what may happen when excitatory neurotransmission causes **too much neurotransmission**. This may possibly occur during the production of various symptoms mediated by the brain, including **panic attacks**. It could also occur during mania, positive symptoms of psychosis, seizures, and other neuronally-mediated disease symptoms. In this case, **too much glutamate** is being released by the red neuron, causing **too much excitation** of the postsynaptic blue neuron's dendrite. Extra release of glutamate causes additional occupancy of postsynaptic glutamate receptors, opening more calcium channels and allowing more calcium to enter the blue dendrite (*see box*). Although this degree of excessive neurotransmission may be associated with psychiatric symptoms, it does not actually damage the neuron (but see Figs. 4–20 and 4–21).

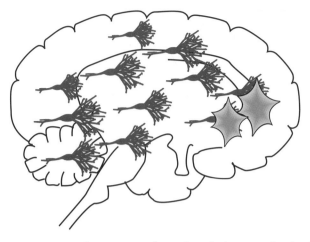

FIGURE 4–20. This figure represents the concept of an **electrical storm** in the brain in which **overexcitation** and **too much neurotransmission** are occurring during the production of various psychiatric symptoms, including those which occur during a panic attack. This may also be a model for other disorders of excessive behavioral symptoms that imply too much neurotransmission, including mania, positive manifestation of psychosis, and seizures.

methodical undercover assassin, eliminating a whole subpopulation of predesignated neurons over a prolonged period of time. Such a systematic process would be consistent with the pace of these slow neurodegenerative disorders. In catastrophic brain diseases such as stroke and global ischemia associated with cardiac arrest, drowning, etc., a whole army of glutamate "hit men" may be hired as mass murderers. In this case, glutamate causes the massacre of an entire region of brain neurons by suddenly subjecting them to molecular mayhem.

Thus, glutamate's actions can range across a vast spectrum. It can be a friendly neuronal conversationalist or a screaming hypothetical mediator of neurological and psychiatric disorders. How might the symptoms and clinical course of various psychiatric disorders fit this model of excitotoxicity? Psychosis possibly shares some analogies with a seizure, in that excessive transmission of dopamine in the mesolimbic areas of brain may lead to symptoms of delusions, hallucinations, and thought disorder in various psychiatric disorders. Panic disorder may be analogous to a seizure in areas of the brain controlling emotions (such as the parahippocampal gyrus), leading to clinical symptoms characterized by a massive emotional discharge of panic, shortness of breath, chest pain, dizziness, feelings of impending death, or fear of losing control. Thus, disorders such as psychosis, epilepsy and panic disorder appear to involve excessive neurotransmission, which may help explain the mechanism by which they produce acute symptoms (Figs. 4–19 and 4–20).

Furthermore, these disorders seem to become more resistant to treatment the longer the disorder persists and the more poorly the symptoms are controlled, as if there were an underlying mechanism of destruction accompanying symptoms that are out of control (Figs. 4–21 through 4–23). Thus, excessive neurotransmission may itself be a cause of deficient neurotransmission. If seizures beget seizures, panic

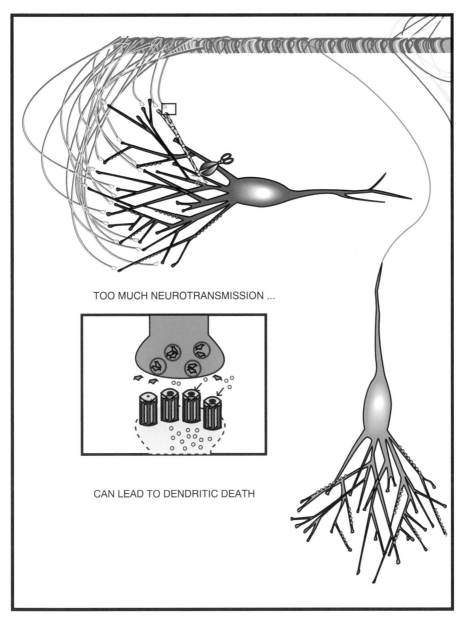

TOO MUCH NEUROTRANSMISSION ...

CAN LEAD TO DENDRITIC DEATH

FIGURE 4–21. If too much neurotransmission occurs for too long, it is hypothetically possible that this would lead to **dendritic death**. The mechanism for this may be tantamount to inappropriately activating the normal dendritic pruning process (indicated schematically as scissors snipping off the dendrite; see Figure 1–23 for a diagram of normal pruning). Thus, far **too much glutamate** release can cause too much opening of the gates of the **calcium** channel, activating an **excitotoxic** demise of the dendrite (*see box*).

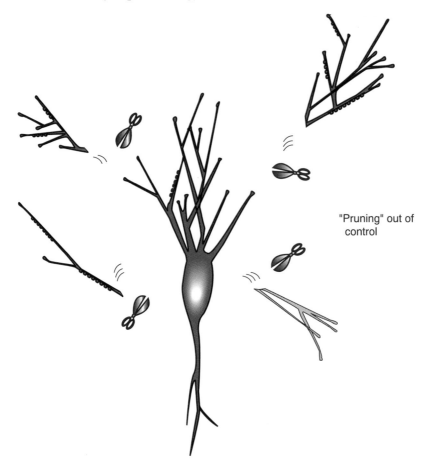

"Pruning" out of
control

A disease may let the normal process of pruning get out of control.  The disease can
cause the neuron to be "pruned to death."

FIGURE 4–22. Neurons appear to have a normal maintenance mechanism for their dendritic tree by
which they are able to prune, or remove, old, unused, or useless synapses and dendrites (normal
mechanism shown in Fig. 1–23). One postulated mechanism for some degenerative diseases is that
this otherwise normal **pruning mechanism** may get **out of control**, eventually rendering the neuron
useless or even killing it by "**pruning it to death.**"

begets panic, psychosis begets psychosis, and mania begets mania, these symptoms
are obviously not good for the brain. The psychopharmacologist must therefore act
to prevent symptoms, not only because symptom control may harness the disruptive
influences of excessive neurotransmission on behavior, but also because symptom
control may ultimately prevent the demise of the neurons mediating these very
behaviors (Figs. 4–20 to 4–23). If these disorders of excessive neurotransmission are
analogous to the brain "burning" during symptomatic crises such as a seizure, psychosis, panic attack, or mania, treatments might not only "put out the fire" but also
salvage the underlying neuronal substrates, which are burning as the fuel for the
fire.

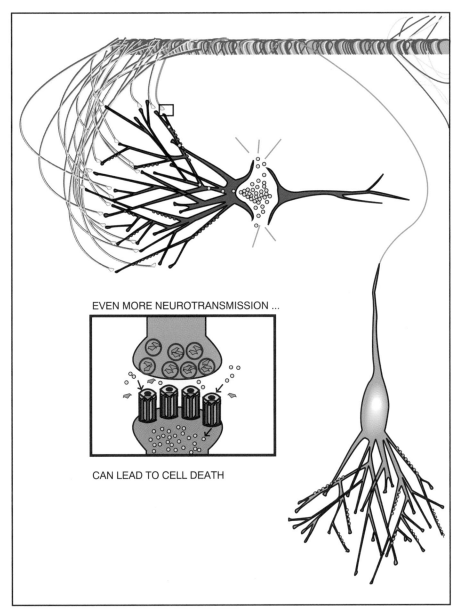

EVEN MORE NEUROTRANSMISSION ...

CAN LEAD TO CELL DEATH

FIGURE 4–23. **Catastrophic overexcitation** can theoretically lead to so much **calcium** flux into a neuron due to dangerous, wide-ranging opening of calcium channels by glutamate (*see box*) that not only is the dendrite destroyed, but so is the entire neuron. This scenario is one in which the neuron is literally **excited to death**. The same idea was represented more simplistically in Figure 4–17. **Excitotoxicity** is a major current hypothesis to explain the mechanism of neuronal death in neuro-degenerative disorders, including aspects of schizophrenia, Alzheimer's disease, Parkinson's disease, amyotrophic lateral sclerosis, and ischemic cell damage from stroke.

Discovery of antagonists to excitotoxicity, such as exemplified by the glutamate antagonists, may portend the possibility of developing new drug therapies for neurodegenerative disorders. At least two approaches to controlling glutamate are showing promise. The first is to protect the neuron from drinking too much calcium by blocking glutamate receptors directly with antagonists. Thus, neurons are only allowed to quench their thirst in normal excitatory neurotransmission but not to guzzle so much calcium that they become excitotoxically inebriated. If such compounds worked, they would be neuroprotective, since they would arrest glutamate before it could assassinate any more neurons. Another approach to developing treatments for illnesses that may be mediated by excitotoxicity is to rescue the cellular machinery once glutamate's cascade of doom has been activated. Thus, free-radical scavengers are being developed that neutralize the troublesome free radicals. Certain chemicals can do this, including vitamin E and experimental agents called lazaroids (so named because they purport to raise neurons from the dead, as the biblical Lazarus was raised).

## No Neurotransmission

There are a myriad of known and suspected mechanisms by which diseases can modify chemical neurotransmission. These can vary from no transmission, as in the case of a degenerated or absent neuron, to too much neurotransmission from a malfunction of the synapse. One of the key consequences of loss of neurons in neurodegenerative disorders such as Parkinson's disease, Huntington's disease, amyotrophic lateral sclerosis (Lou Gehrig's disease), and Alzheimer's disease, is the fact that no neurotransmission occurs subsequent to neuronal loss (Fig. 4–24). This is a conceptually simple mechanism of disease action with profound consequences. It is also at least in part the mechanism of other disorders, such as stroke, multiple sclerosis, and virtually any disorder in which neurons are irreversibly damaged.

One of the earliest attempts to compensate for the dropout of neurons and the consequent loss of neurotransmission (Fig. 4–24) was simply to replace the neurotransmitter (Fig. 4–25). Indeed, this can happen in certain conditions such as Parkinson's disease, where loss of the neurotransmitter dopamine can be replaced. Even in this conceptually simple example, however, therapeutic replacement is in fact not so simple. Dopamine given orally or intravenously cannot get into the brain. Its precursor, L-DOPA, can reach the brain and be converted into dopamine. However, even the precursor needs help in practice, since coadministration of an inhibitor of L-dopa destruction is necessary for L-DOPA to work optimally.

## Other Mechanisms of Abnormal Neurotransmission

Several other mechanisms can be conceptualized. These include the *imbalance* between two neurotransmitters required to regulate a single process. This has been theorized as the mechanism of many of the movement disorders, in which balance between the two neurotransmitters dopamine and acetylcholine is not normal. Another possible aberrancy is that of the *wrong rate* of neurotransmission, possibly disrupting functions such as sleep or biorhythms. We have already discussed how degenerative disorders involve loss of neurons and synapses, and the net result of the loss of key synapses is abnormality of the remaining wiring system of the brain.

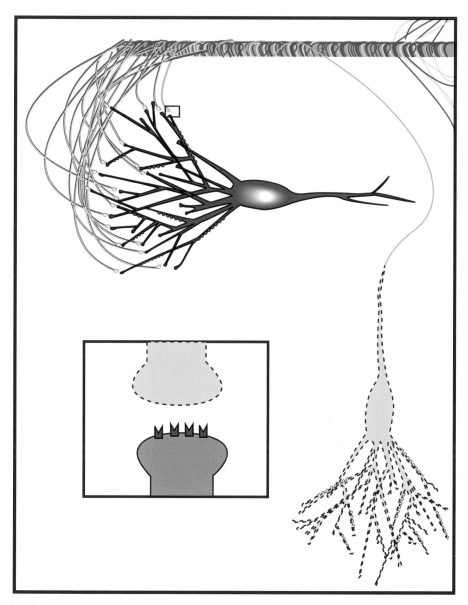

FIGURE 4–24. This figure illustrates what happens in a conceptually simple disease in which a neuron dies, leaving behind **no neurotransmission**. The loss of the red neuron means that neuro-transmission at the former site between the red and the blue neuron is now lost (but see Fig. 4–25).

New neurotransmitter is given as a drug to take over the
functions of the dead neuron

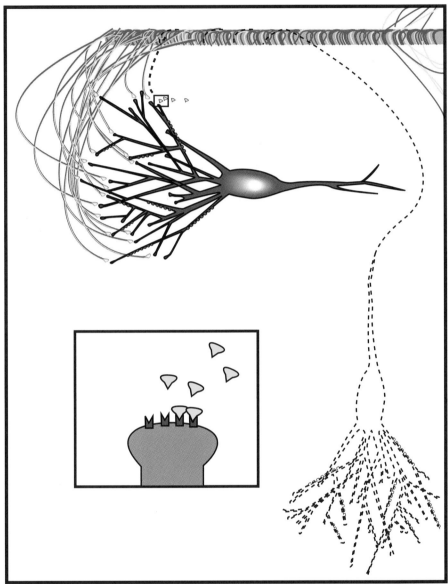

FIGURE 4–25. One of the simplest pharmacological remedies for replacing the function of the lost
neurotransmission from a degenerated neuron is to **replace the neurotransmitter** with a drug that
mimics the former neuron's neurotransmitter. This is shown here with the yellow drug replacing the
natural neurotransmitter that was formerly present when the red neuron was present and functioning
(Fig. 4–11). This strategy is used, for example, when L-DOPA is used to replace the lost neurotransmission in Parkinson's disease when nigrostriatal dopamine neurons degenerate and die.

## Summary

This chapter has reviewed how enzymes and receptors are not only the targets of drug actions but also the sites of disease actions. We have discussed how diseases of the CNS are approached by three disciplines: neurobiology, biological psychiatry, and psychopharmacology. We have also discussed how disease actions in the brain modify neurotransmission by at least eight mechanisms: (1) modifications of molecular neurobiology; (2) loss of neuronal plasticity; (3) excitotoxicity; (4) absence of neurotransmission; (5) excess neurotransmission; (6) an imbalance among neurotransmitters; (7) the wrong rate of neurotransmission; and (8) the wrong neuronal wiring.

# CHAPTER 5

# Depression and Bipolar Disorders

In this chapter, the reader will develop a foundation of knowledge about the mood disorders characterized by depression, mania, or both. Included here are descriptions of the leading hypotheses that attempt to explain the biological basis of mood disorders, especially depression. To understand these hypotheses, this chapter will formulate key pharmacological principles that apply to neurons using specific mono-amine neurotransmitters, namely norepinephrine (NE; also called noradrenaline or NA), dopamine (DA), and serotonin (also called 5-hydroxytryptamine or 5HT). We will also briefly introduce neuropeptides related to substance P. This will set the stage for understanding the pharmacological concepts underlying the use of antide-pressant and mood-stabilizing drugs, which will be reviewed in Chapters 6 and 7.

Clinical descriptions and criteria for diagnosis of disorders of mood will only be mentioned in passing. The reader should consult standard reference sources for this material. Here we will discuss how discoveries of various antidepressants have im-pacted the diagnostic criteria for depression and how they may have modified the natural history and course of this illness. The goal of this chapter is to acquaint the reader with current ideas about the clinical and biological aspects of mood disorders in order to be prepared to understand how the various antidepressants and mood stabilizers work.

## Clinical Features of Mood Disorders

### Description of Mood Disorders

Problems with mood are often called affective disorders. Depression and mania are often seen as opposite ends of an affective or mood spectrum. Classically, mania and depression are "poles" apart, thus generating the terms *unipolar* depression, in which patients just experience the *down* or depressed pole and *bipolar* disorder, in which patients at different times experience either the *up* (manic) pole or the *down* (de-pressed) pole. In practice, however, depression and mania may occur simultaneously, which is called a "mixed" mood state. Mania may also occur in lesser degrees, known as "hypomania," or may switch so fast between mania and depression that it is called "rapid cycling."

Depression is an emotion that is universally experienced by virtually everyone at some time in life. Distinguishing the "normal" emotion of depression from an illness requiring medical treatment is often problematic for those who are not trained in the mental health sciences. Stigma and misinformation in our culture create the widespread popular misconception that mental illness such as depression is not a disease but a deficiency of character, which can be overcome with effort. For example, a survey in the early 1990s of the general population revealed that 71% thought that mental illness was due to emotional weakness; 65% thought it was caused by bad parenting; 45% thought it was the victim's fault and could be willed away; 43% thought that mental illness was incurable; 35% thought it was the consequence of sinful behavior; and only 10% thought it had a biological basis or involved the brain (Table 5–1).

Stigma and misinformation can also extend into medical practice, where many depressed patients present with medically unexplained symptoms. "Somatization" is the term used for such use of physical symptoms to express emotional distress, which may be a major reason for misdiagnosis of mental illness by medical and psycho-

Table 5–1. *Public perceptions of mental illness*

| | |
|---|---|
| 71% | Due to emotional weakness |
| 65% | Caused by bad parenting |
| 45% | Victim's fault; can will it away |
| 43% | Incurable |
| 35% | Consequence of sinful bahavior |
| 10% | Has a biological basis; involves the brain |

logical practitioners. Many depressed patients with somatic complaints are considered to have no real or treatable illness and thus are not treated for a psychiatric disorder once medical illnesses are evaluated and ruled out. In reality, however, most patients with diffuse unexplained somatic symptoms in primary care settings either have a treatable psychiatric illness (e.g., anxiety or depressive disorder) or are responding to stressful life events. Such patients do not generally have a genuine somatization disorder in which "their symptoms are really all in their mind."

Given how frequent and treatable the affective illnesses are, if there are a few most important points to make in this textbook, one of them is the need for the reader to know how to recognize and treat these illnesses.

## Diagnostic Criteria

Accepted, standardized diagnostic criteria are used to separate "normal" depression caused by disappointment or "having a bad day" from the disorders of mood. Such criteria also are used to distinguish feeling good from feeling "better then good" and so expansive and irritable that the feelings amount to mania. Diagnostic criteria for mood disorders are in constant evolution, with current nosologies being set by the Diagnostic and Statistical Manual of Mental Disorders, Fourth Edition (DSM-IV) (Tables 5–2 and 5–3) in the United States and the International Classification of Diseases, Tenth Edition (ICD-10) in other countries. The reader is referred to these references for the specifics of currently accepted diagnostic criteria.

For our purposes, it is sufficient to recognize that the affective disorders are actually *syndromes*. That is, they are *clusters of symptoms*, only one symptom of which is an abnormality of mood. Certainly the quality of mood, the degree of mood change from the normal (up—mania, or down—depression), and the duration of the abnormal mood are all key features of an affective disorder. In addition, however, clinicians must assess *vegetative features* such as sleep, appetite, weight, and sex drive; *cognitive features* such as attention span, frustration tolerance, memory, negative distortions; *impulse control* such as suicide and homicide; *behavioral features* such as motivation, pleasure, interests, fatigability; and *physical (or somatic) features* such as headaches, stomach aches, and muscle tension (Table 5–4).

## Epidemiology and Natural History

In the 1990s, diagnostic criteria for depression began to be applied increasingly to describing the epidemiology and natural history of mood disorders so that the effects

Table 5–2. DSM IV *diagnostic criteria for a major depressive episode*

A. Five (or more) of the following symptoms have been present during the same 2-week period and represent a change from previous functioning; at least one of the symptoms is either (1) depressed mood or (2) loss of interest or pleasure. *Note:* Do not include symptoms that are clearly due to a general medical condition, or mood-incongruent delusions or hallucinations.
   1. Depressed mood most of the day, nearly every day, as indicated by either subjective report (e.g., feels sad or empty) or observation made by others (e.g., appears tearful). *Note:* In children and adolescents, can be irritable mood.
   2. Markedly diminished interest or pleasure in all, or almost all, activities most of the day, nearly every day (as indicated by either subjective account or observation made by others).
   3. Significant weight loss when not dieting or weight gain (e.g., a change of more than 5% of body weight in a month), or decrease or increase in appetite nearly every day. *Note:* In children, consider failure to make expected weight gains.
   4. Insomnia or hypersomnia nearly every day.
   5. Psychomotor agitation or retardation nearly every day (observable by others, not merely subjective feelings of restlessness or being slowed down).
   6. Fatigue or loss of energy nearly every day.
   7. Feelings of worthlessness or excessive or inappropriate guilt (which may be delusional) nearly every day (not merely self-reproach or guilt about being sick).
   8. Diminished ability to think or concentrate, or indecisiveness, nearly every day (either by subjective account or as observed by others).
   9. Recurrent thoughts of death (not just fear of dying), recurrent suicidal ideation without a specific plan, or a suicide attempt or a specific plan for committing suicide.
B. The symptoms do not meet criteria for a mixed episode.
C. The symptoms cause clinically significant distress or impairment in social, occupational, or other important areas of functioning.
D. The symptoms are not due to the direct physiological effects of a substance (e.g., a drug of abuse, a medication, or other treatment) or a general medical condition (e.g., hyperthyroidism).
E. The symptoms are not better accounted for by bereavement (i.e., after the loss of a loved one); the symptoms persist for longer than 2 months or are characterized by marked functional impairment, morbid preoccupation with worthlessness, suicidal ideation, psychotic symptoms, or psychomotor retardation.

of treatments could be better measured. Key questions are: What is the incidence of major depressive disorder versus bipolar disorder? How many people have the condition at the present time, and how many in their lifetimes? Are individuals with mood disorders being identified and treated, and if so, how? Also: What is the outcome of their treatment? What is the natural history of their mood disorder without treatment and how is this affected by treatment?

Answers to these questions are just beginning to evolve (Tables 5–5 through 5–10). For example, the incidence of depression is about 5% of the population, whereas the incidence of bipolar disorder is about 1%. Thus, up to 15 million individuals are currently suffering from depression and another 2 to 3 million from bipolar disorders in the United States. Unfortunately, only about one-third of individuals with depression are in treatment, not only because of underrecognition by health care providers but also because individuals often conceive of their depression as a type of moral deficiency, which is shameful and should be hidden. Individuals often feel as if they could get better if they just "pulled themselves up by the bootstraps"

Table 5–3. *DSM IV diagnostic criteria for a manic episode*

A. A distinct period of abnormally and persistently elevated, expansive, or irritable mood, lasting at least 1 week (or any duration if hospitalization is necessary).

B. During the period of mood disturbance, three (or more) of the following symptoms have persisted (four if the mood is only irritable) and have been present to a significant degree:
1. Inflated self-esteem or grandiosity.
2. Decreased need for sleep (e.g., feels rested after only 3 hours of sleep).
3. More talkative than usual or pressure to keep talking.
4. Flight of ideas or subjective experience that thoughts are racing.
5. Distractability (i.e., attention too easily drawn to unimportant or irrelevant external stimuli).
6. Increase in goal-directed activity (either socially, at work or school, or sexually) or psychomotor agitation.
7. Excessive involvement in pleasurable activities that have a high potential for painful consequences (e.g., engaging in unrestrained buying sprees, sexual indiscretions, or foolish business investments).

C. The symptoms do not meet criteria for a mixed episode.

D. The mood disturbance is sufficiently severe to cause marked impairment in occupational functioning or in usual social activities or relationships with others, or to necessitate hospitalization to prevent harm to self or others, or there are psychotic features.

E. The symptoms are not due to the direct physiological effects of a substance (e.g., a drug of abuse, a medication, or other treatment) or a general medical condition (e.g., hyperthyroidism). *Note*: Manic-like episodes that are clearly caused by somatic antidepressant treatment (e.g., medication, electroconvulsive therapy, light therapy) should not count toward a diagnosis of bipolar I disorder.

Table 5–4. *Depression is a syndrome*

Clusters of symptoms in depression:
  Vegetative
  Cognitive
  Impulse control
  Behavioral
  Physical (somatic)

and tried harder. The reality is that depression is an illness, not a choice, and is just as socially debilitating as coronary artery disease and more debilitating than diabetes mellitus or arthritis. Furthermore, up to 15% of severely depressed patients will ultimately commit suicide. Suicide attempts are up to ten per hundred subjects depressed for a year, with one successful suicide per hundred subjects depressed for a year. In the United States for example, there are approximately 300,000 suicide attempts and 30,000 suicides per year, most, but not all, associated with depression.

The conclusions are impressive: mood disorders are common, debilitating, life-threatening illnesses, which can be successfully treated but which commonly are not treated. Public education efforts are ongoing to identify cases and provide effective treatment.

Table 5–5. *Patient education*

The effectiveness of any treatment rests on a cooperative effort by patient and practitioner.
The patient should be told of the diagnosis, prognosis, and treatment options, including costs,
  duration, and potential side effects. In educating patient and family about the clinical
  management of depression, it is useful to emphasize the following information:
Depression is a medical illness, not a character defect or weakness.
Recovery is the rule, not the exception.
Treatments are effective, and there are many options for treatment. An effective treatment can be
  found for nearly all patients.
The aim of treatment is complete symptom remission, not just getting better but getting and
  staying well.
The risk of recurrence is significant: 50% after one episode, 70% after two episodes, 90% after
  three episodes.
Patient and family should be alert to early signs and symptoms of recurrence and seek treatment
  early if depression returns.

Table 5–6. *Risk factors for major depression*

| Risk factor | Association |
|---|---|
| Sex | Major depresson is twice as likely in women |
| Age | Peak age on onset is 20–40 years |
| Family history | 1.5 to 3 times higher risk with positive history |
| Marital status | Separated and divorced persons report higher rates |
| | Married males lower rates than unmarried males |
| | Married females higher rates than unmarried females |
| Postpartum | An increased risk for the 6-month period following childbirth |
| Negative life events | Possible association |
| Early parental death | Possible association |

Table 5–7. *Depression in the United States*

High rate of occurence
  5–11% lifetime prevalence
  10–15 million in United States depressed in any year
Episodes can be of long duration (years)
Over 50% rate of recurrence following a single episode; higher if patient
    has had multiple episodes
Morbidity comparable to angina and advanced coronary artery disease
High mortality from suicide if untreated

Table 5–8. *Facts about suicide and depression*

20–40% of patients with an affective disorder exhibit nonfatal suicidal behaviors, including thoughts of suicide

Estimates associate 16,000 suicides in the United States annually with depressive disorder

15% of those hospitalized for major depressive disorder attempt suicide

15% of patients with severe primary major depressive disorder of at least 1 month's duration eventually commit suicide

Table 5–9. *Suicide and major depression: the rules of sevens*

One out of seven with recurrent depressive illness commits suicide

70% of suicides have depressive illness

70% of suicides see their primary care physician within 6 weeks of suicide

Suicide is the seventh leading cause of death in the United States

Table 5–10. *The hidden cost of not treating major depression*

Mortality
    30,000 to 35,000 suicides per year
    Fatal accidents due to impaired concentration and attention
    Death due to illnesses that can be sequelae (e.g., alcohol abuse)
Patient morbidity
    Suicide attempts
    Accidents
    Resultant illnesses
    Lost jobs
    Failure to advance in career and school
    Substance abuse
Societal costs
    Dysfunctional families
    Absenteeism
    Decreased productivity
    Job-related injuries
    Adverse effect on quality control in the workplace

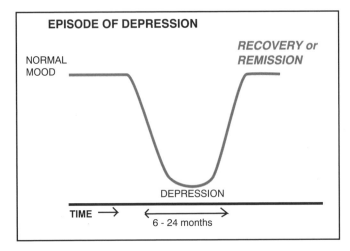

**EPISODE OF DEPRESSION**

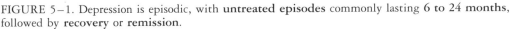

FIGURE 5−1. Depression is episodic, with **untreated episodes** commonly lasting **6 to 24 months**, followed by **recovery** or **remission**.


## Effects of Treatments on Mood Disorders

### Long-Term Outcomes of Mood Disorders and the Five R's of Antidepressant Treatment

Until recently very little was really known about what happens to depression if it is not treated. It is now thought that most untreated episodes of depression last 6 to 24 months (Fig. 5−1). Perhaps only 5 to 10% of untreated sufferers have their episodes continue for more than 2 years. However, the very nature of this illness includes recurrent episodes. Many individuals who present for the first time for treatment will have a history of one or more prior unrecognized and untreated episodes of this illness, dating back to adolescence.

Three terms beginning with the letter "R" are used to describe the improvement of a depressed patient after treatment with an antidepressant, namely response, remission, and recovery. The term *response* generally means that a depressed patient has experienced at least a 50% reduction in symptoms as assessed on a standard psychiatric rating scale such as the Hamilton Depression Rating Scale (Fig. 5−2). This also generally corresponds to a global clinical rating of the patient as much improved or very much improved. *Remission*, on the other hand, is the term used when essentially all symptoms go away, not just 50% of them (Fig. 5−3). The patient is not better; the patient is actually well. If this lasts for 6 to 12 months, remission is then considered to be *recovery* (Fig. 5−3).

Two terms beginning with the letter "R" are used to describe worsening in a patient with depression, relapse and recurrence. If a patient worsens before there is a complete remission or before the remission has turned into a recovery, it is called a *relapse* (Fig. 5−4). However, if a patient worsens a few months after complete recovery, it is called a *recurrence*. The features that predict relapse with greatest accuracy are: (1) multiple prior episodes; (2) severe episodes; (3) long-lasting episodes; (4) episodes with bipolar or psychotic features; and (5) incomplete recovery between two consecutive episodes, also called poor interepisode recovery (Table 5−11).

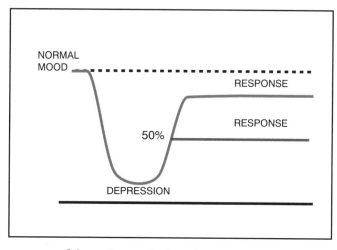

FIGURE 5–2. When treatment of depression results in at least 50% improvement in symptoms, it is called a **response**. Such patients are better, but not well.

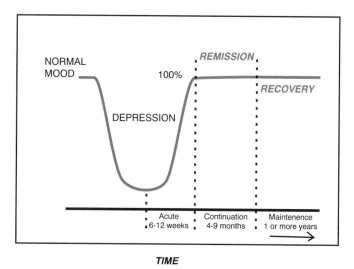

**TIME**

FIGURE 5–3. When treatment of depression results in removal of essentially all symptoms, it is called **remission** for the first several months, and then **recovery** if it is sustained for longer than 6 to 12 months. Such patients are not just better—they are well.

The longitudinal course of bipolar illness is also characterized by many recurrent episodes, some predominantly depressive, some predominantly manic or hypomanic, some mixed with simultaneous features of both mania and depression (Fig. 5–5); some may even be rapid cycling, with at least four ups and/or downs in 12 months (Fig. 5–6). There is worrisome evidence that bipolar disorders may be somewhat progressive, especially if uncontrolled. That is, mood fluctuations become more frequent, more severe, and less responsive to medications as time goes on, especially in cases where there has been little or inadequate treatment.

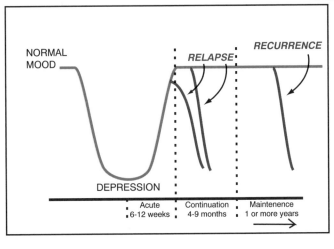

**TIME**

FIGURE 5–4. When depression returns before there is a full remission of symptoms or within the first several months following remission of symptoms, it is called a **relapse**. When depression returns after a patient has recovered, it is called a **recurrence**.

Table 5–11. *Biggest risk factors for a recurrent episode of depression*

| |
| --- |
| Multiple prior episodes |
| Incomplete recoveries from prior episodes |
| Severe episode |
| Chronic episode |
| Bipolar or psychotic features |

Dysthymia is a low-grade but very chronic form of depression, which lasts for more than 2 years (Fig. 5–7). It may represent a relatively stable and unremitting illness of low-grade depression, or it may indicate a state of partial recovery from an episode of major depressive disorder. When major depressive episodes are superimposed on dysthymia, the resulting condition is sometimes called "double depression" (Fig. 5–8) and may account for many of those with poor interepisode recovery.

### Search for Subtypes of Depression That Predict Response to Antidepressants

Although effective for depression in general, antidepressants do not help everyone with depression. In fact, only about two out of three patients with depression will respond to any given antidepressant (Fig. 5–9), whereas only about one out of three will respond to placebo (Fig. 5–10). Follow-up studies of depressed patients after 1 year of clinical treatment show that approximately 40% still have the same diagnosis, 40% have no diagnosis, and the rest either recover partially or develop the diagnosis of dysthymia (Fig. 5–9). In the 1970s and 1980s, the diagnostic criteria

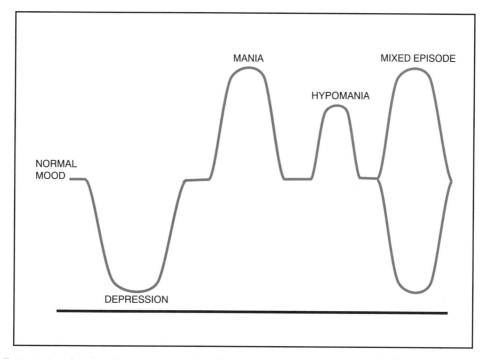

FIGURE 5–5. Bipolar disorder is characterized by various types of episodes of affective disorder, including **depression**, full **mania**, lesser degrees of mania called **hypomania**, and even **mixed episodes** in which mania and depression seem to coincide.

for depression began to focus in part on trying to identify those depressed patients who were the best candidates for the various antidepressant treatments that had become available.

During this era, the idea evolved that there might be one subgroup of unipolar depressives that was especially responsive to antidepressants and another that was not. The first group was hypothesized to have a serious, even melancholic clinical form of depression, which had a biological basis and a high degree of familial occurrence, was episodic in nature, and was likely to respond to tricyclic antidepressants and monoamine oxidase (MAO) inhibitors. Opposed to this was a second form of depression hypothesized to be neurotic and characterological in origin, less severe but more chronic, not especially responsive to antidepressants, and possibly amenable to treatment by psychotherapy. This was called depressive neurosis, or dysthymia.

The search for any biological markers of depression, let alone those that might be predictive of antidepressant treatment responsiveness has been disappointing. It is currently not possible to predict which patient will respond to antidepressants in general or to any specific antidepressant drug. However, it is well established that no matter what the subtype, some patients with any known form of unipolar depression will respond to antidepressants, including those individuals with melancholia as well as those with dysthymia.

Although it is therefore not yet possible to predict who will and who will not respond to a given antidepressant drug, several approaches that fail to predict this are known. These include the concepts of biological versus nonbiological, endogenous

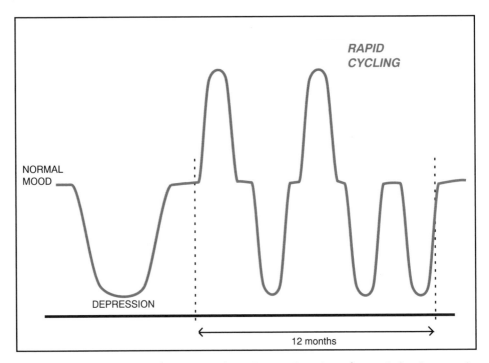

FIGURE 5-6. Bipolar disorder can become **rapid cycling**, with at least four switches into mania, hypomania, depression, or mixed episodes within a 12-month period. This is a particularly difficult form of bipolar disorder to treat.

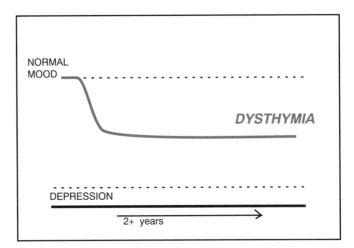

FIGURE 5-7. **Dysthymia** is a low-grade but very chronic form of depression, which lasts for more than 2 years.

146

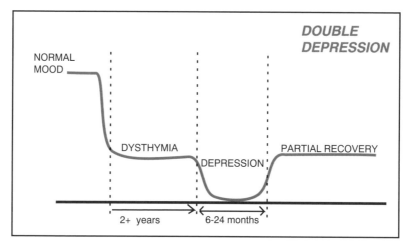

FIGURE 5–8. **Double depression** is a syndrome characterized by oscillation between episodes of major depression and periods of partial recovery or dysthymia.

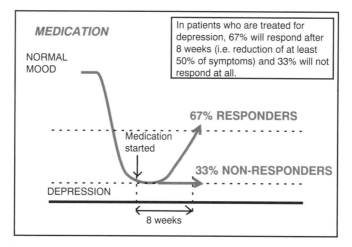

FIGURE 5–9. Virtually every known antidepressant has the same **response rate**, namely 67% of depressed patients respond to a given medication and 33% fail to respond.

versus reactive, melancholic versus neurotic, acute versus chronic, and familial versus nonfamilial depression, and others as well.

## The Good News and the Bad News about Antidepressant Treatments

One can look at the effects of antidepressant treatments on the long-term outcome from depression as either good news or bad news, depending on whether it is seen from the perspective of *response* or from the perspective of *remission*. The news looks good if mere response to an antidepressant is the standard (i.e., getting better), but if one "raises the bar" and asks about remission (i.e., getting well), the news does not look nearly as good (Tables 5–12 and 5–13).

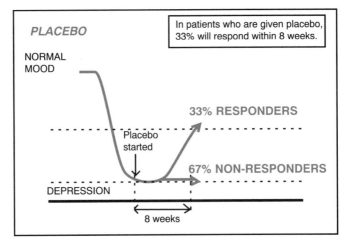

FIGURE 5−10. In controlled clinical trials, 33% of patients respond to **placebo** treatment and 67% fail to respond.

Table 5−12. *Limitations of response definition*

Response is a reduction in the signs and symptoms of depression of
    more than 50% from baseline.
Responders have residual symptoms.
Response is the end point for clinical trials, *not* clinical practice.

Table 5−13. *Remission*

Remission is defined as a Hamilton Depression Score less than 8 to 10 and a clinical global
    impression rating of normal, not mentally ill.
A patient who is in remission may be considered asymptomatic.
Remission is a more relevant end point than response for clinicians, as it signifies that the
    patient is "well."

For example, the good news side of the story is that half to two-thirds of patients respond to any given antidepressant, as mentioned above (Fig. 5−9 and Table 5−14). Even better news is the finding that 90% or more may eventually respond if a number of different antidepressants or combinations of antidepressants are tried in succession. Other good news is that some studies suggest that up to half of responders may go on to experience a complete remission from their depression within 6 months of treatment, and possibly two-thirds or more of the responders will remit within 2 years.

Some of the best news of all is that antidepressants significantly reduce relapse rates during the first 6 to 12 months following initial response to the medication (Figs. 5−11 and 5−12). That is, about half of patients may relapse within 6 months

Table 5–14. *The good news in the treatment of depression*

Half of depressed patients may recover within 6 months of an index episode of depression, and three-fourths may recover within 2 years.

Up to 90% of depressed patients may respond to one or a combination of therapeutic interventions if multiple therapies are tried.

Antidepressants reduce relapse rates.

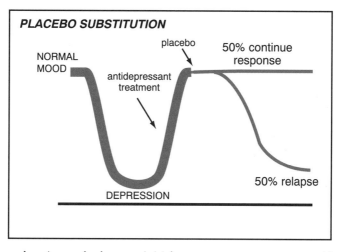

FIGURE 5–11. Depressed patients who have an initial treatment response to an antidepressant will **relapse at the rate of 50%** within 6 to 12 months if their medication is withdrawn and a **placebo substituted.**

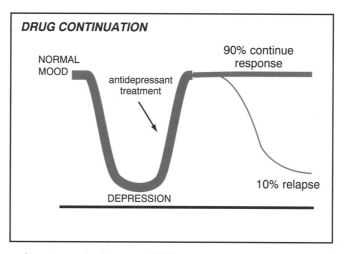

FIGURE 5–12. Depressed patients who have an initial treatment response to an antidepressant will **only relapse at the rate of about 10 to 20%** if their **medication is continued for a year** following recovery.

Table 5–15. *Probability of recurrence as a function of the number of previous episodes*

| Number of Prior Episodes | Recurrence Risk |
|---|---|
| 1 | <50% |
| 2 | 50–90% |
| 3 or more | >90% |

Table 5–16. *Who needs maintenance therapy?*

Patients with:
  Two or more prior episodes
  One prior episode (elderly, youth)
  Chronic episodes
  Incomplete remission

Table 5–17. *The bad news in the treatment of depression*

"Pooping out" is common: the percentage of patients who remain well during the 18-month period following successful treatment for depression is disappointingly low, only 70 to 80%.

Many patients are "treatment-refractory": the percentage of patients who are nonresponders and who have a very poor outcome during long-term follow-up evaluation after a diagnosis of depression is disappointingly high, up to 20%.

Up to half of patients may fail to attain remission, including both those with "apathetic" responses and those with "anxious" responses.

of response if they are switched to placebo (Fig. 5–11), but only about 10 to 25% relapse if they are continued on the drug that made them respond (Fig. 5–12).

On the basis of these findings, treatment guidelines have recently evolved so that depression is not just treated until a response is seen but treatment is continued after attaining a response, so that relapses are prevented (Tables 5–15 and 5–16). Those with their first episode of depression may need treatment for only 1 year following response, unless they had a very prolonged or severe episode, were elderly, were psychotic, or had a response but not a remission. Those with more than one episode may require lifelong treatment with an antidepressant, as the risk of relapse skyrockets the more episodes that a patient experiences (Tables 5–15 and 5–16). Antidepressant treatment reduces these relapse rates, especially in the first year after successful treatment (Figs. 5–11 and 5–12).

The bad news in the treatment of depression (Table 5–17) is that a common experience of antidepressant responders is that their treatment response will "poop out." That is, the percentage of patients who fail to maintain their response during the first 18 months following successful treatment for depression is disappointingly

Table 5–18. *Features of partial remission*

Apathetic responders:
  Reduction of depressed mood
  Continuing anhedonia, lack of motivation, decreased libido, lack of interest, no zest
  Cognitive slowing and decreased concentration
Anxious responders:
  Reduction of depressed mood
  Continuing anxiety, especially generalized anxiety
  Worry, insomnia, somatic symptoms

high, up to 20 to 30%. "Pooping out" may be even more likely in patients who only responded and never remitted (i.e., they never became well).

Although clinical trials conducted under ideal conditions for up to 1 year have high compliance and low dropout rates, this may not reflect what happens in actual clinical practice. Thus, the effectiveness of drugs (how well they work in the real world) may not approximate the efficacy of these same drugs (how well they work in clinical trials). For example, the median time of treatment with an antidepressant in clinical practice is currently only about 78 days, not 1 year, and certainly not a lifetime. Can you imagine treating hypertension or diabetes for only 78 days? Depression is a chronic, recurrent illness, which requires long-term treatment to maintain response and prevent relapses, just like hypertension and diabetes. Therefore, antidepressant *effectiveness* in reducing relapses in clinical practice will likely remain lower than antidepressant *efficacy* in clinical trials until long-term compliance can be increased.

Other bad news in the treatment of depression is that many responders never remit (Table 5–17). In fact, some studies suggest that up to half of patients who respond nevertheless fail to attain remission, including those with either "apathetic responses" or "anxious responses" (Table 5–18). The apathetic responder is one who experiences improved mood with treatment, but has continuing lack of pleasure (anhedonia), decreased libido, lack of energy, and no "zest." The anxious responder, on the other hand, is one who had anxiety mixed with depression and who experiences improved mood with treatment but has continuing anxiety, especially generalized anxiety characterized by excessive worry, plus insomnia and somatic symptoms. Both types of responders are better, but neither is well.

Why settle for silver when you can go for gold? Settling for mere response, whether apathetic or anxious, rather than pushing for full remission and wellness may be partly the fault of antidepressant prescribers, who have been taught that the end point for clinical research in journal publications and for approval by governmental regulatory agencies such as the U.S. Food and Drug Administration (FDA) is response, that is, a minimum of 50% improvement in symptoms (Table 5–12). Although response rates may be appropriate for research, remission rates are more relevant for clinical practice (Table 5–13). Responders may represent continuing illness in a milder form, as well as inadequate treatment, since matching the right antidepressant or combination of antidepressants to each patient will greatly increase the chance of delivering a full remission rather than a mere response (Table 5–19). Failure to push for remission means that the patient is left with an increased risk

Table 5−19. *Implications of partial response in patients who do not attain remission*

Represents continuing illness in a milder form
Can be due to inadequate early treatment
Can also be due to underlying dysthymia or personality disorders
Leads to increased relapse rates
Causes continuing functional impairment
Associated with increased suicide rate

Table 5−20. *Dual mechanism hypothesis*

Remission rates are higher with antidepressants or with combinations of antidepressants having dual serotonin and norepinephrine actions, as compared with those having serotonin selective actions.
*Corollary*: Patients unresponsive to a single-action agent may respond, and eventually remit, with dual-action strategies.

of relapse, continuing functional impairment, and a continuing increase in the risk of suicide (Table 5−19). A patient who is in remission, on the other hand, may be considered asymptomatic or well (Table 5−13).

Another bit of bad news is that many patients are treatment-refractory (Table 5−17). That is, the percentage of nonresponders with a very poor outcome is disturbingly high—about 15 to 20% of all patients treated with antidepressants but perhaps a majority of patients selectively referred to a modern psychiatrist's practice.

Fortunately, there is hope for eliminating the bad news stories listed here, namely dual pharmacological mechanisms (Table 5−20). Data are increasingly showing that the percentage of patients who remit is higher for antidepressants or combinations of antidepressants acting synergistically on both serotonin and norepinephrine than for those acting just on serotonin alone. Exploiting this strategy may help increase the number of remitters, prevent or treat more cases of poop out, and convert treatment-refractory cases into successful outcomes. This will be discussed in more detail in Chapter 7.

It is potentially important to treat symptoms of depression "until they are gone" for reasons other than the obvious reduction of current suffering. Depression may be part of an emerging theme for many psychiatric disorders today, namely, that uncontrolled symptoms may indicate some ongoing pathophysiological mechanism in the brain, which if allowed to persist untreated may cause the ultimate outcome of illness to be worse. Depression seems to beget depression. Depression may thus have a long-lasting or even irreversible neuropathological effect on the brain, rendering treatment less effective if symptoms are allowed to progress than if they are removed by appropriate treatment early in the course of the illness.

In summary, the natural history of depression indicates that this is a life-long illness, which is likely to relapse within several months of an index episode, especially if untreated or under-treated or if antidepressants are discontinued, and is prone to multiple recurrences that are possibly preventable by long-term antidepressant treatment. Antidepressant response rates are high, but remission rates are disappointingly low unless mere response is recognized and targeted for aggressive management, possibly by single drugs or combinations of drugs with dual serotonin-norepinephrine pharmacological mechanisms when selective agents are not fully effective.

### Longitudinal Treatment of Bipolar Disorder

The mood stabilizer lithium was developed as the first treatment for bipolar disorder. It has definitely modified the long-term outcome of bipolar disorder because it not only treats acute episodes of mania, but it is the first psychotropic drug proven to have a prophylactic effect in preventing future episodes of illness. Lithium even treats depression in bipolar patients, although it is not so clear that it is a powerful antidepressant for unipolar depression. Nevertheless, it is used to augment antidepressants for treating resistant cases of unipolar depression.

Other mood stabilizers are arising from the group of drugs that were first developed as anticonvulsants and have also found an important place in the treatment of bipolar disorder. Several anticonvulsants are especially useful for the manic, mixed, and rapid cycling types of bipolar patients and perhaps for the depressive phase of this illness as well. Mood stabilizers will be discussed in detail in Chapter 7. Antipsychotics, especially the newer atypical antipsychotics, are also useful in the treatment of bipolar disorders.

Antidepressants modify the long-term course of bipolar disorder as well. When given with lithium or other mood stabilizers, they may reduce depressive episodes. Interestingly, however, antidepressants can flip a depressed bipolar patient into mania, into mixed mania with depression, or into chaotic rapid cycling every few days or hours, especially in the absence of mood stabilizers. Thus, many patients with bipolar disorders require clever mixing of mood stabilizers and antidepressants, or even avoidance of antidepressants, in order to attain the best outcome.

Without consistent long-term treatment, bipolar disorders are potentially very disruptive. Patients often experience a chronic and chaotic course, in and out of the hospital, with psychotic episodes and relapses. There is a significant concern that intermittent use of mood stabilizers, poor compliance, and increasing numbers of episodes will lead to even more episodes of bipolar disorder, and with less responsiveness to lithium. Thus, stabilizing bipolar disorders with mood stabilizers, atypical antipsychotics, and antidepressants is increasingly important not only in returning these patients to wellness but in preventing unfavorable long-term outcomes.

### Mood Disorders Across the Life Cycle: When Do Antidepressants Start Working?

*Children.* Despite classical psychoanalytic notions suggesting that children do not become depressed, recent evidence is quite to the contrary. Unfortunately, very little controlled research has been done on the use of antidepressants to treat depression in children, so no antidepressant is currently approved for treatment of depression in children. However, many of the newer antidepressants have been extensively tested in children with other conditions. For example, some antidepressants are approved for the treatment of children with obsessive-compulsive disorder. Thus, the safety of some antidepressants is well established in children even if their efficacy for depression is not. Nevertheless, antidepressant treatment studies in children are in progress, and extensive anecdotal observations suggest that antidepressants, particularly the newer, safer ones (see Chapters 6 and 7), are in fact useful for treating depressed children. Changes in FDA regulations have extended patent lives for new drugs in the United States if such drugs are also approved to treat children. Thankfully, this is now providing incentives for doing the research necessary to prove the safety and efficacy of antidepressants to treat depression in children, a long neglected area of psychopharmacology.

Perhaps even more important in children is the issue of bipolar disorder. Mania and mixed mania have not only been greatly underdiagnosed in children in the past but also have been frequently misdiagnosed as attention deficit disorder and hyperactivity. Furthermore, bipolar disorder misdiagnosed as attention deficit disorder and treated with stimulants can produce the same chaos and rapid cycling state as antidepressants can in bipolar disorder. Thus, it is important to consider the diagnosis of bipolar disorder in children, especially those unresponsive or apparently worsened by stimulants and those who have a family member with bipolar disorder. These children may need their stimulants and antidepressants discontinued and treatment with mood stabilizers such as valproic acid or lithium initiated.

*Adolescents.* Documentation of the safety and efficacy of antidepressants and mood stabilizers is better for adolescents than for children, although not at the standard for adults. That is unfortunate, because mood disorders often have their onset in adolescence, especially in girls. Not only do mood disorders frequently begin after puberty, but children with onset of a mood disorder prior to puberty often experience an exacerbation in adolescence. Synaptic restructuring dramatically increases after age 6 and throughout adolescence. Onset of puberty also occurs at this time of the life cycle. Such events may explain the dramatic rise in the incidence of the onset of mood disorders, as well as the exacerbation of preexisting mood disorders, during adolescence.

Unfortunately, mood disorders are frequently not diagnosed in adolescents, especially if they are associated with delinquent antisocial behavior or drug abuse. This is indeed unfortunate, as the opportunity to stabilize the disorder early in its course and possibly even to prevent adverse long-term outcomes associated with lack of adequate treatment can be lost if mood disorders are not aggressively diagnosed and treated in adolescence. The modern psychopharmacologist should have a high index of suspicion and increased vigilance to the presence of a mood disorder in adolescents, because treatments may well be just as effective in adolescents as they are in adults and perhaps more critical to preserve normal development of the individual.

## Biological Basis of Depression

### Monoamine Hypothesis

The first major theory about the biological etiology of depression hypothesized that depression was due to a deficiency of monoamine neurotransmitters, notably norepinephrine (NE) and serotonin (5-hydroxytryptamine [5HT]) (Figs. 5–13 through

## MONOAMINE HYPOTHESIS

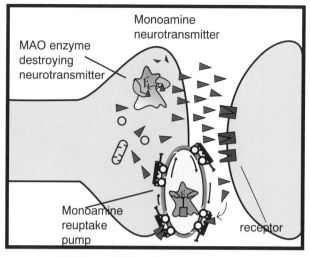

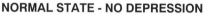

**NORMAL STATE - NO DEPRESSION**

FIGURE 5–13. This figure represents the **normal state** of a monoaminergic neuron. This particular neuron is releasing the neurotransmitter **norepinephrine (NE)** at the normal rate. All the regulatory elements of the neuron are also normal, including the functioning of the enzyme **monoamine oxidase (MAO)**, **which destroys NE**, the **NE reuptake pump** which terminates the action of NE, and the **NE receptors** which react to the release of NE.

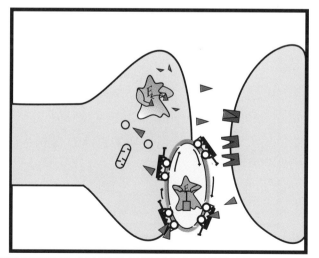

**DEPRESSION: CAUSED BY NEUROTRANSMITTER DEFICIENCY**

FIGURE 5–14. According to the monoamine hypothesis, in the case of **depression** the neurotransmitter is depleted, causing **neurotransmitter deficiency**.

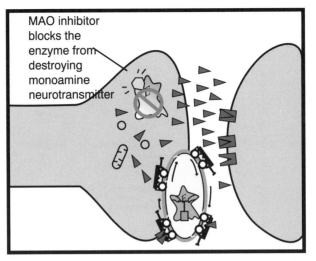

**INCREASE IN NEUROTRANSMITTERS CAUSES RETURN TO NORMAL STATE**

FIGURE 5–15. **Monoamine oxidase inhibitors** act as antidepressants, since they block the enzyme MAO from destroying monoamine neurotransmitters, thus allowing them to accumulate. This accumulation theoretically reverses the prior neurotransmitter deficiency (see Fig. 5–14) and according to the monoamine hypothesis, relieves depression by returning the monoamine neuron to the normal state.

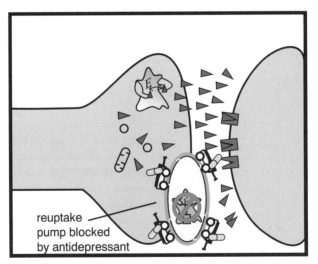

**INCREASE IN NEUROTRANSMITTERS CAUSES RETURN TO NORMAL STATE**

FIGURE 5–16. **Tricyclic antidepressants** exert their antidepressant action by blocking the neurotransmitter reuptake pump, thus causing neurotransmitter to accumulate. This accumulation, according to the monoamine hypothesis, reverses the prior neurotransmitter deficiency (see Fig. 5–14) and relieves depression by returning the monoamine neuron to the normal state.

5–16). Evidence for this was rather simplistic. Certain drugs that depleted these neurotransmitters could induce depression, and the known antidepressants at that time (the tricyclic antidepressants and the MAO inhibitors) both had pharmacological actions that boosted these neurotransmitters. Thus, the idea was that the "normal" amount of monoamine neurotransmitters (Fig. 5–13) became somehow depleted, perhaps by an unknown disease process, by stress, or by drugs (Fig. 5–14), leading to the symptoms of depression. The MAO inhibitors increased the monoamine neurotransmitters, causing relief of depression due to inhibition of MAO (Fig. 5–15). The tricyclic antidepressants also increased the monoamine neurotransmitters, resulting in relief from depression due to blockade of the monoamine transport pumps (Fig. 5–16). Although the monoamine hypothesis is obviously an overly simplified notion about depression, it has been very valuable in focusing attention on the three monoamine neurotransmitter systems norepinephrine, dopamine, and serotonin. This has led to a much better understanding of the physiological functioning of these three neurotransmitters and especially of the various mechanisms by which all known antidepressants act to boost neurotransmission at one or more of these three monoamine neurotransmitter systems.

## Monoaminergic Neurons

In order to understand the monoamine hypothesis, it is necessary first to understand the normal physiological functioning of monoaminergic neurons. The principal monoamine neurotransmitters in the brain are the catecholamines norepinephrine (NE, also called noradrenaline) and dopamine (DA) and the indoleamine serotonin (5HT).

*Noradrenergic neurons.* The noradrenergic neuron uses NE for its neurotransmitter. Monoamine neurotransmitters are synthesized by means of enzymes, which assemble neurotransmitters in the cell body or nerve terminal. For the noradrenergic neuron, this process starts with tyrosine, the amino acid precursor of NE, which is transported into the nervous system from the blood by means of an active transport pump (Fig. 5–17). Once inside the neuron, the tyrosine is acted on by three enzymes in sequence, the first of which is tyrosine hydroxylase (TOH), the rate-limiting and most important enzyme in the regulation of NE synthesis. Tyrosine hydroxylase converts the amino acid tyrosine into dihydroxyphenylalanine (DOPA). The second enzyme DOPA decarboxylase (DDC), then acts, converting DOPA into dopamine (DA), which itself is a neurotransmitter in some neurons. However, for NE neurons, DA is just a precursor of NE. In fact, the third and final NE synthetic enzyme, dopamine beta-hydroxylase (DBH), converts DA into NE. The NE is then stored in synaptic packages called *vesicles* until released by a nerve impulse (Fig. 5–17).

Not only is NE created by enzymes, but it can also be destroyed by enzymes (Fig. 5–18). Two principal destructive enzymes act on NE to turn it into inactive metabolites. The first is MAO, which is located in mitochondria in the presynaptic neuron and elsewhere. The second is catechol-O-methyl transferase (COMT), which is thought to be located largely outside of the presynaptic nerve terminal (Fig. 5–18).

The action of NE can be terminated not only by enzymes that destroy NE, but also cleverly by a transport pump for NE, which removes it from acting in the synapse without destroying it (Fig. 5–18). In fact, such inactivated NE can be re-

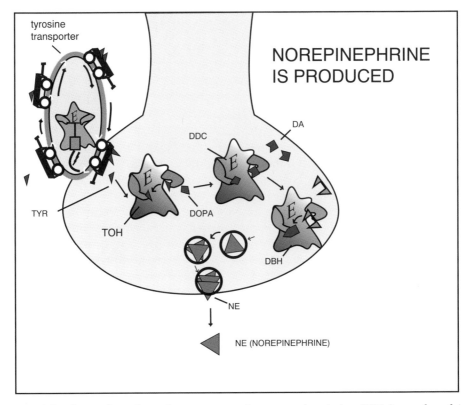

FIGURE 5–17. This figure shows how the neurotransmitter **norepinephrine (NE) is produced** in noradrenergic neurons. This process starts with the amino acid precursor of NE, **tyrosine (tyr)**, being transported into the nervous system from the blood by means of an active transport pump (tyrosine transporter). This active transport pump for tyrosine is separate and distinct from the active transport pump for NE itself (see Fig. 5–18). Once pumped inside the neuron, the tyrosine is acted on by three enzymes in sequence, the first of which, tyrosine hydroxylase (**TOH**), is the rate-limiting and most important enzyme in the regulation of NE synthesis. Tyrosine hydroxylase converts the amino acid tyrosine into **DOPA**. The second enzyme, namely DOPA decarboxylase (**DDC**), then acts by converting DOPA into dopamine (**DA**). The third and final NE synthetic enzyme, dopamine beta hydroxylase (**DBH**), converts DA into NE. The NE is then stored in synaptic packages called vesicles until released by a nerve impulse.

stored for reuse in a later neurotransmitting nerve impulse. The transport pump that terminates the synaptic action of NE is sometimes called the NE "transporter" and sometimes the NE "reuptake pump." This NE reuptake pump is located as part of the presynaptic machinery, where it acts as a vacuum cleaner, whisking NE out of the synapse and off the synaptic receptors and stopping its synaptic actions. Once inside the presynaptic nerve terminal, NE can either be stored again for subsequent reuse when another nerve impulse arrives, or it can be destroyed by NE-destroying enzymes (Fig. 5–18).

The noradrenergic neuron is regulated by a multiplicity of receptors for NE (Fig. 5–19). In the classical subtyping of NE receptors, they were classified as either alpha or beta, depending on their preference for a series of agonists and antagonists. Next, the NE receptors were subclassified into alpha 1 and alpha 2 as well as beta 1 and

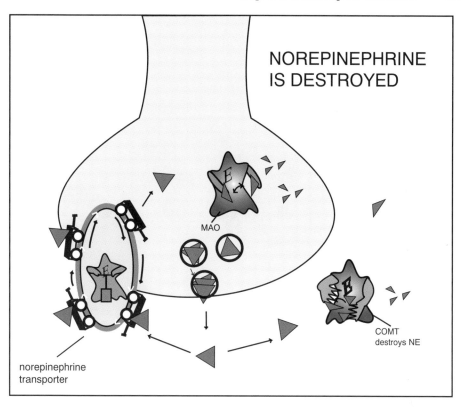

NOREPINEPHRINE
IS DESTROYED

MAO

COMT
destroys NE

norepinephrine
transporter

FIGURE 5–18. **Norepinephrine** (NE) can also be **destroyed** by enzymes in the NE neuron. The principal destructive enzymes are monoamine oxidase (**MAO**) and catechol-O-methyl transferase (**COMT**). The action of NE can be terminated not only by enzymes that destroy NE, but also by a transport pump for NE, called the **norepinephrine transporter**, which prevents NE from acting in the synapse without destroying it. This transport pump is separate and distinct from the transport pump for tyrosine used in carrying tyrosine into the NE neuron for NE synthesis (see Fig. 5–17). The transport pump that terminates the synaptic action of NE is sometimes called the "NE transporter" and sometimes the "NE reuptake pump." There are molecular differences among the transporters for the NE, dopamine, and serotonin neurons. These differences can be exploited by drugs so that the transport of one monoamine can be blocked independently of another. The NE transporter is part of the presynaptic machinery, where it acts as a "vacuum cleaner," whisking NE out of the synapse, and off the synaptic receptors and stopping its synaptic actions. Once inside the presynaptic nerve terminal, NE can either be stored again for subsequent reuse when another nerve impulse arrives, or it can be destroyed by enzymes.

beta 2. More recently, adrenergic receptors have been even further subclassified on the basis of both pharmacologic and molecular differences.

For a general understanding of NE receptors, the reader should begin with an awareness of three key receptors that are postsynaptic, namely beta 1, alpha 1, and alpha 2 receptors (Fig. 5–19). The postsynaptic receptors for NE convert occupancy of an alpha 1, alpha 2, or beta 1 receptor into a physiological function and ultimately result in changes in gene expression in the postsynaptic neuron.

On the other hand, alpha 2 receptors are the only presynaptic noradrenergic receptors on noradrenergic neurons. They regulate NE release and so are called *auto-receptors*. Presynaptic alpha 2 autoreceptors are located both on the axon terminal,

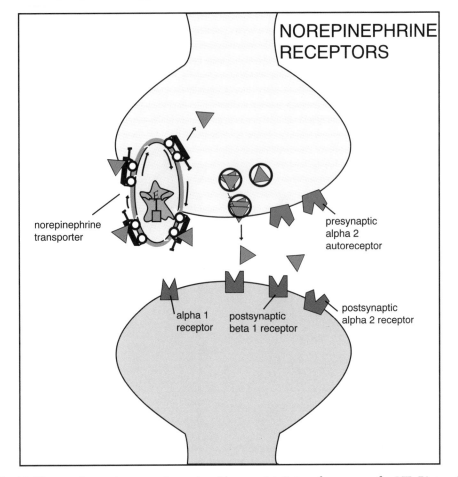

NOREPINEPHRINE
RECEPTORS

norepinephrine
transporter

presynaptic
alpha 2
autoreceptor

alpha 1
receptor

postsynaptic
beta 1 receptor

postsynaptic
alpha 2 receptor

FIGURE 5–19. The noradrenergic neuron is regulated by a multiplicity of **receptors for NE**. Pictured here are the **NE transporter** and several NE receptors, including the presynaptic alpha 2 autoreceptor as well as the postsynaptic alpha 1, alpha 2 and beta 1 adrenergic receptors. The **presynaptic alpha 2 receptor** is important because it is an autoreceptor. That is, when the presynaptic alpha 2 receptor recognizes synaptic NE, it turns off further release of NE. Thus, the presynaptic alpha 2 terminal autoreceptor acts as a brake for the NE neuron. Stimulating this receptor (i.e., stepping on the brake) stops the neuron from firing. This probably occurs physiologically to prevent too much firing of the NE neuron, since it can shut itself off once the firing rate gets too high and the autoreceptor becomes stimulated. Postsynaptic NE receptors generally act by recognizing when NE is released from the presynaptic neuron and react by setting up a molecular cascade in the postsynaptic neuron, thereby causing neurotransmission to pass from the presynaptic to the postsynaptic neuron.

(terminal alpha 2 receptors) (Fig. 5–19) and at the cell body (soma) and nearby dendrites (somatodendritic alpha 2 receptors) (Fig. 5–20). Presynaptic alpha 2 receptors are important because both the terminal and the somatodendritic receptors are autoreceptors. That is, when presynaptic alpha 2 receptors recognize NE, they turn off further release of NE (Figs. 5–21 and 5–22). Thus, presynaptic alpha 2 autoreceptors act as a brake for the NE neuron and also cause what is known as a negative feedback regulatory signal. Stimulating this receptor (i.e., stepping on the brake) stops the neuron from firing. This probably occurs physiologically to prevent

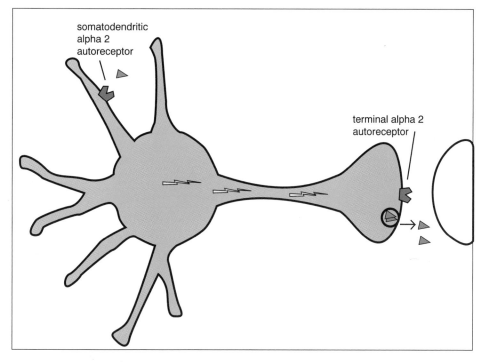

somatodendritic
alpha 2
autoreceptor

terminal alpha 2
autoreceptor

FIGURE 5–20. Both types of presynaptic alpha 2 autoreceptors are shown here. They are located either on the axon terminal, where they are called **terminal alpha 2 receptors**, or at the cell body (soma) and nearby dendrites, where they are called **somatodendritic alpha 2 receptors**.

overfiring of the NE neuron, since it can shut itself off once the firing rate gets too high and the autoreceptor becomes stimulated. It is worthy of note that not only can drugs mimic the natural functioning of the NE neuron by stimulating the presynaptic alpha 2 neuron, but drugs that antagonize this same receptor will have the effect of cutting the brake cable and enhancing the release of NE

Most of the cell bodies for noradrenergic neurons in the brain are located in the brainstem in an area known as the *locus coeruleus* (Fig. 5–23). The principal function of the locus coeruleus is to determine whether attention is being focused on the external environment or on monitoring the internal milieu of the body. It helps to prioritize competing incoming stimuli and fixes attention on just a few of these. Thus, one can either react to a threat from the environment or to signals such as pain coming from the body. Where one is paying attention will determine what one learns and what memories are formed as well.

Norepinephrine and the locus coeruleus are also thought to have an important input into the central nervous system's control of cognition, mood, emotions, movements, and blood pressure. Malfunction of the locus coeruleus is hypothesized to underlie disorders in which mood and cognition intersect, such as depression, anxiety, and disorders of attention and information processing. A norepinephrine deficiency syndrome (Table 5–21) is theoretically characterized by impaired attention, problems in concentrating, and difficulties specifically with working memory and the speed of information processing, as well as psychomotor retardation, fatigue, and

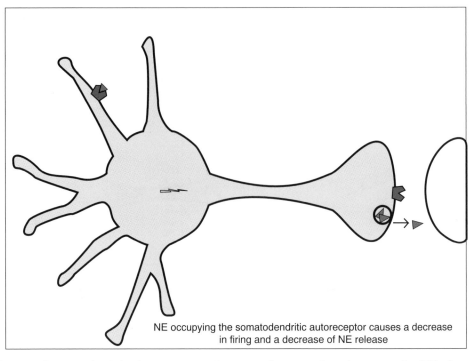

NE occupying the somatodendritic autoreceptor causes a decrease
in firing and a decrease of NE release

FIGURE 5–21. Presynaptic alpha 2 receptors are important because when they recognize NE, they turn off further release of NE. Shown here is the function of **presynaptic somatodendritic autore-ceptors**, namely to act as a brake for the NE neuron and also to cause what is known as a negative feedback regulatory signal. Stimulating this receptor (i.e., "**stepping on the brake**") stops the neuron from firing. This probably occurs physiologically to prevent excessive firing of the NE neuron, since NE can shut itself off once the firing rate gets too high and the autoreceptor becomes stimulated.

apathy. Such symptoms can commonly accompany depression as well as other disorders with impaired attention and cognition, such as attention deficit disorder, schizophrenia, and Alzheimer's disease.

There are many specific noradrenergic pathways in the brain, each mediating a different physiological function. For example, one projection from the locus coeruleus to frontal cortex is thought to be responsible for the regulatory actions of NE on mood (Fig. 5–24); another projection to prefrontal cortex mediates the effects of NE on attention (Fig. 5–25). Different receptors may mediate these differential effects of norepinephrine in frontal cortex, postsynaptic beta 1 receptors for mood (Fig. 5–24) and postsynaptic alpha 2 for attention and cognition (Fig. 5–25).

The projection from the locus coeruleus to limbic cortex may regulate emotions, as well as energy, fatigue, and psychomotor agitation or psychomotor retardation (Fig. 5–26). A projection to the cerebellum may regulate motor movements, especially tremor (Fig. 5–27). Brainstem norepinephrine in cardiovascular centers controls blood pressure (Fig. 5–28). Norepinephrine from sympathetic neurons leaving the spinal cord to innervate peripheral tissues control heart rate (Fig. 5–29) and bladder emptying (Fig. 5–30).

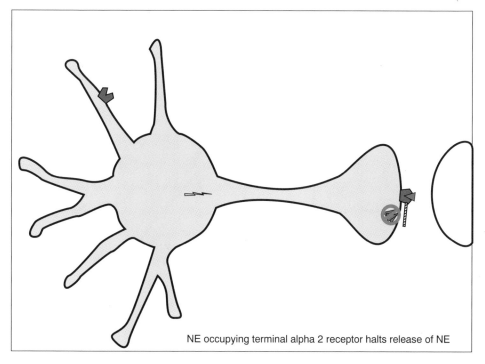

NE occupying terminal alpha 2 receptor halts release of NE

FIGURE 5–22. Shown here is the action of the **presynaptic axon terminal alpha 2 receptors,** which have the same function as the somatodendritic autoreceptors shown in Figure 5–21.

*Dopaminergic neurons.* Dopaminergic neurons utilize the neutotransmitter DA, which is synthesized in dopaminergic nerve terminals by two out of three of the same enzymes that also synthesize NE (Fig. 5–31). However, DA neurons lack the third enzyme, namely, dopamine beta hydroxylase, and thus cannot convert DA to NE. Therefore, it is DA that is stored and used for neurotransmitting purposes.

The DA neuron has a presynaptic transporter (reputake pump), which is unique for DA neurons (Fig. 5–32) but works analogously to the NE transporter (Fig. 5–33). On the other hand, the same enzymes that destroy NE (Fig. 5–18) also destroy DA (MAO and COMT) (Fig. 5–31).

Receptors for dopamine also regulate dopaminergic neurotransmission (Fig. 5–33). A plethora of dopamine receptors exist, including at least five pharmacological subtypes and several more molecular isoforms. Perhaps the most extensively investigated dopamine receptor is the dopamine 2 receptor, as it is stimulated by dopaminergic agonists for the treatment of Parkinson's disease and blocked by dopamine antagonist antipsychotics for the treatment of schizophrenia. Dopamine 1, 2, 3, and 4 receptors are all blocked by some atypical antipsychotic drugs, but it is not clear to what extent dopamine 1, 3, or 4 receptors contribute to the clinical properties of these drugs. Dopamine receptors can be presynaptic, where they function as autoreceptors. They provide negative feedback input, or a braking action on the release of dopamine from the presynaptic neuron. (Fig. 5–33).

*Serotonergic neurons.* Analogous enzymes, transport pumps, and receptors exist in the 5HT neuron (Figs. 5–34 through 5–42). For synthesis of serotonin in serotonergic

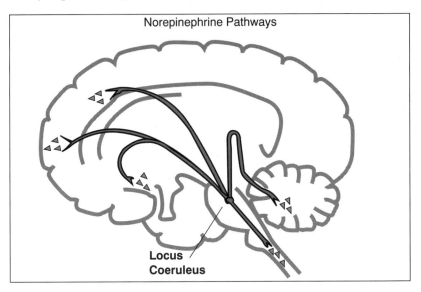

FIGURE 5–23. Most of the cell bodies for noradrenergic neurons in the brain are located in the brainstem in an area known as the **locus coeruleus**. This is the headquarters for most of the important noradrenergic pathways mediating behavior and other functions such as cognition, mood, emotions, and movements. Malfunction of the locus coeruleus is hypothesized to underlie disorders in which mood and cognition intersect, such as depression, anxiety, and disorders of attention and information processing.

Table 5–21. *Norepinephrine deficiency syndrome*

Impaired attention
Problems concentrating
Deficiencies in working memory
Slowness of information processing
Depressed mood
Psychomotor retardation
Fatigue

neurons, however, a different amino acid, tryptophan, is transported into the brain from the plasma to serve as the 5HT precursor (Fig. 5–34). Two synthetic enzymes then convert tryptophan into serotonin: first tryptophan hydroxylase converts tryptophan into 5-hydroxytryptophan, which is then converted by aromatic amino acid decarboxylase into 5HT (Fig. 5–34). Like NE and DA, 5HT is destroyed by MAO and converted into an inactive metabolite (Fig. 5–35). Also, the 5HT neuron has a presynaptic transport pump for serotonin called the serotonin transporter (Fig. 5–35), which is analogous to the NE transporter in NE neurons (Fig. 5–18) and to the DA transporter in DA neurons (Fig. 5–32).

Receptor subtyping for the serotonergic neuron has proceeded at a very rapid pace, with several major categories of 5HT receptors, each further subtyped

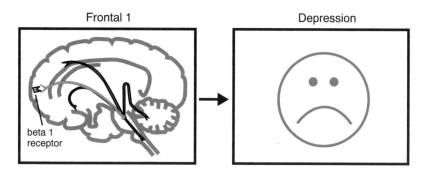

FIGURE 5–24. Some noradrenergic projections from the locus coeruleus to **frontal cortex** are thought to be responsible for the regulatory actions of norepinephrine on **mood. Beta 1** postsynaptic receptors may be important in transducing noradrenergic signals regulating mood in postsynaptic targets.

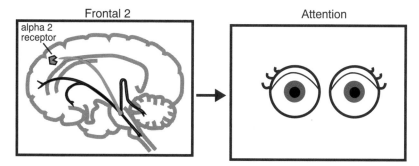

FIGURE 5–25. Other noradrenergic projections from the locus coeruleus to **frontal cortex** are thought to mediate the effects of norepinephrine on **attention**, concentration, and other **cognitive functions**, such as working memory and the speed of information processing. **Alpha 2** postsynaptic receptors may be important in transducing postsynaptic signals regulating attention in postsynaptic target neurons.

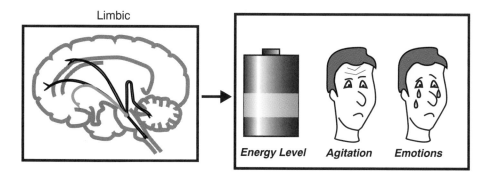

FIGURE 5–26. The noradrenergic projection from the locus coeruleus to **limbic cortex** may mediate emotions, as well as **energy**, fatigue, and psychomotor agitation or psychomotor retardation.

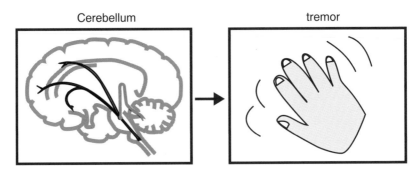

FIGURE 5–27. The noradrenergic projection from the locus coeruleus to the **cerebellum** may mediate motor movements, especially **tremor**.

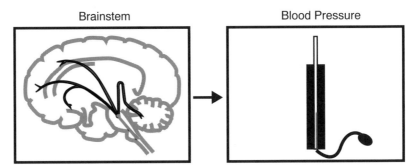

FIGURE 5–28. Brainstem norepinephrine in cardiovascular centers controls **blood pressure**.

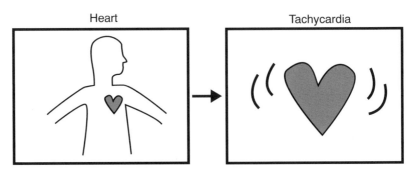

FIGURE 5–29. Noradrenergic innervation of the **heart** via sympathic neurons leaving the spinal cord regulates cardiovascular function, including **heart rate**, via beta 1 receptors.

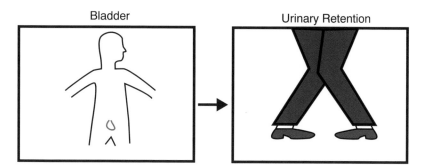

FIGURE 5–30. Noradrenergic innervation of the urinary tract via sympathetic neurons leaving the spinal cord regulates **bladder** emptying via alpha 1 receptors.

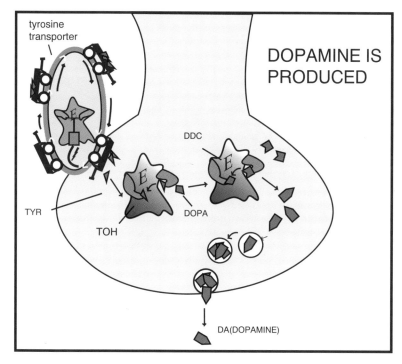

FIGURE 5–31. **Dopamine (DA)** is produced in dopaminergic neurons from the precursor **tyrosine (tyr)**, which is transported into the neuron by an active transport pump, called the tyrosine transporter, and then converted into DA by two of the same three enzymes that also synthesize norepinephrine (Fig. 5–17). The DA-synthesizing enzymes are tyrosine hydroxylase (**TOH**), which produces **DOPA**, and DOPA decarboxylase (**DDC**), which produces DA.

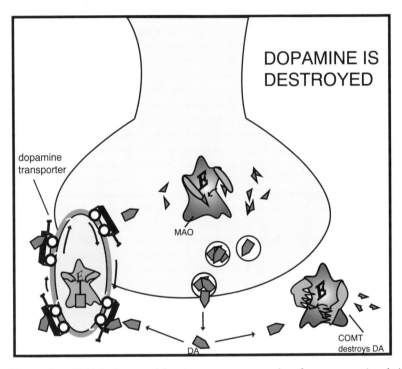

FIGURE 5–32. **Dopamine (DA)** is destroyed by the same enzymes that destroy norepinephrine (see Fig. 5–18), namely monoamine oxidase (**MAO**) and catechol-O-methyl-transferase (**COMT**). The DA neuron has a presynaptic transporter (**reuptake pump**), which is unique to the DA neuron but works analogously to the NE transporter (Fig. 5–18).

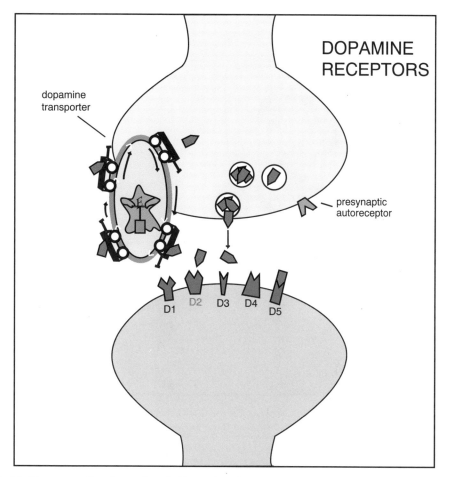

FIGURE 5–33. **Receptors for dopamine** (DA) regulate dopaminergic neurotransmission. A plethora of dopamine receptors exist, including at least five pharmacological subtypes and several more molecular isoforms. Perhaps the most extensively investigated dopamine receptor is the dopamine 2 (D2) receptor, as it is stimulated by dopaminergic agonists for the treatment of Parkinson's disease and blocked by dopamine antagonist neuroleptics and atypical antipsychotics for the treatment of schizophrenia.

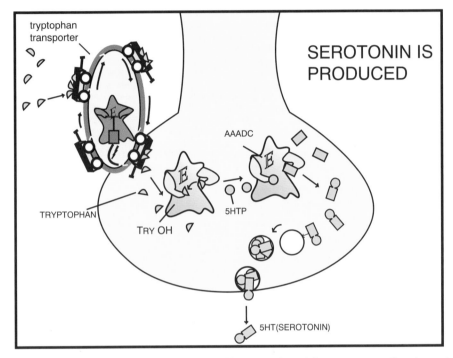

FIGURE 5–34. **Serotonin** (5-hydroxytryptamine [5HT]) is **produced** from enzymes after the amino acid precursor tryptophan is transported into the serotonin neuron. The **tryptophan transport pump** is distinct from the serotonin transporter (see Fig. 5–35). Once transported into the serotonin neuron, tryptophan is converted into 5-hydroxytryptophan (**5HTP**) by the enzyme tryptophan hydroxylase (**TryOH**) which is then converted into 5HT by the enzyme aromatic amino acid decarboxylase (**AAADC**). Serotonin is then stored in synaptic vesicles, where it stays until released by a neuronal impulse.

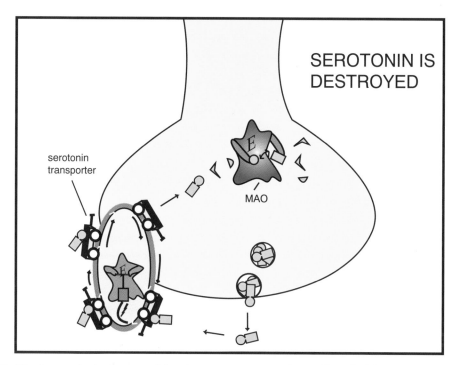

FIGURE 5–35. **Serotonin is destroyed** by the enzyme monoamine oxidase (**MAO**) and converted into an inactive metabolite. The 5HT neuron has a presynaptic transport pump selective for serotonin, which is called the **serotonin transporter** and is analogous to the norepinephrine (NE) transporter in NE neurons (Fig. 5–18) and to the DA transporter in DA neurons (Fig. 5–32).

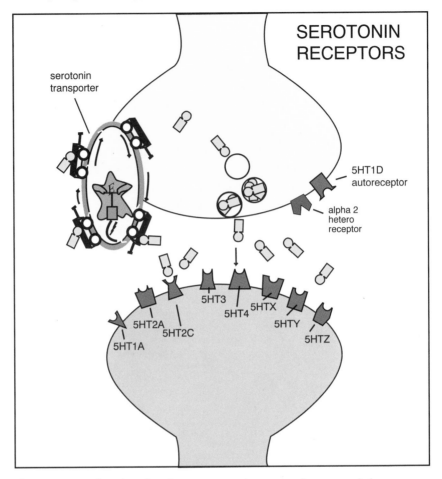

FIGURE 5–36. **Receptor subtyping for the serotonergic neuron** has proceeded at a very rapid pace, with at least four major categories of 5HT receptors, each further subtyped depending on pharmacological or molecular properties. In addition to the serotonin transporter, there is a key pre-synaptic serotonin receptor (the 5HT1D receptor) and another key presynaptic receptor, the alpha 2 noradrenergic heteroreceptor. This organization allows serotonin release to be controlled not only by serotonin but also by norepinephrine, even though the serotonin neuron does not itself release nor-epinephrine. Several postsynaptic serotonin receptors (5HT1A, 5HT1D, 5HT2A, 5HT2C, 5HT3, 5HT4, and many others denoted by 5HT X, Y, and Z) are shown as well. They convey messages from the presynaptic serotonergic neuron to the target cell postsynaptically.

depending on pharmacologic or molecular properties (Fig. 5–36). The 5HT receptors are a good example of how the description of neurotransmitter receptors is in constant flux and is constantly being revised. For a general understanding of the 5HT neuron, the reader can begin with an understanding that there are two key receptors that are presynaptic (5HT1A and 5HT1D) (Figs. 5–36 through 5–42) and several that are postsynaptic (5HT1A, 5HT1D, 5HT2A, 5HT2C, 5HT3, and 5HT4) (Fig. 5–36).

Presynaptic 5HT receptors are autoreceptors and detect the presence of 5HT, causing a shutdown of further 5HT release and 5HT neuronal impulse flow. When

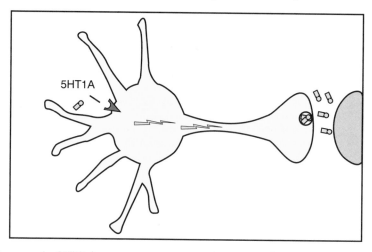

FIGURE 5–37. Presynaptic **5HT1A receptors** are autoreceptors, are located on the cell body and dendrites, and are therefore called somatodendritic autoreceptors.

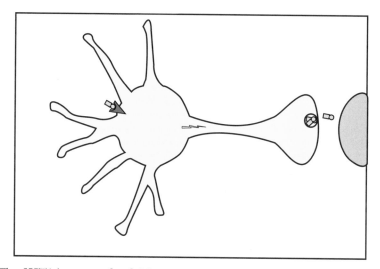

FIGURE 5–38. The **5HT1A somatodendritic autoreceptors** depicted in Figure 5–37 act by detecting the presence of 5HT and causing a **shutdown of 5HT neuronal impulse flow**, depicted here as decreased electrical activity and a reduction in the color of the neuron.

5HT is detected at the dendrites and cell body, this occurs via a 5HT1A receptor, which is also called a *somatodendritic* autoreceptor (Figs. 5–37 and 5–38). This causes a slowing of neuronal impulse flow through the serotonin neuron (Fig. 5–38). When 5HT is detected in the synapse by presynaptic 5HT receptors on axon terminals, this occurs via a 5HT1D receptor, also called a *terminal autoreceptor* (Fig. 5–39). In the case of the 5HT1D terminal autoreceptor, 5HT occupancy of this receptor inhibits 5HT release (Figs. 5–39 through 5–42). On the other hand, drugs that block the 5HT1D autoreceptor can promote 5HT release (Fig. 5–42).

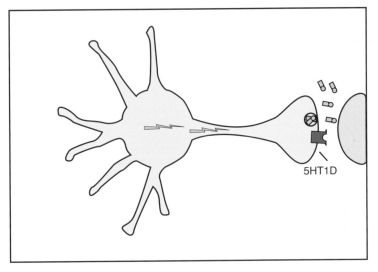

FIGURE 5–39. Presynaptic **5HT1D receptors** are also a type of autoreceptor, but they are located on the presynaptic axon terminal and are therefore called terminal autoreceptors.

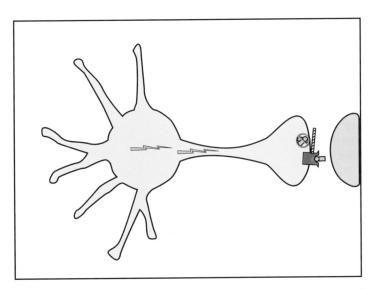

FIGURE 5–40. Depicted here is the consequence of the 5HT1D terminal autoreceptor being stimulated by serotonin. The terminal autoreceptor of Figure 5–39 is occupied here by 5HT, causing the **blockade of 5HT release**, as also shown in Fig. 5–41.

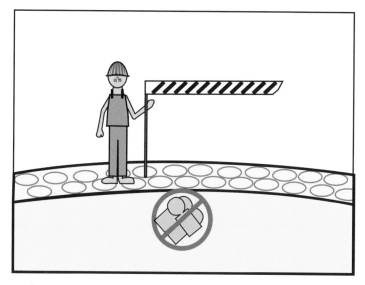

FIGURE 5–41. Depicted here is an enlargement of the 5HT1D terminal autoreceptor being stimulated by serotonin. The terminal autoreceptor of Figure 5–40 is occupied here by 5HT, causing the **blockade of 5HT release**.

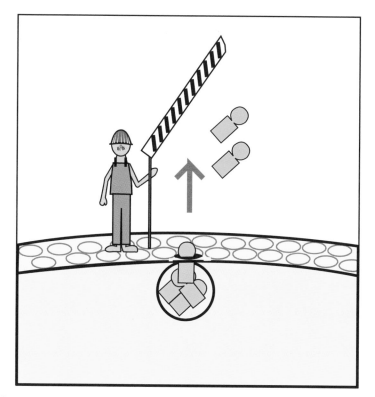

FIGURE 5–42. If a drug blocks a presynaptic **5HT1D terminal autoreceptor**, it would promote the release of 5HT by not allowing 5HT to block its own release. Some 5HT1D antagonists are being tested for the treatment of depression.

175

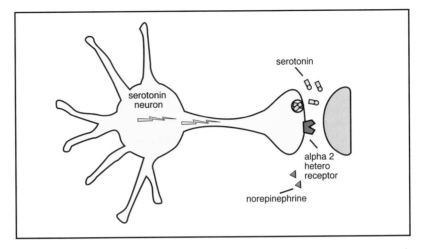

FIGURE 5-43. Shown here are the **alpha 2 presynaptic heteroreceptors** on serotonin axon terminals.

The serotonin neuron not only has serotonin receptors located presynaptically, but also has presynaptic noradrenergic receptors that regulate serotonin release (Figs. 5–36 and 5–43 through 5–46). On the axon terminal of serotonergic receptors are located presynaptic alpha 2 receptors (Figs. 5–35, 5–42, and 5–43), just as they are on noradrenergic neurons (Figs. 5–19 through 5–22). When norepinephrine is released from nearby noradrenergic neurons, it can diffuse to alpha 2 receptors, not only to those on noradrenergic neurons but also to the same receptors on serotonin neurons. Like its actions on noradrenergic neurons, norepinephrine occupancy of alpha 2 receptors on serotonin neurons will turn off serotonin release. Thus, serotonin release can be inhibited by serotonin and by norepinephrine. Alpha 2 receptors on a norepinephrine neuron are called *autoreceptors*, but alpha 2 receptors on serotonin neurons are called *heteroreceptors*.

Another type of presynaptic norepinephrine receptor on serotonin neurons is the alpha 1 receptor, located on the cell bodies (Figs. 5–45 and 5–46). When norepinephrine interacts with this receptor, it *enhances* serotonin release. Thus, norepinephrine can act as both an accelerator and a brake for serotonin release (Table 5–22 and Figs. 5–47 and 5–48).

The anatomic sites of noradrenergic control of serotonin release are shown in Figure 5–47, and include the "brake" at the axon terminals in the cortex and the "accelerator" at the cell bodies in the brainstem. This is shown schematically in Figure 5–48.

Postsynaptic 5HT receptors such as 5HT2A receptors (Fig. 5–49) regulate the translation of 5HT release from the presynaptic nerve into a neurotransmission in the postsynaptic nerve (Fig. 5–50). The 5HT2A, 5HT2C, and 5HT3 receptors are especially important postsynaptic 5HT receptor subtypes because they are implicated in the several physiological actions of serotonin in various serotonin pathways in the central nervous system. More is being learned about the importance of postsynaptic 5HT1A receptors in the brain and 5HT4 receptors in the gastrointestinal tract.

The headquarters for the cell bodies of serotonergic neurons is in the brainstem area called the *raphe nucleus* (Fig. 5–51). Projections from the raphe to the frontal

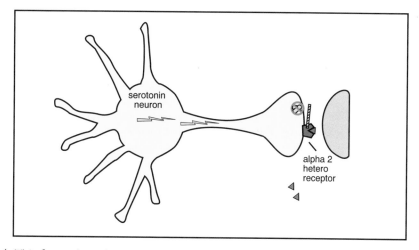

FIGURE 5–44. This figure shows how norepinephrine can function as a **brake for serotonin release**. When norepinephrine is released from nearby noradrenergic neurons, it can diffuse to alpha 2 receptors, not only to those on noradrenergic neurons but as shown here, also to these same receptors on serotonin neurons. Like its actions on noradrenergic neurons, norepinephrine occupancy of alpha 2 receptors on serotonin neurons will turn off serotonin release. Thus, serotonin release can be inhibited not only by serotonin but, as shown here, also by norepinephrine. Alpha 2 receptors on a norepinephrine neuron are called autoreceptors, but alpha 2 receptors on serotonin neurons are called **heteroreceptors**.

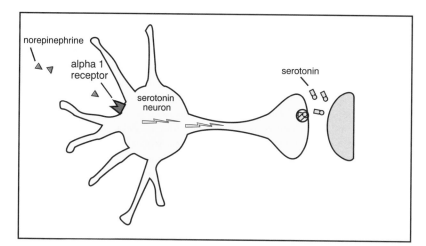

FIGURE 5–45. Another type of presynaptic norepinephrine receptor on serotonin neurons is the **alpha 1 receptor**, located on the cell bodies and dentrites.

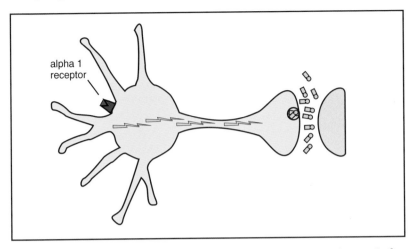

FIGURE 5–46. Shown here is how norepinephrine can act as a facilitator or "**accelerator**" of serotonin release. When norepinephrine interacts with the somatodendritic alpha 1 receptor on serotonin neurons, it enhances serotonin release.

Table 5–22. *Types of noradrenergic interactions with serotonin*

Inhibitory
    Axoaxonic interactions (noradrenergic axons with serotonergic axon terminals)
    Inhibitory alpha 2 heteroreceptors (negative feedback)
    "Brakes"
Excitatory
    Axodendritic interactions (noradrenergic axons with serotonergic cell bodies and
        dendrites)
    Excitatory alpha 1 receptors (positive feedback)
    "Accelerators"

cortex may be important for regulating mood (Fig. 5–52). Projections to basal ganglia, especially on 5HT2A receptors, may help control movements and obsessions and compulsions (Fig. 5–53). Projections from the raphe to the limbic area, especially on 5HT2A and 5HT2C postsynaptic receptors, may be involved in anxiety and panic (Fig. 5–54). Projections to the hypothalamus especially on 5HT3 receptors may regulate appetite and eating behavior (Fig. 5–55). Brainstem sleep centers, especially with 5HT2A postsynaptic receptors, regulate sleep, especially slow-wave sleep (Fig. 5–56). Serotonergic neurons descending down the spinal cord may be responsible for controlling certain spinal reflexes that are part of the sexual response, such as orgasm and ejaculation (Fig. 5–57). The brainstem chemoreceptor trigger zone can mediate vomiting, especially via 5HT3 receptors (Fig. 5–58). Peripheral 5HT3 and 5HT4 receptors may also regulate appetite as well as other gastrointestinal functions, such as gastrointestinal motility (Fig. 5–59). Putting all these pathways and their functions together, a hypothetical serotonin deficiency syndrome (Table 5–23) might comprise depression, anxiety, panic, phobias, obsessions, compulsions, and food craving.

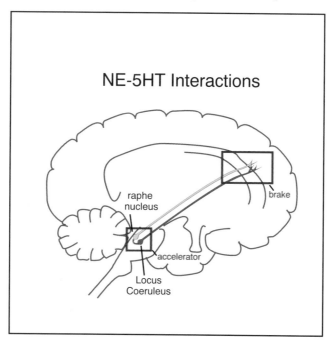

FIGURE 5–47. Two types of **norepinephrine interaction with serotonin** are shown here. In the brainstem, a pathway from locus coeruleus to raphe interacts with serotonergic cell bodies there and **accelerates** serotonin release. A second noradrenergic pathway to target areas in the cortex also interacts with serotonin axon terminals there and **brakes** serotonin release.

### Classical Antidepressants and the Monoamine Hypothesis

The first antidepressants to be discovered came from two classes of agents, namely, the tricyclic antidepressants, so named because their chemical structure has three rings, and the MAO inhibitors, so named because they inhibit the enzyme MAO, which destroys monoamine neurotransmitters. When tricyclic antidepressants block the NE transporter, they increase the availability of NE in the synapse, since the "vacuum cleaner" reuptake pump can no longer sweep NE out of the synapse (Figs. 5–16 and 5–18). When tricyclic antidepressants block the DA pump (Fig. 5–32) or the 5HT pump (Fig. 5–35), they similarly enhance the synaptic availability of DA or 5HT, respectively, and by the same mechanism. When MAO inhibitors block NE, DA, and 5HT breakdown, they boost the levels of these neurotransmitters (Fig. 5–15).

Since it was recognized by the 1960s that all the classical antidepressants boost NE, DA, and 5HT in one manner or another (Figs. 5–15 and 5–16), the original idea was that one or another of these neurotransmitters, also chemically known as monoamines, might be deficient in the first place in depression (Fig. 5–14). Thus, the "monoamine hypothesis" was born. A good deal of effort was expended, especially in the 1960s and 1970s, to identify the theoretically predicted deficiencies of the monoamine neurotransmitters. This effort to date has unfortunately yielded mixed and sometimes confusing results.

Some studies suggest that NE metabolites are deficient in some patients with depression, but this has not been uniformly observed. Other studies suggest that

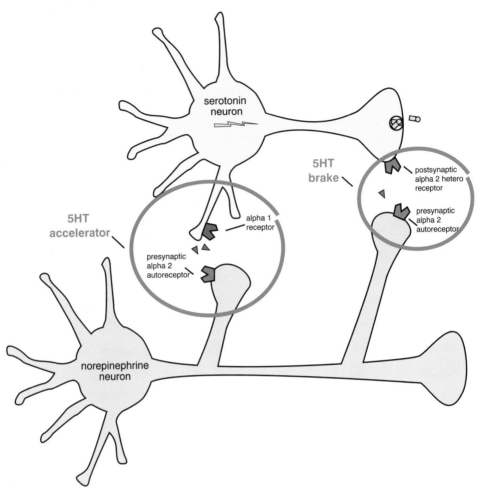

FIGURE 5–48. A schematic representation of both the **excitatory and inhibitory actions of norepinephrine on serotonin release** is shown here. This is the same action shown in Figure 5–47.

the 5HT metabolite 5-hydroxy-indole acetic acid (5HIAA) is reduced in the cerebrospinal fluid (CSF) of depressed patients. On closer examination, however, it has been found that only some of the depressed patients have low CSF 5HIAA, and these tend to be the patients with impulsive behaviors, such as suicide attempts of a violent nature. Subsequently, it was also reported that CSF 5HIAA is decreased in other populations who were subject to violent outbursts of poor impulse control but were not depressed, namely, patients with antisocial personality disorder who were arsonists, and patients with borderline personality disorder with self-destructive behaviors. Thus, low CSF 5HIAA may be linked more closely with impulse control problems than with depression.

Another problem with the monoamine hypothesis is the fact that the timing of antidepressant effects on neurotransmitters is far different from the timing of the antidepressant effects on mood. That is, antidepressants boost monoamines *immedi-*

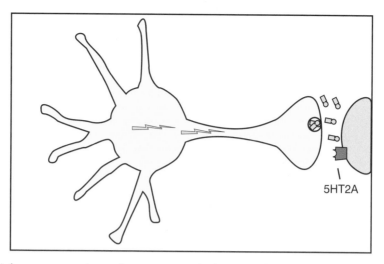

FIGURE 5–49. A key postsynaptic regulatory receptor is the **5HT2A receptor**.

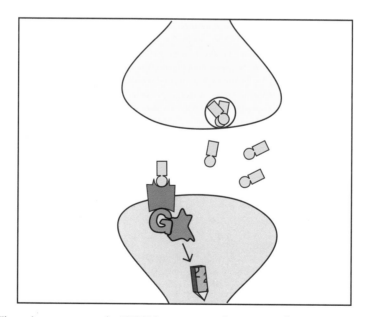

FIGURE 5–50. When the **postsynaptic 5HT2A receptor** of Figure 5–49 is occupied by 5HT, it causes neuronal impulses in the postsynaptic neuron to be transduced via the production of **second messengers**.

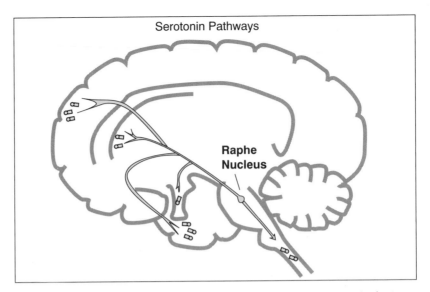

FIGURE 5–51. The headquarters for the cell bodies of serotonergic neurons is in the brainstem area called the **raphe nucleus**.

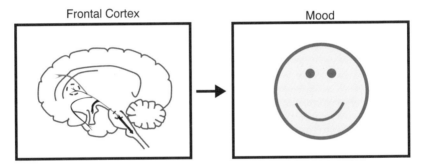

FIGURE 5–52. Serotonergic projections from raphe to **frontal cortex** may be important for regulating mood.

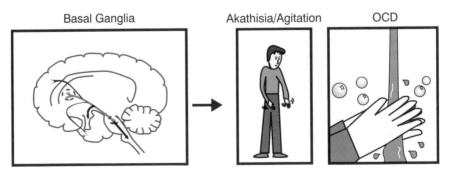

FIGURE 5–53. Serotonergic projections from raphe to **basal ganglia** may help control movements as well as **obsessions and compulsions**.

182

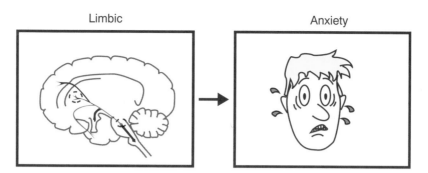

FIGURE 5–54. Serotonergic projections from raphe to **limbic** areas may be involved in **anxiety** and panic.

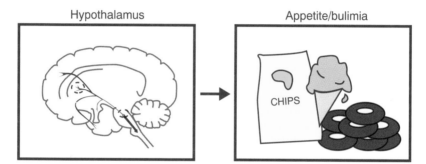

FIGURE 5–55. Serotonergic projections to the **hypothalamus** may regulate appetite and **eating** behavior.

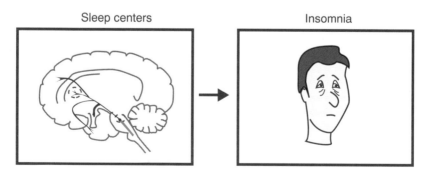

FIGURE 5–56. Serotonergic neurons in brainstem **sleep centers** regulate sleep, especially slow-wave sleep.

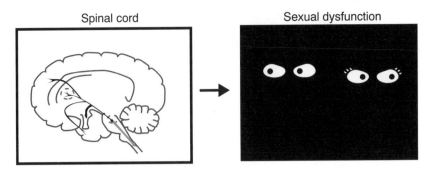

FIGURE 5–57. Serotonergic neurons descending down the **spinal cord** may be responsible for controlling certain spinal reflexes that are part of the **sexual response**, such as orgasm and ejaculation.

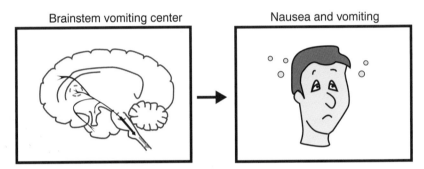

FIGURE 5–58. The chemoreceptor trigger zone in the **brainstem** can mediate **vomiting**, especially via 5HT3 receptors.

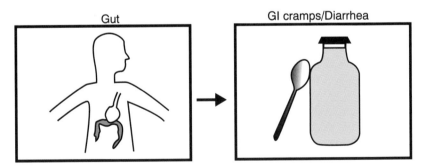

FIGURE 5–59. Peripheral 5HT3 and 5HT4 receptors in the **gut** may regulate appetite as well as other **gastrointestinal functions**, such as gastrointestinal motility.

Table 5–23. *Serotonin deficiency syndrome*

| |
|---|
| Depressed mood |
| Anxiety |
| Panic |
| Phobia |
| Anxiety |
| Obsessions and compulsions |
| Food craving; bulimia |

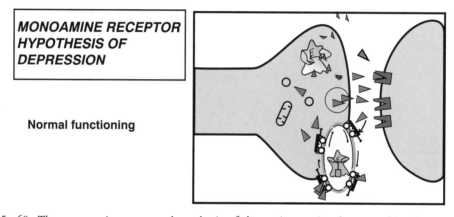

**MONOAMINE RECEPTOR HYPOTHESIS OF DEPRESSION**

**Normal functioning**

FIGURE 5–60. The monoamine receptor hypothesis of depression posits that something is wrong with the receptors for the key monoamine neurotransmitters. Thus, according to this theory, an abnormality in the receptors for monoamine neurotransmitters leads to depression. Such a disturbance in neurotransmitter receptors may be caused by depletion of monoamine neurotransmitters, by abnormalities in the receptors themselves, or by some problem with signal transduction of the neurotransmitter's message from the receptor to other downstream events. Depicted here is the **normal monoamine neuron** with the normal amount of monoamine neurotransmitter and the normal amount of correctly functioning monoamine receptors.

*ately*, but as mentioned earlier, there is a significant *delay* in the onset of their therapeutic actions, which in fact occurs many days to weeks *after* they have already boosted the monoamines. Because of these and other difficulties, the focus of hypotheses for the etiology of depression began to shift from the monoamine neurotransmitters themselves to their receptors. As we shall see, contemporary theories have shifted past the receptors to the molecular events that regulate gene expression.

## Neurotransmitter Receptor Hypothesis

The neurotransmitter receptor theory posits that something is wrong with the receptors for the key monoamine neurotransmitters (Figs. 5–60 through 5–62). According to this theory, an abnormality in the receptors for monoamine neurotransmitters leads to depression (Fig. 5–62). Such a disturbance in neurotransmitter receptors may itself be caused by depletion of monoamine neurotransmitters (Fig. 5–61).

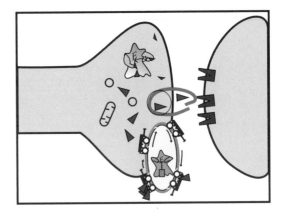

**Decrease in NT**

FIGURE 5–61. In this figure, **monoamine neurotransmitter is depleted** (see red circle), just as previously shown in Figure 5–14.

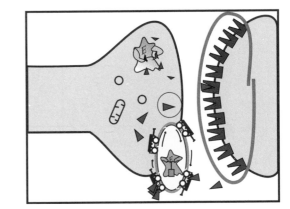

**Receptors up-regulate
due to lack of NT**

FIGURE 5–62. The consequences of monoamine neurotransmitter depletion, of stress, or of some inherited abnormality in neurotransmitter receptor could cause the **postsynaptic receptors to abnormally up-regulate** (indicated in red circle). This up-regulation or other receptor dysfunction is hypothetically linked to the cause of depression.

Depletion of monoamine neurotransmitters (cf. Fig. 5–60 and Fig. 5–61) has already been discussed as the central theme of the monoamine hypothesis of depression (see Figs. 5–13 and 5–14). The neurotransmitter receptor hypothesis of depression takes this theme one step further—namely, that the depletion of neurotransmitter causes compensatory up regulation of postsynaptic neurotransmitter receptors (Fig. 5–62).

Direct evidence of this is generally lacking, but postmortem studies do consistently show increased numbers of serotonin 2 receptors in the frontal cortex of patients who commit suicide. Indirect studies of neurotransmitter receptor functioning in patients with major depressive disorders suggest abnormalities in various neurotransmitter receptors when using neuroendocrine probes or peripheral tissues such as platelets or lymphocytes. Modern molecular techniques are exploring for abnormalities in gene expression of neurotransmitter receptors and enzymes in families with depression but have not yet been successful in identifying molecular lesions.

## The Monoamine Hypothesis of Gene Expression

So far, there is no clear and convincing evidence that monoamine deficiency accounts for depression; that is, there is no "real" monoamine deficit. Likewise, there is no clear and convincing evidence that excesses or deficiencies of monoamine receptors account for depression; that is, there is no pseudomonoamine deficiency due to the monoamines being there but not the monoamine receptors. On the other hand, there is growing evidence that despite apparently normal levels of monoamines and their receptors, these systems do not respond normally. For instance, probing monoaminergic receptors with drugs that stimulate them can lead to deficient output of neuroendocrine hormones. It can also lead to deficient changes in neuronal firing rates, as demonstrated on positron emission tomography (PET).

Such observations have led to the idea that depression may be a pseudomonoamine deficiency due to a deficiency in signal transduction from the monoamine neurotransmitter to its postsynaptic neuron in the presence of normal amounts of neurotransmitter and receptor. If there is a deficiency in the molecular events that cascade from receptor occupancy by neurotransmitter, it could lead to a deficient cellular response and thus be a form of pseudomonoamine deficiency (i.e., the receptor and the neurotransmitter are normal, but the transduction of the signal from neurotransmitter to its receptor is somehow flawed). Such a deficiency in molecular functioning has been described for certain endocrine diseases such as hypoparathyroidism (parathyroid hormone deficiency), pseudohypoparathyroidism (parathyroid receptors deficient but parathyroid hormone levels normal), and pseudo-pseudohypoparathyroidism (signal transduction deficiency leading to hypoparathyroid clinical state despite normal levels of hormone and receptor).

Perhaps a similar situation exists for depression due to a hypothesized problem within the molecular events distal to the receptor. Thus, second messenger systems leading to the formation of intracellular transcription factors that control gene regulation could be the site of deficient functioning of monoamine systems. This is the subject of much current research into the potential molecular basis of affective disorders. This hypothesis suggests some form of molecularly mediated deficiency in monoamines that is distal to the monoamines themselves and their receptors despite apparently normal levels of monoamines and numbers of monoamine receptors.

One candidate mechanism that has been proposed as the site of a possible flaw in signal transduction from monoamine receptors is the target gene for brain-derived neurotrophic factor (BDNF). Normally, BDNF sustains the viability of brain neurons, but under stress, the gene for BDNF is repressed (Fig. 5–63), leading to the atrophy and possible apoptosis of vulnerable neurons in the hippocampus when their BDNF is cut off (Fig. 5–64). This in turn leads to depression and to the consequences of repeated depressive episodes, namely, more and more episodes and less and less responsiveness to treatment. This possibility that hippocampal neurons are decreased in size and impaired in function during depression is supported by recent clinical imaging studies showing decreased brain volume of related structures. This provides a molecular and cellular hypothesis of depression consistent with a mechanism distal to the neurotransmitter receptor and involving an abnormality in gene expression. Thus, stress-induced vulnerability decreases the expression of genes that make neurotrophic factors such as BDNF critical to the survival and function of key neurons (Fig. 5–63). A corollary to this hypothesis is that antidepressants act to

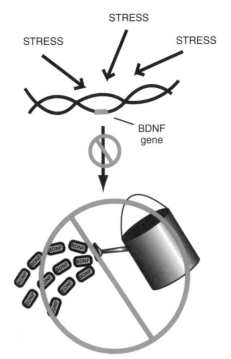

FIGURE 5–63. The monoamine hypothesis of gene action in depression, part 1. One candidate mechanism that has been proposed as the site of a possible flaw in signal transduction from monoamine receptors is the target gene for **brain-derived neurotrophic factor** (BDNF). Normally, BDNF sustains the viability of brain neurons. Shown here, however, is the gene for BDNF under situations of stress. In this case, the gene for BDNF is repressed, and BDNF is not being synthesized.

reverse this by causing the genes for neurotrophic factors to be activated (see Chapter 6).

### Neurokinin Hypothesis of Emotional Dysfunction

Another hypothesis for the pathophysiology of depression and other states of emotional dysfunction relates to the actions of a relatively new class of peptide neurotransmitters known as *neurokinins* (also sometimes called *tachykinins*). This hypothesis was generated by some rather serendipitous observations that an antagonist to one of the neurokinins, namely substance P, may have antidepressant actions. Classically, substance P was thought to be involved in the pain response because it is released from neurons in peripheral tissues in response to inflammation, causing "neurogenic" inflammation and pain (Fig. 5–65). Furthermore, substance P is present in spinal pain pathways, suggesting a role in central nervous system-mediated pain (Fig. 5–65). Unfortunately, however, antagonists to substance P's receptors have so far been unable to reduce neurogenic inflammation or pain of many types in human testing.

On the other hand, suggestions that substance P antagonists may have improved mood, if not pain, in migraine patients led to controlled trials of such drugs in patients with depression. Although these are still early days and not all studies confirm antidepressant effects of substance P antagonists, the possibility that such

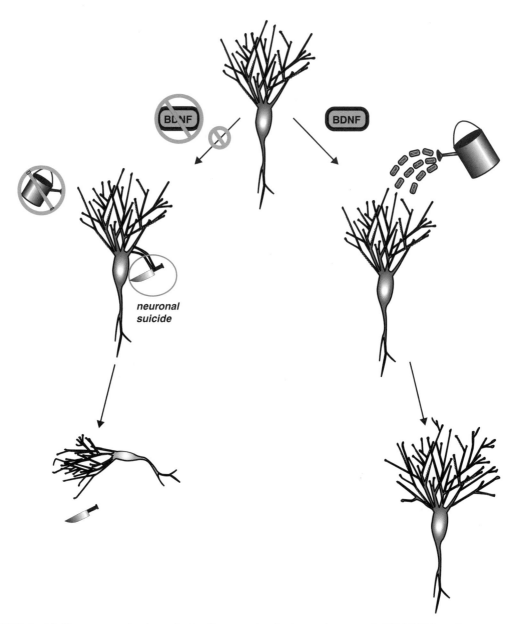

FIGURE 5–64. The monoamine hypothesis of gene action in depression, part 2. If BDNF is no longer made in appropriate amounts, instead of the neuron prospering and developing more and more synapses (right), **stress** causes vulnerable neurons in the hippocampus to **atrophy** and possibly undergo **apoptosis** when their neurotrophic factor is cut off (left). This, in turn, leads to depression and to the consequences of repeated depressive episodes, namely, more and more episodes and less and less responsiveness to treatment. This may explain why hippocampal neurons seem to be decreased in size and impaired in function during depression on the basis of recent clinical neuroimaging studies.

189

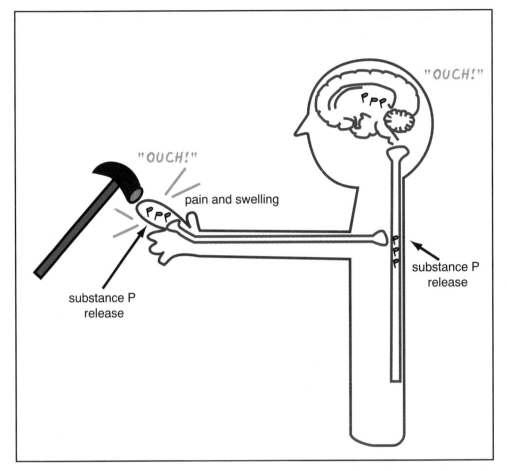

FIGURE 5–65. Classically, **substance P** was thought to be involved in the **pain** response because it is released from neurons in peripheral tissues in response to inflammation, causing "neurogenic" inflammation and pain. Furthermore, substance P is present in spinal pain pathways, which suggests a role in central nervous system–medicated pain. Unfortunately, however, antagonists to substance P's receptors were unable to reduce neurogenic inflammation or pain of many types in human testing.

drugs might be effective in reducing emotional distress has nevertheless spawned a race to find antagonists for all three of the known neurokinins to see if they would have therapeutic actions in a wide variety of psychiatric disorders. Substance P and its related neurokinins are present in areas of the brain such as the amygdala that are thought to be critical for regulating emotions (Fig. 5–66). The neurokinins are also present in areas of the brain rich with monoamines, which suggests a potential regulatory role of neurokinins for monoamine neurotransmitters already known to be important in numerous psychiatric disorders and in the mechanisms of action of numerous psychotropic drugs. Thus, antagonists to all three important neurokinins are currently in clinical testing of various states of emotional dysfunction, including depression, anxiety, and schizophrenia. Over the next few years it should become apparent whether this strategy can be exploited to generate truly novel psychotropic drugs acting on an entirely new neurotransmitter system, namely, the neurokinins.

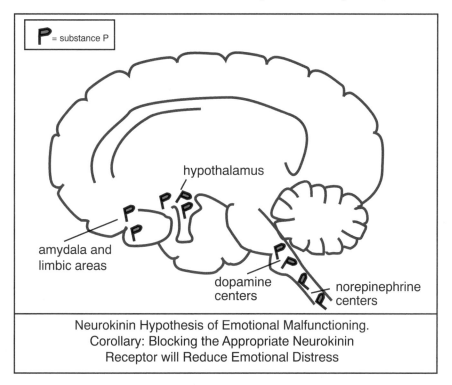

FIGURE 5–66. **Substance P** and its related neurokinins are present in areas of the brain such as the amygdala that are thought to be critical for regulating **emotions**. The neurokinins are also present in areas of the brain rich in monoamines, which suggests a potential regulatory role of monoamine neurotransmitters, which are already known to be important in numerous psychiatric disorders and in the mechanisms of action of numerous psychotropic drugs.

*Substance P and neurokinin 1 receptors.* The first neurokinin was discovered in the 1930s in extracts of brain or intestine. Since it was prepared as a "powder," it was called substance P. This molecule is now known to be a string of 11 amino acids (an undecapeptide) (Fig. 5–67). This is in sharp contrast to monoamine neurotransmitters, which are modifications of a single amino acid.

The following are some of the differences between the synthesis of neurotransmitter by a monoaminergic neuron and by a peptidergic neuron. Whereas monoamines are made from dietary amino acids, peptide neurotransmitters are made from proteins that are direct gene products. However, genes are not translated directly into peptide neurotransmitters but into precursors of the peptide neurotransmitters. These precursors are sometimes called "grandparent" proteins, or pre-propeptides. Further modifications convert these grandparent proteins into the direct precursors of peptide neurotransmitters, sometimes called the "parents" of the neuropeptide, or the propeptides. Finally, modifications of the parental peptide produces the neuropeptide progeny itself.

For neurons utilizing substance P, synthesis starts with the gene called preprotachykinin A (PPT-A) (Fig. 5–68). This gene is transcribed into RNA, which is then "edited," or revised by cutting and pasting, like revising a manuscript or a

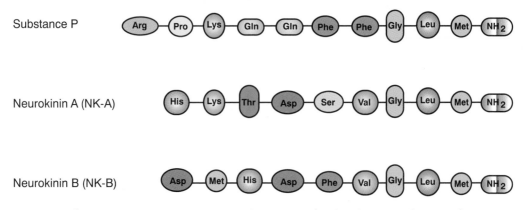

Substance P

Neurokinin A (NK-A)

Neurokinin B (NK-B)

FIGURE 5–67. Shown here are the amino acid sequences for the three neurokinins **substance P**, **neurokinin A** (NK-A) and **neurokinin B** (NK-B). Substance P has 11 amino acid units and NK-A and NK-B each have 10. Several of the amino acids are the same in these three peptides.

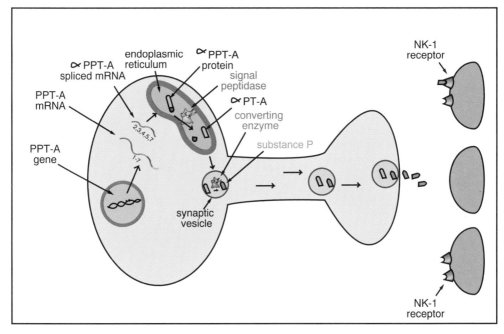

FIGURE 5–68. Substance P neurons and neurokinin 1 receptors, part 1. For neurons utilizing **substance P**, synthesis starts with the gene called pre-protachykinin A (**PPT-A**). This gene is transcribed into RNA, which is then "edited" to form three alternative mRNA splice variants, alpha, beta, and gamma. The actions of the mRNA version called alpha-PPT-A mRNA are shown here. This mRNA is then transcribed into a protein called alpha-PPT-A, which is substance P's "grandparent." It is converted in the endoplasmic reticulum into the "parent" of substance P, called protachykinin A (alpha-PT-A). Finally, this protein is clipped even shorter by another enzyme, called a converting enzyme, in the synaptic vesicle and forms substance P itself.

videotape. Thus, this process is sometimes called "splicing" of the RNA. This leads to different versions of RNA called *alternative mRNA splice variants*.

The mRNA version called alpha-PPT-A mRNA goes on to be transcribed into a protein called alpha-PPT-A, which is substance P's grandparent (Fig. 5–68). It is much longer than substance P itself, as it contains a longer string of amino acids. The alpha-PPT-A grandparent protein needs to be cut down to size by an enzyme in the endoplasmic reticulum called a *signal peptidase*. Thus, pro-tachykinin A (alpha-PT-A) protein is formed, the parent of substance P. Finally, alpha PT-A is clipped even shorter by another enzyme in the synaptic vesicle called a *converting enzyme*, and forms substance P itself (Fig. 5–68).

Substance P can also be formed from two other proteins, called beta-PPT-A and gamma PPT-A (Figs. 5–69 and 5–70). These proteins come from different mRNA splice variants, but the same precursor PPT-A gene. Not only can substance P be formed from these proteins, but so can another important neurokinin, called neurokinin A (NK-A) (Figs. 5–71 and 5–72). Thus, substance P can be formed from three proteins derived from the PPT-A gene, namely, alpha, beta, and gamma PPT-A (Figs. 5–68 to 5–70), and NK-A can be formed from two of these, beta and gamma PPT-A (Figs. 5–71 and 5–72).

Substance P is released from neurons and prefers to interact selectively with the neurokinin 1 (NK-1) subtype of neurokinin receptor (Figs. 5–68 to 5–70). Inter-

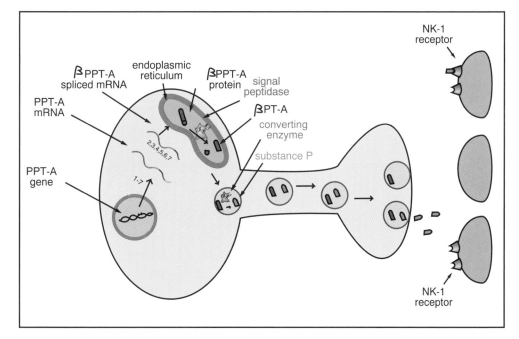

FIGURE 5–69. Substance P and neurokinin 1 receptors, part 2. **Substance P** can also be formed from two other proteins, called **beta-PPT-A**, shown here, and gamma PPT-A, shown in Figure 5–70. These proteins come from different mRNA splice variants but the same precursor PPT-A gene.

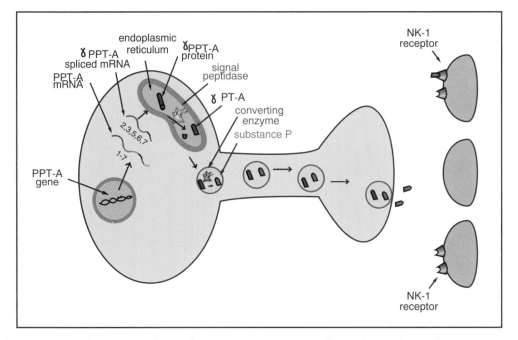

FIGURE 5–70. Substance P and neurokinin 1 receptors, part 3. Shown here is how **substance P** is formed from **gamma PPT-A**. Thus, substance P can be formed from three proteins derived from the PPT-A gene, namely, alpha, beta, and gamma PPT-A (see also Figs. 5–68 and 5–69). When substance P is released from neurons, it prefers to interact selectively with the **neurokinin 1** subtype of neurokinin receptor (Figs. 5–68 to 5–70). However, there is a mismatch in the brain between the locations of substance P and the NK-1 receptors, suggesting that substance P acts preferentially by volume neurotransmission at sites remote from its axon terminals rather than by classical synaptic neurotransmission.

estingly, however, there is a bit of a mismatch in the brain between where substance P is located and where the NK-1 receptors are located. This may suggest that substance P acts preferentially by volume neurotransmission at sites remote from its axon terminals rather than by classical synaptic neurotransmission.

*Neurokinin A and neurokinin 2 receptors.* Neurokinin A (NK-A) is another member of the neurokinin family of peptide neurotransmitters. It is a peptide containing 10 amino acid units (decapeptide), with 5 amino acid units the same as in substance P, including 4 of the last 5 on its N-terminal tail (Fig. 5–67). As mentioned above, it is formed both from the beta and the gamma PPT-A proteins derived from the PPT-A gene (Figs. 5–71 and 5–72). The beta and gamma PPT-A proteins are the grandparents of NK-A and are cut down to size just as described for substance P, eventually forming the peptide neurotransmitter NK-A.

This neurokinin prefers a different receptor than does substance P. Thus, NK-A specifically binds the NK-2 receptor (Figs. 5–71 and 5–72). There are few NK-A receptors in the brain of rats, so the guinea pig is a closer model to humans, with

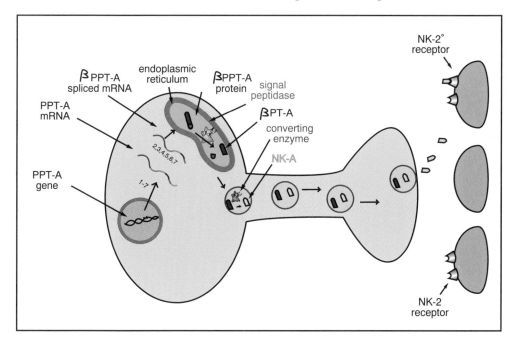

FIGURE 5–71. Neurokinin A and neurokinin 2 receptors, part 1. **Neurokinin A** can be formed from two of the same proteins that form substance P, namely beta and gamma PPT-A. The formation of neurokinin A from **beta PPT-A** is shown here.

NK-A receptors also in peripheral tissues such as the lung. As for substance P, there is a mismatch between the neurotransmitter and its receptor anatomically, which suggests the important role of nonsynaptic volume neurotransmission for NK-A as well. However, the anatomical distribution of NK-A is different from that of substance P, and the anatomical distribution of NK-2 receptors is different from that of NK-1 receptors.

*Neurokinin B and neurokinin B receptors.* The third important member of the neurokinin neurotransmitter family is neurokinin B (NK-B). Like NK-A, it is a ten amino acid peptide (decapeptide). Six of the ten amino acids in NK-B are the same as in NK-A, and four of the last five amino acids in the N-terminal tail of NK-B are identical to substance P (Fig. 5–67).

Neurokinin B is formed from a gene called PPT-B, which is different from that from which substance P and NK-A are derived. However, the process of converting the PPT-B protein into NK-B is analogous to that already described for substance P and NK-A (Fig. 5–73). NK-B prefers its own unique receptors, called NK-3 receptors (Fig. 5–73). Neurokinin B and its NK-3 receptors are also mismatched, and in different anatomical areas from substance P, NK-A, and their NK-1 and NK-2 receptors, respectively.

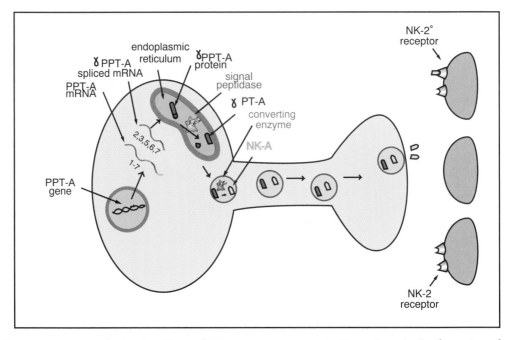

FIGURE 5–72. Neurokinin A and neurokinin 2 receptors, part 2. Shown here is the formation of **NK-A from the gamma PPT-A protein**. The beta and gamma PPT-A proteins are the "grandparents" of NK-A and are cut down to size just as described for substance P, eventually forming the peptide neurotransmitter NK-A. Neurokinin A specifically binds to the **NK-2 receptor**. As for substance P, there is a mismatch between this neurotransmitter and its receptor anatomically, suggesting the important role of nonsynaptic volume neurotransmission for NK-A as well. However, the anatomical distribution of NK-A is different from that of substance P, and the anatomical distribution of NK-2 receptors is different from that of NK-1 receptors.

## Summary

In this chapter we have introduced two major psychopharmacological themes, namely, the affective disorders and the monoamine and neuropeptide neurotransmitters. We have described the clinical features, epidemiology, and longitudinal course of various types of depression, including the impact that treatments are having on the long-term outcome of affective disorders. We have also described the three monoamine neurotransmitter systems—noradrenergic, dopaminergic, and serotonergic. Specifically, the synthesis, metabolism, transport systems, and receptors for each monoaminergic system have been outlined and then applied to the leading theories for the biological basis of depression. These theories of depression are the monoamine hypothesis, the neurotransmitter hypothesis, and the pseudomonoamine hypothesis of defective signal transduction and gene expression. Finally, we have introduced a new family of neurotransmitters and their receptors, called neurokinins, of which substance P is the most prominent member.

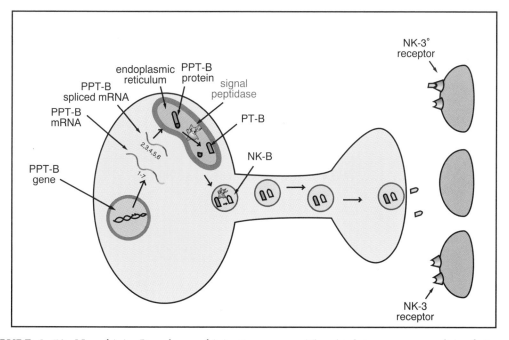

FIGURE 5–73. Neurokinin B and neurokinin 3 receptors. The third important member of the neurokinin neurotransmitter family is **NK-B**, which is formed from a gene, called **PPT-B**, which is different from the gene from which either substance P or NK-A is derived. However, the process of converting the PPT-B protein into NK-B is analogous to that already described for substance P and NK-A. Neurokinin B prefers its own unique receptors, called **NK-3 receptors**. Neurokinin B and its NK-3 receptors are also mismatched and are located in different anatomical areas from substance P, NK-A, and their NK-1 and NK-2 receptors, respectively.

The material in this chapter should provide the reader with the basis for understanding the pharmacologic basis of the treatment of depression discussed in the following two chapters. It should also provide useful background information about the monoamine neurotransmitter systems that serve as the pharmacological basis for several other classes of psychotropic drugs.

# CHAPTER 6

# CLASSICAL ANTIDEPRESSANTS, SEROTONIN SELECTIVE REUPTAKE INHIBITORS, AND NORADRENERGIC REUPTAKE INHIBITORS

In this chapter, we will review pharmacological concepts underlying the use of several classes of antidepressant drugs, including the classical monoamine oxidase (MAO) inhibitors, the classical tricyclic antidepressants, the popular serotonin selective reuptake inhibitors (SSRIs), and the new selective noradrenergic reuptake inhibitors, as well as norepinephrine and dopamine reuptake inhibitors. The goal of this chapter is to acquaint the reader with current ideas about how these antidepressants work. We will explain the mechanisms of action of these drugs by building on general pharmacological concepts. We will also introduce pharmacokinetic concepts for the antidepressants, namely, how the body acts on these drugs through the cytochrome P450 enzyme system.

Our treatment of antidepressants in this chapter is at the conceptual level and not at the pragmatic level. The reader should consult standard drug handbooks for details of doses, side effects, drug interactions, and other issues relevant to the prescribing of these drugs in clinical practice.

## Theories of Antidepressant Drug Action

### Classifications Based on Acute Pharmacological Actions

We do not currently have a complete and adequate explanation of how antidepressant drugs work. What we do know is that all effective antidepressants have identifiable immediate interactions with one or more monoamine neurotransmitter receptor or enzyme. These immediate actions provide the pharmacological foundation for the current classification of the different antidepressants.

According to this classification scheme, there are at least eight separate pharmacological mechanisms of action and more than two dozen antidepressants. Most antidepressants block monoamine reuptake, but some block alpha 2 receptors and others the enzyme monoamine oxidase (MAO). Some antidepressants have direct actions on only one monoamine neurotransmitter system; others have direct actions on more than one monoamine neurotransmitter system. As discussed in Chapter 5, the immediate pharmacological actions of all antidepressants eventually have the effect of boosting the levels of monoamine neurotransmitters (Figs. 5–15 and 5–16; see also Fig. 6–1). This chapter and the following chapter will review those specific receptors and enzymes that are influenced by each of the various antidepressants immediately after administration to a depressed patient. Just how all these different immediate pharmacological actions result ultimately in an antidepressant response a few weeks after administration of an antidepressant agent—that is, the final common pathway of antidepressant treatment response—is the subject of intense research interest and debate (Fig. 6–1). Currently, there is intense focus on the gene expression that is triggered by antidepressants. The monoamine hypothesis of antidepressant action on gene expression suggests that gene expression is ultimately the most important action of antidepressants.

### The Neurotransmitter Receptor Hypothesis of Antidepressant Action

One theory to explain the ultimate mechanism of delayed therapeutic action of antidepressants is the neurotransmitter receptor hypothesis of antidepressant action (Figs. 6–1 through 6–6). This is a hypothesis related to the neurotransmitter receptor hypothesis of depression discussed in Chapter 5 (Figs. 5–60 through 5–62). As previously discussed, this latter hypothesis proposes that depression itself is linked to abnormal functioning of neurotransmitter receptors.

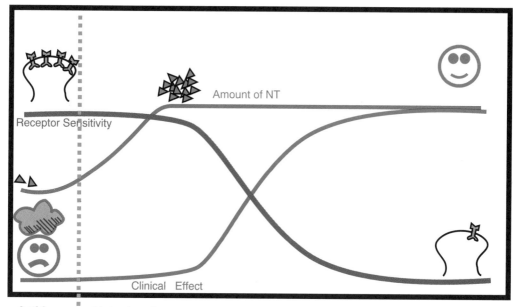

FIGURE 6–1. This figure depicts the different time courses for three effects of antidepressant drugs, namely clinical changes, neurotransmitter (NT) changes, and receptor sensitivity changes. Specifically, the **amount of NT** changes relatively rapidly after an **antidepressant is introduced**. However, the **clinical effect** is delayed, as is the desensitization, or down regulation, of neurotransmitter **receptors**. This temporal correlation of clinical effects with changes in receptor sensitivity has given rise to the hypothesis that changes in neurotransmitter receptor sensitivity may actually mediate the clinical effects of antidepressant drugs. These clinical effects include not only antidepressant and anxiolytic actions but also the development of tolerance to the acute side effects of antidepressant drugs.

Whether or not neurotransmitter receptors are abnormal in depression, the neurotransmitter receptor hypothesis of antidepressant action proposes that antidepressants, no matter what their initial actions on receptors and enzymes, eventually cause a desensitization, or down regulation, of key neurotransmitter receptors in a time course consistent with the delayed onset of antidepressant action of these drugs (Figs. 6–1 through 6–6).

This time course coincides with other events, including the time it takes for a patient to become tolerant to the side effects of antidepressants. Thus, desensitization of some neurotransmitter receptors may lead to the delayed therapeutic actions of antidepressants, whereas desensitization of other neurotransmitter receptors may lead to the decrease of side effects over time.

An overly simplistic view of the neurotransmitter receptor hypothesis of depression is that the normal state becomes one of depression as neurotransmitter is depleted and postsynaptic receptors then up-regulate (Fig. 6–2). Boosting neurotransmitters by MAO inhibition (Figs. 6–3 and 6–4) or by blocking reuptake pumps for monoamine neurotransmitters (Figs. 6–5 and 6–6) eventually results in the down regulation of neurotransmitter receptors in a delayed time course more closely related to the timing of recovery from depression (Figs. 6–1, 6–4, and 6–6).

### NEUROTRANSMITTER RECEPTOR
### HYPOTHESIS OF
### ANTIDEPRESSANT ACTION

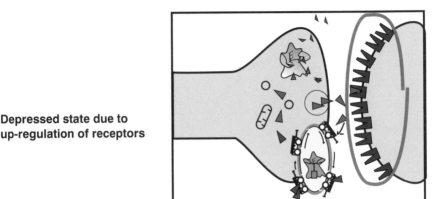

**Depressed state due to
up-regulation of receptors**

FIGURE 6–2. *The neurotransmitter receptor hypothesis of antidepressant action*—part 1. Shown here is the monoaminergic neuron in the **depressed state**, with **up regulation of receptors** (indicated in the red circle).

### NEUROTRANSMITTER RECEPTOR
### HYPOTHESIS OF
### ANTIDEPRESSANT ACTION

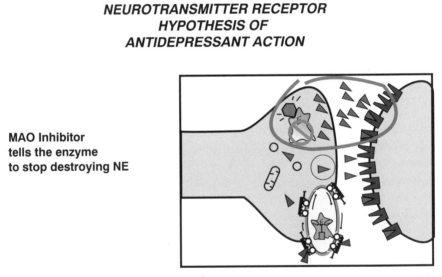

**MAO Inhibitor
tells the enzyme
to stop destroying NE**

FIGURE 6–3. *The neurotransmitter receptor hypothesis of antidepressant action*—part 2. Here, a monoamine oxidase (**MAO**) **inhibitor** is blocking the enzyme and thereby stopping the destruction of neurotransmitter. This causes **more neurotransmitter to be available** in the synapse (indicated in the red circle).

Originally, it was hypothesized that desensitization of postsynaptic receptors may be responsible for the therapeutic actions of antidepressants. It is now clear that desensitization of some postsynaptic receptors is responsible for the development of tolerance to the acute side effects of antidepressants. Attention is currently being

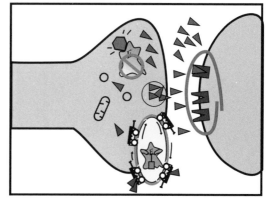

**Increase in NT causes receptors to down-regulate**

FIGURE 6–4. *The neurotransmitter receptor hypothesis of antidepressant action*—part 3. The consequence of **long-lasting blockade** of monoamine oxidase (**MAO**) by an MAO inhibitor is that the neurotransmitter **receptors are desensitized or down-regulated** (indicated in the red circle).

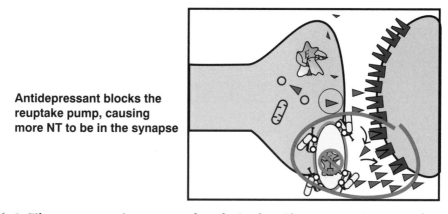

**Antidepressant blocks the reuptake pump, causing more NT to be in the synapse**

FIGURE 6–5. *The neurotransmitter receptor hypothesis of antidepressant action*—part 4. Here, a **tricyclic antidepressant** blocks the reuptake pump, causing **more neurotransmitter** to be available in the synapse (indicated in the red circle). This is very similar to what happens after MAO is inhibited (Fig. 6–3).

focused on the presynaptic receptors and their desensitization in order to explain the therapeutic actions of antidepressants. This will be discussed in more detail in the section on serotonin selective reuptake inhibitors (SSRIs).

## The Monoamine Hypothesis of Antidepressant Action on Gene Expression

As discussed in Chapter 5 (Figs. 5–63 and 5–64), the monoamine hypothesis of gene expression proposes that depression itself is linked to abnormal functioning of neurotransmitter-inducible gene expression, particularly neurotrophic factors such as

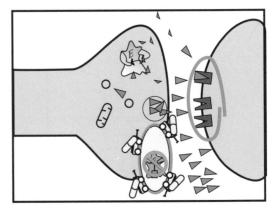

**Increase in NT causes receptors to down-regulate**

FIGURE 6–6. *The neurotransmitter receptor hypothesis of antidepressant action*—part 5. The consequence of **long-lasting blockade** of the reuptake pump by a **tricyclic antidepressant** is to cause the neurotransmitter **receptors to become desensitized or down-regulated** (indicated in the red circle). This is the same outcome as with long-lasting blockade of MAO (see Fig. 6–4).

brain-derived neurotrophic factor (BDNF), leading to atrophy and apoptosis of critical hippocampal neurons. Whether or not the transduction of a monoaminergic neuronal impulse into gene expression is actually abnormal in depression, the monoamine hypothesis of antidepressant action on gene expression proposes that antidepressants, no matter what their initial actions on receptors and enzymes, eventually cause critical genes to be activated or inactivated. One of these may indeed be BDNF, although many others are undoubtedly involved as well (Fig. 6–7). Changes in the genetic expression of monoamine neurotransmitter receptors have already been discussed (Figs. 6–1 through 6–6). Thus, the gene expression hypothesis is consistent with the monoamine receptor hypothesis of antidepressant action but is broader in scope.

Delayed actions of antidepressants may not only explain the delay in onset of therapeutic action of antidepressants; they may also explain why some patients fail to respond to antidepressants, since it is possible that in such patients the initial pharmacological actions are not translated into the required delayed pharmacologic and genetic actions. Knowing the biological basis for treatment nonresponse may lead to a greatly needed advance in the pharmacotherapy of depression, namely an effective treatment for refractory or nonresponding depressed patients, as discussed in Chapter 5. Also, if one understands the key pharmacologic events that are linked to the therapeutic actions of the drugs, it may be possible to accelerate them with future drugs. If so, it could lead to another highly desired advance in the pharmacotherapy of depression, namely a rapid-onset antidepressant.

In summary, all antidepressants have a common action on monoamine neurotransmitters—they boost monoamine neurotransmission, leading to changes in gene expression in the neurons targeted by the monoamines. This includes desensitization of neurotransmitter receptors, leading to both therapeutic action and tolerance to side effects. Although antidepressants are classified on the basis of those actions on neurotransmitter receptors and enzymes that are immediate, attention is increasingly being paid to how these initial and immediate actions translate into delayed actions.

**Monoamine Hypothesis of Antidepresssant Action on Gene Expression**

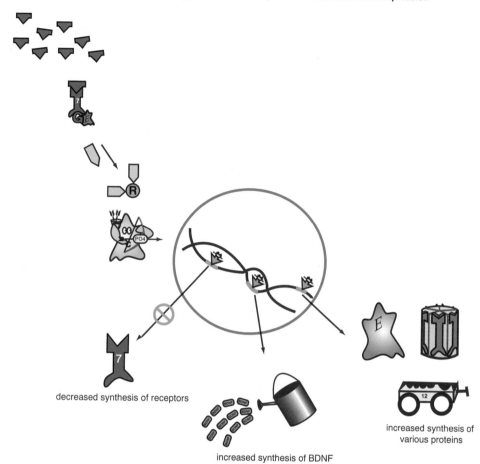

FIGURE 6–7. The **monoamine hypothesis of antidepressant action on gene expression** is shown here. The neurotransmitter at the top is presumably increased by an antidepressant. The cascading consequence of this is ultimately to change the expression of critical genes in order to effect an antidepressant response. This includes down-regulating some genes so that there is decreased synthesis of receptors, as well as up-regulating other genes so that there is increased synthesis of critical proteins, such as brain-derived neurotrophic factor (BDNF).

## Pharmacokinetics of Antidepressants

Recently, there has been a rapid increase in our knowledge about how antidepressants and mood stabilizers are metabolized and about drug interactions with antidepressants and mood stabilizers. *Pharmacokinetics* is the study of how the body acts on drugs, especially to absorb, distribute, metabolize, and excrete them. These pharmacokinetic actions are mediated through the hepatic and gut drug-metabolizing system known as the cytochrome P450 (CYP450) enzyme system.

The CYP450 enzymes and the *pharmacokinetic* actions they represent must be contrasted with the *pharmacodynamic* actions of antidepressants, which were discussed in the previous section on the mechanism of action of antidepressants. Although

Table 6–1. *Pharmacokinetics and pharmacodynamics*

**PHARMACOKINETICS:**
How the body acts on drugs
**PHARMACODYNAMICS:**
How drugs act on the body, especially the brain

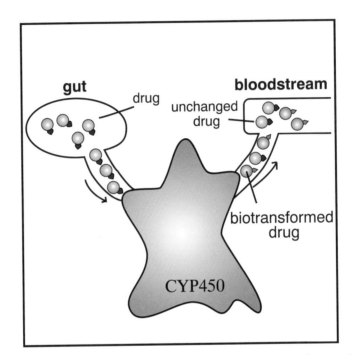

FIGURE 6–8. A **drug** is absorbed and delivered through the gut wall to the liver to be **biotransformed** so that it can be excreted. Specifically, the **cytochrome P450 (CYP450)** enzyme in the gut wall or liver converts the drug substrate into a biotransformed product in the bloodstream. After passing through the gut wall and liver (left), the drug will exist partly as unchanged drug and partly as biotransformed drug (right).

most of this book deals with the *pharmacodynamics* of psychopharmacological agents, especially how these drugs act on the brain, the following section will discuss the *pharmacokinetics* of antidepressants and mood stabilizers, or how the body acts on these drugs (Table 6–1).

The CYP450 enzymes follow the principle of transforming substrates into products. Figure 6–8 shows how an antidepressant is absorbed and delivered through the gut wall to the liver to be biotransformed so that it can be excreted from the body. Specifically, the CYP450 enzyme in the gut wall or liver converts the drug substrate into a biotransformed product in the bloodstream. After passing through the gut wall and liver, the drug will exist partly as unchanged drug and partly as biotransformed product (Fig. 6–8).

There are several known CYP450 systems. Five of the most important enzymes for antidepressant drug metabolism are shown in Figure 6–9. There are over 30

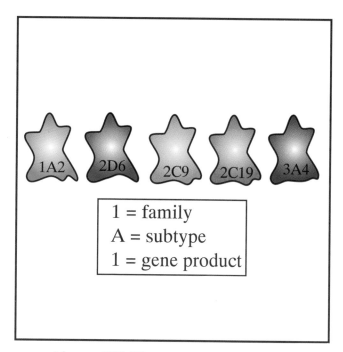

FIGURE 6–9. There are several known **CYP450 enzyme systems**. Five of the most important for antidepressant and mood stabilizer metabolism are shown here.

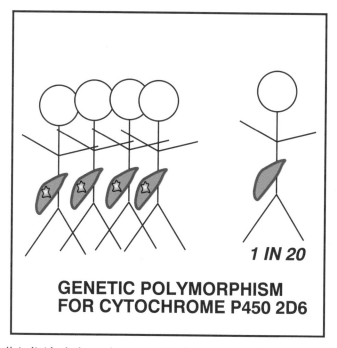

FIGURE 6–10. Not all individuals have the same CYP450 enzymes. For example, about 1 in 20 Caucausians is a **poor metabolizer via 2D6** and must metabolize drugs by an alternative route, which may not be as efficient.

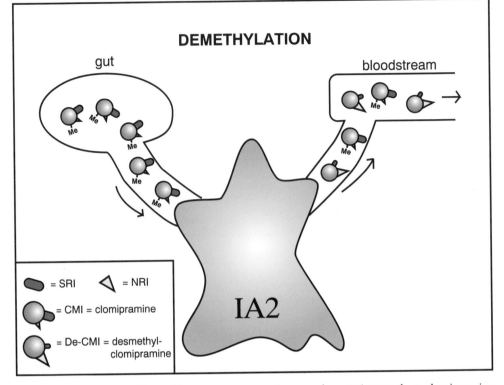

FIGURE 6–11. Certain tricyclic antidepressants, especially secondary amines such as clomipramine and imipramine, are substrates for **CYP450 1A2**. This enzyme converts the tricyclics into active metabolites by demethylation to form desmethylclomipramine and desipramine, respectively.

known CYP450 enzymes, and probably many more awaiting discovery and classi- fication. Not all individuals have all the same CYP450 enzymes. In such cases, the enzyme is said to be polymorphic. For example, about 5 to 10% of Caucasians are poor metabolizers via the enzyme CYP450 2D6 (Fig. 6–10). They must metabolize drugs by alternative routes, which may not be as efficient as the CYP450 2D6 route. Another CYP450 enzyme, 2C19, has reduced activity in approximately 20% of Japanese and Chinese individuals and in 3 to 5% of Caucasians.

### CYP450 1A2

One CYP450 enzyme of relevance to antidepressants is 1A2 (Figs. 6–11 and 6–12). Certain tricyclic antidepressants (TCAs) are *substrates* for this enzyme, espe- cially the secondary amines such as clomipramine and imipramine (Fig. 6–11). CYP450 1A2 demethylates such TCAs, but does not thereby inactivate them. In these cases, the desmethyl metabolite of the TCA (e.g., desmethylclomipramine and desipramine) is still an active drug (Fig. 6–12).

CYP450 1A2 is *inhibited* by the serotonin selective reuptake inhibitor fluvoxamine (Fig. 6–12) Thus, when fluvoxamine is given concomitantly with other drugs that use 1A2 for their metabolism, those drugs can no longer be metabolized as efficiently.

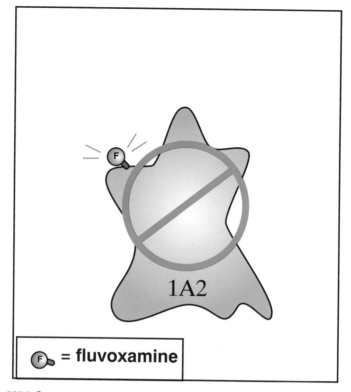

FIGURE 6–12. The SSRI **fluvoxamine** is a potent **inhibitor** of the enzyme CYP450 1A2.

An example of a potentially important drug interaction is that which occurs when fluvoxamine is given along with theophyllin (Figure 6–13). In that case, the theophyllin dose must be lowered or else the blood levels of theophyllin will rise and possibly cause side effects, even toxic side effects such as seizures. The same may occur with caffeine. Fluvoxamine also affects the metabolism of atypical antipsychotics.

### CYP450 2D6

Another important CYP450 enzyme for antidepressants is 2D6. Tricyclic antidepressants are *substrates* for 2D6, which hydroxylates and thereby inactivates them (Fig. 6–14). Several antidepressants from the SSRI class are *inhibitors* of CYP2D6 (Fig. 6–15). There is a wide range of potency for 2D6 inhibition by the five SSRIs, with paroxetine and fluoxetine the most potent and fluvoxamine, sertraline, and citalopram the least potent.

One of the most important drug interactions that SSRIs can cause through inhibition of 2D6 is to raise plasma levels of tricyclic antidepressants (TCAs) if these TCAs are given concomitantly with SSRIs or if there is switching between TCAs and SSRIs. Since TCAs are substrates for 2D6 (Fig. 6–14) and SSRIs are inhibitors of 2D6 (Fig. 6–15), concomitant administration will raise TCA levels, perhaps to toxic levels (Fig. 6–16). Concomitant administration of an SSRI and a TCA thus

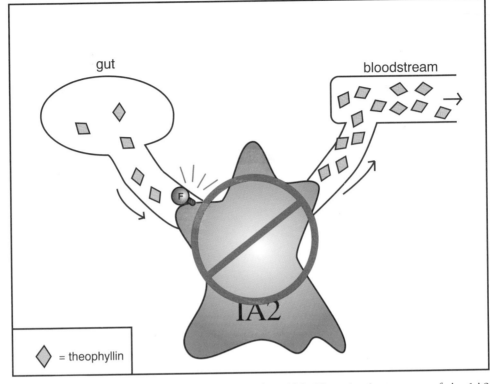

FIGURE 6–13. **Theophyllin** is a **substrate** for CYP450 1A2. Thus, in the presence of the 1A2 inhibitor **fluvoxamine**, theophyllin levels rise. The theophyllin dose must be lowered when it is given with fluvoxamine in order to avoid side effects.

requires monitoring of the plasma drug concentrations of the TCA and probably a reduction in its dose. CYP450 2D6 also interacts with atypical antipsychotics.

## CYP450 3A4

A third important CYP450 enzyme for antidepressants and mood stabilizers is 3A4. Some benzodiazepines (e.g., alprazolam and triazolam) are *substrates* for 3A4 (Fig. 6–17). Some antidepressants are 3A4 *inhibitors*, including the SSRIs fluoxetine and fluvoxamine and the antidepressant nefazodone (Fig. 6–18). Administration of a 3A4 substrate with a 3A4 inhibitor will raise the level of the substrate. For example, fluoxetine, fluvoxamine, or nefazodone will raise the levels of alprazolam or triazolam, requiring dose reduction of the benzodiazepine (Fig. 6–18).

Other nonpsychotropic drugs are also substrates (Fig. 6–17) or inhibitors of 3A4 (Fig. 6–18). It is important to understand the consequences of concomitant administration of psychotropic drugs that are either substrates or inhibitors of 3A4 with nonpsychotropic drugs that are also either substrates or inhibitors of 3A4. Notably, some 3A4 substrates such as cisapride, terfenidine, and astemazole must be metabolized, or else toxic levels of the drug can accumulate, with cardiovascular consequences such as prolonged QT interval and sudden death. Thus, they cannot be

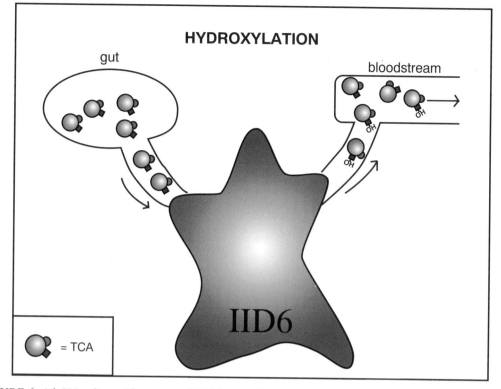

FIGURE 6–14. Tricyclic antidepressants (TCAs) are **substrates** for CYP450 **2D6**, which hydroxylates and thereby inactivates them.

given with a 3A4 inhibitor because of this potential danger, and use of fluoxetine, fluvoxamine, and nefazodone with such 3A4 substrates must be avoided. Changes in 3A4 activity also affect atypical antipsychotic drug levels.

### CYP450 Inducers

Finally, not only can drugs be substrates or inhibitors for CYP450 enzymes; they can also be *inducers*. An inducer increases the activity of the enzyme over time because it induces the synthesis of more copies of the enzyme. One example of this is the effects of the anticonvulsant and mood stabilizer carbamazepine, which induces 3A4 over time (Fig. 6–19). Another example of CYP450 enzyme induction is cigarette smoking, which induces 1A2 over time (Fig. 6–20). The consequence of such enzyme induction is that substrates for the induced enzyme will be more efficiently metabolized over time, and thus their levels in the plasma will fall. Doses of such substrate drugs may therefore need to be increased over time to compensate for this.

For example carbamazepine is both a substrate and an inducer of 3A4. Thus as treatment becomes chronic, 3A4 is induced and carbamazepine blood levels fall (Fig. 6–19). Failure to recognize this effect and to increase carbamazepine dosage to compensate for it may lead to a failure of anticonvulsant or mood-stabilizing efficacy, with breakthrough symptoms.

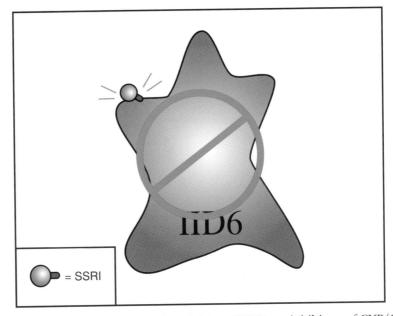

FIGURE 6–15. Some serotonin selective reuptake inhibitors (SSRIs) are **inhibitors** of CYP450 2D6. Fluoxetine and paroxetine are potent **inhibitors** of 2D6, and fluvoxamine, sertaline, and citalopram are weak inhibitors of 2D6.

Another important thing to remember about a CYP450 inducer is what happens if the inducer is stopped. Thus, if one stops smoking, 1A2 substrate levels will rise. If one stops carbamazepine, the plasma concentrations will rise for any concomitantly administered drug that is a 3A4 substrate.

An overview of some actions of antidepressants at various CYP450 enzyme systems is given in Table 6–2. This is not a comprehensive list, and the discussion here has only been at the conceptual level, leaving out many important details that the prescriber will need to know. In this rapidly evolving area of therapeutics, the only way to keep up is to continually consult updated standard reference materials on drug interactions and the specific dosing implications that such interactions cause. In summary (Table 6–3), many drug interactions require dosage adjustment of one of the drugs. A few combinations must be strictly avoided. Many drug interactions are statistically significant but not clinically significant. By following the principles outlined here, the skilled practitioner and antidepressant prescriber must learn whether any given drug interaction is clinically relevant.

## Classical Antidepressants: Monoamine Oxidase Inhibitors and Tricyclic Antidepressants

### Monoamine Oxidase Inhibitors

The first clincially effective antidepressants to be discovered were immediate inhibitors of the enzyme monoamine oxidase (MAO) (Table 6–4 and Figs. 5–15, 6–3, and 6–4). They were discovered by accident when an antituberculosis drug was

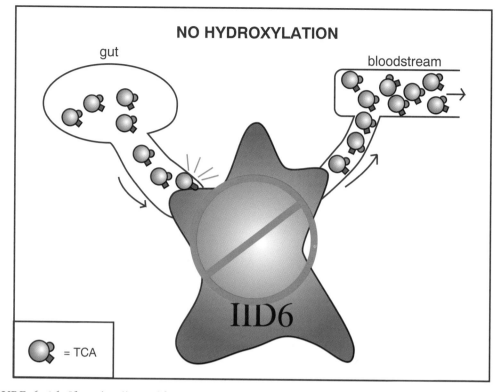

FIGURE 6–16. If a **tricyclic antidepressant** (TCA) is given together with a **serotonin selective reuptake inhibitor** (SSRI), the SSRI will prevent TCA metabolism. This causes TCA levels to increase, which can be toxic. Therefore either monitoring of TCA plasma concentration with dose reduction of the TCA, or avoidance of the combination, is required.

observed to help depression that coexisted in some of the tuberculosis patients. This antituberculosis drug, which was also an antidepressant, was soon discovered to inhibit the enzyme MAO. It was soon thereafter shown that inhibition of MAO was unrelated to its antitubercular actions but was the immediate biochemical event that caused its ultimate antidepressant actions. This discovery soon led to the synthesis of more drugs in the 1950s and 1960s that inhibited MAO but lacked unwanted additional properties, such as antituberculosis properties. Although best known as powerful antidepressants, the MAO inhibitors are also therapeutic agents for certain anxiety disorders, such as panic disorder and social phobia.

The original MAO inhibitors are all irreversible enzyme inhibitors, which bind to MAO irreversibly and destroy its function forever. Enzyme activity returns only after new enzyme is synthesized (see Figs. 5–15, 6–3 and 6–4). Sometimes such inhibitors are called "suicide inhibitors" because once the enzyme binds the inhibitor, the enzyme essentially commits suicide in that it can never function again until a new enzyme protein is synthesized by the neuron's DNA in the cell nucleus.

Monoamine oxidase exists in two subtypes, A and B. Both forms are inhibited by the original MAO inhibitors, which are therefore nonselective. The A form metabolizes the neurotransmitter monoamines most closely linked to depression (serotonin and norepinephrine).

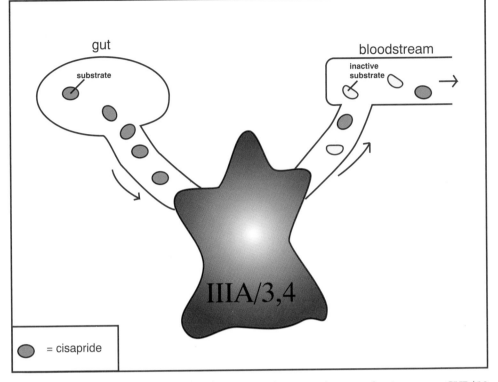

FIGURE 6–17. The benzodiazepines alprazolam and triazolam are **substrates** for the enzyme CYP450 3A4. The nonpsychotropic drugs cisapride and astemazole are also substrates for 3A4.

It thereby also metabolizes the amine most closely linked to control of blood pressure (norepinephrine). The B form is thought to convert some amine substrates, called protoxins, into toxins that may cause damage to neurons. Because of these observations, MAO A inhibition is linked both to antidepressant action and to the troublesome hypertensive side effects of the MAO inhibitors. Inhibition of MAO B is linked to prevention of neurodegenerative processes, such as those in Parkinson's disease.

Two developments have occurred with MAO inhibitors in recent years. One is the production of selective inhibitors of MAO A or of MAO B. The other advance is the production of selective MAO A inhibitors that are reversible. The implications of these advances are multiple. One of the most troublesome properties of the original nonselective, irreversible MAO inhibitors is the fact that after they inhibit MAO, amines taken in from the diet can cause dangerous elevations in blood pressure. Normally, such dietary amines are safely metabolized by MAO before they can cause blood pressure elevations (Figs. 6–21 and 6–22). However, when MAO A is inhibited, blood pressure can rise suddenly and dramatically and can even cause intracerebral hemorrhage and death after consumption of certain tyramine-containing foods or beverages (Fig. 6–23). This risk can be controlled by restricting the diet so that dangerous foods are eliminated and also restricting the simultaneous dangerous use of certain medications (e.g., the pain killer meperidine [Demerol]; the

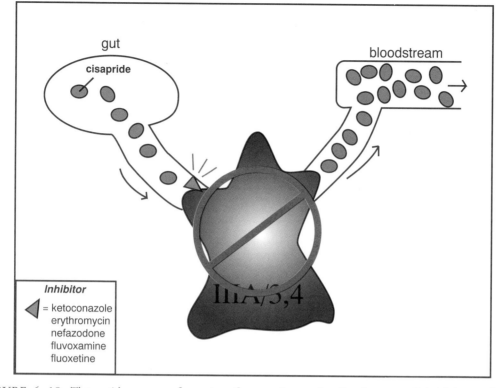

FIGURE 6–18. The antidepressants fluoxetine, fluvoxamine, and nefazodone are all **inhibitors** of CYP450 3A4. More potent inhibitors of this enzyme include the nonpsychotropic drugs ketoconazole, erythromycin, and protease inhibitors. If a 3A4 inhibitor is given with cisapride or astemazole, levels of these substrates can rise to toxic levels. Thus, fluoxetine, fluvoxamine, and nefazodone cannot be given with cisapride or astemazole.

serotonin selective reuptake inhibitors; sympathomimetic agents). The risk of hypertensive crisis and the hassle of restricting diet and medications have generally been the price that a patient has had to pay for the therapeutic benefits of the MAO inhibitors.

In the case of MAO B inhibitors, no significant amount of MAO A is inhibited, and there is very little risk of hypertension from dietary amines. Patients taking MAO B inhibitors to prevent progression of Parkinson's disease, for example, do not require any special diet. On the other hand, MAO B inhibitors are not effective antidepressants at doses that are selective for MAO B.

A newer class of MAO inhibitors, which has entered clinical practice for the treatment of depression, is known as reversible inhibitors of MAO A (RIMAs). This is a very welcome development in new drug therapeutics for depression, because it has the potential of making MAO A inhibition for the treatment of depression much safer. That is, the "suicide inhibitors" are associated with the dangerous hypertensive episodes mentioned above, which are caused when patients eat food rich in tyramine (such as cheese). This so-called cheese reaction occurs when the tyramine in the diet releases norepinephrine and other sympathomimetic amines (Fig. 5–23). When MAO is inhibited irreversibly, the levels of these amines rise to a dangerous level

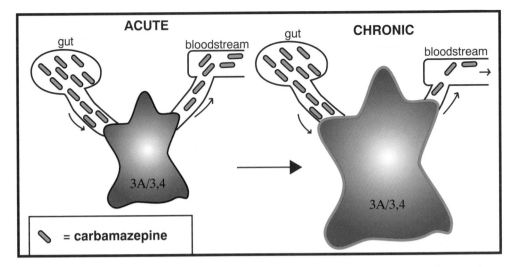

FIGURE 6–19. The anticonvulsant and mood stabilizer carbamazepine is a **substrate** for CYP450 3A4. It can also **induce** the metabolism of 3A4 by inducing more copies of the enzyme to be formed, thereby raising the enzyme activity of 3A4. Over time, therefore, carbamazepine doses may need to be increased to compensate for this increased metabolism.

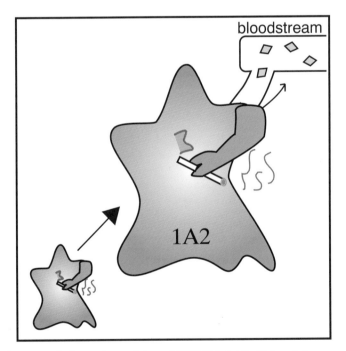

FIGURE 6–20. **Smoking** can **induce** the activity of CYP450 **1A2**. This might require that 1A2 substrates administered to a smoker be given in a higher dose. It may also require such 1A2 substrates to have their doses decreased if a smoker stops smoking.

Table 6–2. *Inhibition potential of antidepressants at CYP450 enzyme systems*

| Relative rank | 1A2 | 2C9/19 | 2D6 | 3A4 |
|---|---|---|---|---|
| High | fluvoxamine | fluvoxamine fluoxetine | paroxetine fluoxetine | fluvoxamine nefazodone fluoxetine |
| Moderate to low | tertiary TCAs fluoxetine paroxetine | sertraline fluoxetine | secondary TCAs | sertraline TCAs paroxetine |
| Low to minimal | venlafaxine bupropion citalopram reboxetine mirtazapine sertraline nefazodone | venlafaxine bupropion citalopram reboxetine mirtazapine nefazodone paroxetine | venlafaxine bupropion citalopram reboxetine mirtazapine sertraline nefazodone fluvoxamine | venlafaxine bupropion citalopram reboxetine mirtazapine |

Table 6–3. *Pharmacokinetics summary*

A few combinations must be avoided.
Several combinations require dosage adjustment of one of the drugs.
Many drug interactions are statistically significant but clinically insignificant.

Table 6–4. *Monoamine oxidase (MAO) inhibitors*

Classical MAO inhibitors—irreversible and nonselective
  phenelzine (Nardil)
  tranylcypromine (Parnate)
  isocarboxazid (Marplan)
Reversible inhibitors of MAO A (RIMAS)
  moclobemide (Aurorix)
Selective inhibitors of MAO B
  deprenyl (Selegiline; Eldepryl)

because they are not being destroyed by MAO. Blood pressure soars, even causing blood vessels to rupture in the brain.

Enter the reversible MAO inhibitors. If someone eats cheese, tyramine will still release sympathomimetic amines, but these amines will chase the reversible inhibitor off the MAO enzyme, allowing the dangerous amines to be destroyed (Fig. 6–24). This is sort of like having your cake—or cheese—and eating it, too. The reversible MAO inhibitors have the same therapeutic effects as the suicide inhibitors of MAO, but without the likelihood of a cheese reaction if a patient inadvertently takes in otherwise dangerous dietary tyramine.

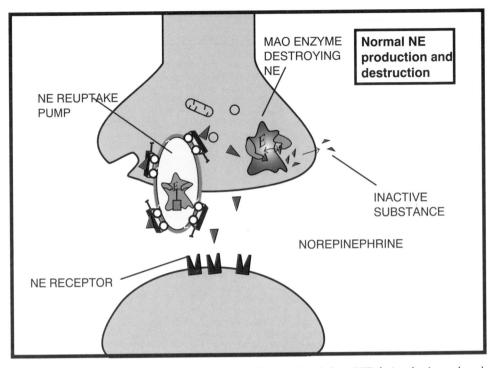

FIGURE 6–21. This figure shows the normal process of **norepinephrine (NE)** being both produced and **destroyed. Monoamine oxidase (MAO)** is the enzyme that normally acts to destroy NE to keep it in balance.

As MAO inhibitors have applications as second-line treatment for anxiety disorders, such as panic disorder and social phobia, in addition to depression, the RIMAs have the potential to make the treatment of these additional disorders by MAO A inhibition much safer as well.

In terms of the new MAO inhibitors that may become available in the future, it is possible that some new RIMAs may be approved as antidepressants. Moclobemide, available in many countries, is unlikely, for commercial reasons, to become available in the United States. Another promising RIMA, brofaramine, is also unlikely to be developed for any country. However, befloxatone is progressing in clinical trials, and other RIMAs are also potential drug development candidates, including RS-8359, cimoxatone, and toloxatone.

## Tricyclic Antidepressants

The tricyclic antidepressants (Table 6–5) were so named because their organic chemical structure contains three rings (Fig. 6–25). The tricyclic antidepressants were synthesized about the same time as other three-ringed molecules that were shown to be effective tranquilizers for schizophrenia (i.e., the early antipsychotic neuroleptic drugs such as chlorpromazine) (Fig. 6–26). The tricyclic antidepressants were a disappointment when tested as antipsychotics. Even though they have a three-ringed structure, they were not effective in the treatment of schizophrenia and were almost

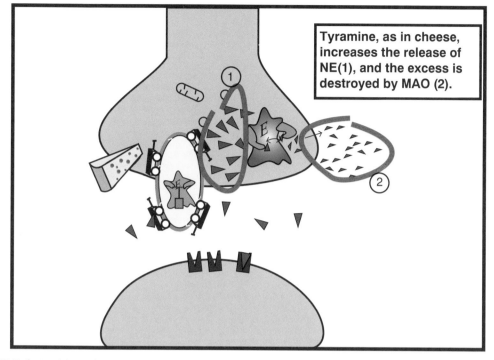

**Tyramine, as in cheese, increases the release of NE(1), and the excess is destroyed by MAO (2).**

FIGURE 6–22. **Tyramine** is an amine present in food such as **cheese**. Indicated in this figure is how tyramine (depicted as cheese) acts to **increase the release of norepinephrine (NE)** (red circle 1). However, in normal circumstances, the enzyme **monoamine oxidase (MAO) readily destroys the excess NE** released by tyramine, and no harm is done (see red circle 2).

discarded. However, during testing for schizophrenia, they were discovered to be antidepressants. That is, careful clinicians detected antidepressant properties, although not antipsychotic properties, in the schizophrenic patients. Thus, the antidepressant properties of the tricyclic antidepressants were serendipitously observed in the 1950s and 1960s, and eventually these compounds were marketed for the treatment of depression.

Long after their antidepressant properties were observed, the tricyclics were discovered to block the reuptake pumps for both serotonin and norepinephrine, and to a lesser extent, dopamine (Figs. 5–16, 6–5, and 6–6). Some tricyclics have more potency for inhibition of the serotonin reuptake pump (e.g., clomipramine); others are more selective for norepinephrine over serotonin (e.g., desipramine, maprotilene, nortriptyline, protriptyline). Most, however, block both serotonin and norepinephrine reuptake.

In addition, essentially all the tricyclic antidepressants have at least three other actions: blockade of muscarinic cholinergic receptors, blockade of H1 histamine receptors, and blockade of alpha 1 adrenergic receptors (Fig. 6–27). Whereas blockade of the serotonin and norepinephrine reuptake pumps is thought to account for the *therapeutic actions* of these drugs (Figs. 6–28 and 6–29), the other three pharmacologic properties are thought to account for their *side effects* (Figs. 6–30, 6–31, and

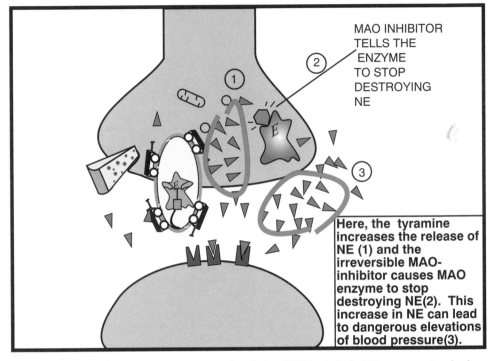

FIGURE 6–23. Here, tyramine is releasing norepinephrine (NE) (red circle 1) just as previously shown in Figure 6–9. However, this time **monoamine oxidase (MAO)** is also being **inhibited** by a typical, irreversible MAO inhibitor. This results in MAO **stopping its destruction of norepinephrine (NE)** (arrow 2). As already indicated in Figure 6–3, such MAO inhibition in itself causes **accumulation of NE**. However, when MAO inhibition is taking place in the presence of tyramine, the combination can lead to a very large accumulation of NE (red circle 3). Such a great NE accumulation can cause dangerous elevations of blood pressure.

6–32). Some of the tricyclic antidepressants also have the ability to block serotonin 2A receptors, which may contribute to the therapeutic actions of those agents with this property. Blockade of serotonin 2A receptors is discussed in Chapter 7. Tricyclic antidepressants also block sodium channels in the heart and brain, which can cause cardiac arrhythmias and cardiac arrest in overdose, as well as seizures.

In terms of the *therapeutic actions* of tricyclic antidepressants, they essentially work as allosteric modulators of the neurotransmitter reuptake process. Specifically, they are negative allosteric modulators. After the neurotransmitter norepinephrine or serotonin binds to its own selective receptor site, it is normally transported back into the presynaptic neuron as discussed in Chapter 5 (Fig. 5–16). However, when certain antidepressants bind to an allosteric site close to the neurotransmitter transporter, this causes the neurotransmitter to no longer be able to bind there, thus blocking synaptic reuptake of the neurotransmitter (Figs. 6–28 and 6–29). Therefore, norepinephrine and serotonin cannot be shuttled back into the presynaptic neuron.

In terms of side effects of the tricyclic antidepressants (Table 6–5), blockade of alpha 1 adrenergic receptors causes orthostatic hypotension and dizziness (Fig. 6–30). Anticholinergic actions at muscarinic cholinergic receptors cause dry mouth, blurred vision, urinary retention, and constipation and memory disturbances (Fig.

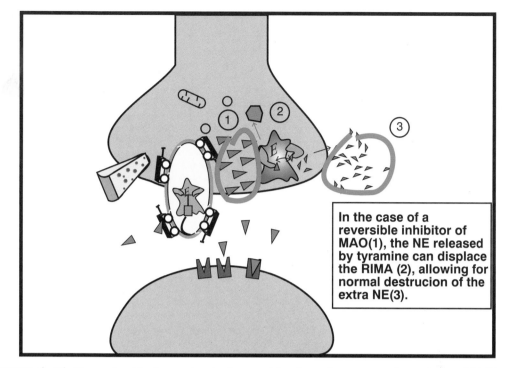

In the case of a reversible inhibitor of MAO(1), the NE released by tyramine can displace the RIMA (2), allowing for normal destrucion of the extra NE(3).

FIGURE 6–24. Shown in this figure also is the **combination of a monoamine oxidase (MAO) inhibitor and tyramine**. However, in this case the MAO inhibitor is of the **reversible** type (reversible inhibitor of MAO A, or **RIMA**). In contrast to the situation shown in the previous figure (Fig. 6–23), the accumulation of norepinephrine (NE) caused by tyramine (indicated in red circle 1) can actually strip the RIMA off MAO (arrow 2). MAO, now devoid of its inhibitor, can merrily do its job, which is to destroy the NE (red circle 3) and thus prevent the dangerous accumulation of NE. Such a reversal of MAO by NE is only possible with a RIMA and not with the classical MAO inhibitors, which are completely irreversible.

Table 6–5. *Tricyclic antidepressants*

clomipramine (Anafranil)
imipramine (Tofranil)
amitriptyline (Elavil; Endep; Tryptizol; Loroxyl)
nortriptyline (Pamelor; Noratren)
protriptyline (Vivactil)
maprotiline (Ludiomil)
amoxapine (Asendin)
doxepin (Sinequan; Adapin)
desipramine (Norpramin; Pertofran)
trimipramine (Surmontil)

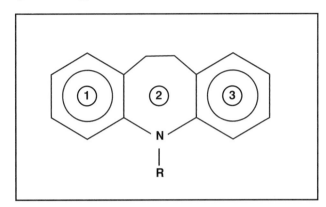

FIGURE 6–25. This is the **chemical structure of a tricyclic antidepressant (TCA)**. The three rings show how this group of drugs got its name.

6–31). Blockade of H1 histamine receptors causes sedation and weight gain (Fig. 6–32).

The term *tricyclic antidepressant* is archaic by today's pharmacology. First, the antidepressants that block biogenic amine reuptake are no longer all tricyclic; the new agents can have one, two, three, or four rings in their structures. Second, the tricyclic antidepressants are not merely antidepressant since some of them have anti-obsessive compulsive disorder effects and others have antipanic effects.

Like the MAO inhibitors, tricyclic antidepressants have fallen into second-line use for depression in North America and much of Europe. However, there still remains considerable use of these agents, and they are even among the most frequently prescribed antidepressants in certain countries, including Germany and countries in Latin America, as well as in the Third World, where generic pricing makes these agents less expensive than the newer antidepressants that are still under patent protection.

## Selective Serotonin Reuptake Inhibitors

### What Five Drugs Share in Common

The SSRIs comprise a class of drugs with five prominent members, which together account for the majority of prescriptions for antidepressants in the United States and several other countries. These are fluoxetine, sertraline, paroxetine, fluvoxamine, and citalopram (Table 6–6). Although each of these five SSRIs belongs to a chemically distinct family, all have a single major pharmacologic feature in common, namely, selective and potent inhibition of serotonin reuptake, which is more powerful than their actions on norepinephrine reuptake or on alpha 1, histamine 1, or muscarinic cholinergic receptors, and with virtually no ability to block sodium channels, even in overdose. This simple concept is shown in Figs. 6–33 and 6–34.

Thus, the SSRIs all share important differentiating features from the tricyclic antidepressants, which they have largely replaced in clinical practice. That is, SSRIs have more powerful and selective serotonin reuptake inhibiting properties than the tricyclic antidepressants. By removing undesirable pharmacologic properties of the

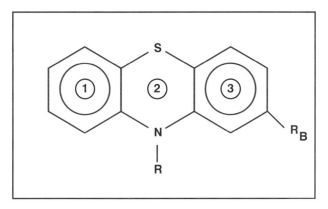

FIGURE 6–26. This is a general **chemical formula for the phenothiazine type of antipsychotic drugs**. These drugs also have three rings, and the first antidepressants were modeled after such drugs.

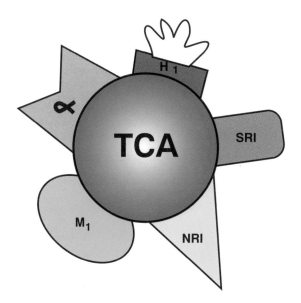

The **Tricyclic Antidepressant** has five actions: blocking the reuptake of serotonin, blocking the reuptake of norepinephrine, blockade of alpha 1 adrenergic receptors, blockade of H1 histamine receptors, and blockade of muscarinic cholinergic receptors.

FIGURE 6–27. Shown here is an icon of a **tricyclic antidepressant (TCA)**. These drugs are actually **five drugs in one:** (1) a serotonin reuptake inhibitor (SRI); (2) a norepinephrine reuptake inhibitor (NRI); (3) an anticholinergic/antimuscarinic drug (M1); (4) an alpha adrenergic antagonist (alpha); and (5) an antihistamine (H1).

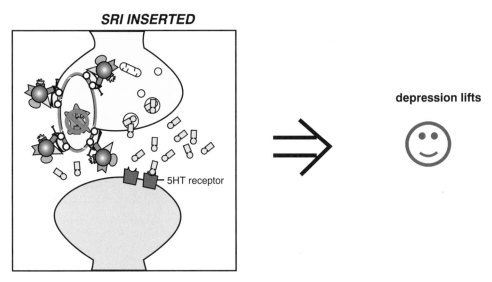

FIGURE 6–28. *Therapeutic actions of the tricyclic antidepressants*—**part 1.** In this diagram, the icon of the **TCA** is shown with its serotonin reuptake inhibitor (**SRI**) portion inserted into the serotonin reuptake pump, blocking it and causing an **antidepressant effect**.

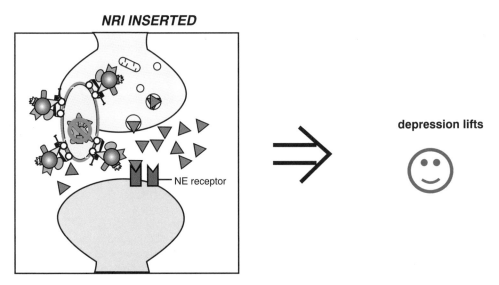

FIGURE 6–29. *Therapeutic actions of the tricyclic antidepressants*—**part 2.** In this diagram, the icon of the **TCA** is shown with its norepinephrine reuptake inhibitor (**NRI**) portion inserted into the norepinephrine reuptake pump, blocking it and causing an **antidepressant effect**. Thus, both the serotonin reuptake portion (see Fig. 6–28) and the NRI portion of the TCA act pharmacologically to cause an antidepressant effect.

224

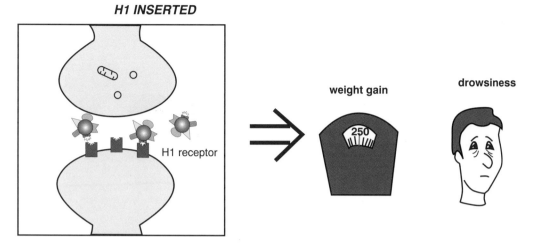

FIGURE 6–30. *Side effects of the tricyclic antidepressants*—part 1. In this diagram, the icon of the **TCA** is shown with its antihistamine (**H1**) portion inserted into histamine receptors, causing the side effects of **weight gain and drowsiness**.

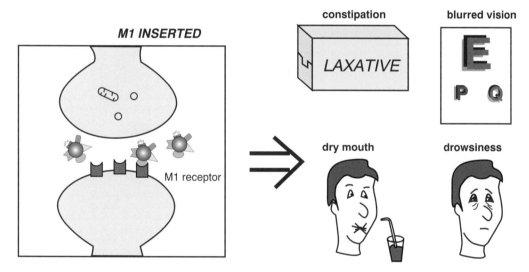

FIGURE 6–31. *Side effects of the tricyclic antidepressants*—part 2. In this diagram, the icon of the **TCA** is shown with its anticholinergic/antimuscarinic (**M1**) portion inserted into acetylcholine receptors, causing the side effects of **constipation, blurred vision, dry mouth, and drowsiness**.

tricyclics, the SSRIs also eliminated the undesirable side effects associated with them (Figs. 6–30 to 6–32). In particular, SSRIs lack the danger in overdose that the tricyclics all share. Whereas a 15-day supply of a tricyclic antidepressant can be a lethal dose, SSRIs, by contrast, rarely if ever cause death in overdose by themselves.

## *Pharmacologic and Molecular Mechanism of Action of the SSRIs*

Although the action of SSRIs at the *presynaptic axon terminal* has classically been emphasized (Figs. 6–1 through 6–6), research has more recently determined that

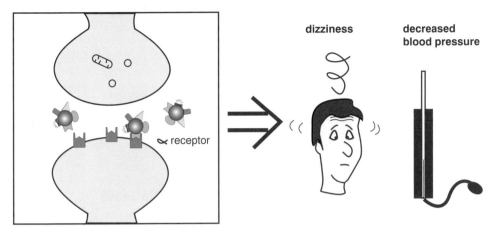

FIGURE 6–32. *Side effects of the tricyclic antidepressants*—part 3. In this diagram, the icon of the **TCA** is shown with its alpha adrenergic antagonist (alpha) portion inserted into alpha adrenergic receptors, causing the side effects of **dizziness, decreased blood pressure, and drowsiness**.

Table 6–6. *Serotonin selective reuptake inhibitors (SSRIs)*

| |
|---|
| fluoxetine (Prozac) |
| sertraline (Zoloft) |
| paroxetine (Paxil) |
| fluvoxamine (Luvox, Feverin, Dumirox, Floxyfral) |
| citalopram (Celexa, Cipramil, Serostat, Cipram) |

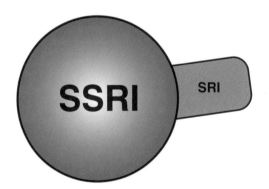

FIGURE 6–33. Shown here is the icon of a selective **serotonin** reuptake inhibitor (**SSRI**). In this case, four of the five pharmacological properties of the tricyclic antidepressants (**TCAs**) (Fig. 6–27) were removed. Only the serotonin reuptake inhibitor (**SRI**) portion remains; thus the SRI action is selective, which is why these agents are called **selective SRIs**.

## SSRI ACTION

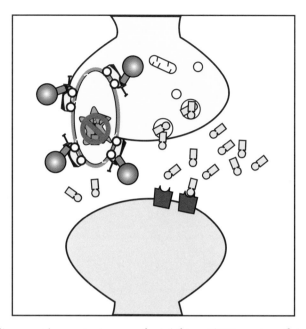

FIGURE 6–34. In this diagram, the serotonin reuptake inhibitor (**SRI**) portion of the **SSRI** molecule is shown inserted into the serotonin reuptake pump, blocking it and causing an **antidepressant effect**. This is analogous to one of the dimensions of the tricyclic antidepressants (TCAs), already shown in Figure 6–28.

events occurring at the *somatodendritic* end of the serotonin neuron (near the cell body) may be more important in explaining their therapeutic actions (Figs. 6–35 through 6–38). It may be that the events occurring at postsynaptic serotonin neurons mediate the acute side effects and the development of tolerance to these side effects over time (Fig. 6–39).

The monoamine hypothesis of depression states that in the depressed state (Fig. 6–35), serotonin may be deficient, both at presynaptic somatodendritic areas near the cell body and in the synapse itself near the axon terminal. Neuronal firing rates may be diminished. Also, the neurotransmitter receptor hypothesis states that pre- and postsynaptic receptors may be up-regulated. The monoamine hypothesis of delayed gene action suggests that these receptors may not be able to transduce receptor occupancy by serotonin into the necessary regulation of postsynaptic genes, such as those for the neurotrophic factor BDNF (see Figs. 5–63 and 6–7). These ideas are shown in Figure 6–35 and may be the starting point for the serotonin neuron and its targets when SSRIs are first administered to a depressed patient. On the other hand, it is also possible that the serotonin neuron is actually normal but that the events triggered by SSRIs compensate for neurochemical deficiencies elsewhere in the brain.

When an SSRI is given acutely, serotonin rises owing to blockade of its transport pump. What was surprising to discover, however, is that blocking the presynaptic reuptake pump does *not* immediately lead to a great deal of serotonin in the synapse.

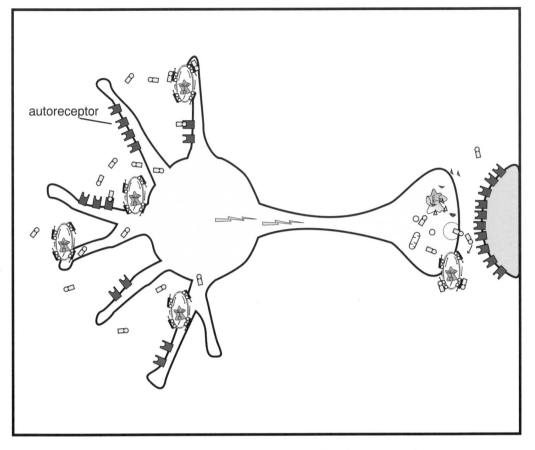

*Depressed State: Low 5HT, up-regulated receptors, low amount*
*of signals in the neuron to release more 5HT*

FIGURE 6–35. *Mechanism of action of serotonin selective reuptake inhibitors (SSRIs)—part 1.*
Depicted here is a **serotonin neuron in a depressed patient**. In depression, the serotonin neuron is
conceptualized as having a relative **deficiency of the neurotransmitter serotonin**. Also, the number
of **serotonin receptors** is **up-regulated**, or increased, including presynaptic **autoreceptors** as well
as **postsynaptic receptors**.

In fact, when SSRI treatment is initiated, 5HT rises to a much higher level at the
cell body area in the midbrain raphe than in the areas of the brain where the axons
terminate (Fig. 6–36). The somatodendritic area of the serotonin neuron is where
the serotonin (5HT) first increases, and the serotonin receptors there have 5HT1A
pharmacology. Such immediate pharmacologic actions obviously cannot explain the
delayed therapeutic actions of the SSRIs. However, these immediate actions may
explain the side effects that are caused by the SSRIs when treatment is initiated.

Over time, the increased 5HT at the somatodendritic 5HT1A autoreceptors causes
them to down-regulate and become desensitized (Fig. 6–37). When the increase in
serotonin is recognized by these presynaptic 5HT1A receptors, this information is
sent to the cell nucleus of the serotonin neuron. The genome's reaction to this
information is to issue instructions that cause these same receptors to become de-

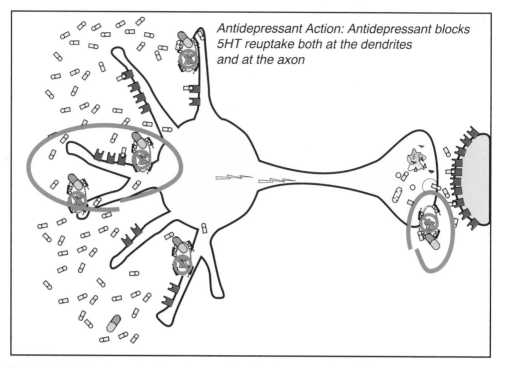

FIGURE 6–36. *Mechanism of action of serotonin selective reuptake inhibitors (SSRIs)*—part 2. When an SSRI is administered, it immediately blocks the serotonin reuptake pump (see icon of an SSRI drug capsule blocking the reuptake pump). However, this causes **serotonin to increase initially only in the somatodendritic area** of the serotonin neuron (left) and not in the axon terminals (right).

sensitized over time. The time course of this desensitization correlates with the onset of the therapeutic actions of the SSRIs.

Once the 5HT1A somatodendritic autoreceptors are desensitized, 5HT can no longer effectively inhibit its own release, and the serotonin neuron is therefore disinhibited. This results in a flurry of 5HT release from axons due to an increase in neuronal impulse flow (Fig. 6–38). This is just another way of saying that the serotonin release is "turned on" at the axon terminals. The serotonin that now pours out of the various projections of serotonin pathways in the brain theoretically mediates the various therapeutic actions of the SSRIs.

While the presynaptic somatodendritic 5HT1A autoreceptors are desensitizing, serotonin is building up in synapses, causing the postsynaptic serotonin receptors to desensitize as well. This happens because the increase in synaptic serotonin is recognized by postsynaptic serotonin 2A, 2C, 3, and other receptors. These receptors in turn send this information to the cell nucleus of the *postsynaptic* neuron that serotonin is targeting. The reaction of the genome in the postsynaptic neuron is also to issue instructions to down-regulate or desensitize these receptors. The time course of this desensitization correlates with the onset of tolerance to the side effects of the SSRIs (Fig. 6–39).

This theory thus suggests a pharmacological cascading mechanism, whereby the SSRIs exert their therapeutic actions, namely, powerful disinhibition of serotonin

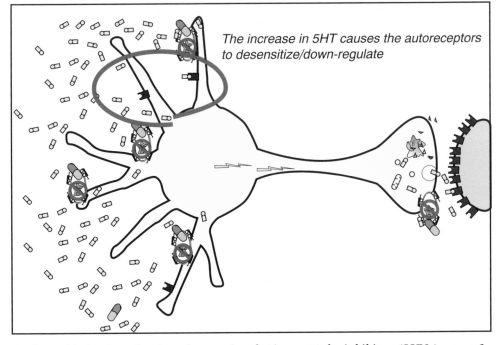

The increase in 5HT causes the autoreceptors to desensitize/down-regulate

FIGURE 6–37. *Mechanism of action of serotonin selective reuptake inhibitors (SSRIs)—*part 3. The consequence of serotonin increasing in the somatodentritic area of the serotonin neuron, as depicted in the Figure 6–36, is to cause the **somatodendritic serotonin 1A autoreceptors to desensitize or down-regulate** (red circle).

release in key pathways throughout the brain. Furthermore, side effects are hypothetically caused by the acute actions of serotonin at undesirable receptors in undesirable pathways. Finally, side effects may attenuate over time by desensitization of the very receptors that mediate them.

There are potentially exciting corollaries to this hypothesis. First, if the ultimate increase in serotonin at critical synapses is required for therapeutic actions, then its failure to occur may explain why some patients respond to an SSRI and others do not. Also, if new drugs could be designed to increase serotonin at the right places at a faster rate, it could result in a much needed rapid-acting antidepressant. Such ideas are mere research hypotheses at this time but could lead to additional studies clarifying the molecular events that are key mediators of depressive illness as well as of antidepressant treatment responses.

### Serotonin Pathways and Receptors That Mediate Therapeutic Actions and Side Effects of SSRIs

As mentioned above, the SSRIs cause both their therapeutic actions and their side effects by increasing serotonin at synapses, where reuptake is blocked and serotonin release is disinhibited. In general, increasing serotonin in desirable pathways and at targeted receptor subtypes leads to the well-known therapeutic actions of these drugs. However, since SSRIs increase serotonin in virtually every serotonin pathway

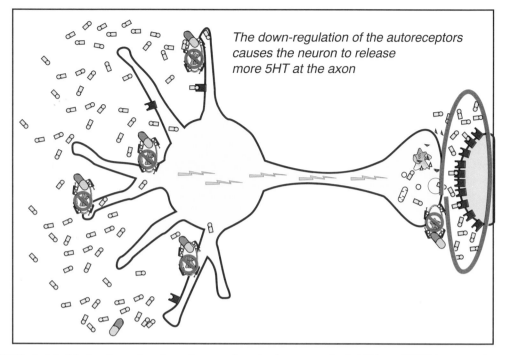

FIGURE 6–38. *Mechanism of action of serotonin selective reuptake inhibitors (SSRIs)*—part 4. Once the somatodendritic autoreceptors down-regulate as depicted in Figure 6–37, there is no longer inhibition of impulse flow in the serotonin neuron. Thus, **neuronal impulse flow is turned on**. The consequence of this is **release of serotonin in the axon terminal** (red circle). However, **this increase is delayed** as compared with the increase of serotonin in the somatodendritic areas of the serotonin neuron, depicted in Figure 6–36. This delay is the result of the time it takes for somatodendritic serotonin to down-regulate the serotonin 1A autoreceptors and turn on neuronal impulse flow in the serotonin neuron. This delay may explain why antidepressants do not relieve depression immediately. It is also the reason why the mechanism of action of antidepressants may be linked to increasing neuronal impulse flow in serotonin neurons, with serotonin levels increasing at axon terminals before an SSRI can exert its antidepressant effects.

and at virtually every serotonin receptor, some of these serotonin actions are undesirable and therefore account for side effects. By understanding the functions of the various serotonin pathways and the distribution of the various serotonin receptor subtypes, it is possible to gain insight into both the therapeutic actions and the side effects that the SSRIs share as a class.

In terms of antidepressant actions, evidence points to the projection of serotonin neurons from the midbrain raphe to frontal cortex as the substrate of this therapeutic action (Fig. 5–51). Therapeutic actions in bulimia, binge eating, and various other eating disorders may be mediated by serotonin's pathway from raphe to hypothalamic feeding and appetite centers (Fig. 5–55).

Because different pathways seem to mediate the different therapeutic actions of SSRIs, it would not be surprising if serotonin's therapeutic roles differed from one therapeutic indication to another. This, indeed, seems to be the case and may be the basis for the different therapeutic profiles of SSRIs from one therapeutic indication to another. Contrasting antidepressant and antibulimic actions, for example, are in-

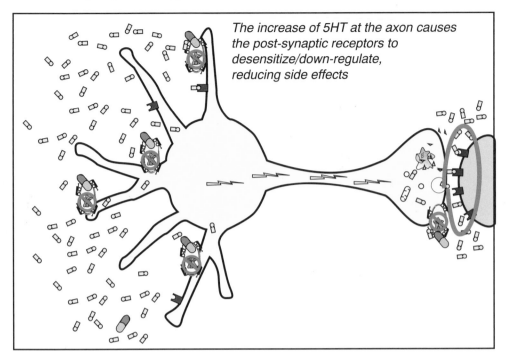

*The increase of 5HT at the axon causes the post-synaptic receptors to desensitize/down-regulate, reducing side effects*

FIGURE 6–39. *Mechanism of action of serotonin selective reuptake inhibitors (SSRIs)*—part 5. Finally, once the SSRIs have blocked the reuptake pump (Fig. 6–36), increased somatodendritic serotonin (Fig. 6–36), desensitized somatodendritic serotonin 1A autoreceptors (Fig. 6–37), turned on neuronal impulse flow (Fig. 6–38), and increased release of serotonin from axon terminals (Fig. 6–38), the final step shown here may be the desensitization of postsynaptic serotonin receptors. This has also been shown in previous figures demonstrating the actions of monoamine oxidase (MAO) inhibitors (Fig. 6–4) and the actions of tricyclic antidepressants (Fig. 6–6). This desensitization may mediate the reduction of side effects of SSRIs as tolerance develops.

Table 6–7. *Antidepressant profile of SSRIs*

| |
| --- |
| Starting dose usually the same as the maintenance dose |
| Onset of response usually 3 to 8 weeks |
| Response is frequently complete remission of symptoms |
| Target symptoms do not worsen when treatment initiated |

dicated by differing doses, onsets of action, and documentation of long-term actions, as summarized in Tables 6–7 and 6–8.

In terms of side effects of SSRIs, acute stimulation of at least four serotonin receptor subtypes may be responsible for mediating these undesirable actions. These include the 5HT2A, 5HT2C, 5HT3, and 5HT4 receptors. Since SSRI side effects are generally acute, starting from the first dose and if anything attenuate over time, it may be that the acute increase in synaptic serotonin is sufficient to mediate side effects but insufficient to mediate therapeutic effects until the much more robust disinhibition of the neuron "kicks in" once autoreceptors are down regulated. If the

Table 6–8. *Antibulimic profile of SSRIs*

| |
|---|
| Usual starting dose is higher than for other indications |
| Onset of response may be faster than for other indications |
| May not be as effective as for other indications in maintaining acute effects chronically |
| Fluoxetine has best efficacy data to date and also serotonin 2C properties |
| Target symptoms do not worsen on initiation of treatment |

postsynaptic receptors that theoretically mediate side effects down regulate or de-sensitize, the side effects attenuate or go away. Presumably, the signal of receptor occupancy of serotonin to the postsynaptic receptor is detected by the genome of the target neuron, and decreasing the genetic expression of these receptors that mediate the side effects causes the side effects to go away.

The undesirable side effects of SSRIs seem to involve not only specific serotonin receptor subtypes but also the action of serotonin at the receptors in specific areas of the body, including brain, spinal cord, and gut. The topography of serotonin receptor subtypes in different serotonin pathways may thus help to explain how side effects are mediated. Thus, acute stimulation of serotonin 2A and 2C receptors in the projection from raphe to limbic cortex may cause the acute mental agitation, anxiety, or induction of panic attacks that can be observed with early dosing of an SSRI (Fig. 5–54). Acute stimulation of the 2A receptors in the basal ganglia may lead to changes in motor movements due to serotonin's inhibition of dopamine neurotransmission there (Fig. 5–53). Thus, akathisia (restlessness), psychomotor re-tardation, or even mild parkinsonism and dystonic movements can result. Stimula-tion of serotonin 2A receptors in the brainstem sleep centers may cause rapid muscle movements called *myoclonus* during the night; it may also disrupt slow-wave sleep and cause nocturnal awakenings (Fig. 5–56). Stimulation of serotonin 2A receptors in the spinal cord may inhibit the spinal reflexes of orgasm and ejaculation and cause sexual dysfunction (Fig. 5–57). Stimulation of serotonin 2A receptors in mesocortical pleasure centers may reduce dopamine activity there and cause apathy (e.g., apathetic recoveries discussed in Chapter 5; see Table 5–18) or decreased libido.

Stimulation of serotonin 3 receptors in the hypothalamus or brainstem may cause nausea or vomiting, respectively (Fig. 5–58). Stimulation of serotonin 3 and 4 re-ceptors in the gastrointestinal tract may cause increased bowel motility, gastrointes-tinal cramps and diarrhea (Fig. 5–59).

Thus, virtually all side effects of the SSRIs can be understood as undesirable actions of serotonin in undesirable pathways at undesirable receptor subtypes. This appears to be the "cost of doing business," as it is not possible for a systemically administered SSRI to act only at the desirable receptors in the desirable places; it must act everywhere it is distributed, which means all over the brain and all over the body. Fortunately, SSRI side effects are more of a nuisance than a danger, and they generally attenuate over time, although they can cause an important subset of patients to discontinue an SSRI prematurely.

Although several SSRIs other than the five listed in Table 6–6 have been syn-thesized, with the exception of the active enantiomers of currently marketed SSRIs such as fluoxetine and citalopram, it is unlikely any new SSRI will be developed as an antidepressant, as many other novel mechanisms are now available for clinical testing. Extended-release formulations of currently marketed SSRIs such as paroxe-tine and fluvoxamine may also become available. One novel and distinct mechanism related to the SSRIs is exemplified by tianeptine. This agent is in clinical testing and available in France as a counterintuitive serotonin reuptake *enhancer*. Whether this will develop into a well-documented antidepressant worldwide is still unknown.

### Not-So-Selective Serotonin Reuptake Inhibitors: Five Unique Drugs or One Class with Five Members?

Although the SSRIs clearly share the same mechanism of action, therapeutic profiles, and overall side effect profiles, individual patients often react very differently to one SSRI versus another. This is not generally observed in large clinical trials, where group differences between two SSRIs either in efficacy or in side effects are very difficult to document. Rather, such differences are seen by prescribers treating pa-tients one at a time, with some patients experiencing a therapeutic response to one SSRI and not another and other patients tolerating one SSRI but not another.

Although there is no generally accepted explanation that accounts for these com-monly observed clinical phenomena, it makes sense to consider the pharmacologic characteristics of the five SSRIs that differ one from another as candidates for ex-plaining the broad range of individual patient reactions to different SSRIs. Now that the SSRIs have been in widespread clinical use for over a decade, pharmacolo-gists have discovered that these five drugs have actions at receptors other than the serotonin transporter and at various enzymes that may be important to their overall actions, both therapeutically and in terms of tolerability.

The reality is that one or another of the SSRIs has pharmacologic actions within one or two orders of magnitude of their potencies for serotonin reuptake inhibition at a wide variety of receptors and enzymes. Furthermore, no two SSRIs have identical secondary pharmacological characteristics. These actions can include norepinephrine reuptake blockade, dopamine reuptake blockade, serotonin 2C agonist actions, mus-carinic cholinergic antagonist actions, interaction with the sigma receptor, inhibition of the enzyme nitric oxide synthetase, and inhibition of the cytochrome P450 en-zymes 1A2, 2D6, and 3A4 (Fig. 6–40). Whether these secondary binding profiles can account for the differences in efficacy and tolerability in individual patients remains to be proved. However, it does lead to provocative hypothesis generation and gives a rational basis for physicians not to be denied access to one or another of the SSRIs by payors claiming "they are all the same."

The candidate secondary pharmacologic mechanisms for each of the five SSRIs are shown in Figures 6–41 to 6–45. These may lead to variations from one drug to another that could prove potentially more advantageous or less advantageous for different patient profiles. However, these are hypotheses that as yet are unconfirmed. Nevertheless, there are real differences among the five SSRIs for many individual patients, and sometimes only an empirical trial of different SSRIs will lead to the best match of a drug to an individual patient.

### Selective Noradrenergic Reuptake Inhibitors

Although some tricyclic antidepressants (e.g., desipramine, maprotilene) block nor-epinephrine reuptake more potently than serotonin reuptake, even these tricyclics

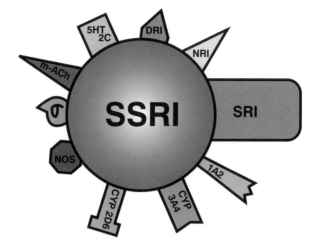

FIGURE 6–40. Icon of various **secondary pharmacologic properties** that may be associated with one or more of the five different **SSRIs**. This includes not only serotonin reuptake inhibition (SRI), but also lesser degrees of actions at other neurotransmitter receptors and enzymes, including norepinephrine reuptake inhibition (NRI), dopamine reuptake inhibition (DRI), serotonin 2C agonist actions (5HT2C), muscarinic/cholinergic antagonist actions (m-ACH), sigma actions (sigma), and inhibition of nitric oxide synthetase (NOS), CYP450 2D6, 3A4, or 1A2.

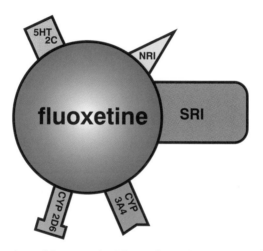

FIGURE 6–41. Icon of **fluoxetine** with serotonin 2C agonist action, norepinephrine reuptake inhibition (NRI), and 2D6 and 3A4 inhibition, in addition to serotonin reuptake inhibition (SRI).

are not really selective, since they still block alpha 1, histamine 1, and muscarinic cholinergic receptors, as do all tricyclics. The first truly selective noradrenergic reuptake inhibitor (NRI) is reboxetine, which lacks these undesirable binding properties (Figs. 6–46 and 6–47).

Thus, reboxetine is the logical pharmacological complement to the SSRIs—since it provides selective *noradrenergic* reuptake inhibition greater than serotonin reuptake inhibition but without the undesirable binding properties of the tricyclic antidepressants. The discovery of reboxetine has given rise to the questions: What is the

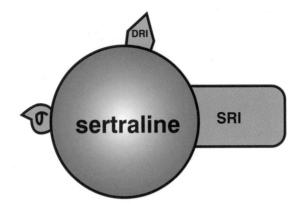

FIGURE 6–42. Icon of **sertraline** with dopamine reuptake inhibition (DRI) and sigma actions, in addition to serotonin reuptake inhibition (SRI).

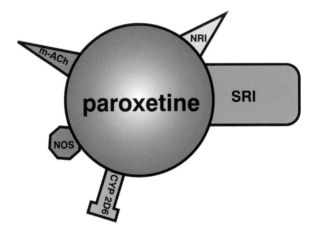

FIGURE 6–43. Icon of **paroxetine** with muscarinic/cholinergic antagonist actions (mACH), norepinephrine reuptake inhibition (NRI), and serotonin 2D6 and 3A4 inhibition, in addition to serotonin reuptake inhibition (SRI).

clinical difference between increasing noradrenergic neurotransmission and increasing serotonergic neurotransmission? Since norepinephrine and serotonin are intimately interrelated, does it make any difference which reuptake pump is inhibited?

Although norepinephrine and serotonin have overlapping functions in the regulation of mood, the hypothetical noradrenaline deficiency syndrome is not identical to the hypothetical serotonin deficiency syndrome (Tables 5–21 and 5–23). Furthermore, not all patients with depression respond to an SSRI nor do all respond to a selective NRI, although more may respond to agents or combinations of agents that block both serotonin and norepinephrine reuptake. Moreover, many patients who respond to serotonin reuptake blockers do not remit completely and seem to have improved mood but an enduring noradrenergic deficiency syndrome, which is sometimes called an apathetic response to the SSRI (e.g., Table 5–18).

Although it is not yet possible to determine who will respond to a serotonergic agent and who to a noradrenergic agent prior to empirical treatment, there is the

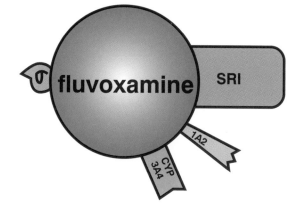

FIGURE 6–44. Icon of **fluvoxamine** with sigma actions and serotonin 1A2 and 3A4 inhibition, in addition to serotonin reuptake inhibition (SRI).

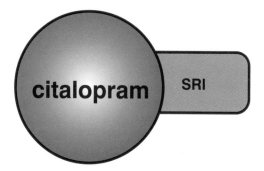

FIGURE 6–45. Icon of **citalopram**, relatively selective for serotonin reuptake inhibition (SRI).

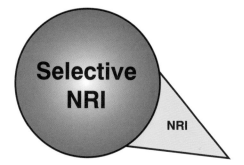

FIGURE 6–46. Icon of a **selective norepinephrine reuptake inhibitor** (NRI).

notion that those with the serotonin deficiency syndrome (i.e., depression associated with anxiety, panic, phobias, posttraumatic stress disorder, obsessions, compulsions, or eating disorders) might be more responsive to serotonergic antidepressants. This is supported by the fact that serotonergic antidepressants are efficacious not only in depression but also in obsessive-compulsive disorder, eating disorders, panic, social phobia, and even posttraumatic stress disorder, whereas noradrenergic antidepressants

## *Selective NRI ACTION*

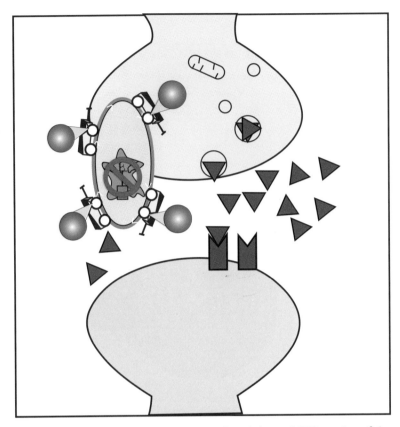

FIGURE 6–47. In this diagram, the norepinephrine reuptake inhibitor (**NRI**) portion of the selective NRI molecule is shown inserted in the norepinephrine reuptake pump, blocking it and causing an **antidepressant effect**.

are not well documented to improve generalized anxiety, panic, phobias, obsessive-compulsive disorder, or eating disorders.

On the other hand, patients with the noradrenergic deficiency syndrome (i.e., those whose depression is associated with fatigue, apathy, and notable cognitive disturbances, particularly impaired concentration, problems with sustaining and focusing attention, slowness in information processing, and deficiencies in working memory) may theoretically be more responsive to noradrenergic agents. Since the selective noradrenergic reuptake inhibitors have only recently become available, this theory is based on animal research. Confirmation of the usefulness of this approach in clinical practice awaits the results of ongoing research. Nevertheless, just as the SSRIs, first introduced for the treatment of depression, expanded their therapeutic uses to a host of anxiety disorders and other applications, so will the selective NRIs undoubtedly expand their therapeutic uses beyond the treatment of depression. For example, other theoretical considerations from preclinical work suggest that norad-

Table 6–9. *Potential therapeutic profile of reboxetine*

Depression
Fatigue
Apathy
Psychomotor retardation
Attention deficit and impaired concentration
Disorders (not limited to depression) characterized by cognitive slowing, especially
    deficiencies in working memory and in the speed of information processing

renergic enhancement should improve overall social functioning and work capacity by targeting psychomotor retardation, fatique, and apathy (Table 6–9). Noradrenergic enhancement might even boost cognitive functioning in disorders other than depression that are characterized by deficits in attention and memory, such as Alzheimer's disease, attention deficit disorder, and the cognitive disturbances associated with schizophrenia (Table 6–9).

Early indications from the use of reboxetine show that its efficacy is at least comparable to that of the tricyclic antidepressants and the SSRIs. In addition, reboxetine may specifically enhance social functioning, perhaps by converting apathetic responders into full remitters. Furthermore, reboxetine may be useful for severe depression, for depression unresponsive to other antidepressants, and as an adjunct to serotonergic antidepressants when dual neurotransmitter mechanisms are necessary to treat the most difficult cases.

Several specific noradrenergic pathways and receptors mediate both the therapeutic actions and the side effects of selective noradrenergic reuptake inhibitors (NRIs). As discussed above for the SSRIs, an analogous set of actions by norepinephrine in various noradrenergic pathways and at various noradrenergic receptors throughout the brain and the body may explain both the therapeutic actions and the side effects of the selective NRIs. That is, increasing norepinephrine at desirable synapses and at desirable noradrenergic receptors would lead to the therapeutic properties of the selective NRIs. Side effects would be due to increasing norepinephrine at undesirable places at the "cost of doing business," since selective NRIs increase norepinephrine in virtually every noradrenergic pathway and at virtually every noradrenergic receptor. By understanding the functions of the various norepinephrine pathways and the distribution of the various noradrenergic receptor subtypes, it is possible to gain insight into both the therapeutic actions and the side effects of the selective NRIs, such as reboxetine (Fig. 5–23).

In terms of antidepressant actions, evidence points to the projection of noradrenergic neurons from the locus coeruleus to the frontal cortex as the substrate of this therapeutic action (Fig. 5–24). The noradrenergic receptor subtype that may mediate norepinephrine's antidepressant actions there is the beta 1 postsynaptic receptor. Therapeutic actions in cognition are not yet established but could theoretically be mediated by norepinephrine's pathway from the locus coeruleus to other areas of the frontal cortex (Fig. 5–25). Postsynaptic receptors thought to mediate cognitive actions of norepinephrine in animal models are especially the alpha 2 noradrenergic receptor subtype. Therapeutic actions in improving apathy, fatigue, and psychomotor retardation could theoretically be mediated by the noradrenergic pathway from the locus coeruleus to the limbic cortex (Fig. 5–26).

Experience with the SSRIs predicts that as therapeutic actions of selective NRIs expand beyond antidepressant actions, the doses of drug, onsets of action, degrees of efficacy, and tolerability profiles may differ from one therapeutic use to another (Table 6–7 and 6–8).

In terms of side effects of the selective NRIs, acute stimulation of at least four clinically important noradrenergic receptor subtypes in various parts of the brain and body may be responsible for mediating these undesirable actions. This includes alpha 1 postsynaptic receptors, alpha 2 presynaptic receptors, alpha 2 postsynaptic receptors, and beta 1 postsynaptic noradrenergic receptors. As with the SSRIs, the side effects of selective NRIs are generally acute, starting from the first dose and if anything, attenuate over time. If the receptors that mediate side effects down regulate or desensitize, the side effects attenuate or go away.

Side effects of selective NRIs seem to involve not only specific noradrenergic receptor subtypes but also the action of norepinephrine at its receptors in specific areas of the body, including brain, spinal cord, heart, gastrointestinal tract, and urinary bladder. The topography of noradrenergic receptor subtypes in different norepinephrine pathways may thus help to explain how such side effects are mediated (Fig. 5–23). Thus, acute stimulation of beta 1 receptors in the cerebellum or peripheral sympathetic nervous system may cause motor activation or tremor (Fig. 5–27). Acute stimulation of noradrenergic receptors in the limbic system may cause agitation (Fig. 5–26). Acute stimulation of noradrenergic receptors in the brainstem cardiovascular centers and descending into the spinal cord may alter blood pressure (Fig. 5–28).

Stimulation of beta 1 noradrenergic receptors in the heart may cause changes in heart rate (Fig. 5–29). Stimulation of noradrenergic receptors in the sympathetic nervous system may also cause a net reduction of parasympathetic cholinergic tone, since these systems often have reciprocal roles in peripheral organs and tissues. Thus, increased norepinephrine may produce symptoms reminiscent of anticholinergic side effects. This is not due to direct blockade of muscarinic cholinergic receptors but to indirect reduction of net parasympathetic tone resulting from increased sympathetic tone. Thus, a "pseudo-anticholinergic" syndrome of dry mouth, constipation, and urinary retention (Fig. 5–30) may be caused by selective NRIs, even though they have no direct actions on cholinergic receptors. Usually, however, the indirect reduction of cholinergic tone yields milder and shorter lasting symptoms than does direct blockade of muscarinic cholinergic receptors.

Thus, virtually all side effects of the selective NRIs can be understood as undesirable actions of norepinephrine in undesirable pathways at undesirable receptor subtypes. Just as for the SSRIs, this occurs because it is not possible for a systemically administered drug to act only at the desirable receptors in the desirable places; it must act everywhere it is distributed, which means all over the brain and all over the body. Fortunately, selective NRI side effects are more of a nuisance than a danger, and they generally attenuate over time, although they can cause an important subset of patients to discontinue treatment.

In addition to reboxetine, which is currently marketed, other selective NRIs are in clinical testing at present for depression or attention deficit disorder. These include

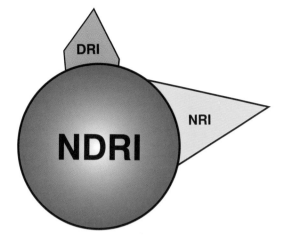

FIGURE 6–48. Shown here is the icon of a **norepinephrine and dopamine** reuptake inhibitor (**NDRI**). In this case, four of the five pharmacological properties of the tricyclic antidepressants (TCAs) (Fig. 6–27) were removed. Only the norepinephrine reuptake inhibitor (**NRI**) portion remains; to this is added a dopamine reuptake inhibitor action (DRI).

1555U88 and tomoxetine, although Org4428 was dropped from further clinical development.

## Norepinephrine and Dopamine Reuptake Blockers

Bupropion is the prototypical agent of the norepinephrine and dopamine reuptake inhibitors (Fig. 6–48). For many years, its mechanism of action was unclear. Bupropion itself has weak reuptake properties for dopamine, and weaker yet reuptake properties for norepinephrine. The action of the drug on norepinephrine and dopamine neurotransmission, however, has always appeared to be more powerful than these weak properties could explain, which has led to proposals that bupropion acts rather vaguely as an adrenergic modulator of some type. Bupropion is metabolized to an active metabolite, which is not only a more powerful norepinephrine reuptake blocker than bupropion itself but is also concentrated in the brain. In some ways, therefore, bupropion is more of a pro-drug (i.e., precursor) than a drug itself. That is, it gives rise to the "real" drug, namely its hydroxylated active metabolite, and it is this metabolite that is the actual mediator of antidepressant efficacy via norepinephrine and dopamine reuptake blockade (Fig. 6–49).

A sustained release formulation of bupropion (bupropion SR) has largely replaced immediate-release bupropion, not only because dosing frequency is reduced to only twice daily but also because of increased tolerability, especially an apparent reduction in the frequency of seizures associated with the immediate-release formulation.

Bupropion SR is generally activating or even stimulating. Interestingly, bupropion SR does not appear to be associated with production of the bothersome sexual dysfunction that can occur with the SSRIs, probably because bupropion lacks a significant serotonergic component to its mechanism of action. Thus, it may be a useful antidepressant not only for patients who cannot tolerate the serotonergic side effects of SSRIs, but also for patients whose depression does not respond to boosting

## NDRI ACTION

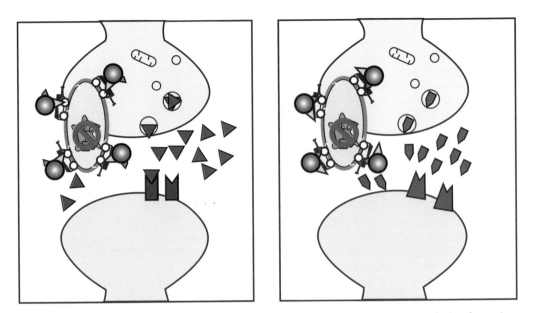

FIGURE 6—49. In this diagram, the norepinephrine reuptake inhibitor (**NRI**) and the dopamine reuptake inhibitor (**DRI**) portions of the **NDRI** molecule are shown inserted in the norepinephrine and the dopamine reuptake pumps, respectively, blocking them and causing an **antidepressant effect**.

serotonin by SSRIs. Bupropion SR is also useful in decreasing the craving associated with smoking cessation.

Other prodopaminergic agents are available as antidepressants in some countries, for example, amineptine in France and Brazil. Brasofensine, a dopamine reuptake blocker, is in clinical testing. Another vaguely prodopaminergic agent is modafanil, recently approved for the treatment of narcolepsy but not depression. It may act in part as a dopamine reuptake inhibitor but not a dopamine releaser like amphetamine. It may have theoretical antidepressant actions, but this has not been established in clinical trials. One potential worry that keeps pharmaceutical sponsors away from testing dopamine reuptake inhibitors as antidepressants is the possibility that they may be reinforcing and lead to abuse similar to stimulant abuse.

## Summary

In this chapter, we have discussed the mechanisms of action of the major antidepressant drugs. The acute pharmacological actions of these agents on receptors and enzymes have been described, as well as the major hypothesis that attempts to explain how all current antidepressants ultimately work. That hypothesis is known as the neurotransmitter receptor hypothesis of antidepressant action. We have also introduced pharmacokinetic concepts relating to the metabolism of antidepressants and mood stabilizers by the cytochrome P450 enzyme system.

Specific antidepressant agents that the reader should now understand include the monoamine oxidase inhibitors, tricyclic antidepressants, serotonin selective reuptake inhibitors, and noradrenergic reuptake inhibitors, including both selective norepinephrine reuptake inhibitors and norepinephrine–dopamine reuptake inhibitors.

Although the specific pragmatic guidelines for use of these various therapeutic agents for depression have not been emphasized, the reader should now have a basis for the rational use of these antidepressant drugs founded on application of principles discussed earlier in this chapter, namely, drug actions on neurotransmission via actions at key receptors and enzymes. Other antidepressants and mood stabilizers, as well as how to combine them, are discussed in Chapter 7.

# CHAPTER 7

# NEWER ANTIDEPRESSANTS AND MOOD STABILIZERS

In this chapter, we will continue our review of pharmacological concepts underlying the use of antidepressant and mood-stabilizing drugs. The goal of this chapter is to acquaint the reader with current ideas about how several of the newer antidepressants work. We will also introduce ideas about the pharmacologic mechanism of action of the mood stabilizers. As in Chapter 6, we will explain the mechanisms of action of these drugs by building on general pharmacological concepts.

Our treatment of antidepressants in this chapter continues at the conceptual level, and not at the pragmatic level. The reader should consult standard drug handbooks for details of doses, side effects, drug interactions, and other issues relevant to the prescribing of these drugs in clinical practice.

Discussion of antidepressants and mood stabilizers will begin with the antidepressants that act by a dual pharmacological mechanism, including dual reuptake blockade, alpha 2 antagonism and dual serotonin 2A antagonism/serotonin reuptake blockade. We will also explore several antidepressants under development but not

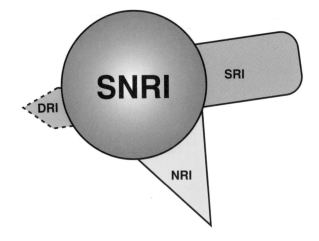

The **Serotonin-Norepinephrine reuptake inhibitor**
blocks the reuptake of norepinephrine and of serotonin.

FIGURE 7–1. Shown here is the icon of a dual reuptake inhibitor, which combines the actions of both a **serotonin** reuptake inhibitor (**SRI**) and a **norepinephrine** reuptake inhibitor (**NRI**). In this case, three of the five pharmacological properties of the tricyclic antidepressants (TCAs) (Fig. 6–27) were removed. Both the SRI portion and the NRI portion of the TCA remain; however the alpha, antihistamine, and anticholinergic portions are removed. These **serotonin/norepinephrine reuptake inhibitors** are called **SNRIs** or **dual inhibitors**. A small amount of dopamine reuptake inhibition (DRI) is also present in some of these agents, especially at high doses.

yet introduced into clinical practice. Next, we will introduce the use of lithium and anticonvulsants as mood stabilizers. Finally, we will discuss the use of combinations of drugs and briefly mention electroconvulsive therapy (ECT) and psychotherapy for the treatment of mood disorders.

## Dual Serotonin and Norepinephrine Reuptake Inhibitors

One class of antidepressants that combines the actions of both the selective serotonin reuptake inhibitors (SSRIs) and the selective noradrenergic reuptake inhibitors (NRIs) is the class of dual serotonin and noradrenergic reuptake inhibitors (SNRIs) (Fig. 7–1). The designation "dual reuptake inhibitors" can be confusing because many tricyclic antidepressants (TCAs) are also dual reuptake inhibitors of both norepinephrine (NE) and serotonin (5-hydroxytryptamine [5HT]). What is unique about venlafaxine, the prototypical SNRI, is that it shares the NE and 5HT, and to a lesser extent dopamine (DA) reuptake inhibitory properties of the classical TCAs (Fig. 7–1), but without alpha 1, cholinergic, or histamine receptor blocking properties (see Figs. 6–30 to 6–32). Thus, SNRIs are not only dual-action agents, but they are **selective** for this dual action. Dual-action SNRIs thus have the properties of an SSRI and a selective NRI added together in the same molecule.

Venlafaxine is the only dual-action SNRI currently marketed. Depending on the dose, it has different degrees of inhibition of 5HT reuptake (most potent and therefore present at low doses), NE reuptake (moderate potency and therefore present at higher doses) and DA reuptake (least potent and therefore present only at highest doses) (Fig. 7–2). However, there are no significant actions on other receptors. Venlafaxine is now available in an extended-release formulation (venlafaxine XR), which not only allows once daily administration but also significantly reduces side effects, especially nausea. The increased tolerability of venlafaxine in this new formulation is important, especially considering the trend in psychiatry to use higher doses of venlafaxine XR to exploit both the NE and the 5HT mechanism.

Additional dual 5HT-NE reuptake inhibitors include sibutramine, which is approved for the treatment of obesity but not depression. Tramadol is a kappa opiate agonist approved for the treatment of pain, but it also has serotonin and norepinephrine reuptake inhibitor properties. Dual reuptake inhibitors in clinical testing as antidepressants include milnacipran and duloxetine.

Are two antidepressant mechanisms better than one? The original tricyclic antidepressants have multiple pharmacological mechanisms and are termed "dirty drugs" because many of these mechanisms were undesirable, as they cause side effects (Fig. 7–3). The idea was then to "clean up" these agents by making them selective, and thus the SSRI era was born. Indeed, developing such selective agents made them devoid of pharmacologic properties that mediated anticholinergic, antihistaminic, and antiadrenergic side effects (Fig. 7–3). However, selectivity may sometimes be less desired than multiple pharmacologic mechanisms, as in difficult cases that are

## SNRI ACTIONS

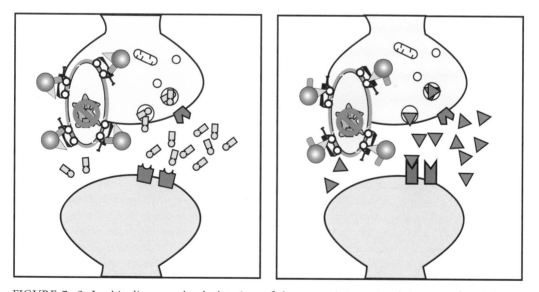

FIGURE 7–2. In this diagram, the dual actions of the serotonin/norepinephrine reuptake inhibitors (SNRIs) are shown. Both the norepinephrine reuptake inhibitor (NRI) portion of the SNRI molecule (left panel) and the serotonin reuptake inhibitor (SRI) portion of the SNRI molecule are inserted into their respective reuptake pumps. Consequently, both reuptake pumps are blocked, and the drug mediates an **antidepressant effect**. This is analogous to two of the dimensions of the tricyclic antidepressants (TCAs), already shown in Figures 6–28 and 6–29. It is also analogous to the single action of SSRIs (Fig. 6–33) added to the single action of the selective NRIs (Figure 6–46).

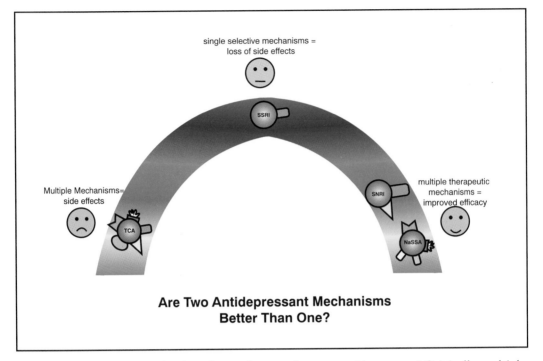

single selective mechanisms =
loss of side effects

SSRI

Multiple Mechanisms=
side effects

TCA

multiple therapeutic
mechanisms =
improved efficacy

SNRI

NaSSA

**Are Two Antidepressant Mechanisms
Better Than One?**

FIGURE 7–3. Are **two mechanisms** better than one for some antidepressants? Originally, multiple mechanisms were synonymous with "dirty drugs" because they implied unwanted side effects. This is shown as tricyclic antidepressants on the left. The trend to develop selective drugs (center) led to removal of unwanted side effects. More recently, the trend has again been to add multiple mechanisms together to improve tolerability and enhance efficacy. **Enhanced efficacy** from synergistic pharmacological mechanisms can apparently increase therapeutic responses in some patients, especially those resistant to single-mechanism agents.

resistant to treatment with drugs having a selective serotonergic mechanism. Thus, more recently psychotropic drug development has been trending back to multiple pharmacologic mechanisms in the hope that this would exploit potential synergies among two or more independent therapeutic mechanisms. For antidepressants, this has led to the development of drugs that exhibit "intramolecular polypharmacy," such as the dual SNRIs discussed here (Fig. 7–3). It has also led to the increasing use of two antidepressants together for treatment-resistant cases, combining two or more synergistic therapeutic mechanisms, as discussed below.

Thus, not only are dual-reuptake inhibitors effective antidepressants, but they may have some therapeutic advantages over the SSRIs. Theoretically, the addition of NE, and to a lesser extent DA, reuptake blockade to 5HT reuptake blockade (Fig. 7–2) might lead to pharmacological synergy among these neurotransmitter systems and thus boost efficacy. Synergy is the working together of two or more mechanisms so that the total efficacy is greater than the sum of its parts (in other words, 1 + 1 = 10).

The molecular basis of this synergy may be manifest at the level of genetic expression. Thus, beta-adrenergic receptor stimulation by NE results in gene expression, as discussed previously and shown in Figure 7–4. However, in the presence of

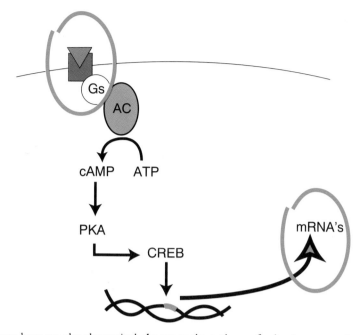

FIGURE 7–4. Shown here are the theoretical **therapeutic actions** of selective serotonin antidepressants on **gene expression**. The purple norepinephrine (NE) at the top (top red circle) is causing a cascade of biochemical events resulting in the transcription of a neuron's genes (mRNAs in the bottom circle). The noradrenergic receptor is linked to a stimulatory G protein (Gs), which is linked in turn to the enzyme adenylate cyclase (AC), which converts ATP into the second messenger cAMP. Next, cAMP activates protein kinase A (PKA), which then activates a transcription factor such as cyclic AMP response element binding (CREB) protein.

simultaneous serotonin 2A receptor stimulation by serotonin, gene expression is amplified synergistically (Fig. 7–5). Thus, norepinephrine and serotonin may work together to produce critical expression of genes in a manner that does not occur when either works alone. This could theoretically explain why dual 5HT-NE reuptake blockade may produce synergistic antidepressant effects in some patients.

Indications that there may be antidepressant synergy from dual 5HT-NE actions that correspond with these theoretical molecular events comes from studies in which venlafaxine has produced increased remission rates in major depressive disorders as compared with SSRIs. Increased remission rates with the TCAs over the SSRIs have also been reported and support the concept of dual action being more efficacious than SSRI action alone for remission of depression in some patients.

Another indication that the dual mechanisms may lead to more efficacy is the finding that venlafaxine seems to have greater efficacy as the dose increases, whereas other antidepressants seem to have little difference in efficacy at higher doses. Since the noradrenergic (and dopaminergic) action of venlafaxine is greater at higher doses, this suggests that there is more and more efficacy as the second mechanism becomes active (i.e., the noradrenergic "boost"). This also supports the rationale for using dual mechanisms for the most difficult patients, (i.e., those who are treatment-resistant to SSRIs and other antidepressants and those who are responders but not remitters to SSRIs or other antidepressants).

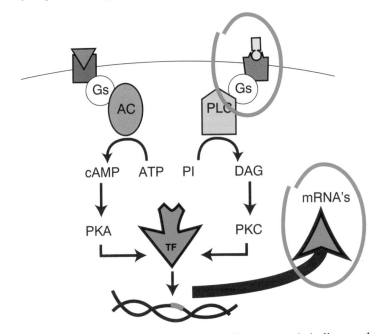

FIGURE 7–5. When serotonin (5HT) and norepinephrine (NE) act synergistically to **enhance gene expression** (compare with Fig. 7–4), this theoretically results in enhanced therapeutic efficacy in depression. Thus, the cascade on the left (shown also in Fig. 7–4) here is occurring simultaneously with the activation of the cascade on the right. Serotonin (top red circle) is thus working with NE on the left to cause even more gene activation (mRNAs in the bottom red circle) than NE can cause by itself in Figure 7–4. This is **synergy**. The 5HT receptor here is coupled to a stimulatory G protein (Gs), which activates the enzyme phospholipase C (PLC) to convert phosphatidyl inositol (PI) to diacylglycerol (DAG) and activate calcium flux, so that protein kinase C (PKC) can increase the transcription of neuronal genes by working synergistically at the level of transcription factors (TF).

Other information suggesting therapeutic advantages for dual mechanisms is the finding that the SNRI venlafaxine XR is an effective generalized anxiolytic. That is, among the known antidepressants only venlafaxine XR is approved as a generalized anxiolytic as well as an antidepressant. Such actions might have the favorable therapeutic consequences of converting anxious depression into complete remission of *both* depression and anxiety. Additional support for the role of dual SNRI action yielding enhanced efficacy in both depression and anxiety comes from evidence that the dual-action but nonselective tricyclic antidepressants also appear to be effective as generalized anxiolytics but have never been marketed for this indication. Dual-action mirtazapine may also have some generalized anxiolytic effects (see below).

There are a number of ways to implement this dual mechanism strategy beyond just using higher doses of venlafaxine XR. One of these is to use other dual 5HT/ NE–acting antidepressants, such as mirtazapine, discussed below, or possibly even going back to certain tricyclic antidepressants or monoamine oxidase inhibitors (MAOIs). Another would be to use pharmacologically rational combinations of drugs with potentially synergistic mechanisms. An obvious example of how to deliver dual serotonin and noradrenergic reuptake inhibition would be to add reboxetine to an SSRI. This and other dual mechanism strategies will be discussed in further detail in the section on antidepressant combinations.

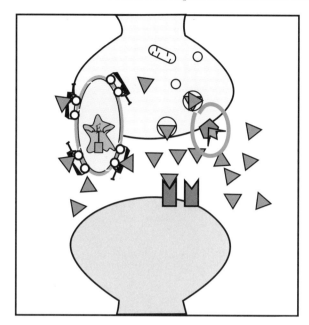

FIGURE 7–6. **Alpha 2 antagonists** (red circle) can increase noradrenergic neurotransmission by "cutting the brake cable" for noradrenergic neurons. That is, alpha 2 antagonists block presynaptic alpha 2 autoreceptors (red circle), which are the "brakes" on noradrenergic neurons. This causes noradrenergic neurons to become disinhibited, since norepinephrine (NE) can no longer block its own release. Thus, **noradrenergic** neurotransmission is **enhanced**.

### Dual Serotonin and Norepinephrine Actions Via Alpha 2 Antagonism

Blocking the reuptake pump for monoamines or the enzyme monoamine oxidase (MAO) are not the only mechanisms to increase serotonin and norepinephrine. Another way to raise both serotonin and norepinephrine levels is to block alpha 2 receptors. Recall that norepinephrine turns off its own release by interacting with presynaptic alpha 2 autoreceptors on noreadrenergic neurons (Fig. 5–21); norepinephrine also turns off serotonin release by interacting with presynaptic alpha 2 heteroreceptors on serotonergic neurons (Fig. 5–44). If an alpha 2 antagonist is administered, norepinephrine can no longer turn off its own release, and noradrenergic neurons are thus disinhibited (Fig. 7–6). That is, the alpha 2 antagonist "cuts the brake cable" of the noradrenergic neuron, and norepinephrine release is thereby increased.

Similarly, alpha 2 antagonists do not allow norepinephrine to turn off serotonin release. Therefore, serotonergic neurons become disinhibited (Fig. 7–7). Similarly to their actions at noradrenergic neurons, alpha 2 antagonists act at serotonergic neurons to "cut the brake cable" of noradrenergic inhibition norepinephrine brake on serotonin shown in Figs. 5–47 and 5–48. Serotonin release is therefore increased (Fig. 7–7).

A second mechanism to increase serotonin release after administration of an alpha 2 antagonist may be even more important. Recall that norepinephrine neurons from the locus coeruleus innervate the cell bodies of serotonergic neurons in the midbrain raphe (Figs. 5–47 and 5–48). This noradrenergic input enhances serotonin release

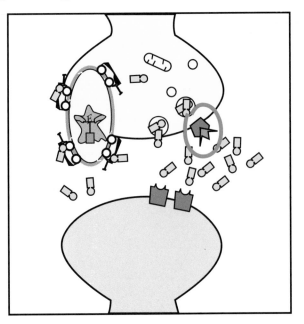

FIGURE 7–7. **Alpha 2 antagonists** can also increase serotonergic neurotransmission by "cutting the brake cable" for serotonergic neurons (compare with Fig. 7–6). That is, alpha 2 antagonists block presynaptic alpha 2 heteroreceptors (red circle), the "brakes" on serotonergic neurons. This causes serotonergic neurons to become disinhibited, since norepinephrine (NE) can no longer block serotonin (5HT) release. Thus, **serotonergic** neurotransmission is **enhanced**.

via a postsynaptic alpha 1 receptor. Thus, when norepinephrine is disinhibited in the noradrenergic pathway to the raphe, the norepinephrine release there will increase and cause alpha 1 receptors to be stimulated, thereby provoking more serotonin release (Fig. 7–8). This is like stepping on the serotonin accelerator. Thus, alpha 2 antagonists both cut the brake cable and step on the accelerator for serotonin release (Fig. 7–9).

Alpha 2 antagonist actions thus yield dual enhancement of both serotonin and norepinephrine release (Fig. 7–10). Although no selective alpha 2 antagonist is available for use as an antidepressant, one drug with prominent alpha 2 properties, namely mirtazapine, is available worldwide as an antidepressant (Fig. 7–10). Mirtazapine does not block any monoamine transporter, but in addition to its potent antagonist actions on alpha 2 receptors it also has antagonist actions at serotonin 2A, 2C, and 3 receptors and histamine 1 receptors (Fig. 7–10). The 5HT2A antagonist properties may contribute to mirtazapine's antidepressant actions (Fig. 7–11), and these serotonin 2A antagonist properties as well as serotonin 2C antagonist and H1 antihistamine properties may contribute to its anxiolytic and sedative hypnotic properties (Figs. 7–11 to 7–13). By blocking serotonin 2A, 2C, and 3 receptors, the side effects associated with stimulating them, especially anxiety, nausea, and sexual dysfunction are avoided (Fig. 7–11). However, blocking serotonin 2A and H1 antihistamine receptors accounts for the side effect of sedation, and blocking serotonin 2C and H1 receptors accounts for the side effect of weight gain (Fig. 7–12).

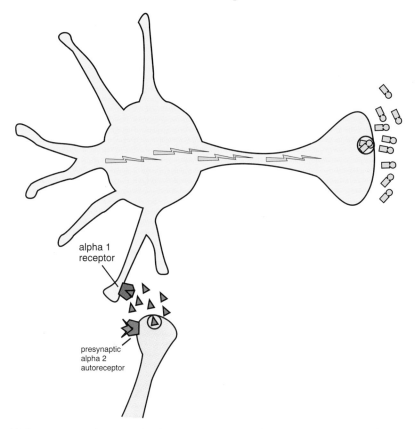

FIGURE 7–8. **Alpha 2 antagonists** can also **increase serotonergic neurotransmission** by "stepping on the serotonin (5HT) accelerator." That is, norepinephrine (NE) input for the locus coeruleus (bottom) to the cell bodies of serotonergic neurons in the midbrain raphe synapse on postsynaptic excitatory alpha 1 receptors. This **increases** serotonergic neuronal firing and serotonin release from the serotonin nerve terminal on the right.

The therapeutic actions of mirtazapine are thought to be mainly mediated through its alpha 2 antagonist properties. As mentioned above, by blocking presynaptic alpha 2 receptors, mirtazapine cuts the brake cable and disinhibits both serotonin and norepinephrine release; by disinhibiting norepinephrine release, alpha 1 receptors are stimulated by norepinephrine, and serotonin release is enhanced by stepping on the serotonin accelerator (Fig. 7–13). An integrated view of all of mirtazapine's pharmacologic actions is shown in Figure 7–13.

In addition to its efficacy as a first-line antidepressant, mirtazapine may have enhanced efficacy due to its dual mechanism of action (Fig. 7–3), especially in combination with other antidepressants that block serotonin and/or norepinephrine reuptake. This will be discussed below in the section on antidepressant combinations. Mirtazapine may also have utility in panic disorder, generalized anxiety disorder, and other anxiety disorders, but has not been intensively studied for these indications.

Two other alpha 2 antagonists are marketed as antidepressants in some countries (but not the United States), namely, mianserin (worldwide except in the United

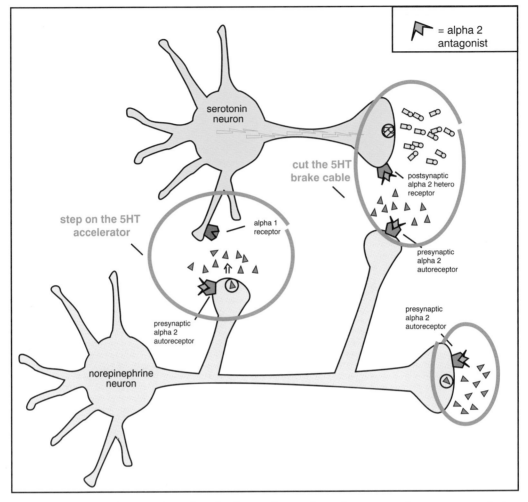

FIGURE 7–9. This diagram shows how **both noradrenergic and serotonergic neurotransmission are enhanced by alpha 2 antagonists.** The noradrenergic neuron at the bottom is interacting with the serotonergic neuron at the top. The noradrenergic neuron is disinhibited at all of its axon terminals because an alpha 2 antagonist is blocking all of its presynaptic alpha 2 autoreceptors. Thus, this has the effect of "cutting the brake cables" for norepinephrine (NE) release at all of its noradrenergic nerve terminals (NE released in all three red circles). Serotonin (5HT) release is enhanced by NE via two distinct mechanisms. First, alpha 2 antagonists "step on the 5HT accelerator" when NE stimulates alpha 1 receptors on the 5HT cell body and dendrites (left red circle). Second, alpha 2 antagonists "cut the 5HT brake cable" when alpha 2 presynaptic heteroreceptors are blocked on the 5HT axon terminal (middle red circle).

States) and setiptilene (Japan). Mianserin has alpha 1 antagonist properties, which mitigate the effects of enhancing serotonergic neurotransmission, so that this drug enhances predominantly noradrenergic neurotransmission, yet with associated 5HT2A, 5HT2C, 5HT3, and H1 antagonist properties. Yohimbine is also an alpha 2 antagonist, but its alpha 1 antagonist properties similarly mitigate its pro-monoaminergic actions. Several selective alpha 2 antagonists, including idazoxan and fluparoxan, have been tested, but they have not yet demonstrated robust antide-

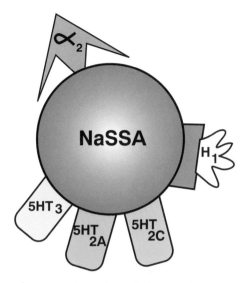

FIGURE 7–10. Icon for **mirtazapine**, sometimes also called a noradrenergic and specific serotonergic antidepressant (NaSSA). Its primary therapeutic action is alpha 2 antagonism as shown in Figures 7–6 through 7–9. It also blocks three serotonin receptors: 5HT2A, 5HT2C, and 5HT3. Finally, it blocks H1 histamine receptors.

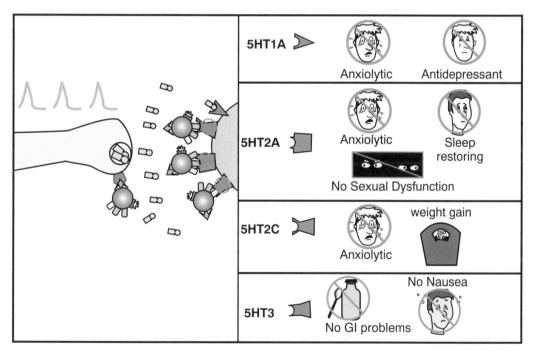

FIGURE 7–11. **Mirtazapine** actions at **serotonin** (5HT) synapses. When presynaptic alpha 2 heteroreceptors are blocked, 5HT is released, but it is directed to the 5HT1A receptor because 5HT actions at 5HT2A, 5HT2C, and 5HT3 receptors are blocked. The result is that antidepressant and anxiolytic actions are preserved but the side effects associated with stimulating 5HT2A, 5HT2C, and 5HT3 receptors are blocked. However, sedation and weight gain may result from these actions.

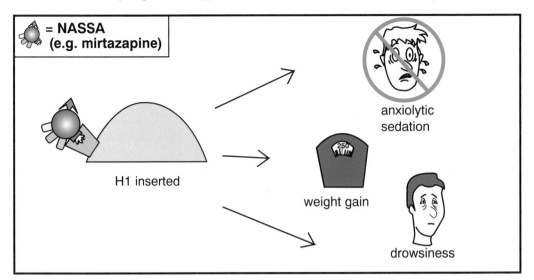

FIGURE 7–12. When **mirtazapine** blocks **histamine** 1 receptors, it can cause anxiolytic actions, but also sedation and weight gain as side effects.

pressant efficacy and also are not always well tolerated because they can provoke panic, anxiety, and prolonged erections in men.

## Dual Serotonin 2 Antagonists/Serotonin Reuptake Inhibitors

Several antidepressants share the ability to block serotonin 2A receptors as well as serotonin reuptake. In fact, some of the tricyclic antidepressants, such as amitriptyline, nortriptyline, doxepine, and especially amoxapine, have this combination of actions at the serotonin synapse. Since the potency of blockade of serotonin 2A receptors varies considerably among the tricyclics, it is not clear how important this action is to the therapeutic actions of tricyclic antidepressants in general.

However, there is another chemical class of antidepressants known as phenylpiperazines, which are more selective than the tricyclic antidepressants and whose most powerful pharmacological action is to block serotonin 2A receptors (Fig. 7–14). This includes the agents nefazodone and trazodone. Both of these agents also block serotonin reuptake but do so in a less potent manner than either the tricyclic antidepressants or the SSRIs (Fig. 7–15). Since the pharmacological mechanism of action of dual serotonin 2A antagonist/serotonin reuptake inhibitors derives from a combination of powerful antagonism of serotonin 2A receptors with less powerful blockade of serotonin reuptake, these agents are classified separately as serotonin 2A antagonists/reuptake inhibitors (*SARIs*) (Figs. 7–14 and 7–15).

Nefazodone is the prototypical member of the SARI class of antidepressants. It is a powerful serotonin 2A antagonist with secondary actions as a serotonin and norepinephrine reuptake inhibitor (Figs. 7–14 and 7–15). Nefazodone also blocks alpha 1 receptors, but the clinical consequences of this are generally not important, perhaps because its norepinephrine reuptake inhibition reduces this action *in vivo*.

The major distinction between the SARIs and other classes of antidepressants is that SARIs are predominantly 5HT2A antagonists. A lesser but important amount

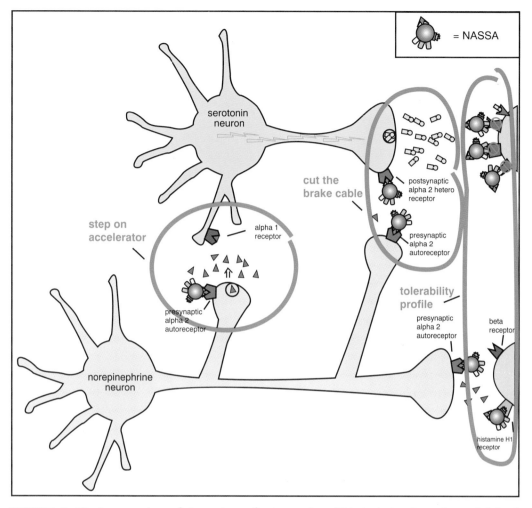

FIGURE 7–13. An **overview** of the actions of **mirtazapine**. This includes the actions of alpha 2 antagonists already shown in Figure 7–9, that is, the therapeutic actions of cutting the NE brake cable while stepping on the 5HT accelerator (left circle), as well as cutting the 5HT brake cable (middle circle). This increases both 5HT and NE neurotransmission. On the right are the additional actions of mirtazapine beyond alpha 2 antagonism. These postsynaptic actions mainly account for the tolerability profile of mirtazapine.

of 5HT reuptake inhibition also occurs. That is, the SARI nefazodone may exploit the natural antagonism between 5HT1A and 5HT2A receptors by increasing 5HT through reuptake blockade while simultaneously blocking its actions at 5HT2A receptors. Normally, stimulation of 5HT2A receptors mitigates the stimulation of 5HT1A receptors (Figs. 7–16 and 7–17). This may also play out at the level of gene expression, where gene expression by 5HT1A stimulation alone (Fig. 7–18) is opposed by simultaneous stimulation of 5HT2A receptors (Fig. 7–19).

On the other hand, if 5HT2A receptors are blocked rather than stimulated, the normal inhibiting influence on 5HT1A receptor stimulation is lost. This may indirectly boost the effects of stimulating 5HT1A receptors, since it is no longer

## Serotonin Antagonist/Reuptake Inhibitors (SARIs)

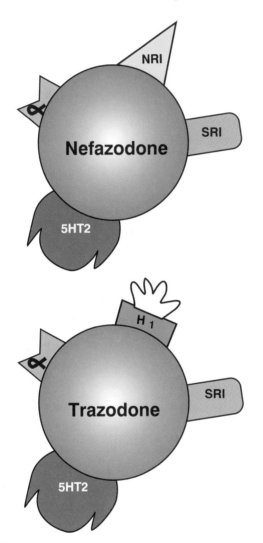

FIGURE 7–14. Shown here are icons for two of the serotonin 2A antagonist/reuptake inhibitors (**SARIs**). Nefazodone is the prototype agent in this class, which also includes trazodone. These agents also have a **dual action**, but the two mechanisms are different from the dual actions of the serotonin norepinephrine reuptake inhibitors (SNRIs). The SARIs act by potent **blockade of serotonin 2A (5HT2A) receptors, combined with less potent serotonin reuptake inhibitor (SRI) actions.** Nefazodone also has weak norepinephrine reuptake inhibition (NRI) as well as weak alpha 1 adrenergic blocking properties. Trazodone also contains antihistamine properties and alpha 1 antagonist properties but lacks the NRI properties of nefazodone.

## SARI (NEFAZODONE) ACTIONS AT 5HT SYNAPSES

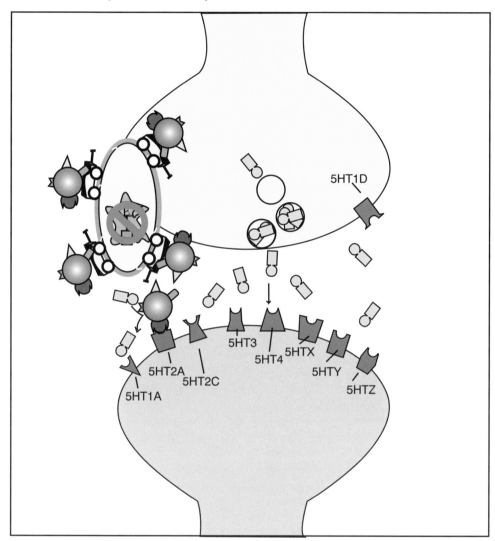

FIGURE 7–15. This diagram shows the dual actions of the **serotonin 2A antagonist/reuptake inhibitor (SARI) nefazodone**. This agent acts both presynaptically and postsynaptically. Presynaptic actions are indicated by the serotonin reuptake inhibitor (**SRI**) portion of the icon, which is inserted into the serotonin reuptake pump, blocking it. Postsynaptic actions are indicated by the **serotonin 2A receptor antagonist** portion of the icon (5HT2A), inserted into the serotonin 2 receptor, blocking it. It is believed that both actions contribute to the antidepressant actions of nefazodone. Blocking serotonin actions at 5HT2A receptors may also diminish side effects mediated by stimulation of 5HT2A receptors when the SRI acts to increase 5HT at all receptor subtypes. The serotonin 2A antagonist properties are stronger than the serotonin reuptake properties, so serotonin antagonism predominates at the 5HT2A receptor.

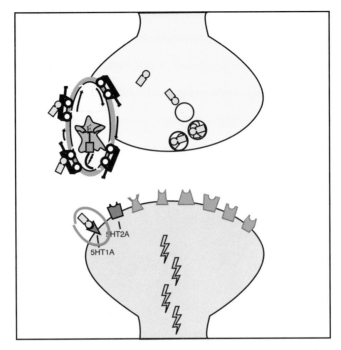

FIGURE 7–16. *Synergy between 5HT1A stimulation and 5HT2A antagonism*–part 1. Shown here is the pharmacologic action of 5HT1A stimulation alone (red circle).

mitigated by 5HT2A stimulation (Fig. 7–20). This same phenomenon may occur at the gene level as well (Fig. 7–21).

The SARI nefazodone may therefore not mediate its therapeutic actions merely by blocking 5HT2A receptors. In fact, selective 5HT2A antagonists have been tested in depression and have not been shown to be particularly efficacious antidepressants. The action of increasing 5HT via reuptake inhibition, leading to stimulation of 5HT1A receptors, may therefore be an important part of nefazodone's action. Without 5HT1A stimulation, 5HT2A antagonism would have nothing to potentiate. This principle will be discussed in further detail in the section on antidepressant combinations in which SSRIs are combined with other 5HT2A antagonists such as the atypical antipsychotics for resistant cases of depression. Combining indirect 5HT1A agonism with direct 5HT2A antagonism is another example of "intramolecular polypharmacy," exploiting the synergy that exists between these two mechanisms and again suggesting that two antidepressant mechanisms may sometimes be better than one.

When 5HT reuptake is inhibited selectively, as with the SSRIs, it causes essentially all serotonin receptors to be stimulated by the increased levels of 5HT that result. Although this has proved to be quite useful for treating depression and other disorders, it also has its costs. For example, we have discussed how stimulation of 5HT1A receptors in the raphe may help depression (Fig. 5–52), but how stimulating 5HT2A and 5HT2C receptors in the limbic cortex may cause agitation or anxiety (Figs. 5–53 and 5–54), and how stimulating 5HT2A receptors in the spinal cord may lead to sexual dysfunction (Fig. 5–57). Thus, an agent that combines 5HT

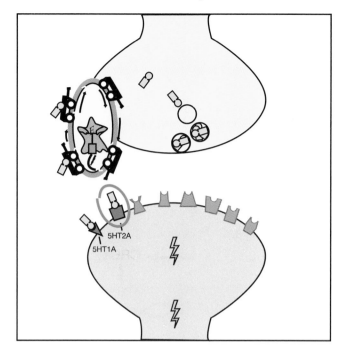

FIGURE 7–17. *Synergy between 5HT1A stimulation and 5HT2A antagonism*–part 2. Stimulation of 5HT2A receptors by 5HT (red circle) reduces the actions of 5HT at 5HT1A receptors (compare with Fig. 7–16).

reuptake blockade with stronger 5HT2A antagonism would theoretically reduce the undesired actions of 5HT when it stimulates 5HT2A receptors. In this case, competition between 5HT reuptake blockade and stronger 5HT2A antagonism results in net antagonism at the 5HT2A receptor. In fact, the SARI nefazodone thus theoretically lacks the potential to cause sexual dysfunction, and usually also insomnia and anxiety, associated with the SSRIs.

Clinical experience suggests that nefazodone may also be useful in panic disorder, posttraumatic stress disorder, and generalized anxiety disorder, but without the 5HT2A-activating side effects associated with the SSRIs.

Trazodone is the original member of the SARI group of antidepresssants. It also blocks alpha 1 receptors and histamine receptors (Fig. 7–14). Perhaps because of its histamine receptor blocking properties, it is extremely sedating. For this reason, its antidepressant use tends to be limited, yet it is well accepted as an excellent non-dependence-forming hypnotic, but it was never actually marketed for this indication. Its sedative hypnotic doses are generally lower than its effective antidepressant doses. Trazodone is used mostly as an adjunct to antidepressants because it not only increases the tolerability of SSRIs by blocking their side effects associated with stimulating 5HT2A receptors, such as insomnia and agitation, but it also can enhance the therapeutic efficacy of SSRIs, perhaps by exploiting the synergy of blocking 5HT2A receptors while stimulating 5HT1A receptors as discussed above. A rare but troublesome side effect of trazodone is priapism (prolonged erections in men, usually painful), which is treated by injecting alpha adrenergic agonists into the penis to reverse the priapism and prevent vascular damage to the penis.

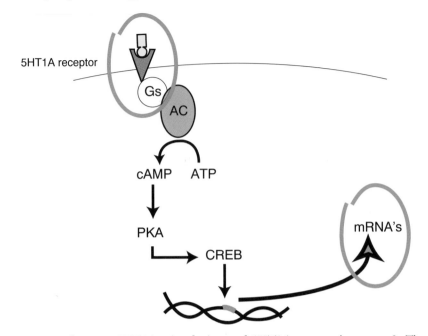

FIGURE 7–18. *Synergy between 5HT1A stimulation and 5HT2A antagonism*–part 3. The molecular consequences of 5HT1A stimulation alone, shown here, result in a certain amount of gene expression corresponding to the pharmacological actions shown in Figure 7–16. Serotonin (5HT) occupancy of its 5HT1A receptor (top red circle) causes a certain amount of gene transcription (see bottom red circle on the right). The 5HT1A receptor is coupled to a stimulatory G protein (Gs) and adenylate cyclase (AC), which produces the second messenger cyclic AMP from ATP. This in turn activates protein kinase A (PKA), so that transcription factors such as cyclic AMP response element binding protein (CREB) can activate gene expression (mRNAs).

Nefazodone is in clinical testing as an extended-release formulation, which will reduce its administration to once daily and may also reduce its side effects. YM992 is another serotonin 2A antagonist with serotonin reuptake inhibition properties that is in testing as an antidepressant. Other more selective 5HT2 antagonists have been tested and discarded as potential antidepressants, including ritanserin and amesergide. However, MDL-100907 and SR46349 are selective 5HT2A antagonists in testing for schizophrenia. Furthermore, drugs with serotonin 2A antagonist properties but also dopamine antagonist properties, called serotonin-dopamine antagonists, or atypical antipsychotics, are in testing for bipolar disorder and for treatment-resistant depression. They will be discussed in further detail in the sections of this chapter below on bipolar disorder/antidepressant combinations. Agents with 5HT2A antagonist properties but also 5HT1A agonist properties are in testing as potential novel antidepressants; these include flibanserin, and possibly adatanserin and BMS181,101.

## New Antidepressants in Development

Currently, what is needed is an antidepressant that has onset of action faster than 2 to 8 weeks and has efficacy in more than two out of three patients. That efficacy

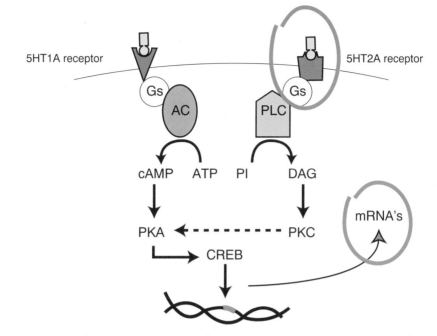

FIGURE 7–19. *Synergy between 5HT1A stimulation and 5HT2A antagonism*–part 4. The molecular consequences of 5HT2A receptor stimulation concomitant with 5HT1A receptor stimulation is to reduce the gene expression of 5HT1A stimulation alone (i.e., that shown in Fig. 7–18). These molecular consequences correlate with the pharmacologic actions of simultaneous 5HT1A and 5HT2A stimulation shown in Figure 7–17. Simultaneous activation of the 5HT2A receptor by serotonin (on the right) will alter the consequences of activating 5HT1A receptors in a negative way and reduce the gene expression of 5HT1A receptors acting alone (Fig. 7–18). Thus, occupancy of the 5HT2A receptor (top circle) causes coupling of a stimulatory G protein (Gs) with the enzyme phospholipase C (PLC). This, in turn, activates calcium flux and converts phosphatidylinositol (PI) into diacylglycerol (DAG). This activates the enzyme phosphokinase C (PKC), which has an inhibitory action on phosphokinase A (PKA). This reduces the activation of transcription factors such as cyclic AMP response element binding protein (CREB) and leads to a decrease in gene expression (bottom red circle).

should be robust, causing remission, not response, and sustaining that remission for longer periods of time and in a larger proportion of patients than current antidepressants. Several theoretical candidates are in development, and some related to the mechanisms discussed above have already been mentioned. A sampling of other potential candidate antidepressants is given below. Most are variations on the theme of modulating either adrenergic neurons or serotonergic neurons with novel pharmacological mechanisms. Others attempt to achieve antidepressant actions by modulating peptide systems.

## Monoaminergic Modulators

*Beta agonists.* Beta adrenergic receptors can be rapidly down regulated by agonists and if this is desired for an antidepressant action, beta agonists may be useful. To date, it has not been possible to identify beta 1 or beta 2 agonists that successfully penetrate the brain and yet are not cardiotoxic. Pursuing safer beta 1 and beta 2

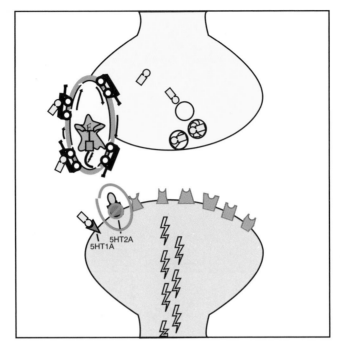

FIGURE 7–20. *Synergy between 5HT1A stimulation and 5HT2A antagonism*–part 5. If 5HT2A receptors are pharmacologically blocked rather than stimulated, they can no longer inhibit 5HT1A actions. Thus, 5HT1A receptors are disinhibited (compare with Figs. 7–16 and 7–17).

agonists, perhaps as partial agonists, may optimize the pharmacological properties. However, beta 3 agonists such as SR58611 show preclinical efficacy as antidepressants and are in preliminary clinical testing.

*Second messenger systems.* Enhancing adrenergic functioning distal to the receptor occupancy site can theoretically be accomplished by targeting either the G proteins or the adenylate cyclase enzyme. Both types of agents are under development. Rolipram has shown promise in the past as an antidepressant that blocks the destruction of cyclic adenosine monophospate (cAMP) second messengers. Lithium mimetics that act on monoamine receptor G proteins or on enzymes regulating phosphatidyl inositol second messenger systems are being tested preclinically. It may turn out fortuitously that some of the anticonvulsants known or suspected to be useful for bipolar disorder, including depression, act on second messenger systems. Further exploitation of this approach may have to await clarification of the biochemical cascade that regulates critical gene expression in monoaminergic neurons and their targets.

*5HT1A agonists, partial agonists and antagonists.* Although many 5HT1A agonists have been extensively tested in clinical trials, none has made it to the market as an antidepressant, and only one has been approved as a generalized anxiolytic. Several 5HT1A agonists and partial agonists have been dropped from clinical development, but others still survive in clinical research. Gepirone ER, a chemical cousin of bus-

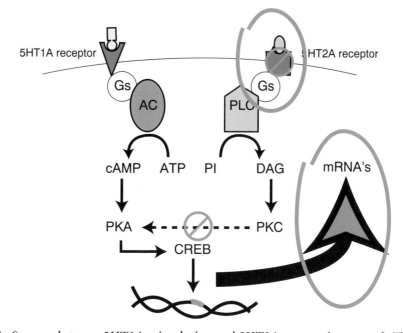

FIGURE 7–21. *Synergy between 5HT1A stimulation and 5HT2A antagonism*–part 6. The molecular consequences of 5HT1A receptor disinhibition by 5HT2A receptor blockade is shown here, namely enhanced gene expression. These molecular events are the consequence of the pharmacological actions shown in Figure 7–20. Simultaneous inhibition of the 5HT2A receptor on the right can stop the negative consequences that 5HT2A receptor stimulation by 5HT can have on gene expression, as shown in Figure 7–19. Thus, gene expression of the 5HT1A receptor (Fig. 7–18) is enhanced when 5HT2A receptors are blocked (bottom red circle) rather than diminished when they are stimulated (Fig. 7–19). The molecular basis of these effects is best reviewed by comparing Figures 7–18, 7–19, and 7–21. The pharmacological basis of these effects is best reviewed by comparing Figures 7–16, 7–17, and 7–20.

pirone, is continuing in clinical development in the United States and tandospirone in Japan. Ipsapirone, sunepitron, transdermal buspirone, and others have been dropped from clinical development, although there may be some continuing interest in flesinoxan or others.

Theoretically, a 5HT1A antagonist might be a rapid-onset antidepressant owing to immediate disinhibition of the serotonin neuron. This has been demonstrated preclinically, but no selective 5HT1A antagonist has undergone clinical testing in depression.

*Serotonin and dopamine reuptake inhibition.* Dual reuptake blockers of both serotonin and dopamine are in clinical testing. Although the SSRI sertraline has some dopamine reuptake inhibition as well as more potent serotonin reuptake inhibition, minaprine and bazinaprine have more potent dopamine actions and are thus dual serotonin/dopamine agents.

*Serotonin 1D antagonists.* Theoretically, a 5HT1A antagonist should rapidly disinhibit the serotonin neuron and be a rapid-onset antidepressant. One such compound CP-448,187 is entering clinical development.

## Neurokinin Antagonists

As explained in Chapter 5, theoretical considerations and some serendipitous clinical observations suggest that neurokinin antagonists, especially NK1 antagonists (i.e., substance P antagonists) may be novel antidepressants. Thus clinical testing is underway on NK1 antagonists including SR140333, MK-869, L-760,735, L-733,060, CP-96,345, and CP-122,721, as well as several others; NK2 antagonists such as SR48968 and GR-159,897; and NK3 antagonists such as SR142801.

## Novel Neurotransmitter Mechanisms

Other potentially novel antidepressants in clinical testing target different neurotransmitter systems, including sigma receptors, peptides such as neurotensin or cholecystokinin, and endogenous reward systems such as anandamide. These are in their very early testing phase.

## Herbs

Herbal medicines such as hypericum, the active ingredient in St. John's wort, are used widely throughout the world, although never proven to be antidepressants by the same level of scrutiny as drugs marketed as antidepressants, such as TCAs and SSRIs. However, legitimate high-standard clinical testing is in progress to see whether herbs, especially St. John's wort, will prove to be antidepressants when held up to the same scrutiny that any drug undergoes prior to being marketed as an antidepressant. Recent reports that St. John's wort may have some toxic effect on reproductive functioning may mitigate the enthusiasm for this approach, however. One study suggests that it negatively affects fertility in both men and women. In addition, there is some evidence for mutation of the gene in sperm cells that may possibly increase risk to the developing fetus. Therefore, pregnancy is not currently recommended while taking these herbs.

## Mood-Stabilizing Drugs

### Lithium, the Classical Mood Stabilizer

Mood disorders characterized by elevations of mood above normal as well as depressions below normal are classically treated with lithium, an ion whose mechanism of action is not certain. Candidates for its mechanism of action are sites beyond the receptor in the second messenger system, perhaps either as an inhibitor of an enzyme, called inositol monophosphatase, involved in the phosphatidyl inositol system as a modulator of G proteins, or even as a regulator of gene expression by modulating protein kinase C (Fig. 7–22).

Lithium not only treats acute episodes of mania and hypomania but was the first psychotropic agent shown to prevent recurrent episodes of illness. Lithium may also be effective in treating and preventing episodes of depression in patients with bipolar disorder. It is least effective for rapid cycling or mixed episodes. Overall, lithium is effective in only 40 to 50% of patients. Furthermore, many patients are unable to tolerate it because of numerous side effects, including gastrointestinal symptoms

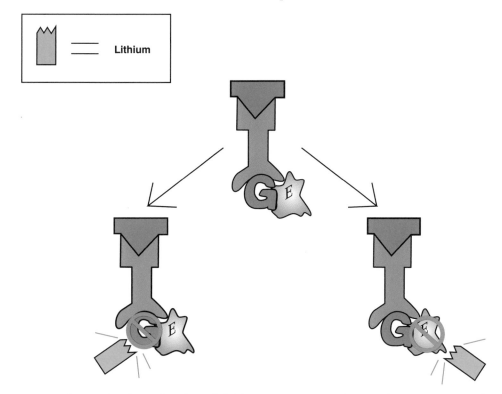

FIGURE 7–22. The **mechanism of action of lithium** is not well understood but is hypothesized to involve **modifying second messenger systems**. One possibility is that lithium alters **G proteins** and their ability to transduce signals inside the cell once the neurotransmitter receptor is occupied by the neurotransmitter. Another theory is that lithium alters **enzymes** that interact with the second-messenger system, such as inositol monophosphatase, or others.

such as dyspepsia, nausea, vomiting, and diarrhea, as well as weight gain, hair loss, acne, tremor, sedation, decreased cognition, and incoordination. There are also long-term adverse effects on the thyroid and kidney. Lithium has a narrow therapeutic window, requiring monitoring of plasma drug levels.

### Anticonvulsants as Mood Stabilizers

Based on theories that mania may "kindle" further episodes of mania, a logical parallel with seizure disorders was drawn, since seizures can kindle more seizures. Thus, trials of several anticonvulsants, beginning with carbamazepine, have been conducted, and several are showing indications of efficacy in treating the manic phase of bipolar disorder (Table 7–1). Only valproic acid, however, is actually approved for this indication.

The mechanism of action of anticonvulsants remains poorly characterized, both in terms of their anticonvulsant effects or their antimanic/mood stabilizing effects. They may even have multiple mechanisms of action. At the cell membrane, anti-convulsants appear to act on ion channels, including sodium, potassium, and calcium channels. By interfering with sodium movements through voltage-operated sodium

Table 7–1. *Anticonvulsants used
to treat bipolar disorder*

valproic acid (Depakote)
carbamazepine
lamotrigine
gabapentin
topiramate

channels, for example, several anticonvulsants cause use-dependent blockade of sodium inflow. That is, when the sodium channels are being "used" during neuronal activity such as seizures, anticonvulsants can prolong their inactivation, thus providing anticonvulsant action. Whether such a mechanism is also the cause of the mood-stabilizing effects of anticonvulsants is yet unknown.

When ion channels are inactivated, this may result in changes of both excitatory and inhibitory neurotransmission. Glutamate is the universal excitatory neurotransmitter and gamma-aminobutyric acid (GABA) is the universal inhibitory neurotransmitter. In particular, anticonvulsants appear to modulate the effects of the inhibitory neurotransmitter GABA by augmenting its synthesis, augmenting its release, inhibiting its breakdown, reducing its reuptake into GABA neurons, or augmenting its effects at GABA receptors. Some of these actions may be the consequence of anticonvulsant actions at ion channels.

Anticonvulsants may also interfere with neurotransmission by the excitatory neurotransmitter glutamate, in particular by reducing its release. Simply put, inhibitory neurotransmission with GABA may be enhanced and excitatory neurotransmission with glutamate may be reduced by anticonvulsants.

Other actions of some anticonvulsants include inhibition of the enzyme carbonic anhydrase, negative modulation of calcium channel activity, and actions on second messenger systems, including inhibition of phosphokinase C. Beyond the second messenger, there is the possibility that second messenger systems may be affected, analogously to what is hypothesized for lithium.

*Valproic acid.* Although its exact mechanism of action remains uncertain, valproic acid (also valproate sodium, or valproate) may inhibit sodium and/or calcium channel function and perhaps thereby boost GABA inhibitory action as well as reduce glutamate excitatory action (Fig. 7–23). A unique and patented pharmaceutical formulation of valproic acid, called Depakote, reduces gastrointestinal side effects.

The Depakote form of valproic acid is approved for the acute phase of bipolar disorder. It is also commonly used on a long-term basis, although its prophylactic effects have not been as well established. Valproic acid is now frequently used as a first-line treatment for bipolar disorders, as well as in combination with lithium for patients refractory to lithium monotherapy and especially for patients with rapid cycling and mixed episodes. Oral loading can lead to rapid stabilization, and plasma levels must be monitored to keep drug levels within the therapeutic range.

Valproic acid can have unacceptable side effects, such as hair loss, weight gain, and sedation. Certain problems can limit valproic acid's usefulness in women of child-bearing potential, including the fact that it can cause neural tube defects in

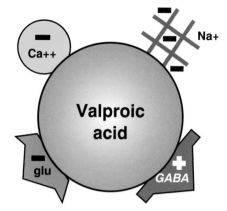

FIGURE 7–23. Shown here is an icon of **valproic acid**'s pharmacologic actions. By interfering with calcium channels and sodium channels, valproate is thought both to enhance the inhibitory actions of gamma aminobutyric acid (GABA) and to reduce the excitatory actions of glutamate.

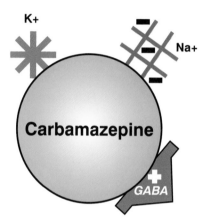

FIGURE 7–24. Shown here is an icon of **carbamazepine**'s pharmacologic actions. By interfering with sodium and potassium, carbamazepine is thought to enhance the inhibitory actions of gamma aminobutyric acid (GABA).

the developing fetus. Menstrual disturbances, polycystic ovaries, hyperandrogenism, obesity, and insulin resistance may also be associated with valproic acid therapy.

*Carbamazepine.* The anticonvulsant carbamazepine was actually the first to be shown to be effective in the manic phase of bipolar disorder, but it has not been approved for this use by regulatory authorities such as the U.S. Food and Drug Administration (FDA). Its mechanism of action may be to enhance GABA function, perhaps in part by actions on sodium and/or potassium channels (Fig. 7–24). Because its efficacy is less well documented and its side effects can include sedation and hematological abnormalities, it is not as well accepted for first-line use in the treatment of mood disorders as either lithium or valproic acid.

*Lamotrigine.* Lamotrigine is approved as an anticonvulsant but not as a mood stabilizer. It is postulated to inhibit sodium channels and to inhibit the release of glu-

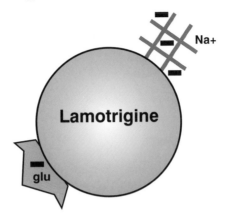

FIGURE 7–25. Shown here is an icon of **lamotrigine**'s pharmacologic actions. By interfering with sodium channels, lamotrigine is thought to reduce the excitatory actions of glutamate.

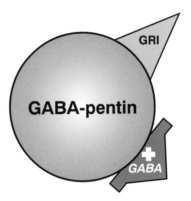

FIGURE 7–26. Shown here is an icon of **gabapentin**'s pharmacologic actions. Gabapentin is thought to act by inhibiting the reuptake of gamma aminobutyric acid (GABA) into GABA terminals (shown as GRI for GABA reuptake inhibition). This enhances the inhibitory actions of GABA.

tamate (Fig. 7–25). Numerous reports suggest that lamotrigine is not only able to stabilize bipolar manic and mixed episodes but it may also be useful for the depressive episodes of this disorder. Further testing of lamotrigine's safety and efficacy in mood disorders is ongoing.

*Gabapentin.* This compound was synthesized as a GABA analogue but turned out not to directly modulate the GABA receptor. It may well interact at the GABA transporter and increase GABA levels (Fig. 7–26). It also decreases glutamate levels. It is approved as an anticonvulsant and was originally observed to improve mood and quality of life in seizure disorder patients. Numerous studies suggest efficacy in the manic phase of bipolar disorder, and further clinical evaluation as a mood stabilizer is ongoing. A gabapentin analogue called pregabalin is also undergoing clinical evaluation as an anticonvulsant and as a mood stabilizer.

*Topiramate.* Topiramate is another compound approved as an anticonvulsant and in clinical testing as a mood stabilizer. Its mechanism of action appears to be to enhance

GABA function and reduce glutamate function by interfering with both sodium and calcium channels. In addition, it is a weak inhibitor of carbonic anhydrase (Fig. 7–27). Topiramate's mood-stabilizing actions may occur at lower doses than its anticonvulsant actions. This compound also has the interesting side effect of weight loss in some patients, a most unique effect among mood stabilizers, which generally cause weight gain.

## Other Mood Stabilizing Drugs

*Benzodiazepines.* Benzodiazepines have anticonvulsant actions, especially intravenous diazepam and oral clonazepam. They are also sedating. Both of these actions have led to the use of benzodiazepines for the treatment of mood disorders, especially as adjunctive treatment for agitation and psychotic behavior during the phase of acute mania. Benzodiazepines are also broadly used in anxiety and sleep disorders.

*Antipsychotics.* Classical neuroleptics (such as haloperidol and the phenothiazine chlorpromazine) have long played a role in the treatment of agitation and the psychosis of mania. More recently, the atypical antipsychotics (such as risperidone, olanzapine and guetiapine) have begun to replace the older neuroleptics and assume an important adjunctive role in the treatment of bipolar disorders. Atypical antipsychotics may also improve mood in schizophrenia. Currently, the atypical antipsychotics are becoming more widely used for management of the manic phase of bipolar disorder Clinical studies are also ongoing to determine the role of these agents in the long-term management of bipolar disorder, including first-line use, maintenance treatment, and use in combination with mood stabilizers for treatment-resistant cases, especially mixed and rapid cycling cases.

## Drug Combinations for Treatment-Resistant Patients— Rational Polypharmacy

So far, we have discussed many individual members of the "depression pharmacy" (Fig. 7–28). More than two dozen different agents acting by eight distinct mechanisms are thus useful for treating the typical case of depression (Fig. 7–29). However, psychopharmacologists are increasingly being called on to provide treatment for patients who do not respond to their initial treatment with one or another of the various antidepressants available from the depression pharmacy (Figs. 7–28 and 7–29). The following section is a somewhat complex discussion of how different drugs are combined to treat depression and bipolar disorders, and may not be of interest to the novice. Thus, some readers may wish to skip this section and jump ahead to the section on electroconvulsive therapy.

The most frequent strategy for managing patients who do not respond to several different antidepressant monotherapies is to augment treatment with a second agent. Such treatment-resistant (sometimes also called treatment-refractory) cases have classically been approached with an algorithm, first trying single agents from different pharmacological classes (Fig. 7–29) and then boosting single agents with a second drug, making for a variety of possible drug combinations (Figs. 7–30 through 7–57). The three augmenting agents that have been most studied are lithium, thyroid hormone, and buspirone. Other augmenting strategies discussed here are commonly

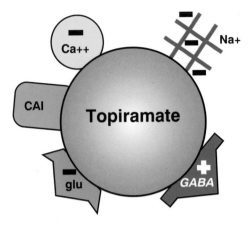

FIGURE 7–27. Shown here is an icon of **topiramate**'s pharmacologic actions. By interfering with calcium channels and sodium channels, topiramate is thought both to enhance the inhibitory actions of gamma aminobutyric acid (GABA) and to reduce the excitatory actions of glutamate. Topiramate is also a carbonic anhydrase inhibitor (CAI) and as such has independent anticonvulsant actions.

employed in practice, but their use is often based more on art and anecdote than on scientific studies.

## Lithium and Mood Stabilizers as Augmenting Agents

Lithium is the classical augmenting agent for unipolar depression resistant to first-line treatment with antidepressants (classic combo in Fig. 7–30). Lithium may boost the antidepressant actions of first-line antidepressants by acting synergistically on second messenger systems. Early studies indicate that the anticonvulsant class of mood stabilizers can also augment inadequate treatment responses to first-line antidepressants. Lithium and anticonvulsants are also used in combination with antidepressants for bipolar depression; however, in this disorder the mood stabilizers are the first-line treatment and antidepressants are given to augment inadequate response to a mood stabilizer rather than the other way around (see discussion of combination treatments for bipolar disorders below).

## Thyroid Hormone as an Augmenting Agent

Since thyroid illness is commonly associated with depression, especially in women, it has long been observed that treating the thyroid abnormalities also can reverse the depression. This is especially true for treating hypothyroidism with thyroid hormone replacement (either T3 or T4). It has even been observed that giving supplemental thyroid hormone to depressed patients unresponsive to first-line antidepressants but without overt hypothyroidism can boost the antidepressant response of the first-line antidepressant (thyroid combo in Fig. 7–30). Thyroid hormone is also commonly administered to bipolar patients resistant to mood stabilizers, particularly those with rapid cycling (see discussion of combinations for bipolar disorders below).

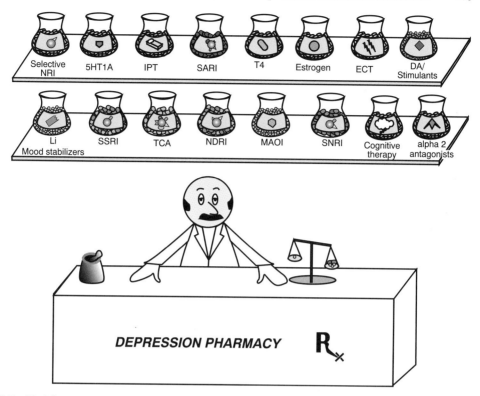

FIGURE 7–28. There are many treatments for depression, indicated here as therapies on the shelf of the depression pharmacy. Many of these treatments are used as single interventions in the treatment of depression. The therapies include **selective norepinephrine reuptake inhibitors** (selective NRIs); serotonin 1A receptor agonists (**5HT1A agents**) interpersonal psychotherapy (IPT); serotonin antagonists/reuptake inhibitors (**SARIs**); thyroid hormone (**TH**) or **estrogen**; electroconvulsive therapy (**ECT**); dopaminergic agonists such as pramipexole and dopamine releasers/stimulants such as amphetamine and methylphenidate **DA/stimulants**; lithium (**Li**) or other mood stabilizers; serotonin selective reuptake inhibitors (**SSRIs**); tricyclic antidepressants (**TCAs**); norepinephrine and dopamine reuptake inhibitors (**NDRIs**); monoamine oxidase inhibitors (**MAOIs**); serotonin norepinephrine reuptake inhibitors (**SNRIs**); **cognitive therapy** (psychotherapy) and **alpha 2 antagonists**.

### Buspirone, the Serotonin 1A Augmenting Agent

The serotonin 1A partial agonist buspirone, whose primary use is in generalized anxiety disorder, is also used as a popular augmenting agent for treatment-resistant depression, particularly in North America (serotonin 1A combo in Fig. 7–30). Its potential mechanism of action as an antidepressant augmenting agent is shown in Figures 7–31 to 7–33.

If serotonin is very low or depleted from serotonergic neurons in depression, there would not be much of it released for an SSRI to block its reuptake (Fig. 7–31). Thus, there would theoretically be inadequate desensitization of somatodendritic 5HT1A autoreceptors. Unlike the SSRIs, which are all dependent for their actions on the endogenous release of serotonin, buspirone is not dependent on serotonin levels because it has direct actions on 5HT1A receptors (Fig. 7–32). Thus, buspirone may be able to "kick start" the desensitization process directly. Initially,

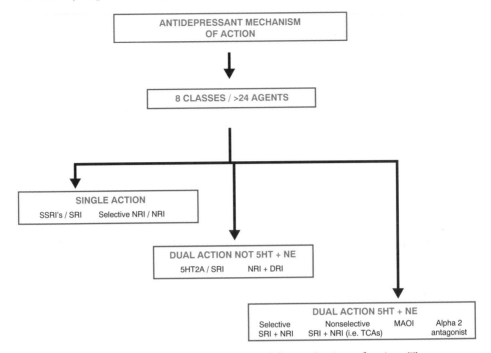

FIGURE 7–29. **Antidepressant monotherapies** organized by mechanism of action. There are over two dozen agents acting by eight distinct pharmacological mechanisms. These include antidepressants that have single neurotransmitter action (the five SSRIs and the selective NRI reboxetine); agents that have dual actions on the same or similar neurotransmitter system (the SARI nefazodone and the NDRI bupropion); and agents that have dual actions (TCAs, MAOIs, the dual SNRI venlafaxine, and the alpha 2 antagonist mirtazapine).

buspirone also slows neuronal impulses, which may also help the neuron to replete its serotonin (Fig. 7–32).

Thus, buspirone is synergistic with the SSRIs (Fig. 7–33). To the extent that buspirone is a partial agonist and thus partially blocks the 5HT1A autoreceptors, it

FIGURE 7–30. Combination treatments for unipolar depression (unipolar combos). The treatment of depression generally begins with a single agent, called a **first-line agent**, as **monotherapy**. If single agents acting by a single neurotransmitter mechanism fail, then single agents acting by multiple neurotransmitter mechanisms may be effective. If these monotherapies also fail, antidepressants are often used in **combination** with other drugs, hormones, or even other antidepressants. For example, the classical combination of agents is a first-line agent with lithium or a mood stabilizer as augmentation (**classic combo**). Another strategy is to augment a first-line agent with thyroid hormone (**thyroid combo**). Yet another approach that has been well documented to work in some cases is addition of the 5HT1A partial agonist buspirone or possibly the 5HT1A antagonist pindolol to a first-line antidepressant, especially an SSRI (**serotonin 1A combo**). A powerful if potentially dangerous combination is to use a tricyclic antidepressant and a monoamine oxidase inhibitor simultaneously (**cautious combo**). Early studies suggest that addition of reproductive hormones, especially estradiol, for women with treatment-resistant depression may be helpful in some cases (**estrogen combo**). Short-term use of sedative-hypnotics or anxiolytics may be necessary if insomnia or anxiety is persistent and cannot be managed by other strategies (**insomnia/anxiety combo**).

# Unipolar Combos

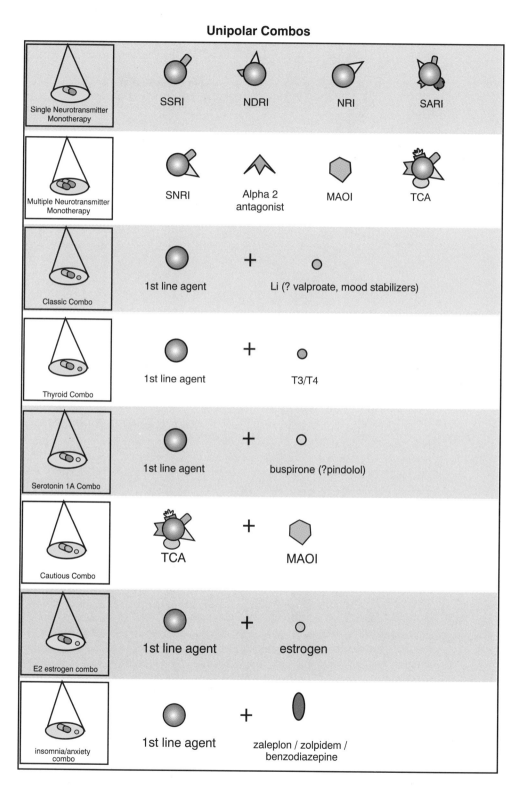

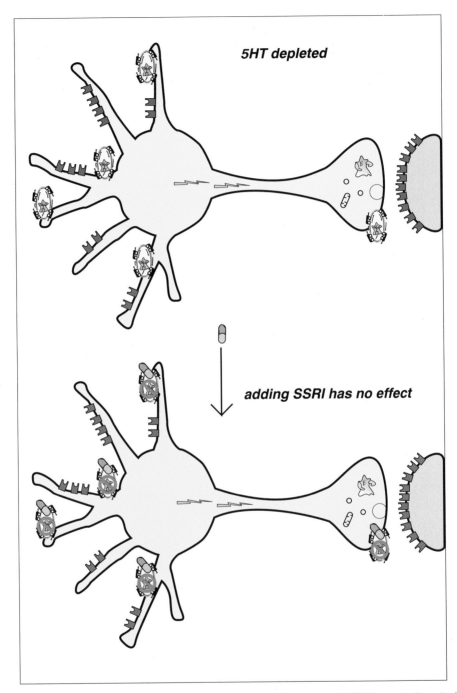

FIGURE 7–31. *Mechanism of action of buspirone augmentation*–part 1. SSRIs act indirectly by increasing synaptic levels of 5HT that has been released there. If 5HT is depleted, there is no 5HT release, and SSRIs are ineffective. This has been postulated to be the explanation for the lack of SSRI therapeutic actions or loss of therapeutic action of SSRI ("poop out") in some patients.

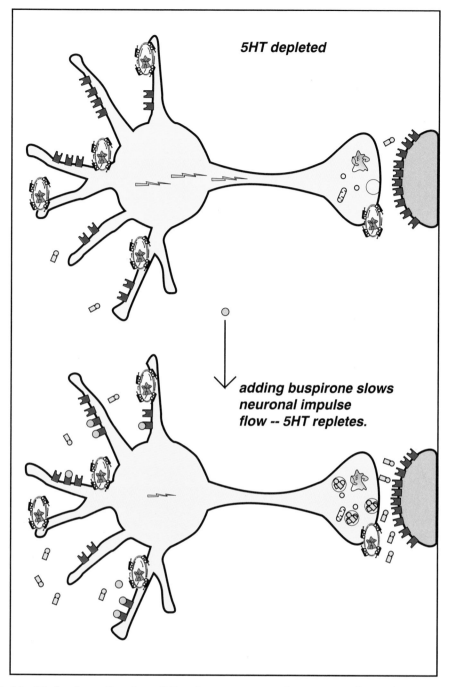

FIGURE 7–32. *Mechanism of action of buspirone augmentation—part* 2. Shown here is how buspirone may augment SSRI action both by repleting 5HT and by directly desensitizing 5HT1A receptors. One theoretical mechanism of how 5HT is allowed to reaccumulate in the 5HT-depleted neuron is the shutdown of neuronal impulse flow. If 5HT release is essentially turned off for a while so that the neuron retains all the 5HT it synthesizes, this may allow repletion of 5HT stores. A 5HT1A partial agonist such as buspirone acts directly on somatodendritic autoreceptors to inhibit neuronal impulse flow, possibly allowing repletion of 5HT stores. Also, buspirone could boost actions directly at 5HT1A receptors to help the small amount of 5HT available in this scenario accomplish the targeted desensitization of 5HT1A somatodendritic autoreceptors that is necessary for antidepressant actions.

277

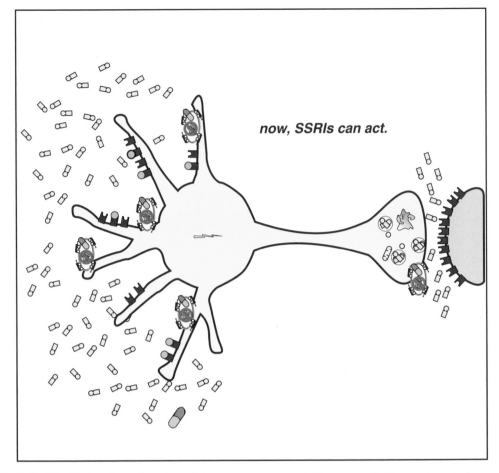

*now, SSRIs can act.*

FIGURE 7–33. *Mechanism of action of buspirone augmentation*–part 3. Shown here is how buspirone potentiates ineffective SSRI action at 5HT1A somatodendritic autoreceptors, resulting in the desired disinhibition of the 5HT neuron. This combination of 5HT1A agonists plus SSRIs may be more effective, not only in depression but also in other disorders treated by SSRIs, such as obsessive-compulsive disorder and panic.

may act even faster than an SSRI. Blockade of these receptors immediately disinhibits them, whereas stimulation of them causes delayed disinhibition due to the time it takes for them to desensitize.

### Pindolol, Another Serotonin 1A Augmenting Agent

The idea of blocking 5HT1A somatodendritic autoreceptors is also exploited by pindolol, a well-known beta adrenergic blocker that also is an antagonist and very partial agonist at 5HT1A receptors. Preclinical studies suggest that pindolol can immediately disinhibit serotonin neurons, leading to the proposal that it may be a rapid onset antidepressant or augmenting agent. Some clinical studies do suggest that pindolol augmentation may speed the onset of action of SSRIs or may boost inadequate response to SSRIs, but not all investigators agree. Nevertheless, 5HT1A antagonists are in development as potential novel and rapid-acting antidepressants.

## Monoamine Oxidase Inhibitor/Tricyclic Antidepressant Combinations

One old-fashioned augmentation strategy that has fallen out of favor in recent years is to combine with great caution a TCA and an MAO inhibitor (the cautious combo in Fig. 7–30). Given its potential dangers (e.g., sudden hypertensive episodes, orthostatic hypotension, drug and dietary interactions, obesity), as well as the wide variety of other antidepressant combinations available today, this combination is rarely necessary or justified.

## Estrogen and Reproductive Hormones as Antidepressant Augmenting Agents

Another hormone combination therapy is to combine a first-line antidepressant, especially an SSRI, with estrogen replacement therapy in perimenopausal or postmenopausal women refractory to treatment with antidepressant monotherapies (the estrogen combo in Fig. 7–30). Unfortunately, there are few if any controlled clinical trials to provide guidance on how to combine estrogen with antidepressants. Numerous case reports and anecdotes from clinicians demonstrate that some women respond to estrogen who do not respond to antidepressants, and other women respond to estrogen plus an antidepressant who do not respond to antidepressants alone. Since estrogen is itself a direct activator of transcription, it may be able to synergize at the genomic level with the transcription activated by SSRIs (Fig. 7–34) to produce a molecular result greater than that which the SSRIs can produce alone.

Other uses of the reproductive hormone approach are to avoid cyclical use of estrogen/progestins, eliminate progestins, add testosterone, or add dihydroepiandrosterone (DHEA). Such approaches remain anecdotal and require controlled studies of how they may be useful augmenting agents for antidepressants both in women and in men.

## Insomnia/Anxiety Combinations

Insomnia is a common comorbid condition with depression, and frequently is made worse by antidepressants, particularly the SSRIs. When insomnia persists despite adequate evaluation and attempts to reduce it by other approaches, it is often necessary to use a concomitant sedative-hypnotic, especially a short-acting nonbenzodiazepine with rapid onset such as zaleplon or zolpidem. At times a benzodiazepine sedative hypnotic such as triazolam or temazepam may be necessary. If anxiety persists during the day and cannot be otherwise managed, it may be necessary to add an anxiolytic benzodiazepine such as alprazolam or clonazepam. Use of sedative-hypnotics and anxiolytics should be short-term whenever possible.

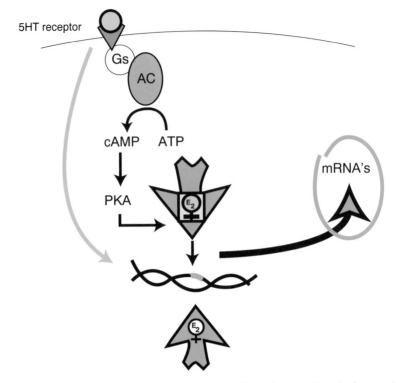

FIGURE 7–34. **Estrogen** acts at receptors in the neuronal cell nucleus to directly **boost the transcription of genes**. This may be synergistic with the antidepressant actions of first-line antidepressant agents in activating transcription factors (TF) in some women.

## Bipolar Combinations

Combination treatment with two or more psychotropic medications is the rule rather than the exception for bipolar disorders (bipolar combos in Fig. 7–35). First-line treatment is with either lithium or valproic acid. When patients fail to stabilize in the acute manic phase on one of these first-line treatments, the preferred second-

FIGURE 7–35. Combination treatments for bipolar disorder (**bipolar combos**). Combination drug treatment is the rule rather than the exception for patients with bipolar disorder. It is best to attempt monotherapy, however, with first-line lithium or valproic acid, with second-line atypical antipsychotics, or with third-line anticonvulsant mood stabilizers. A very common situation in acute treatment of the manic phase of bipolar disorder is to treat with both a mood stabilizer and an atypical antipsychotic (**atypical combo**). Agitated patients may require intermittent doses of sedating benzodiazepines (**benzo assault weapon**), whereas patients out of control may require intermittent doses of tranquilizing neuroleptics (**neuroleptic nuclear weapon**). For maintenance treatment, patients often require combinations of two mood stabilizers (**mood stabilizer combo**) or a mood stabilizer with an atypical antipsychotic (**atypical combo**). For patients who have depressive episodes despite mood stabilizer or atypical combos, antidepressants may be required (**antidepressant combo**). However, antidepressants may also decompensate patients into overt mania, rapid cycling states, or mixed states of mania and depression. Thus, antidepressant combos are used cautiously.

# Bipolar Combos

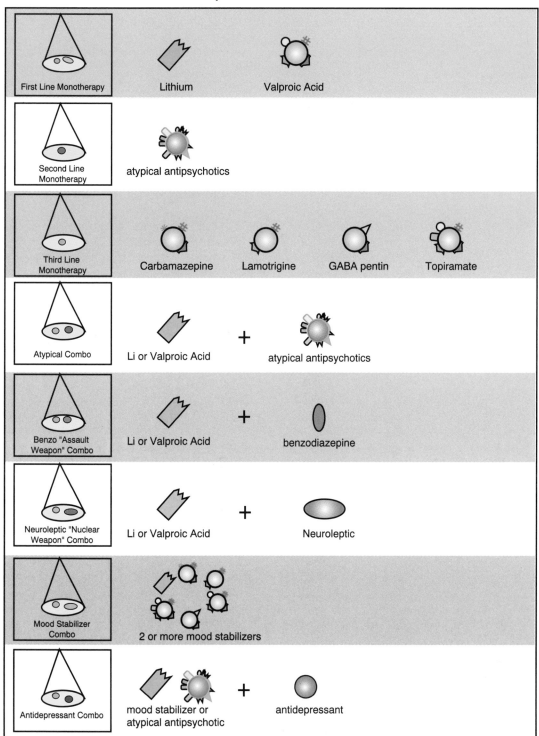

line agent is an atypical antipsychotic. Atypical antipsychotics are even becoming first-line treatments for the manic phase of bipolar disorder.

If lithium, valproic acid, or atypical antipsychotic monotherapies are not effective in the acute situation, they can be used together (atypical combo in Fig. 7–35). If this is not effective, a benzodiazepine or a conventional antipsychotic (i.e., a neuroleptic) can be added to first- or second-line monotherapies, especially for the most disturbed patients (Fig. 7–35). That is, sedating benzodiazepines can be used for lesser degrees of agitation (benzo assault weapon in Fig. 7–35), but neuroleptic antipsychotics may be necessary for the most disturbed and out-of-control patients (nuclear weapon in Fig. 7–35). Neuroleptic antipsychotics should be restricted to the acute phase, and administered sparingly.

For maintenance treatment, failure of first-line mood stabilizers or second-line atypical antipsychotics to control symptoms adequately may lead to monotherapy trials with other anticonvulsants such as carbamazepine, lamotrigine, gabapentin, and topiramate (third-line monotherapy).

Therapeutic recommendations for maintenance treatment of bipolar disorder are undergoing rapid changes. In the recent past, lithium was the hallmark of this treatment, often with antidepressant co-therapy for patients prone to depression as well as mania and not adequately controlled by lithium alone. Now, however, several new therapeutic principles are guiding the treatment of bipolar disorders in the maintenance phase.

First, anticonvulsants, particularly valproic acid, are now considered excellent first-line choices along with lithium, although lithium is the only agent approved for such use.

Second, atypical antipsychotics are clearly second-line choices for maintenance therapy of bipolar disorder when one or more mood stabilizers alone or in combination are not adequate. Furthermore, atypical antipsychotics are also becoming first-line choices for bipolar maintenance as the safety and efficacy data from controlled trials continue to evolve.

Third, antidepressant treatments are not benign in this condition. Although many bipolar patients have been classically maintained on both lithium and an antidepressant, it is now recognized that antidepressants frequently decompensate bipolar patients, causing not only overt mania or hypomania, but also the problems of mixed mania and rapid cycling, which are much more difficult to recognize and treat. The trend today is to use antidepressants sparingly and if necessary, only in the presence of robust mood stabilization with mood stabilizers, atypical antipsychotics, or both. In fact, both mood stabilizers and atypical antipsychotics may prove to be useful for the depressed phase of bipolar illness, reducing or perhaps eliminating the need for potentially destabilizing antidepressants in bipolar patients. Thus, antidepressants are now relegated to third-line use in bipolar disorder, behind lithium or anticonvulsant mood stabilizers and atypical antipsychotics. This is an antidepressant-sparing strategy for the treatment of bipolar disorder.

Combination treatments for maintenance of bipolar disorder can include two or more mood stabilizers; a mood stabilizer and an atypical antipsychotic; a mood stabilizer and/or atypical antipsychotic with a benzodiazepine; a mood stabilizer with thyroid hormone; and even a mood stabilizer and/or atypical antipsychotic with an antidepressant (Fig. 7–35).

## A Rational Approach to Antidepressant Combinations with Other Antidepressants

In the current managed care era, the modern psychopharmacologist/psychiatrist may deal almost exclusively with patients resistant to conventional treatment approaches, since easier cases are handled by lower cost or primary care providers, and these difficult cases are selectively referred. Treating patients resistant to well documented strategies by using less well documented but pharmacologically and molecularly rational strategies is not for the novice, nor for those who wish to work within treatment guidelines for drugs with government regulatory approvals and with the documentation of numerous published controlled clinical trials. First-line monotherapies and combination therapies are summarized in Figure 7–36.

The rationale for proceeding to the use of combinations of two antidepressants is based on a number of factors. First, certain combinations of antidepressants can exploit theoretical pharmacologic and molecular synergies to boost monoaminergic neurotransmission. Second, some combinations of antidepressants have anecdotal and empirical evidence of safety and efficacy from uncontrolled use in clinical practice. Finally, the idea of using multiple pharmacologic mechanisms simultaneously for the most difficult cases is already a recognized therapeutic approach in other areas of medicine, such as the treatment of resistant bacterial and human immunodeficiency virus infections, cancer, and resistant hypertension. Later in this chapter we will describe three specific approaches to the management of patients resistant to first-line monotherapies and typical augmentation strategies, namely, the serotonergic strategy, the adrenergic strategy, and the dual-mechanism or "heroic" strategy.

*Diagnosing treatment resistance.* Many patients have a difficult time with antidepressants, and following a trial with several of drugs, it is easy to conclude that they are treatment-resistant. Prior to concluding that a patient is not responding to antidepressants and therefore truly treatment-resistant, however, it is necessary to carefully review the treatment history to rule out medication intolerance masquerading as medication resistance (e.g., many medications tried, but few adequate trials of full doses for 4 to 8 weeks). The solution to medication intolerance may be to augment with an antidepressant that cancels the side effects of the antidepressant that is not tolerable.

The other situation to rule out when establishing treatment resistance in depression is misdiagnosis as resistant unipolar depression when the patient is actually bipolar. That is, an apparently unipolar patient with drug-induced agitation may actually be a bipolar patient with antidepressant-induced rapid cycling or mixed mania of an unrecognized bipolar disorder. This situation will commonly be exacerbated by combining two antidepressants. The solution to this problem may, in fact, be to discontinue antidepressants and optimize treatment with mood stabilizers and atypical antipsychotics before using any antidepressant agent.

*Principles of antidepressant combinations.* The first principle of combination treatment with antidepressants is to combine mechanisms, not just drugs. That is, the important thing is the pharmacological mechanisms being combined; drugs are just the "mules" that carry mechanisms on their backs. Some drugs have one principal mech-

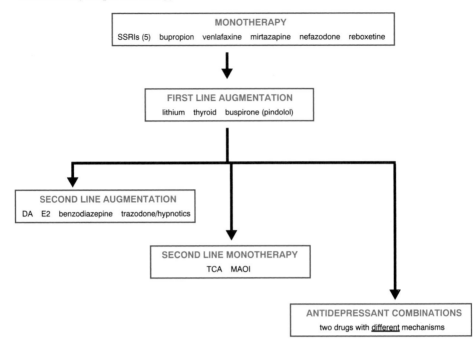

FIGURE 7–36. This figure summarizes both **first-line monotherapies** and the most commonly used **combination therapies** for unipolar depression. Note that antidepressant combinations at the far right and the end of the line are to be used after other strategies fail.

anism, others multiple mechanisms. Thus, combining two drugs may in fact be combining three or more mechanisms. Furthermore, there are many different drug mules that carry the same mechanisms, allowing for multiple approaches to achieving any given mixture of mechanisms by using several different combinations of drugs.

A second principle of antidepressant combination is to promote bad mathematics. That is, successful mixture of drug mechanisms leads to pharmacological synergy for antidepressant therapeutic actions (where 1 + 1 = 10). Furthermore, knowing the mechanism of antidepressant side effects can lead to other successful mixtures of drug mechanisms where opposing side effect profiles promote tolerability (in other words, where 1 + 1 = 0). The cleverest mixtures of antidepressants can yield both forms of bad mathematics at the same time, namely synergistic boost to efficacy along with improved tolerability achieved by canceling mutual side effects.

The third principle of antidepressant combinations is to exploit theoretically important synergies within the serotonin, norepinephrine, and even dopamine monoaminergic systems. Specifically, two independent pharmacologic actions at any one of the monoaminergic systems can be synergistic. Examples of this are combination of either serotonin or norepinephrine reuptake blockade with alpha 2 blockade, or 5HT reuptake blockade with serotonin 2A antagonism, as discussed earlier in this chapter. Specific examples of how to implement this approach for serotonin are given in Figure 7–37. Specific examples of how to implement this approach for norepinephrine and dopamine are given in Figures 7–38 to 7–43.

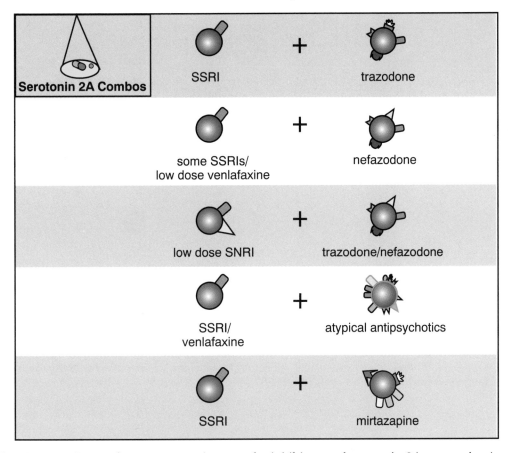

FIGURE 7–37. Synergy between **serotonin reuptake inhibitors** and **serotonin 2A antagonists** is commonly observed. Various specific drug combinations to implement this strategy in unipolar depression are shown here.

The other theoretically important synergy to exploit for treating resistant depression is that between serotonin and norepinephrine (e.g., Figs. 7–39 and 7–44). Thus, boosting neurotransmission at both monoamine systems with either a single drug or combinations of drugs can also boost therapeutic efficacy in treatment-resistant depression. Several specific examples of how to implement this strategy are given in Figures 7–45 to 7–57.

*Synergy within the serotoninergic system.* Boosting serotonin neurotransmission has proved to be useful not only in treatment-resistant depression, but for treatment resistance within the whole family of "serotonin spectrum disorders," such as obsessive-compulsive disorder, panic disorder, social phobia, posttraumatic stress disorder, and bulimia.

A major example of pharmacologic synergy within the serotonin system is the 5HT2A antagonist strategy. This is shown in Figures 7–20 and 7–21 and was discussed earlier in the section on nefazodone and the SARIs. For this strategy, robust inhibition of serotonin reuptake by agents in the left column of Figure 7–37 is

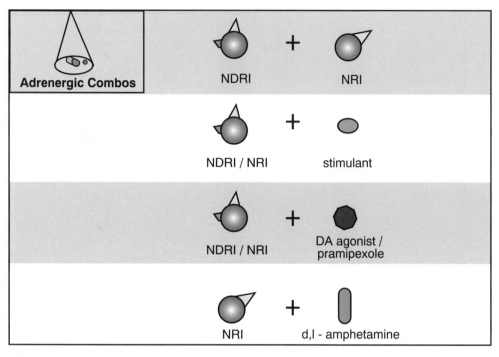

FIGURE 7–38. Shown here are various drug combinations for use in treatment resistant unipolar depression to **boost adrenergic neurotransmission**, which include either norepinephrine, dopamine, or both.

combined with robust inhibition of serotonin 2A receptors in the right column of Figure 7–37. These are not necessarily the only mechanisms combined by the specific agents shown, but this strategy is the common denominator across all pairings.

Perhaps the most commonly used example of the serotonin 2A strategy is the combination of an SSRI with trazodone. Clinicians have long recognized that trazodone will improve the agitation and insomnia often associated with SSRIs, allow high doses of the SSRI to be given, and consequently boost the efficacy of the SSRI not only in depression, but also in obsessive-compulsive disorder and other anxiety disorders. Thus, both types of bad math are in play here.

Perhaps the best documented example showing the enhanced efficacy of this serotonin 2A antagonist strategy is the use of the atypical antipsychotics to boost efficacy in nonpsychotic depression refractory to treatment with an SSRI.

*Norepinephrine and synergy.* Boosting noradrenergic neurotransmission may be useful not only in depression in general, but in partial responders as well, especially those with fatigue, apathy, and cognitive slowing. Several examples of how to boost noradrenergic neurotransmission beyond that of single agents alone are given in Figure 7–38. Thus, selective noradrenergic reuptake inhibitors such as reboxetine or nonselective noradrenergic reuptake inhibitors such as desipramine can be combined with the noradrenergic/dopaminergic agent bupropion. Also, bupropion or a noradrenergic reuptake inhibitor can be combined with a dopamine-releasing stimulant (such as amphetamine, methylphenidate, diethylpropion or phentermine) or with a

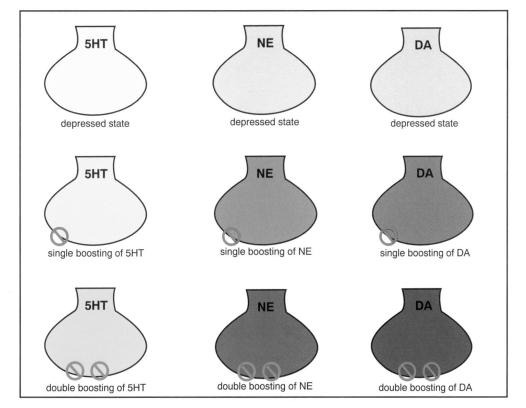

FIGURE 7–39. **Key to combos.** The figures from here to the end of the chapter will employ the visual key shown here. The depressed, unmedicated state is shown by faded colors representing neurotransmitter depletion. If any of the three monoamine neurotransmitters (5HT, NE, or DA) is boosted by one of the drugs in the combination being illustrated, its corresponding color will light up moderately. Thus, single boosting of 5HT will moderately light up yellow; single boosting of NE will moderately light up purple; and single boosting of DA will moderately light up blue. Some of the combos have synergistic actions on the same monoamine neurotransmitter system. In such cases, the colors will be doubly lit up to represent the potential synergy of this approach by the brightest coloring of 5HT (yellow), NE (purple), or DA (blue).

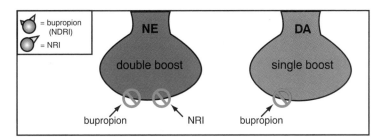

FIGURE 7–40. **Adrenergic combo 1: Bupropion** plus norepinephrine reuptake inhibitor (**NRI**). Here the NE actions of bupropion are double-boosted by the NRI (either selective reboxetine or nonselective desipramine, maprotilene, nortriptyline, or protriptyline). Dopamine is single-boosted by bupropion only.

287

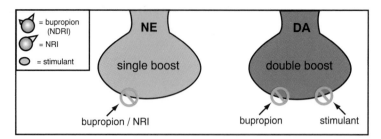

FIGURE 7–41. **Adrenergic combo 2: Bupropion** can be combined with a **stimulant** such as *d*-amphetamine or methylphenidate. The stimulant will add a double dopamine boost to bupropion, which boosts dopamine in its own right. A single boost of norepinephrine from bupropion also is present.

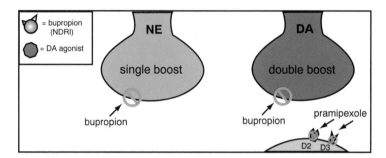

FIGURE 7–42. **Adrenergic combo 3:** The actions of **bupropion** at dopamine neurons can be double-boosted by a direct-acting dopamine **D2 and D3 agonist** such as pramipexole. Norepinephrine is also single-boosted by bupropion.

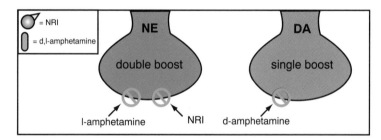

FIGURE 7–43. **Adrenergic combo 4: NRI** plus *d,l*-amphetamine. In this case, the NRI action at NE is double-boosted by a mixture of amphetamine salts containing the *l* as well as the *d* form of amphetamine. The *l*-amphetamine causes NE release. In addition, DA will be single-boosted by the *d*-amphetamine, which causes DA release.

direct dopamine agonist such as pramipexole. Anecdotally, this may be especially useful for patients with retarded or melancholic depression or those who require an antidepressant concomitantly with a mood stabilizer for bipolar depression.

*The heroic strategy: boosting both serotonin and norepinephrine.* In the most refractory of all patients, it may be necessary to use both serotonin and adrenergic combination

# Unipolar Combos

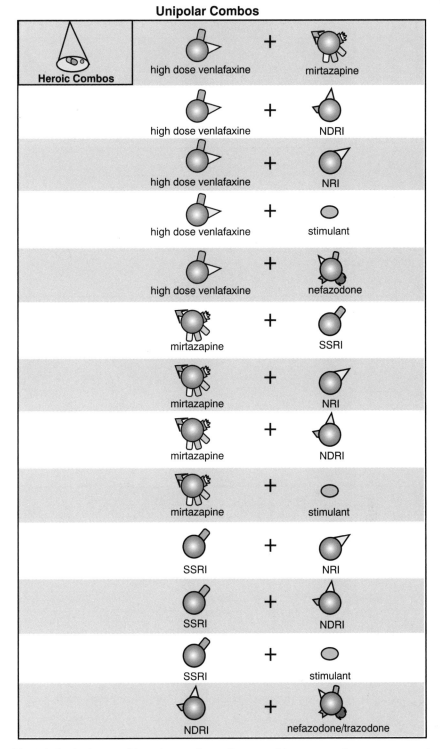

FIGURE 7–44. A baker's dozen of **heroic combos** of two antidepressants for treatment-resistant unipolar depression are shown here. Each individual-combination is explained in the figures that follow (Figs. 7–45 through 7–57).

289

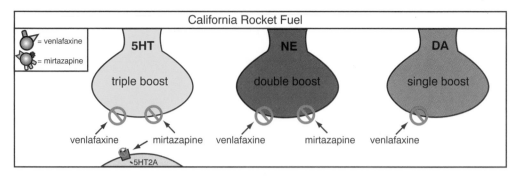

FIGURE 7-45. Heroic combo 1, or "**California rocket fuel**": High-dose venlafaxine plus mirtazapine. This is a combination of antidepressants that has a great degree of theoretical synergy: reuptake
blockade plus alpha 2 blockade; serotonin reuptake plus 5HT2A antagonism; 5HT actions plus NE
actions. Specifically, 5HT is triple-boosted, with reuptake blockade, alpha 2 antagonism, and 5HT2A
antagonism; NE is double-boosted, with reuptake blockade plus alpha 2 antagonism; and there may
even be a bit of single boost to DA from reuptake blockade.

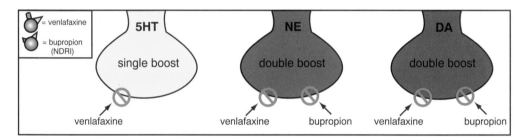

FIGURE 7-46. Heroic combo 2: **High-dose venlafaxine plus NDRI** (bupropion). Here, 5HT is
single-boosted, NE is double-boosted, and DA is double-boosted.

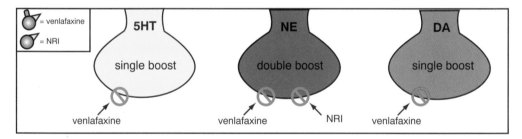

FIGURE 7-47. Heroic combo 3: **High-dose venlafaxine plus NRI**. Here, 5HT is single-boosted,
NE is double-boosted, and DA may be single-boosted. The NRI could be either selective reboxetine
or a nonselective TCA such as desipramine, maprotilene, nortriptyline, or protriptyline.

strategies (heroic combo; Fig. 7-44). A baker's dozen of heroic combos are given in
Figure 7-44 and shown graphically in Figures 7-45 through 7-57. These specific
drug combinations all do the same thing to one extent or another, namely, boost or
double-boost serotonin, norepinephrine, and/or dopamine. The net effects of these
combinations are shown in different shades of color in Figures 7-45 through 7-57,
with light colors representing no boost to the corresponding monoamine's neuro-

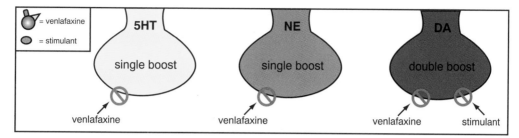

FIGURE 7–48. Heroic combo 4: **High-dose venlafaxine plus stimulant**. Here, 5HT and NE are single-boosted and DA is double-boosted. The stimulants could include *d*-amphetamine, methylphenidate, phentermine, or diethylpropion. It could also include direct-acting dopamine agonists such as pramipexole.

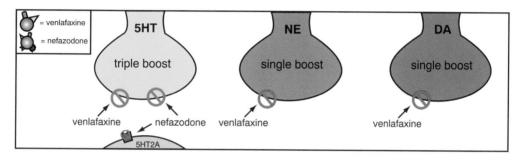

FIGURE 7–49. Heroic combo 5: **Venlafaxine plus nefazodone**. Serotonin will be double-boosted to a certain extent by nefazodone alone. At any dose of venlafaxine, the boosting of serotonin will be considerably enhanced. This enhancement of nefazodone's serotonin action can also be replicated by SSRIs, but citalopram may be the best tolerated. At high doses of venlafaxine, there will be not only boosting of 5HT but also single-boosting of NE and maybe DA.

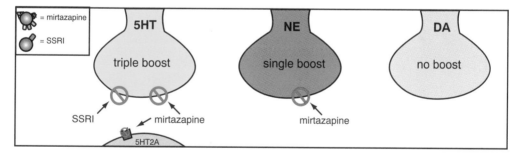

FIGURE 7–50. Heroic combo 6: **Mirtazapine plus SSRI**. Here serotonin is double-disinhibited both by reuptake blockage and by alpha 2 antagonism; NE is also single-boosted.

transmission, medium-intensity colors representing a single boost to that monoamine's neurotransmission, and high-intensity colors representing a double boost (see figure key in Fig. 7–39). One of the most theoretically powerful combinations is that of high-dose venlafaxine with mirtazapine ("California rocket fuel" in Fig. 7–45; also Fig. 7–44). These drugs combine synergies on synergy, that is, reuptake

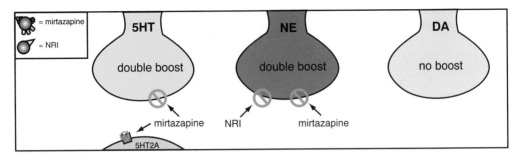

FIGURE 7–51. Heroic combo 7: **Mirtazapine plus NRI.** Here NE is double-disinhibited both by reuptake blockade and by alpha 2 antagonism. Reboxetine is better tolerated with mirtazapine than TCAs for this purpose. Serotonin is also single-boosted.

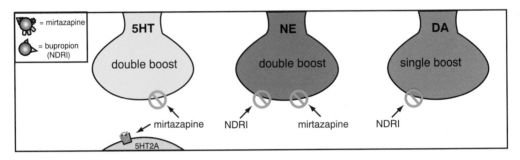

FIGURE 7–52. Heroic combo 8: **Mirtazapine plus NDRI** (bupropion). Here NE is double-boosted, and 5HT and DA are single-boosted.

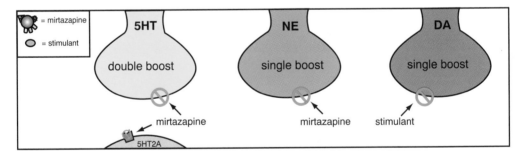

FIGURE 7–53. Heroic combo 9: **Mirtazapine plus stimulant.** Here, 5HT, NE, and DA are all single-boosted. The stimulants could include *d*-amphetamine, methylphenidate, phentermine, or di-ethylpropion. It could also include direct-acting dopamine agonists such as pramipexole.

blockade plus alpha 2 blockade for double disinhibition, actions at 5HT and NE actions boosting 5HT at 5HT1A receptors yet blocking 5HT2A receptors.

The point is to use safe and rational drug combinations that exploit expected pharmacological and molecular synergies while even promoting mutual tolerabilities. Each of the combinations in Figure 7–44 is used clinically and has helped some patients but not others. Unfortunately, little scientific documentation of this empirical usefulness of such rational combinations is yet available, but many studies

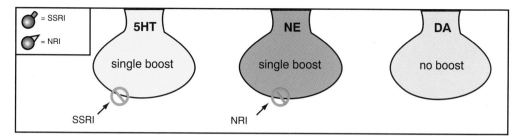

FIGURE 7–54. Heroic combo 10: **SSRI plus NRI.** Here, 5HT and NE are both single-boosted. The preferred NRI is selective reboxetine, as there are no drug interactions. Nonselective TCAs that are preferential NRIs such as desipramine, maprotilene, nortriptyline, or protriptyline can be combined if plasma drug levels of the TCA are monitored, especially if fluoxetine or paroxetine is the SSRI chosen.

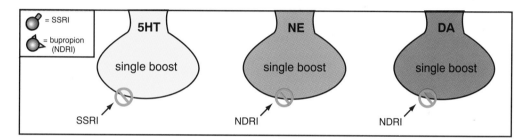

FIGURE 7–55. Heroic combo 11: **SSRI plus NDRI** (bupropion). Here 5HT, NE, and DA are all single-boosted.

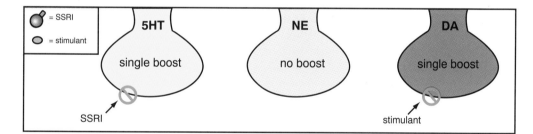

FIGURE 7–56. Heroic combo 12: **SSRI plus stimulant.** Here, 5HT and DA are single-boosted. The stimulants could include *d*-amphetamine, methylphenidate, phentermine, or diethylpropion. The combo could also include direct-acting dopamine agonists such as pramipexole.

are ongoing and should clarify the best options for the most difficult cases in which the benefits of this approach outweigh the risks.

## Electroconvulsive Therapy

Failure to respond to a variety of antidepressants, singly or in combination, is the key factor indicating consideration of electroconvulsive therapy (ECT). This is the only therapeutic agent for the treatment of depression that is rapid in onset and can

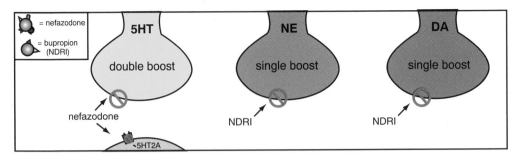

FIGURE 7–57. Heroic combo 13: **Nefazodone plus NDRI** (bupropion). In this case, the serotonergic single boost of nefazodone is added to the NE and DA single boost of bupropion.

start after even a single treatment, typically within a few days. The mechanism is unknown but is thought to be related to the probable mobilization of neurotransmitters caused by the seizure. In experimental animals, ECT down-regulates beta receptors (analogous to antidepressants) but up-regulates 5HT2 receptors (opposite of antidepressants). Memory loss and social stigma are the primary problems associated with ECT and limit its use. There can also be striking regional differences across the various countries in the world in the frequency of ECT use and in ECT techniques. For example, ECT may be more commonly used in Europe and the United Kingdom and on the U.S. East Coast and less commonly used on the U.S. West Coast.

Electroconvulsive therapy is especially useful when rapid onset of clinical effect is desired and when patients are refractory to a number of antidepressant drugs. It is also very helpful in psychotic and bipolar depression and in postpartum psychosis. If the mechanism of the therapeutic action of ECT could be unraveled, it might lead to a new antidepressant drug capable of rapid onset of antidepressant effects or with special value for refractory patients. Until then, ECT will remain a valuable member of the therapeutic armamentarium for depression.

## Psychotherapy

In recent years, modern psychotherapy research has begun to standardize and test selected psychotherapies in a manner analogous to the testing of antidepresssant drugs in clinical trials. Thus, psychotherapies are now being tested by being administered according to standard protocols by therapists receiving standardized training and using standardized manuals, and also in standard "doses" for fixed duration. Such uses of psychotherapies are being compared in clinical trials with placebo or antidepressants. The results have shown that interpersonal psychotherapy and cognitive psychotherapy for depression may be as effective as antidepressants themselves in certain patients. Proof of the efficacy of certain psychotherapies is thus beginning to evolve.

Research is only beginning on how to combine psychotherapy with drugs. Although some of the earliest studies did not indicate any additive benefit of tricyclic antidepressants and interpersonal psychotherapy, recent studies are now demonstrating that there can be an additive benefit between psychotherapy and antidepressants. One recent study of nefazodone suggests that it is particularly effective when combined with cognitive behavioral psychotherapy for patients with chronic depression. Another study of nortriptyline suggests an additive benefit of interpersonal psychotherapy, particularly when looking at long-term outcomes. It is not known whether the addition of psychotherapy to antidepressant responders who are not in full remission might lead to remission and recovery, but this is an interesting possibility. Although psychotherapy is frequently employed on an empirical basis, it is not yet proven that its addition to the psychopharmacological treatment of patients resistant to antidepressant monotherapy treatment (either no response, or a response but not a remission) improves outcomes. As managed care reduces the availability of psychotherapy, mental health professionals are becoming increasingly dependent on a psychopharmacological approach. The rapidly evolving scientific demonstration of the benefit of adjunctive psychotherapy should provide much needed and welcome justification by showing who benefits from what kinds of psychotherapy combined with which specific antidepressants. Cognitive and behavioral psychotherapies are also of value as adjuncts to antidepressants for the treatment of anxiety disorders.

## Summary

In this chapter, we have discussed the mechanisms of action of several of the newer classes of antidepressant drugs and mood stabilizers. The acute pharmacological actions of these agents on neurotransmitter receptors have been described. The reader should now understand the proposed mechanisms of action of dual reuptake inhibitors, alpha 2 antagonists, and serotonin 2A antagonists/serotonin reuptake inhibitors, as well as those of lithium and the anticonvulsant mood stabilizers for the treatment of bipolar disorder, particularly the acute manic phase.

We have reviewed antidepressant augmentation strategies, including the principles and several specific examples. Finally, we have touched on the use of electroconvulsive therapy and psychotherapy for the treatment of depression.

Although the specific pragmatic guidelines for use of these various therapeutic modalities for depression have not been emphasized, the reader should now have a basis for the rational use of antidepressant and mood-stabilizing drugs founded on application of principles of drug action on neurotransmission via actions at key receptors and enzymes.

# CHAPTER 8

# ANXIOLYTICS AND SEDATIVE-HYPNOTICS

In this chapter we will discuss anxiety and the antianxiety drugs (i.e., anxiolytics) as well as insomnia and the sedative-hypnotic drugs (i.e. sleeping pills). We will emphasize generalized anxiety in this chapter and take up specific anxiety disorders such as panic disorder and obsessive-compulsive disorder in the following chapter. Here we will sketch a simple outline of the clinical features and the biological basis of anxiety and insomnia in order to provide background for understanding the actions of anxiolytic as well as sedative-hypnotic drugs. The reader is referred to standard references for details on diagnostic criteria for the various specific disorders of

297

anxiety and sleep because here we will emphasize only general principles and concepts about the emotion of anxiety and the phenomena of sleep.

Our discussion of antianxiety and sedative-hypnotic treatments will attempt to develop the psychopharmacological concepts underlying the functioning of such treatments. We will build on the pharmacological principles already introduced in our earlier discussions of serotonin and norepinephrine neurons and their receptors. We will also describe in some detail the pharmacology of the gamma-aminobutyric acid (GABA) neuron and GABA receptors linked to benzodiazepine receptors. However, we will not provide pragmatic guidelines on the use of anxiolytics or sedative hypnotics in clinical practice. The reader is referred to standard handbooks of drug treatment for specifics of drug dosing and side effects.

## Clinical Description of Anxiety

Anxiety is a normal emotion under circumstances of threat and is thought to be part of the evolutionary "fight or flight" reaction of survival. Whereas it may be normal or even adaptive to be anxious when a sabertooth tiger or its modern day equivalent is attacking, there are many circumstances in which the presence of anxiety is maladaptive and constitutes a psychiatric disorder. The idea of anxiety as a psychiatric disorder, however, has undergone considerable change in recent years.

There are significant prognostic and treatment implications to categorizing anxiety disorders by their diagnostic subtype (obsessive-compulsive disorder, panic disorder, social phobia generalized anxiety disorder [GAD] etc.). Diagnostic criteria for these entities are given in the Diagnostic and Statistical Manual of Mental Disorders, 4th edition (DSM-IV) and the International Classification of Diseases, 10th edition (ICD-10). Anxiety disorder subtypes will be discussed in further detail in Chapter 9. Here we will discuss generalized anxiety disorder (Table 8–1). This is an interesting entity to researchers and nosologists, but it is often not diagnosed in clinical practice. That is, primary care physicians tend to treat *symptoms* of anxiety and/or depression, whether or not they reach diagnostic thresholds (Fig. 8–1). Psychiatrists tend to focus on major depressive disorder or anxiety disorder subtypes that are usually comorbid conditions with GAD and not to address GAD explicitly.

Recent trends, however, suggest that GAD may be more important than originally thought and certainly worthy of diagnostic recognition, because it commonly represents a state of incomplete recovery from any number of anxiety and affective disorders. Incomplete recovery from depression has been discussed in Chapter 5 and called the "anxious responder" to an antidepressant (see Table 5–18). The term *anxious responder* refers to a patient with anxious depression whose disorder improves with antidepressant treatment by elimination of the depressed mood but who is not in complete remission because the generalized anxiety, worry, tension, insomnia, and somatic symptoms persist. As a form of anxious depression continuing in milder form, it continues to cause disability and distress and even worse, may be a harbinger of breakdown into another episode of depression. The same residual state may be the case for incomplete treatment responses to anxiety disorder subtypes such as panic disorder and others. Thus, it is important to take a careful longitudinal history of the patient who presents with generalized anxiety but does not meet diagnostic criteria for major depressive disorder or an anxiety disorder subtype at the time of

Table 8–1. *DSM-IV diagnostic criteria for generalized anxiety disorder*

A. Excessive anxiety and worry (apprehensive expectation), occurring more days than not
   for at least 6 months, about a number of events or activities (such as work or school
   performance)
B. Difficulty in controlling the worry
C. Anxiety and worry associated with three or more of the following six symptoms, with
   at least some symptoms present for more days than not for the past 6 months (*Note*:
   Only one item required for children)
   1. Restless or feeling keyed up or on edge
   2. Easily fatigued
   3. Difficulty in concentrating or mind going blank
   4. Irritability
   5. Muscle tension
   6. Sleep disturbance (difficulty falling asleep or staying asleep, or restless and
      unsatisfying sleep)
D. The focus of the anxiety and worry is not confined to features of an Axis I disorder.
   For example, the anxiety or worry is not about having a panic attack (as in panic
   disorder); being embarrassed in public (as in social phobia); being contaminated (as in
   obsessive-compulsive disorder); being away from home or close relatives (as in
   separation anxiety disorder); gaining weight (as in anorexia nervosa); or having a
   serious illness (as in hypochondriasis); and the anxiety and worry do not occur
   exclusively during posttraumatic stress disorder.
E. The anxiety, worry, or physical symptoms cause clinically significant distress or
   impairment in social, occupational, or other important areas of functioning.
F. The disturbance is not due to the direct physiological effects of a substance (e.g., a
   drug of abuse or a medication) or to a general medical condition (e.g.,
   hyperthyroidism) and does not occur exclusively during a mood disorder, a psychotic
   disorder, or a pervasive developmental disorder.

the interview because chronic anxiety is rarely a stable condition (compare Figs. 8–2 to 8–4).

Generalized anxiety disorder (GAD) is thus not a trivial disorder (Fig. 8–2). In fact, when one defines recovery from either major depressive disorder or GAD as reduction to only one or two symptoms with a subjective sense of returning to normal self, major depressive disorder has an 80% rate of recovery in 2 years, whereas GAD has only a 20% chance of recovery. Some patients with GAD experience a chronic state of symptomatic impairment (Fig. 8–3); other patients with GAD experience a waxing and waning course just above and just below the diagnostic threshold over long periods of time despite current treatment regimens (Fig. 8–4). Long-standing GAD may be a harbinger of panic disorder (Fig. 8–5) or major depressive disorder with or without anxiety (Fig. 8–6).

## Drug Treatments for Anxiety

### Antidepressants or Anxiolytics?

If pathological and generalized anxiety is a state of incomplete recovery from depression or from anxiety disorder subtypes, it would not be surprising if highly

# COMBINATIONS OF SYNDROMES

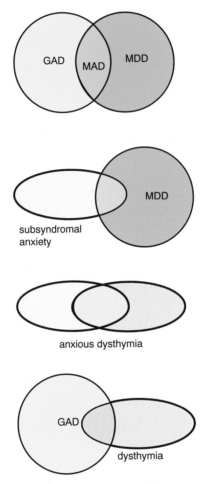

FIGURE 8–1. Anxiety and depression can be combined in a **wide variety of syndromes**. Generalized anxiety disorder (**GAD**) can overlap with major depressive disorder (**MDD**) to form mixed anxiety depression (**MAD**). Subsyndromal anxiety overlapping with subsyndromal depression to form subsyndromal mixed anxiety depression, sometimes also called *anxious dysthymia*. Major depressive disorder can also overlap with subsyndromal symptoms of anxiety to create **anxious depression**; GAD can also overlap with symptoms of depression such as dysthymia to create **GAD with depressive features**. Thus, a **spectrum of symptoms and disorders** is possible, ranging from pure anxiety without depression, to various mixtures of each in varying intensities, to pure depression without anxiety.

effective treatments for depression and anxiety disorders might also be effective for generalized symptoms of anxiety. Indeed, the leading treatments for generalized anxiety today are increasingly drugs originally developed as antidepressants.

Original drug classifications in the 1960s emphasized that there were important distinctions between the *antidepressants* (e.g., tricyclic antidepressants) versus the *anxiolytics* (e.g., benzodiazepines) available at that time. This reflected the diagnostic notions then prevalent, which tended to dichotomize major depressive disorder and

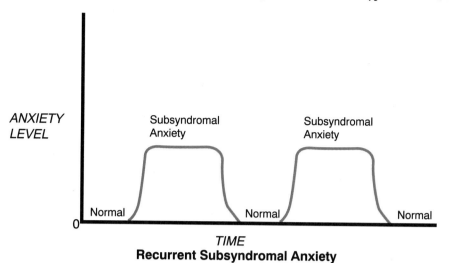

FIGURE 8–2. Some patients with **subsyndromal anxiety** have an intermittent clinical course, which **waxes and wanes over time** between a normal state and a state of subsyndromal anxiety.

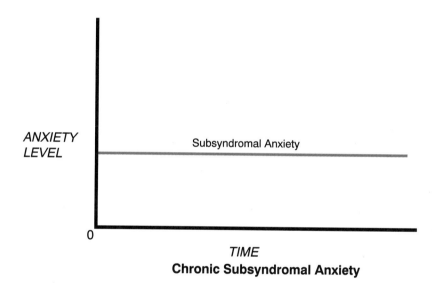

FIGURE 8–3. In contrast to the pattern shown in Figure 8–2, other patients with subsyndromal anxiety have a chronic and relatively stable yet **unremitting clinical course** over time.

generalized anxiety disorder while largely lumping all anxiety disorder subtypes together (Fig. 8–7).

By the 1970s and early 1980s it was recognized that certain tricyclic antidepressants and monoamine oxidase (MAO) inhibitors were effective in treating panic disorder and one tricyclic antidepressant (clomipramine) was effective in treating obsessive-compulsive disorder. Thus, there began to be recognized that some antidepressants overlapped with anxiolytics for the treatment of anxiety disorder subtypes or for mixtures of anxiety and depression (Fig. 8–8). However, *either* anxiolytics

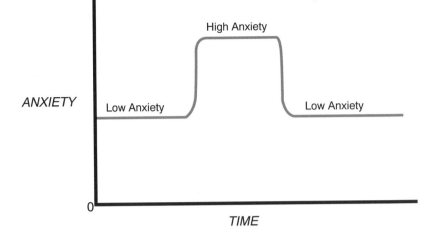

**Double Anxiety Syndrome**

FIGURE 8–4. Subsyndromal anxiety can also be a **harbinger** of an episode of a full generalized anxiety disorder (GAD). Such patients may have an intermittent clinical course, which waxes and wanes over time between subsyndromal anxiety and GAD. Decompensating to full GAD with recovery only to a state of subsyndromal anxiety over time can also be called the **double anxiety syndrome**.

*Subsyndromal Anxiety can be a precursor to GAD or Panic disorder*

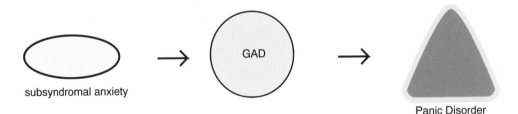

FIGURE 8–5. **Not only may subsyndromal anxiety** be a harbinger for decompensation to generalized anxiety disorder (**GAD**), but GAD in turn may be a harbinger for decompensation to **panic disorder** in some patients.

(such as benzodiazepines or buspirone) *or* antidepressants (such as tricyclic antidepressants or MAO inhibitors) were considered first-line treatments for some anxiety disorder subtypes.

By the 1990s antidepressants from the serotonin selective reuptake inhibitor (SSRI) class became recognized as preferred first-line treatments for anxiety disorder subtypes, ranging from obsessive-compulsive disorder, to panic disorder, and now to social phobia and posttraumatic stress disorder (Fig. 8–9). Not all antidepressants, however, are affacious anxiolytics. For example, desipramine and bupropion seem to be of little help in several anxiety disorder subtypes. Documentation of efficacy

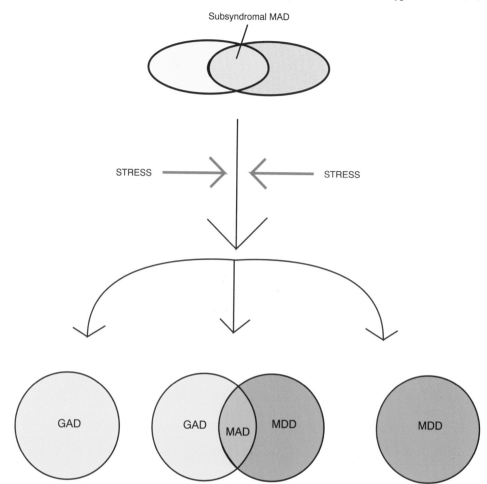

FIGURE 8–6. Subsyndromal mixed anxiety depression (**MAD**) may be an **unstable psychological state**, characterized by **vulnerability under stress to decompensation** to more severe psychiatric disorders, such as generalized anxiety disorder (**GAD**), full-syndrome **MAD**, or major depressive disorder (**MDD**).

for several of the newer antidepressants other than SSRIs in anxiety disorder subtypes is preliminary at best, but there are some positive reports and small trials of nefazodone, mirtazapine, and venlafaxine for the treatment of panic disorder and posttraumatic stress disorder.

Meanwhile, benzodiazepines became second-line treatments or augmentation treatments for these anxiety disorder subtypes in the 1990s. While buspirone continues to be recognized as a first-line general anxiolytic, it has not developed a convincing efficacy profile for anxiety disorder subtypes or for the treatment of major depressive disorder.

Recently, venlafaxine XR became the first agent to be approved both to treat mood in depression and anxiety in GAD. Thus, the final gap in the great divide between antidepressants and anxiolytics has been bridged (Fig. 8–10). It has been

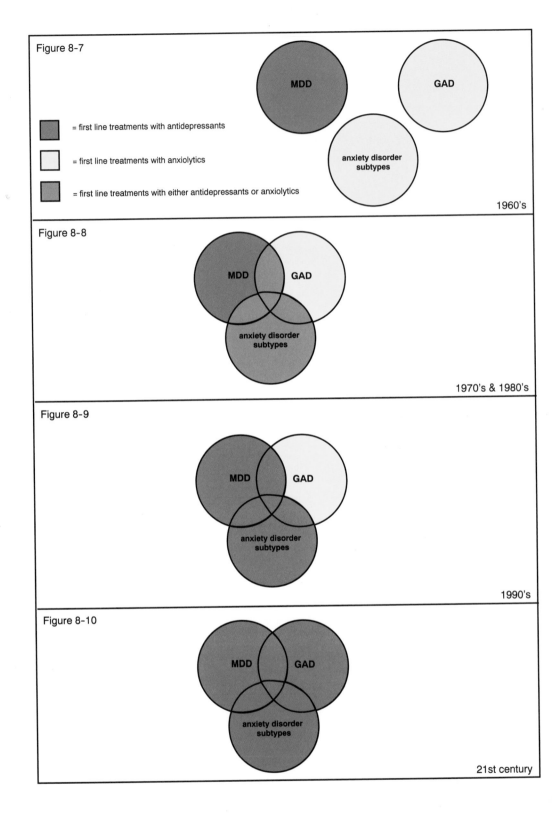

Figure 8-7

= first line treatments with antidepressants

= first line treatments with anxiolytics

= first line treatments with either antidepressants or anxiolytics

MDD

GAD

anxiety disorder subtypes

1960's

Figure 8-8

MDD

GAD

anxiety disorder subtypes

1970's & 1980's

Figure 8-9

MDD

GAD

anxiety disorder subtypes

1990's

Figure 8-10

MDD

GAD

anxiety disorder subtypes

21st century

attempted in the past but without success to obtain approval for numerous agents as both antidepressants and general anxiolytics. Early attempts to show that tricyclic antidepressants were also effective as general anxiolytics were promising but came after the tricyclic antidepressant era was already over. Tricyclic antidepressants appear to be slower in onset but perhaps more efficacious than even benzodiazepines for the treatment of GAD. Currently, mirtazapine and nefazodone have shown positive results in individual cases and small trials in GAD, and similar studies are currently in progress for paroxetine, but venlafaxine XR is widely recognized as effective for GAD.

## Get All the Way Well, Not Just Convert Depression with Anxiety into Anxiety without Depression

Given the high degree of comorbidity of depression and generalized anxiety as well as anxiety disorder subtypes, the "holy grail" sought for a psychotropic drug has been to combine antidepressant with anxiolytic action. Otherwise, patients treated with an antidepressant that is ineffective for their comorbid anxiety states will improve their symptoms of depression and continue to suffer from symptoms of anxiety. Alternatively, two agents must be given concomitantly, one effective for the depression and the other effective for the anxiety disorder.

Depression and anxiety disorder subtypes are treated simultaneously with SSRIs, and this approach often requires only one drug. This is not always true, however, for patients with comorbid major depressive disorder and GAD. In such cases, depression is often targeted first in the hierarchy of symptoms, with the result that some patients may respond by decreasing their overall symptoms of depression but continue to have generalized symptoms of anxiety rather than remitting completely to an asymptomatic state of wellness (Table 5–18). Given the trend showing that some antidepressants are also anxiolytics, it may now be possible, more than ever, to eliminate symptoms of both depressed mood and anxiety in the common situation where patients have both major depressive disorder and GAD. Such a therapeutic result would return patients with comorbid depression and generalized anxiety to a state of wellness without residual symptoms of either depression or anxiety.

---

FIGURE 8–7. In the 1960s depression and its treatments were classified separately from anxiety plus anxiety disorder subtypes and their treatments.

FIGURE 8–8. In the 1970s and 1980s there began to be an overlap between the use of traditional antidepressants and traditional anxiolytics for treatment of some anxiety disorder subtypes and mixtures of depression and anxiety, but *not* for generalized anxiety disorder.

FIGURE 8–9. By the 1990s the serotonin selective reuptake inhibitors (SSRIs) replaced classical anxiolytics as first-line treatments for anxiety disorder subtypes and for mixtures of anxiety and depression but not for generalized anxiety disorder.

FIGURE 8–10. In the late 1990s the antidepressants venlafaxine XR and others have become first-line treatments for generalized anxiety disorder. Thus, antidepressants are now first-line treatments for both depression and anxiety disorders, rendering the classification of antidepressant versus anxiolytic inappropriate for many antidepressants.

## Serotonergic Anxiolytics

Early attempts to account for the roles of serotonin (5-hydroxy-tryptamine [5HT]) in anxiety and depression by formulating the former as a serotonin dysregulation syndrome and the latter as a serotonin deficiency syndrome are naive and very imprecise oversimplifications and certainly do not explain how serotonergic antidepressants could also be treatments for anxiety. Furthermore, a serotonin partial agonist, buspirone, is recognized as a generalized anxiolytic but not as a treatment for depression or for anxiety disorder subtypes. Although some data do indeed suggest that serotonin partial agonists at the 5HT1A receptor may have antidepressant properties, some investigators remain skeptical about how powerful either the anxiolytic or antidepressant effects of this class of drugs are. The single 5HT1A agonist approved for the treatment of anxiety, buspirone, is more widely used in the United States than in many other countries, and despite over a decade of widespread clinical testing, no other 5HT1A agonist has been approved. Gepirone is still progressing as an XR formulation and tandospirone is continuing to be tested in Japan. However, the fate of many other 5HT1A agonists remains tenuous or their clinical testing has been abandoned; these drugs include flesinoxan, sunepitron, adatanserin, and ipsapirone.

Buspirone remains the prototypical agent for the 5HT1A class of anxiolytics. Its advantages as compared with the benzodiazepines include lack of interactions with alcohol, benzodiazepines, or sedative hypnotic agents; absence of drug dependence or withdrawal symptoms with long-term use; and ease of use in patients with prior drug or alcohol abuse history. Its disadvantage as compared with the benzodiazepines is a delay in the onset of action, which is similar to the delay in therapeutic onset for the antidepressants. This has led to the belief that 5HT1A agonists exert their therapeutic effects by virtue of adaptive neuronal events and receptor events rather than simply by the acute occupancy of 5HT1A receptors by the drug, as discussed extensively above (Fig. 8–11). In this way, the presumed mechanism of action of 5HT1A partial agonists appears to be analogous to that of the antidepressants, which are also presumed to act by adaptations in neurotransmitter receptors, and different from that of the benzodiazepine anxiolytics, which act relatively acutely by occupancy of benzodiazepine receptors.

Buspirone tends to be used preferentially in patients with chronic and persistent anxiety, in patients with comorbid substance abuse, and in elderly patients, because it is well tolerated and has no significant pharmacokinetic drug interactions. What is clear is that buspirone shows reproducible efficacy in certain animal models of anxiety and in GAD, which points to a potentially important role of serotonin in mediating anxiety symptoms through 5HT1A receptors. Buspirone also has a role as an augmenting agent for the treatment of resistant depression, as discussed in Chapter 7.

## Noradrenergic Anxiolytics

Electrical stimulation of the locus coeruleus to make it overactive creates a state analogous to anxiety in experimental animals. Thus, overactivity of norepinephrine neurons is thought to underlie anxiety states (Fig. 8–12). Indeed, examples of anx-

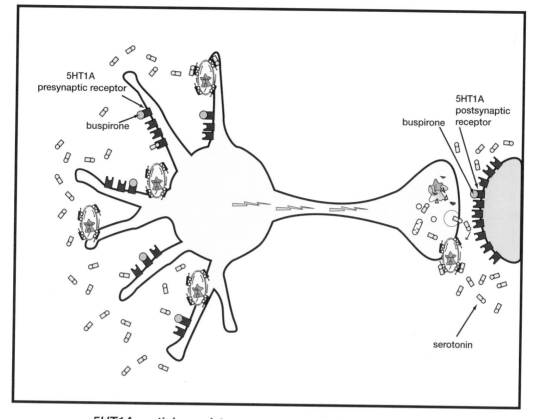

**5HT1A partial agonist causes up-regulation of autoreceptors**

FIGURE 8–11. Serotonin 1A partial agonists such as buspirone may reduce anxiety by actions both at presynaptic somatodendritic autoreceptors (left) and at postsynaptic receptors (right). Presynaptic actions are more likely related to anxiolytic actions, and postsynaptic actions are perhaps more likely linked to side effects such as nausea and dizziness.

iety symptoms consistent with adrenergic overactivity include tachycardia, tremor, and sweating (Fig. 8–12).

If overactivity of the locus coeruleus noradrenergic neurons is associated with anxiety, then administration of an alpha 2 agonist should act in a manner similar to the action of norepinephrine itself on its presynaptic alpha 2 autoreceptors. Thus, anxiety can be thereby reduced because of an alpha 2 agonist stimulating these alpha 2 autoreceptors, thus "stepping on the brake" of norepinephrine release (Fig. 8–13). In fact, the alpha 2 agonist clonidine has some clinically recognized anxiolytic actions. Clonidine is especially useful in blocking the noradrenergic aspects of anxiety (tachycardia, dilated pupils, sweating, and tremor). However, it is less powerful in blocking the subjective and emotional aspects of anxiety. These same adrenergic blocking properties of clonidine due to its stimulation of alpha 2 presynaptic autoreceptors have been successfully applied to reducing the adrenergic symptoms pro-

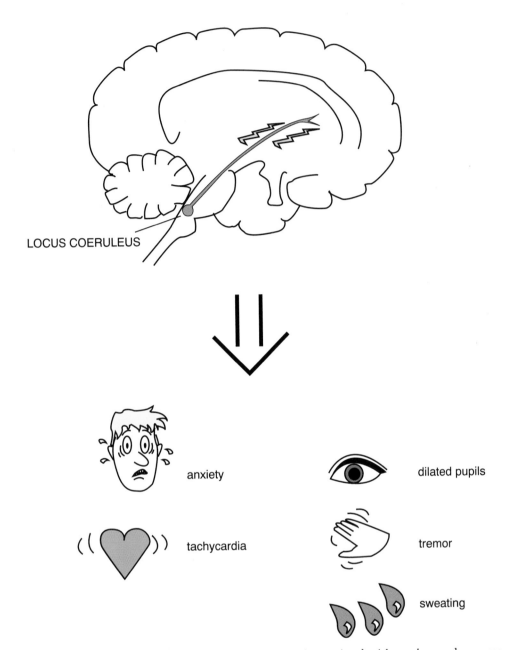

LOCUS COERULEUS

anxiety

dilated pupils

tachycardia

tremor

sweating

FIGURE 8–12. **Overactivity of norepinephrine neurons** is associated with **anxiety** and may mediate the autonomic symptoms associated with anxiety, such as **tachycardia, dilated pupils, tremor,** and **sweating**. Shown here are hyperactive norepinephrine neurons with their axons projecting forward to the cerebral cortex from their cell bodies in the **locus coeruleus**.

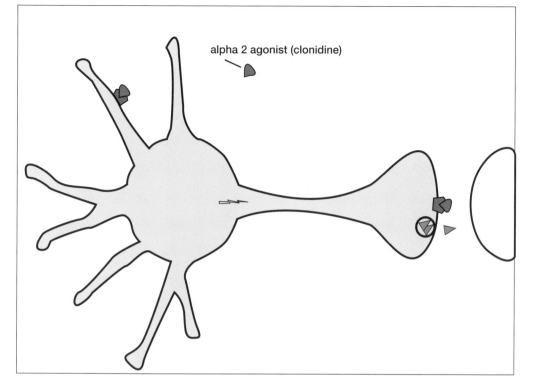

alpha 2 agonist (clonidine)

alpha 2 agonist occupies autoreceptors which decreases firing and decreases release
of NE, which has an anxiolytic effect

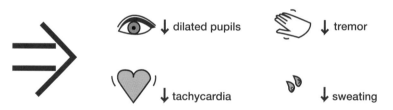

↓ dilated pupils     ↓ tremor

↓ tachycardia     ↓ sweating

FIGURE 8–13. If an **alpha 2 agonist** such as clonidine, is administered, it will have much the same action as norepinephrine (NE) itself both at somatodendritic alpha 2 autoreceptors and at terminal alpha 2 autoreceptors. This action is that of **reducing** both **neuronal impulse in NE neurons** and **release of NE** from noradrenergic axon terminals. Thus, alpha 2 agonists will **decrease** the symptoms associated with **anxiety**, especially the autonomic symptoms of **dilated pupils, tachycardia, tremor,** and **sweating**.

voked during detoxification of patients from alcohol, barbiturates, heroin, or benzodiazepines (see Chapter 13).

Overactivity of noradrenergic neurons creates too much postsynaptic norepinephrine at noradrenergic receptors, particularly beta receptors (Fig. 8–14). As is consistent with the hypothesis of a state of norepinephrine excess in anxiety, it is possible to reduce symptoms of anxiety in some cases by blocking beta receptors with beta

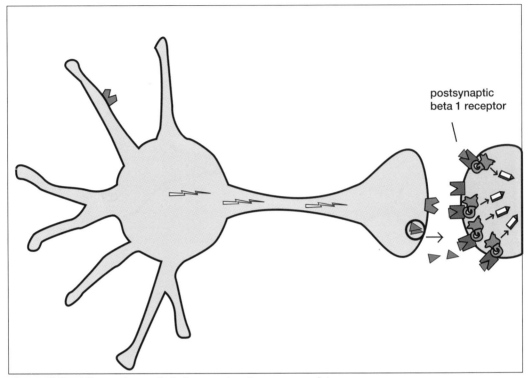

postsynaptic
beta 1 receptor

Overactivity at the postsynaptic beta receptors increases anxiety

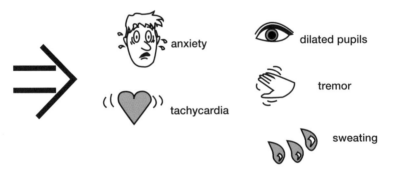

anxiety

dilated pupils

tremor

tachycardia

sweating

FIGURE 8–14. The **overactivity** of norepinephrine (**NE**) neurons and **excess release of NE** from nerve terminals that occurs in **anxiety** also causes events to occur at postsynaptic NE receptors. In this case, excess NE activity causes an excess of NE occupying **postsynaptic beta adrenergic receptors**. This in turn causes an excess in postsynaptic signaling via second and subsequent messenger systems. These excess signals via postsynaptic beta adrenergic receptors mediate the autonomic symptoms associated with anxiety, including **tachycardia, dilated pupils, tremor,** and **sweating.**

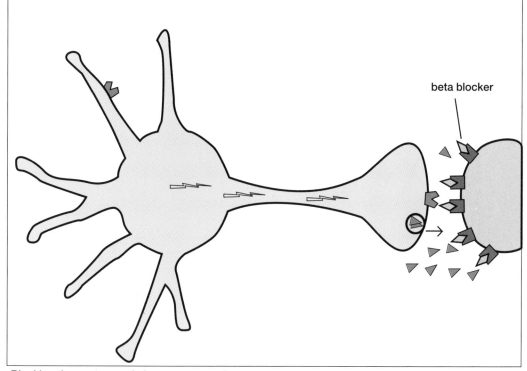

Blocking the postsynaptic beta receptors decreases anxiety

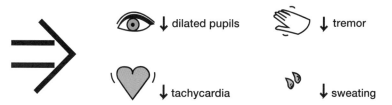

↓ dilated pupils          ↓ tremor

↓ tachycardia          ↓ sweating

FIGURE 8–15. If **excessive activity** of norepinephrine (**NE**) at **postsynaptic beta adrenergic receptors**, shown in Figure 8–14, can be **blocked**, so can the symptoms of anxiety that are mediated by the beta receptors. Shown here is a **beta adrenergic blocker**, or antagonist, which is preventing the excess activity of NE neurons and excess NE release to cause a corresponding excess stimulation of postsynaptic beta adrenergic receptors. This antagonist action at beta receptors can **decrease the autonomic symptoms associated with anxiety**, such as dilated pupils, tremor, tachycardia, and sweating.

blocking drugs (Fig. 8–15). This may be especially useful in cases of social phobia, as will be discussed in Chapter 9.

### GABAergic Neurons and the Benzodiazepine Anxiolytics

Understanding the actions of benzodiazepines requires background knowledge of the pharmacology of GABA-ergic neurotransmission. The neurotransmitter for GABA-

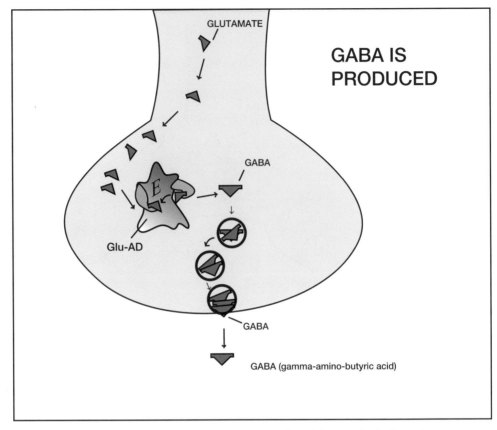

FIGURE 8–16. Gamma-aminobutyric acid (**GABA**) is **produced** by synthesis from the precursor amino acid **glutamate** by the enzyme glutamic acid decarboxylase (**Glu-AD**).

ergic neurons is GABA, which is synthesized from the amino acid precursor glutamate via the enzyme glutamic acid decarboxylase (Glu-AD) (Fig. 8–16). Glutamate (glutamic acid) is derived from intraneuronal stores of amino acids. It is a nonessential amino acid and is the most abundant free amino acid in the central nervous system (CNS). Glutamate also participates in multiple metabolic functions and can be synthesized from numerous precursors (see discussion of glutamate neurons in Chapter 10). The GABA neuron has a presynaptic transporter (reuptake pump) (Fig. 8–17) similar to those of norepinephrine, dopamine, and serotonin and discussed in Chapter 5. This transporter terminates the action of synaptic GABA by removing it from the synaptic cleft for restorage or for destruction by the enzyme GABA transaminase (GABA-T) (Fig. 8–17).

Receptors for GABA also regulate GABA-ergic neurotransmission. There are two known subtypes of GABA receptors, known as GABA A and GABA B (Fig. 8–18). The *GABA A receptors* are the ones that are gatekeepers for a chloride channel (Figs. 8–19 and 8–20). They are *allosterically modulated* by a potpourri of nearby receptors. This includes the well-known benzodiazepine receptor (Fig. 8–19). The concept of allosteric modulation of one receptor by another has already been introduced in Chapter 3.

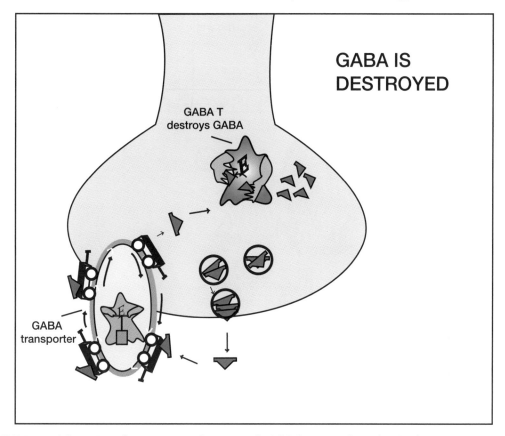

FIGURE 8–17. The action of gamma-aminobutyric acid (**GABA**) is **terminated** either by **enzymatic destruction** by GABA transaminase (**GABA T**) or by removal from the synaptic cleft by the **GABA transporter**. Following transport back into the presynaptic neuron, GABA can be re-stored in synaptic vesicles for reuse during a subsequent neurotransmission, as already pointed out for the norepinephrine, dopamine, and serotonin neurons.

The fundamental neurobiological importance of the GABA A receptor is underscored by observations that even more receptor sites exist at or near this complex (Fig. 8–20). This includes receptor sites for nonbenzodiazepine sedative-hypnotics such as zolpidem and zaleplon, for the convulsant drug picrotoxin, for the anticonvulsant barbiturates, and perhaps even for alcohol. This receptor complex is hypothetically responsible in part for mediating such wide-ranging CNS activities as seizures, anticonvulsant drug effects, and the behavioral effects of alcohol, as well as the known anxiolytic, sedative-hypnotic, and muscle relaxant effects of the benzodiazepines.

A second GABA receptor subtype, the *GABA-B receptor* (Fig. 8–12) is not allosterically modulated by benzodiazepines but binds selectively to the muscle relaxant baclofen. Its physiological role is not well known yet, but does not appear to be closely linked to anxiety disorders or to anxiolytics.

*Benzodiazepine receptors.* There are multiple molecular forms of benzodiazepine receptors, and there is continuing debate about how differences in the amino acid com-

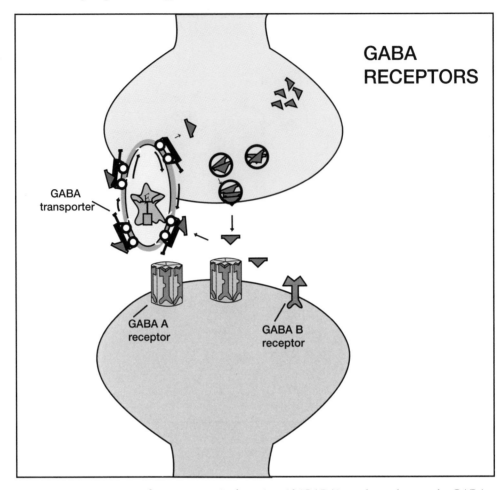

FIGURE 8–18. Various receptors for gamma-aminobutyric acid (GABA) are shown here at the GABA synapse. On the presynaptic side is the **GABA transporter**, the receptor linked to an active transport pump that removes GABA from the synaptic cleft, thus terminating its actions there. On the post-synaptic side, two subtypes of GABA receptors are shown. The first is the **GABA A receptor**, which is a member of the superfamily of ligand-gated ion channel receptors. The second is the **GABA B receptor**.

position of benzodiazepine receptors may lead to pharmacological differences in ligand binding and in functional activity. There may be at least five benzodiazepine receptor subtypes, including three with distinct pharmacologic profiles. For example, benzodiazepine 1 (sometimes called omega 1) receptors are preferentially located in the cerebellum and contain recognition sites with high affinities both for benzodiazepines and for agents with different chemical structures. Anxiolytic action as well as sedative-hypnotic actions seem to be mediated mostly through the benzodiazepine 1 receptor subtype. Benzodiazepine 2 (omega 2) receptors, on the other hand, are located predominantly in the spinal cord and striatum. These receptors may be involved in mediating the muscle relaxant actions of benzodiazepines. Finally, the

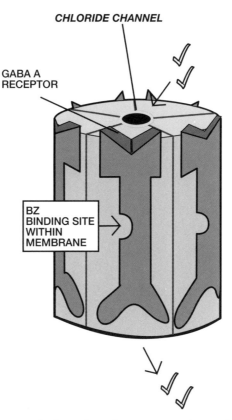

FIGURE 8–19. The **GABA A receptor** is shown here. It acts as a gatekeeper for a **chloride channel**. It also has a key **allosteric modulatory site** nearby, known as the **benzodiazepine (BZ) binding site**.

benzodiazepine 3 receptor, also known as the peripheral (i.e., outside the CNS) type, is abundant in the kidney. Its role in anxiolytic actions remains unclear.

Actions at benzodiazepine receptors are thought to underlie virtually all the pharmacological actions of the benzodiazepines, those that are desirable as well as those that are undesirable. This includes the desirable *therapeutic* actions of benzodiazepines as anxiolytics and sedative-hypnotics, as well as anticonvulsants and muscle relaxants. It also includes their undesirable *side effects* as amnestic agents and as agents that cause adaptations at the benzodiazepine receptor with chronic administration, which are thought to underlie the production of dependence and withdrawal from these agents (see Chapter 13).

Benzodiazepines are listed in the Table 8–2. The fact that they act at a naturally occurring receptor in brain has led to speculation that the brain may make its own benzodiazepine, or "endogenous Valium." Identification of a naturally occurring ligand for the benzodiazepine receptor, however, is yet incomplete. Modulation of the GABA–benzodiazepine receptor complex is therefore not only thought to underlie the pharmacological actions of antianxiety drugs but is also theorized to serve as the vehicle for mediating the emotion of anxiety itself. It has been speculated, for example, that reduced actions of GABA and the postulated endogenous benzodiaze-

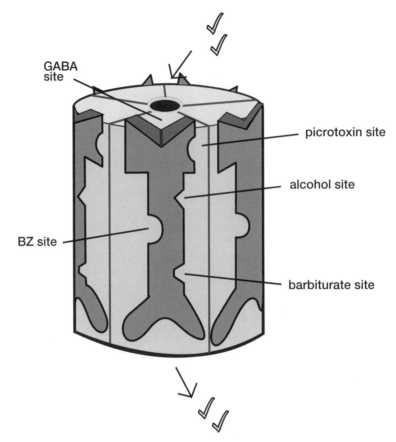

GABA
site

picrotoxin site

alcohol site

BZ site

barbiturate site

FIGURE 8–20. Multiple modulatory sites near the **GABA A receptor** are shown here. These include not only the **benzodiazepine (BZ) receptor** already shown in Figure 8–19, but also sites for the convulsant drug **picrotoxin**, for the anticonvulsant **barbiturate**, and possibly for **alcohol** as well. These nearby receptors suggest how GABA may be involved in modulating such diverse physiological effects as anxiety, seizures, and even the effects of alcohol.

pines at this receptor complex may be associated with the emotion of anxiety, whether the emotion is normal or pathological.

*Positive allosteric interactions between GABA A receptors and benzodiazepine receptors.* In technical language, the benzodiazepines are positive allosteric modulators of fast inhibitory neurotransmission by GABA at GABA A receptors. The inhibitory neurotransmitter GABA is the gatekeeper neurotransmitter that interacts selectively with its GABA A receptor, the primary receptor site of this GABA–benzodiazepine chloride channel receptor complex shown (Fig. 8–19). Thus, this complex is an example of the superfamily of receptors already discussed in Chapter 3 (see Figs. 3–3 through 3–14) and known as *ligand-gated receptor complexes*. In the case of the GABA–benzodiazepine receptor complex, this particular superfamily complex acts to control a chloride ion channel mediating fast neurotransmission (see discussion in Chapter 1 and Fig. 1–6).

Table 8–2. *Some of the major benzodiazepines*

Alprazolam (Xanax)
Clonazepam (Klonopin)
Diazepam (Valium)
Chlordiazepoxide (Librium)
Lorazepam (Ativan)
Oxazepam (Serax)
Prazepam (Centrex)
Clorazepate (Tranxene)
Triazolam (Halcion)
Temazepam (Restoril)
Flurazepam (Dalmane)
Midazolam (Versed)
Quazepam (Doral)
Flumazenil (Romazicon)
Mitrazepam
Lormetazolam
Loprazolam
Clobazam
Flunitrazepam
Brotizolam

The GABA A receptors are arranged as helical columns around a chloride channel, which itself is a column of columns, as mentioned in Chapter 3 and shown in Figures 3–6 through 3–12 as well as in Figures 8–18 through 8–20. Following occupancy of the GABA A receptor site by GABA molecules, the GABA A receptor columns in turn interact with the chloride channel to open it a bit (Fig. 8–21). The resulting increased chloride conductance into the neuron occurs quickly (fast neurotransmission; see Chapter 1 and Fig. 1–6) and is inhibitory to the finding of that neuron.

Near the receptor site for GABA is not only the chloride channel but also another neurotransmitter receptor, namely the benzodiazepine receptor binding site (Fig. 8–19), as already mentioned. Benzodiazepine receptor binding sites also affect the conductance of chloride through the chloride channel. However, the benzodiazepine receptor binding site does not do this by directly modulating the chloride channel but by *allosterically* modulating the GABA A receptor binding site, which in turn modulates the chloride channel. Thus, when a benzodiazepine binds to its own benzodiazepine receptor site, a neighbor of the GABA A receptor binding site, nothing happens if GABA is not also binding to its own GABA A receptor site (Fig. 8–22). On the other hand, when GABA is binding to its GABA A receptor site, the simultaneous binding of benzodiazepine to its benzodiazepine binding site (allosteric, i.e., "other site") causes a large amplification in GABA's ability to increase the conductance of chloride through the channel (Fig. 8–23).

Why is this necessary? It turns out that GABA working by itself can increase chloride conductance through the chloride channel only to a certain extent (Fig. 8–21). Benzodiazepines cannot increase chloride conductance at all when working by themselves (Fig. 8–22). However, allosteric modulation is the mechanism to maximize the chloride conductance beyond that which GABA alone, as in Figure

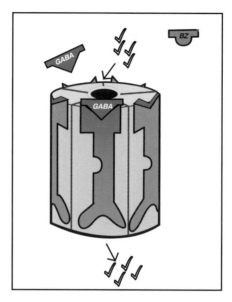

FIGURE 8–21. **GABA** is the ligand that acts at the **GABA A receptor site** to participate in opening the molecular gate for an inhibitory chloride channel. Thus, when GABA alone binds to the GABA A receptor, it **opens the chloride channel** so that more chloride can now enter the cell and cause inhibitory neurotransmission. Also shown is a **benzodiazepine (BZ) ligand**, which is **not** binding to the benzodiazepine receptor in this example (but see Figs. 8–22 and 8–23).

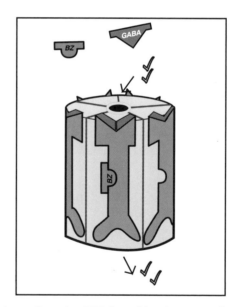

FIGURE 8–22. Shown here is a benzodiazepine **(BZ)** ligand binding to the **benzodiazepine receptor** on the GABA A receptor complex. Note that **GABA** itself is **not** binding to the GABA A receptor site in this example. Note also that the chloride channel is **not opening**. This example is thus in contrast to the previous example (Fig. 8–21), in which GABA alone was binding to the GABA A receptor. In the current example, where **BZ ligand alone** binds to the GABA A receptor, essentially **no more chloride can enter** the cell to cause inhibitory neurotransmission. However, see the contrast in Figure 8–23, in which both GABA and benzodiazepine bind to the GABA A receptor complex.

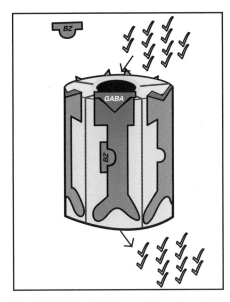

FIGURE 8–23. In this example, **both GABA and benzodiazepine (BZ) ligands** are binding to their respective receptor sites on the **GABA A receptor complex**. This causes **far more opening of the chloride channel** than can be effected by GABA acting alone. Thus, it can be said that benzodiazepine ligands **allosterically modulate** GABA's ability to open the chloride channel. It is this positive allosteric modulation of the BZ receptor by benzodiazepine drugs that is thought to account for their **anxiolytic actions**.

8–21, can accomplish. Thus, GABA can increase chloride conductance through the chloride channel much more dramatically when a benzodiazepine receptor binding site is helping it allosterically than it can when it is working alone to modulate the chloride channel (Fig. 8–23).

In other words, benzodiazepines *allosterically modulate* GABA neurotransmission by potentiating GABA's ability to increase conductance of chloride through its channel. That is, with GABA plus benzodiazepines, 1 + 1 = 10, not 2. This mechanism greatly expands the scope of the neuron to regulate its fast inhibitory neurotransmission with chemical ligands.

*Inverse agonists, partial agonists, and antagonists at benzodiazepine receptors.* For a further degree of regulatory control of GABA neurotransmission, the concept of allosteric modulation can be combined with the concept of inverse agonists. Inverse agonists have already been introduced (see Chapter 3). Thus, *positive* allosteric modulation of benzodiazepines on GABA A receptors occurs because the benzodiazepines are *full agonists* at the benzodiazepine site (Fig. 8–23). However, *negative* allosteric modulation can occur when an *inverse agonist* binds to the benzodiazepine site. Instead of *increasing* the chloride conductance that GABA provokes (Fig. 8–22), the inverse agonist *decreases* it (Fig. 8–24).

This can translate into opposite behavioral actions for agonists versus inverse agonists. For example, benzodiazepine full agonists *reduce* anxiety by increasing chloride conductance, as shown in Figure 8–23. However, a benzodiazepine inverse agonist *causes* anxiety and does this by decreasing chloride conductance, as shown in

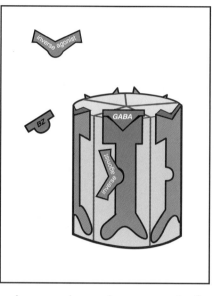

FIGURE 8–24. Shown here is what happens when an **inverse agonist** for the benzodiazepine (BZ) receptor influences GABA binding at the **GABA A receptor**. In this example, the inverse agonist **closes the chloride channel**. Thus, an inverse BZ agonist **allosterically modulates** GABA in the **opposite direction** from a normal BZ full agonist, such as that shown in Figure 8–23. Consequently, a benzodiazepine inverse agonist increases anxiety (i.e., it is **anxiogenic**, rather than anxiolytic).

Figure 8–24. Benzodiazepine inverse agonists would be expected to be not only anxiogenic (creating anxiety) but also proconvulsant (increasing the likelihood of seizures), activating (opposite of sedating) and promnestic (memory promoting, the opposite of amnestic; see Fig. 8–25). The latter promnestic actions have even been considered as a possible therapeutic strategy for memory disorders such as Alzheimer's disease (see Chapter 12). However, these agents are potentially dangerous if they can simultaneously promote anxiety and seizures. Indeed, early clinical testing in humans has produced some severe anxiety reactions to inverse benzodiazepine agonists.

Consequently, the pharmacological properties of agonists and inverse agonists reveal that there can be obvious and dramatic clinical and behavioral distinctions across the agonist–antagonist–inverse agonist spectrum (Figs. 3–14 and 8-25), which can be explained by the principles of allosteric modulation of receptors.

An intermediate in the agonist spectrum (Fig. 8–25) is a partial agonist. Partial agonists have the theoretical possibility of separating the desired (anxiolytic) effects from the undesired effects (daytime sedation, ataxia, memory disturbance, dependency, and withdrawal) (see Fig. 8–25). That is, full agonists theoretically exert the full portfolio of benzodiazepine actions, whereas a partial agonist would separate those actions thought to require only partial agonism (anxiolytic effects) from those thought to require full agonism (sedation, and dependency; see Fig. 8–25). A wide variety of partial agonists for the benzodiazepine receptor have been synthesized and tested. The results to date are generally disappointing, since too much partial agonism fails to distinguish such agents from the full agonists already marketed, and too little partial agonism is associated with too little clinical efficacy in anxiety.

## AGONIST SPECTRUM IN ANXIETY

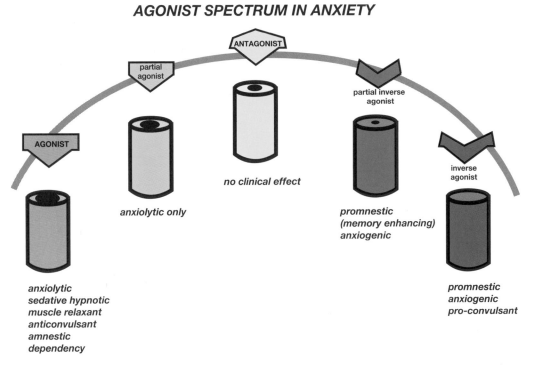

FIGURE 8–25. This figure reveals that there is a whole spectrum of agonist activities at the benzodiazepine receptor, ranging from **full agonist actions** through **antagonist actions** all the way to **inverse agonist actions**. These actions have already been introduced in Figure 3–14. **Full agonists** (far left of the spectrum) not only have **desired** therapeutic actions (anxiolytic, sedative-hypnotic, muscle relaxant, and anticonvulsant), but also **undesired** side effects (amnesia and dependency). Theoretically, a **happy medium** halfway between a full agonist and an antagonist might be provided by a **partial agonist** which might be **anxiolytic without causing dependency**, for example. **Antagonists** (middle of the spectrum) have no clinical effects by themselves but may reverse the actions of any ligand at the benzodiazepine site, including the actions of both agonists and inverse agonists (see Figs. 8–26 and 8–27). **Full inverse agonists** (far right of the spectrum) cause clinical effects essentially **opposite** to those of full agonists and therefore cause potentially **desirable** memory-enhancing (promnestic) effects but also the **undesirable** side effects of increasing anxiety and promoting seizures. Perhaps a **happy medium** could also be attained here by finding a **partial inverse agonist** that could still enhance memory without causing anxiety or seizures.

However, this idea of a partial agonist is a conceptually attractive one, based on the promise of such agents from preclinical testing and from theoretical considerations.

Pharmacologic manipulations of benzodiazepines have advanced to the point that an antagonist, flumazanil, has been developed that can block the actions of the benzodiazepines and reverse their actions, for example, after anesthesia or after an overdose (Fig. 8–26). Interestingly, as predicted from the pharmacology of the agonist spectrum (Fig. 8–25), the benzodiazepine antagonist flumazanil is also able to reverse the actions of inverse agonists (Fig. 8–27). This underscores the pharmacological principles, developed in Chapter 3, showing how drugs can influence a neurotransmitter system over a very broad range when a spectrum of agents can work on the one hand from full agonist through partial agonist to neutral antagonist and

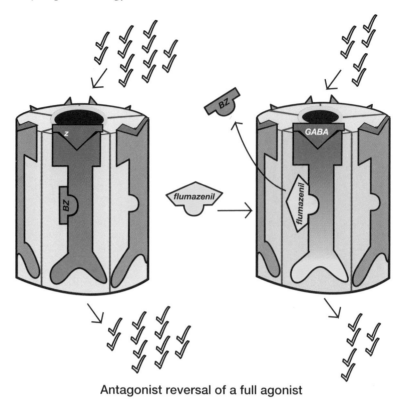

**Antagonist reversal of a full agonist**

FIGURE 8–26. The **benzodiazepine (BZ) receptor antagonist flumazanil** is able to reverse a full agonist benzodiazepine acting at the benzodiazepine receptor of the **GABA A receptor complex.** This may be helpful in **reversing** the sedative effects of full agonist benzodiazepines when administered for aesthetic purposes or when taken in an overdose by a patient.

on the other hand from neutral antagonist to partial inverse agonist to full inverse agonist (Figs. 3–14 and 8–25).

*Benzodiazepines and the treatment of anxiety.* Benzodiazepines grew up in an era when the diagnosis and treatment of anxiety was considered to be quite separate from the diagnosis and treatment of depression (Fig. 8–7). These agents revolutionized the treatment of anxiety when they were introduced in the 1960s, because they were both less sedating and less dependence-forming than the earlier agents, such as barbiturates and meprobamate, that they replaced. Furthermore, benzodiazepines have other properties, including anticonvulsant, muscle relaxant, and sedative-hypnotic actions.

Using benzodiazepines to treat anxiety requires knowledge of how to balance the risks of these agents rationally against their benefits and to compare this with other available therapeutic interventions. For short-term anxiety-related conditions, such as an adjustment disorder with onset after a stressful life event, benzodiazepines can provide rapid relief with little risk of dependence or withdrawal if use is limited to several weeks to a few months. However, for conditions likely to require treatment

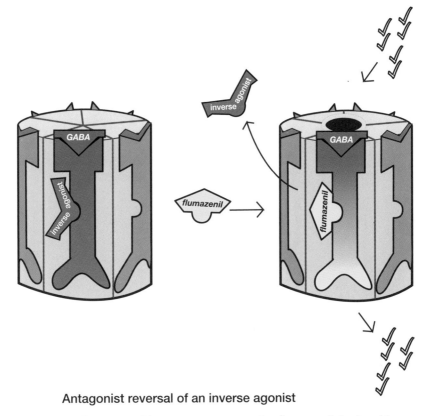

**Antagonist reversal of an inverse agonist**

FIGURE 8–27. The **benzodiazepine (BZ) receptor** antagonist flumazenil is also able to reverse inverse agonist benzodiazepines acting at the benzodiazepine receptors of the **GABA A receptor complex.**

for longer than 4 to 6 months, such as GAD, panic disorder, or anxiety associated with depression, the risks of dependence and withdrawal are greatly increased, and long-term use may not be justified in light of the other treatment options.

Short-term stabilization of symptoms in GAD and use as needed for sudden surges in symptoms are usually well justified uses for benzodiazepines. On the other hand, long-term treatment of GAD must encompass consideration of other interventions first before long-term use of benzodiazepines is generally indicated. Thus, life-style changes can be the cornerstone of long-term treatment for this condition, including stress reduction techniques, exercise, healthy diet, appropriate work situation, and adequate management of interpersonal affairs.

## Other Drug Treatments for Anxiety

*Barbiturates.* The very earliest treatments for generalized anxiety were sedating barbiturates. These agents had little in the way of specific antianxiety action; they merely reduced anxiety in direct proportion to their ability to sedate. Because of serious dependency and withdrawal problems (see Chapter 13) and lack of a favorable safety profile, especially when mixed with other drugs or in overdose, the barbiturates fell out of favor as soon as the much more selective and less dangerous antianxiety agents of the benzodiazepine class were discovered.

*Meprobamate.* Meprobamate (Miltown) and tybamate (no longer available in the United States) are members of a chemical class called propanediols, but which are pharmacologically very similar to the barbiturates. No advantage of meprobamate over barbiturates has been demonstrated, and although popular during the 1950s as an antianxiety agent in the United States, it has fallen into disfavor and is infrequently prescribed owing to its liability to abuse and withdrawal symptoms, similar to that of the barbiturates and much more severe than that of the benzodiazepines.

*Adjunctive treatments.* Numerous adjunctive treatments are available for generalized anxiety disorder. These agents are considered not only to be second-line agents with inferior efficacy but also to work essentially by producing sedation rather than a specific anxiolytic effect. These include the sedating antihistamines, beta adrenergic blockers, and clonidine. The beta blockers may have some efficacy in social phobia (see Chapter 9) and the alpha 2 agonist clonidine may also be helpful in anxiety associated with hyperadrenergic states (Figure 8–13).

## New Prospects

*Partial agonists at benzodiazepine receptors* are under investigation. All of the marketed benzodiazepines are essentially full agonists at the GABA–benzodiazepine receptor complex. It is theoretically possible to improve on the actions of full agonists if a partial agonist of optimal partiality could be identified (Fig. 8–20). Animal models predict that a partial agonist would still be anxiolytic but would cause less sedation and have less propensity for dependence and withdrawal. Attempts to identify a partial agonist for use in humans are still underway, using either benzodiazepine-type agents or other unique chemical structures that are not benzodiazepines.

*Cholecystokinin (CCK) antagonists* are in clinical testing in anxiety disorders, especially panic disorder (see Chapter 9). Corticotropin-releasing factor (CRF) is a neuropeptide, which may mediate some anxiety behaviors in experimental animals. This has led to the proposal that *CRF antagonists* may be anxiolytic. Numerous CRF antagonists being developed and tested for anxiety are in the very earliest stages of development. *Neuroactive steroids* are molecules based on a steroid chemical structure, which interact with the GABA–benzodiazepine receptor complex. As some of these agents are naturally occurring, it is hoped that analogues may be effective anxiolytics, with perhaps more "natural" actions than the marketed benzodiazepine anxiolytics. Such agents are in early development.

## Clinical Description of Insomnia

Insomnia is a complaint, not a disease. The causes of insomnia are classified both in the DSM-IV for psychiatrists and in the International Classification of Sleep Disorders for sleep experts (Table 8–3). Insomnia can be a primary problem, or it can be secondary to medical or psychiatric disorders or to medications. Insomnia can also be due psychophysiological factors such as stress or to circadian rhythm distur-

Table 8–3. *Classification of insomnia*

Primary insomnia, with underlying pathophysiology of sleep
Insomnia secondary to a psychiatric disorder
Insomnia secondary to a medication or drug of abuse
Insomnia secondary to a general medical condition, especially with pain- or sleep-
  disordered breathing
Circadian rhythm disturbance
Periodic limb movement disorder
Restless legs syndrome

bances such as jet lag. The reader is referred to textbooks on the etiology and classification of insomnia and other sleep disorders for details.

Here we will emphasize the use of sedative-hypnotic drugs for the treatment of insomnia. Before prescribing such drugs, however, it is very useful to understand the differential diagnosis of insomnia so that sedative-hypnotic drugs are appropriately used. Thus, if a sleep disorder is secondary to a psychiatric disorder, the ultimate treatment of the sleep disorder is to treat the psychiatric disorder. The same applies to medical disorders that are the primary cause of a sleep disorder. Examples include gastroesophageal reflux, respiratory disorders such as central and obstructive sleep apneas, and medical conditions causing pain. Treating the primary condition often relieves the insomnia, and sedative-hypnotics can be avoided.

If a sleep disorder is due to a medication or to drugs of abuse, changing the medication or stopping the drug of abuse may relieve the problem. If the sleep problem is due to narcolepsy, parasomnias, or a sleep-related movement disorder such as periodic limb movement disorder or restless legs syndrome, treatment aimed at these conditions may alleviate the sleep disturbance. Also, some sleep complaints are due to poor sleep hygiene and amenable to simple behavioral changes such as regular exercise not too late in the day, avoidance of caffeine late in the day, avoidance of naps, and maintaining the bedroom for sleep and sexual activity only.

When these issues are taken into consideration, there is still a high frequency of primary insomnia, as well as secondary insomnia the primary cause of which cannot be satisfactorily treated. Many patients also have both a psychiatric disorder and a primary insomnia. Still others have a psychiatric disorder requiring a sleep-disrupting antidepressant. Here we will discuss the use of sedative-hypnotics for these patients.

Insomnia may also be classified according to its duration as a symptom. Thus, *transient insomnia* occurs in normal sleepers who have traveled to another time zone (jet lag), who are sleeping in an unfamiliar surrounding, or who are under acute situational stress. Often treatment is not required, and insomnia is reversed with time alone. *Short-term insomnia* can be experienced by one who is generally a normal sleeper but is under a stress that does not resolve within a few days, such as divorce, bankruptcy, or a lawsuit. Such individuals may not meet the criteria for a psychiatric disorder other than an adjustment disorder and yet may require short-term symptomatic relief of their insomnia in order to function optimally.

Finally, *long-term insomnia* is not only persistent but disabling. Studies suggest that almost all of these patients have either an associated psychiatric disorder, an associated drug use, abuse, or withdrawal problem, or an associated medical disorder. As mentioned above, treatment of these associated disorders may be sufficient to treat the insomnia as well. However, if the underlying disorder is not treatable or if there is a requirement to relieve the symptom of insomnia before the underlying condition can be relieved, it may be necessary to treat the insomnia symptomatically with a sedative-hypnotic agent.

Product labeling and recommendations from sleep experts suggest that sedative-hypnotic drugs be used for a maximum of several weeks. Short-term insomnia should be treated for no more than three weeks, while long-term insomnia should be treated intermittently whenever possible. Chronic treatment can be one night in three for up to 4 months. However, clinical practice suggests that symptoms of clinically significant insomnia can persist for months to years in many patients. Although there is the risk of developing dependence over long periods of time, there is no evidence that sedative-hypnotics lose their efficacy over long periods. Thus, for patients with continuing symptoms of insomnia, treatment may have to be extended beyond 4 months. In such cases, the continuing need for sedative-hypnotics should be reevaluated every few months.

## Drug Treatments for Insomnia

Assuming that insomnia cannot be adequately treated by addressing directly an underlying problem responsible for causing the insomnia, then sedative-hypnotic drugs can be used to induce sleep pharmacologically. Such treatments can be controversial if they are overused or abused or if treating insomnia symptomatically removes the impetus to diagnose and relieve any underlying condition(s). One cannot deny, however, the widespread incidence of the complaint of insomnia in the general population, the perceived disruption of functioning and the disability that this symptom produces, and the strength of the demands of patients for drug treatments for this complaint.

### Nonbenzodiazepine Short-Acting Hypnotics

The newer sedative-hypnotics that are not benzodiazepines are rapidly becoming the first-line treatment for insomnia. These agents not only have pharmacodynamic advantages over benzodiazepines in terms of their mechanism of action, but perhaps more importantly, pharmacokinetic advantages as well. Three nonbenzodiazepine sedative-hypnotic agents that are now available are zaleplon (a pyrazolopyrimidine), zopiclone (a cyclopyrrolone not available in the United States), and zolpidem (an imidazopyridine) (Figs. 8–28–8–30; Table 8–4).

Zaleplon (Fig. 8–28) and zolpidem (Fig. 8–29) act at selectively at omega 1 benzodiazepine receptors involved in sedation but not at omega 2 benzodiazepine receptors concentrated in brain areas regulating cognition, memory, and motor functioning. Thus, such agents should theoretically have less of the unwanted cognitive, memory, and motor side effects of the benzodiazepines that act on both omega 1 and omega 2 receptors. Also, these three agents all share the ideal profile of a sedative-hypnotic agent, namely, rapid onset and short duration. Even before these

zaleplon

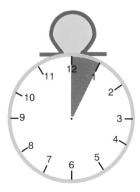

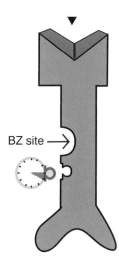

BZ site →

FIGURE 8–28. The hypnotic agent **zaleplon** is a rapid-onset, short-acting nonbenzodiazepine which binds to omega sites near benzodiazepine sites on GABA-A receptors.

drugs were available, there was a shift in emphasis to the fast-onset, shorter-duration benzodiazepines in order to obtain a rapid onset of effect and to prevent carryover effects to the next day and accumulation of carryover effects after several days.

Another advantage of these agents over even fast-onset, short-duration benzodiazepines such as triazolam is that the binding of nonbenzodiazepines to the benzodiazepine receptor is different from benzodiazepine binding to this receptor, and may exhibit partial agonist properties (Fig. 8–28). Perhaps because of this, rebound insomnia (i.e., insomnia caused by withdrawal of the drug), dependence, withdrawal

zolpidem

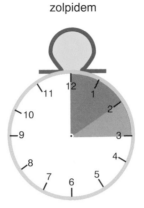

FIGURE 8–29. The hypnotic agent **zolpidem** is relatively short acting nonbenzodiazepine which binds to omega sites near benzodiazepine sites on GABA-A receptors.

zopiclone

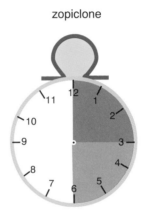

FIGURE 8–30. The hypnotic agent **zopiclone** is an intermediate acting nonbenzodiazepine which binds to omega sites near benzodiazepine sites on GABA-A receptors.

symptoms and loss of efficacy over time are uncommon with the nonbenzodiazepine sedative-hypnotics.

*Zaleplon.* The recently approved agent *zaleplon* (Fig. 8–28) appears to be the ultimate in rapid onset (1-hour peak concentrations) and short duration (1-hour half-life with no active metabolite). The short half-life makes zaleplon ideal for jet lag and for those who require complete drug washout prior to arising. One theoretical concern about a drug with such a short half-life is that its use may be better for patients with sleep onset difficulties than for those with sleep problems in the middle of the night, when zaleplon may have already worn off. In practice, however, the use of a very short acting drug such as zaleplon will treat sleep onset problems and actually facilitate sleep continuity in the middle of the night by allowing natural sleep to unfold. Furthermore, in the case of a patient with middle-of-the-night sleep disruption, zaleplon is short enough in action that taking a first or even a repeat dose on

Table 8–4. *Sedative-hypnotic agents*

| | |
|---|---|
| *Novel nonbenzodiazepines*<br>  Rapid-onset, short-acting<br>    Zaleplon<br>    Zolpidem<br>    Zopiclone | *Sedating antihistamines (may be available<br>    over the counter)*<br>    Diphenhydramine<br>    Doxylamine<br>    Hydroxyzine |
| *Benzodiazepines*<br>  Rapid-onset, short-acting<br>    Triazolam<br>  Delayed onset, intermediate-acting<br>    Temazepam<br>    Estazolam<br>  Rapid onset, long-acting<br>    Flurazepam<br>    Quazepam | *Sedating anticholinergic (over the counter)*<br>    Scopolamine<br><br>*Natural products*<br>    Melatonin<br>    Valerian<br><br>*Older sedative-hypnotics*<br>    Chloral hydrate |
| *Sedating antidepressants*<br>  Tricyclic antidepressants<br>  Trazodone<br>  Mirtazapine<br>  Nefazodone | |

awakening in the middle of the night will still allow the drug to wear off by the time of arising in the morning.

*Zolpidem (Fig. 8–29).* This was the first omega 1 selective nonbenzodiazepine sedative-hypnotic and rapidly replaced benzodiazepines as the preferred agent for many patients and prescribers. It has a somewhat later peak drug concentration (2 to 3 hours) and longer half-life (1.5 to 3 hours) than zaleplon.

*Zopiclone (Fig. 8–30).* This agent is available outside the United States and has a slightly later peak drug concentration than zaleplon but a more rapid peak than zolpidem. However, its half-life (3.5 to 6 hours) is much longer than that of either zaleplon or zolpidem.

## Sedative-Hypnotic Benzodiazepines

The benzodiazepines are still widely prescribed for the treatment of insomnia. These agents have been extensively discussed above in terms of their mechanism of action and use in anxiety. Their mechanism of action in insomnia is the same as for anxiety (see Figs. 8–23 to 8–25). Whether a benzodiazepine is used for sedation or for anxiety is based largely on half-life, with the shorter half-life drugs preferred for insomnia because they are more likely to wear off by morning. However, in practice virtually all the benzodiazepines are used for the treatment of insomnia (Table 8–4).

Pharmacokinetics differ significantly among the most widely used benzodiazepine hypnotics, with some such as triazolam (Fig. 8–31) having rapid onset and short

triazolam

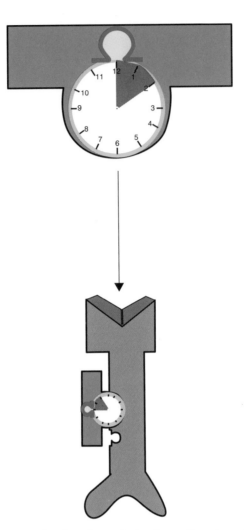

FIGURE 8–31. The hypnotic agent **triazolam** is a sedating benzodiazepine with a short duration of action.

half-life, some such as flurazepam (Fig. 8–32) having relatively rapid onset but prolonged half-life, and others such as temazepam (Fig. 8–33) having somewhat delayed onset but intermediate half-life (Table 8–4). Ideally, the pattern of sleep disturbance should be matched to the sedative-hypnotic, especially since there are so many choices of how to customize a therapy for an individual patient. If a patient has difficulty getting to sleep, a fast-onset, short-acting agent should be considered. If a patient has middle-of-the-night insomnia, an intermediate-onset, intermediate-acting benzodiazepine might be best, especially if the short-acting agents are not effective. If a patient has problems both falling asleep and staying asleep, a fast-onset, intermediate-acting agent might be needed.

flumazepam

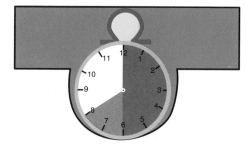

FIGURE 8–32. The hypnotic agent **flumazepam** is a sedating benzodiazepine with a long duration of action.

temazepam

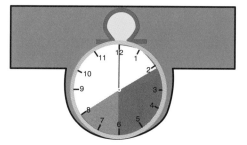

FIGURE 8–33. The hypnotic agent is a sedating **benzodiazepine** with a somewhat delayed onset of action and intermediate duration of action.

There are several problems with using benzodiazepines for the treatment of insomnia. Short-term difficulties associated with benzodiazepine use for insomnia are usually related to giving too high a dose for an individual patient. In such cases, there are carryover effects the morning after administration, including not only a "drugged feeling" and the persistence of sedation when the patient wants to be alert, but also interference with memory formation once the patient is awake. These problems can often be handled by reducing the dose of the benzodiazepine, using a shorter half-life benzodiazepine, or switching to a short-acting nonbenzodiazepine hypnotic, particularly in elderly patients.

Longer-term difficulties associated with benzodiazepine use for insomnia come from observations that many patients develop tolerance for these agents, so that they stop working after a week or two. To avoid this, patients must take a sleeping pill only a few times within several days, or for only about 10 days in a row followed by several days or weeks with no drug treatment. Furthermore, if patients persist in taking benzodiazepines as sedative-hypnotics for several weeks to months, there can be a withdrawal syndrome once the medications are stopped, particularly if they are stopped suddenly. This is discussed in further detail in Chapter 13.

Discontinuance of benzodiazepines as sedative-hypnotics in patients who have been taking them for a prolonged time can cause a condition called *rebound insomnia,* in which a patient's insomnia worsens as soon as benzodiazepines are stopped. Although this condition can be avoided by short-term or only intermittent use of benzodiazepines as sedative-hypnotics, it is often masked in long-term benzodiazepine users until they suddenly stop their medication. Treatment of those grown tolerant to the use of sedative-hypnotic benzodiazepines involves a program of tapered withdrawal, discussed in detail in Chapter 13.

## Antidepressants with Sedative-Hypnotic Properties

There are also numerous antidepressants that have sedative-hypnotic properties (Table 8–4). Some of these antidepressants are sedating owing to anticholinergic-antihistaminic actions. Not surprisingly, the tricyclic antidepressants (TCAs) can therefore be useful hypnotics to induce sleep in some patients. Thus, skillful use of a TCA in a depressed patient with insomnia can turn the liability of unwanted sedation into the asset of relief of insomnia if the TCA is given at bedtime. This property, as discussed in Chapter 6, has nothing to do, however, with the reason that TCAs are antidepressants (shown in Figs. 6–15 and 6–16).

Another antidepressant, namely trazodone, also has significant sedating properties. This may be due to its serotonin 2A antagonist properties, which may act to induce and restore slow-wave sleep (Fig. 7–14). Trazodone can be used safely with most other psychotropic drugs and so is a popular choice when a patient must take another medication that disrupts sleep, such as an SSRI. Other sedating antidepressants that block serotonin 2A receptors include mirtazapine and nefazodone. These agents are occasionally also used for their sedative-hypnotic properties.

## Over-the-Counter Agents

Numerous nonprescription agents (sleeping pills) are popular with the general public (Table 8–4). Although there are trade names that differ widely from time to time and from country to country, essentially all over-the-counter sleeping pills contain one or more of three active ingredients: (1) the anticholinergic agent scopolamine; (2) an antihistamine that also has anticholinergic properties; and (3) a mild pain reliever. Antihistaminergic and anticholinergic properties have already been discussed in relationship to tricyclic antidepressants. Sleep induction by these agents occurs at the expense of side effects such as dry mouth, blurred vision, and constipation. They can even cause confusion or memory problems, particularly in the elderly. However, they are not truly dependence-forming, do not cause severe sleep problems when withdrawn, and are generally safe in the doses available over the counter.

In recent years, natural products such as melatonin and herbs such as valerian have become popular over-the-counter remedies for insomnia. There are no comprehensive evaluations of safety and efficacy of these products. Beyond questions of safety and efficacy, there is no consensus on what their doses should be. Nevertheless, these products continue to be used widely by some patients.

## Other Nonbenzodiazepines as Sedative-Hypnotics

Various older agents have an extensive prior history of use as sedative-hypnotics. These include barbiturates and related compounds such as ethchlorvynol and ethinamate; chloral hydrate and derivatives; and piperidinedione derivatives such as glu-tethimide and methyprylon. Because of problems of tolerance, abuse, dependence, overdose, and several withdrawal reactions far more severe than those associated with the benzodiazepines, barbiturates and piperidinedione derivatives are rarely pre-scribed as sedative-hypnotics today. Chloral hydrate is still somewhat commonly used because it can be an effective short-term sedative-hypnotic and is inexpensive. How-ever, it is generally to be avoided in patients with severe renal, hepatic, and cardiac disease and in those who are taking numerous other drugs because of its ability to affect hepatic drug-metabolizing enzymes. The potential of chloral hydrate to induce tolerance, physical dependence, and addiction requires cautious use in those with histories of drug or alcohol abuse problems and only short-term use in any patient.

## Summary

In this chapter we have provided clinical descriptions of anxiety and insomnia. We have also described the biological basis for anxiety and insomnia, emphasizing three neurotransmitter systems: GABA-benzodiazepines, serotonin, and norepinephrine. Finally, we have discussed the treatments for anxiety and insomnia and how they play on these three neurotransmitter systems.

In discussing the GABA neurotransmitter system, we have shown how benzodi-azepines are allosteric modulators of GABA-A receptors and in turn, of inhibitory chloride channels. The benzodiazepine receptor may be involved in the mediation of the emotion of anxiety as well as in the mechanism of anxiolytic drug action.

In terms of the noradrenergic system, this chapter has described the locus co-eruleus as that part of the brain containing the noradrenergic neurons that mediate some of the symptoms of anxiety through alpha 2 and beta adrenergic receptors. Our discussion has also extended to the role of serotonin in anxiety, which appears to be key, yet quite complex and incompletely understood. One current theory de-veloped in this chapter is the notion that anxiolytic drugs act as partial agonists at serotonin 1A receptors.

We have discussed how various antidepressants, especially venlafaxine XR, are being used increasingly for the treatment of generalized anxiety disorder. Buspirone remains a first-line generalized anxiolytic for chronic anxiety, and benzodiazepines are used largely for short-term treatment of intermittent anxiety symptoms.

The nonbenzodiazepine sedative-hypnotics zaleplon, zolpidem, and zopiclone are replacing benzodiazepine sedative-hypnotics as first-line treatments for insomnia. Some antidepressants, such as sedating tricyclic antidepressants and trazodone, are also used as sedative-hypnotic agents for the treatment of insomnia.

# CHAPTER 9

# DRUG TREATMENTS FOR OBSESSIVE-COMPULSIVE DISORDER, PANIC DISORDER, AND PHOBIC DISORDERS

Impressive advances are being made in the treatment of anxiety disorders. These treatments have largely derived from the new antidepressants, as essentially all new treatments for the anxiety disorders are also antidepressants. Thus, a good deal of the information on the drugs and their mechanisms of action will be found in Chapters 6 and 7 on antidepressants. The adaptation of antidepressants as significant new treatments for anxiety disorders has had a large hand in the remaking of diagnostic criteria for subtypes of anxiety disorder. Thus, the tasks of clarifying the clinical description, epidemiology, and natural history of obsessive-compulsive disorder, panic disorder, social phobia, and posttraumatic stress disorder were greatly facilitated once effective new treatments became available over the past decade.

The anxiety disorders as a group are the most common psychiatric disorders and therefore very important for the psychopharmacologist to understand and treat effectively. Knowledge about the anxiety disorders is advancing at a rapid pace, and new treatments and diagnostic criteria are still evolving. To equip the reader with the necessary foundation to keep up with the pace of change in the anxiety disorders, this chapter will set forth the psychopharmacological principles underlying contemporary treatment strategies for them. The details are likely to change rapidly, so this chapter will emphasize underlying concepts rather than specific facts about drug doses and pragmatic prescribing information. The reader is referred to standard reference sources for such data. Here we will emphasize the therapeutic agents, and their pharmacological mechanisms of action for the treatment of the most prominent anxiety disorders in psychopharmacology, namely, obsessive-compulsive disorder, panic disorder, social phobia, and posttraumatic stress disorder. Generalized anxiety disorder was discussed in Chapter 8.

## Obsessive-Compulsive Disorder

### Clinical Description

Obsessive-compulsive disorder (OCD) is a syndrome characterized by obsessions and/ or compulsions, which together last at least an hour per day and are sufficiently bothersome that they interfere with one's normal social or occupational functioning. *Obsessions* are experienced internally and subjectively by the patient as thoughts, impulses, or images. According to standard definitions in the Diagnostic and Statistical Manual of Mental Disorders, 4th edition (DSM-IV), obsessions are intrusive and inappropriate and cause marked anxiety and distress. Common obsessions are listed in Table 9–1.

Table 9–1. *Common obsessions*

Contamination
Aggression
Religion (scrupulosity)
Safety/harm
Need for exactness or symmetry
Somatic (body) fears

Table 9–2. *Common compulsions*

Checking
Cleaning/washing
Counting
Repeating
Ordering/arranging
Hoarding/collecting

*Compulsions*, on the other hand, are repetitive behaviors or purposeful mental acts that are sometimes observed by family members or clinicians, whereas it is not possible to observe an obsession. Patients are often subjectively driven to act out their compulsions either in response to an obsession or according to rigid rules aimed at preventing distress or some dreaded event. Unfortunately, the compulsions are not realistically able to prevent the distress or the dreaded event, and at some level the patient generally recognizes this. Common compulsions are listed in Table 9–2. The formal DSM-IV diagnostic criteria for OCD are given in Table 9–3. Numerous other psychiatric disorders that are considered by some experts to be related to OCD are listed as OCD Spectrum Disorders in Table 9–4. These include conditions such as pathological gambling, eating disorders, paraphilias, kleptomania, body dysmorphic disorder, and several others.

Interest in OCD skyrocketed once clomipramine was recognized throughout the world to be an effective treatment in the mid-1980s. Originally thought to be a rare condition, recent epidemiological studies now suggest that OCD exists in about 1 out of every 50 adults and in about 1 out of every 200 children. Thus, as news that OCD is common and treatable emerged, intensive research efforts began to document that all five serotonin selective reuptake inhibitors (SSRIs) and certain forms of behavioral therapy are also effective treatments for OCD. The initial euphoria of the 1980s is somewhat balanced today by the sobering realization that treatments ameliorate but do not eliminate OCD symptoms in many patients, and that relapse is very common after discontinuing treatments for OCD.

## Biological Basis

Despite a great deal of work in this area, the biological basis for OCD remains unknown. Some data suggest a genetic component to the etiology of OCD, but

Table 9–3. *DSM IV diagnostic criteria for obsessive-compulsive disorder*

1. Either obsessions or compulsions
   Obsessions defined by
   a. Recurrent and persistent thoughts, impulses, or images that are experienced, at some time during the disturbance, as intrusive and inappropriate and that cause marked anxiety or distress.
   b. The thoughts, impulses, or images are not simply excessive worries about real-life problems.
   c. The person attempts to ignore or suppress such thoughts, impulses, or images or to neutralize them with some other thought or action.
   d. The person recognizes that the obsessional thoughts, impulses, or images are a product of his or her own mind and not imposed from without as in thought insertion.
   Compulsions defined by
   a. Repetitive behaviors (e.g., hand washing, ordering, checking) or mental acts (e.g., praying, counting, repeating words silently) that the person feels driven to perform in response to an obsession or according to rules that must be applied rigidly.
   b. The behaviors or mental acts are aimed at preventing or reducing distress or preventing some dreaded event or situation; however, these behaviors or mental acts either are not connected in a realistic way with what they are designed to neutralize or prevent or they are clearly excessive.
2. At some point during the course of the disorder, the person has recognized that the obsessions or compulsions are excessive or unreasonable (this does not apply to children).
3. The obsessions or compulsions caused marked distress, are time-consuming (take more than 1 hour per day), or significantly interfere with occupational or academic functioning or with usual social activities or relationships.
4. If another Axis I disorder is present, the content of the obsessions or compulsions is not restricted to it (e.g., preoccupation with food in the presence of an eating disorder; hair pulling in the presence of trichotillomania; concern with appearance in the presence of body dysmorphic disorder; preoccupation with drugs in the presence of a substance abuse disorder; preoccupation with having a serious illness in the presence of hypochondriasis; preoccupation with sexual urges or fantasies in the presence of a paraphilia; or guilty ruminations in the presence of major depressive disorder.
5. The disturbance is not due to the direct physiological effects of a substance (e.g., a drug of abuse or a medication) or a general medical condition.

abnormal genes or gene products have yet to be identified. Some evidence implicates abnormal neuronal activity as well as alterations in neurotransmitters in OCD patients, but it is not known whether this is a cause or an effect of OCD. There is also a long-standing belief that there is a neurologic basis for OCD, which derives mainly from data implicating the basal ganglia in OCD plus the relative success of psychosurgery in some patients.

*The serotonin hypothesis.* Although it is unlikely that one neurotransmitter system can explain all the complexities of OCD, recent efforts to elucidate the pathophysiology of OCD have centered largely around the role of the neurotransmitter serotonin

Table 9–4. *OCD spectrum disorders*

Gambling
Paraphilia
Body dysmorphic disorder
Trichotillomania
Hypochondriasis
Somatization disorder
Tourette syndrome
Autism
Asperger's disorder
Kleptomania
Impulse control disorders
Obsessive compulsive personality disorder
Bulimia
Anorexia nervosa

(5HT). The serotonin hypothesis of OCD, which states that OCD is linked to 5HT dysfunction, stems largely from pharmacological treatment studies.

It has been known since the mid-1980s that clomipramine, a potent but nonselective serotonin reuptake inhibitor, is effective in reducing OCD symptoms. Since then, numerous studies have confirmed the superiority of clomipramine over placebo in OCD patients, whereas other antidepressant medications with less potent inhibitory effects on serotonin reuptake (e.g., nortripytline, desipramine) seem to be ineffective in OCD. Demonstration of the anti-OCD actions of all five SSRIs, namely, fluoxetine, sertraline, paroxetine, fluvoxamine, and citalopram, also supports the hypothesis that the antiobsessional effects of these various pharmacologic agents is due to their potent serotonergic reuptake blocking activity.

The hypothesis that SSRIs work in OCD by a serotonergic mechanism is also supported by studies showing a strong positive correlation between improvement in obsessive-compulsive symptoms during clomipramine treatment and drug-induced decreases in cerebrospinal fluid (CSF) levels of the serotonin metabolite 5-hydroxyindoleacetic acid (5-HIAA) and platelet serotonin concentrations. Thus, peripheral markers of 5HT function link the symptomatic improvement in OCD symptoms produced by SSRIs to changes in 5HT function. However, these markers do not consistently highlight a 5HT abnormality in untreated patients with OCD.

*Dopamine and obsessive-compulsive disorder.* Up to 40% of OCD patients do not respond to SSRIs. Thus, at least some OCD patients fail to demonstrate convincing dysregulation in serotonin function. Therefore, other neurotransmitters may be involved in the pathophysiology of OCD in some patients.

Several lines of evidence show that dopamine (DA) is implicated in the mediation of some obsessive-compulsive behavior. Animal studies demonstrate that high doses of various dopaminergic agents, such as amphetamine, bromocriptine, apomorphine, and L-DOPA, induce stereotyped movements in animals, which resemble compulsive behaviors in OCD patients. Increased dopaminergic neurotransmission may be responsible for this. Human studies consistently report that abuse of stimulants such as amphetamine can cause seemingly purposeless, complex, repetitive behaviors, which resemble behaviors occurring in OCD. Cocaine can also worsen compulsive symptoms in patients with chronic motor tic disorders such as Tourette syndrome.

The strongest support for a role of DA in mediating OCD symptoms comes from the relationship between OCD symptoms and several neurological disorders associated with dysfunction of DA in the basal ganglia (Von Economo encephalitis, Tourette syndrome, and Sydenham chorea). There is even recent evidence that autoimmune-mediated damage to the basal ganglia in some vulnerable children may be linked to the development of OCD. The most intriguing relationship between DA in the basal ganglia and OCD may be the link between the Tourette syndrome and obsessive-compulsive symptoms. Tourette syndrome is a chronic neuropsychiatric disorder characterized by multiple motor and vocal tics. Between 45% and 90% of Tourette patients also have obsessions and compulsions. If OCD symptoms were considered alone, a high percentage of Tourette patients would meet diagnostic criteria for OCD. Family genetic studies show that Tourette syndrome and OCD are linked, leading to proposals that a common genetic factor may manifest itself as tics in some individuals and as obsessions and compulsions in others. Put differently, perhaps tics are the behavioral manifestations of a genetically based basal ganglia dysfunction, with Tourette syndrome being manifested as "tics of the body" and OCD as "tics of the mind."

Also supportive of DA involvement in the pathophysiology of OCD are observations that adjunctive therapy with the older conventional antipsychotics-neuroleptics (which block DA receptors) added to ongoing SSRI treatment reduces the severity of OCD symptoms in OCD patients resistant to SSRI treatment alone, especially in those with concomitant Tourette syndrome.

*Serotonin-dopamine hypothesis.* On the basis of the studies of both 5HT and DA in OCD, it seems possible that at least in some forms of OCD (e.g., OCD with a history of Tourette syndrome), both 5HT and DA transmitter systems may be involved in the pathophysiology of symptoms. It is not clear whether the primary abnormality is in 5HT function, DA function, or serotonin-dopaminergic balance. This hypothesis is supported by many preclinical data, which suggest that important anatomic and functional interactions exist between serotonergic and dopaminergic neurons. This will be discussed in detail in Chapter 11 in the sections on antipsychotic drugs that work simultaneously on DA and 5HT receptors.

Thus, it may be that decreases in 5HT tonic inhibitory influences on DA neurons could lead to increased dopaminergic function due to the functional connections between DA and 5HT neurons in the basal ganglia. Thus, OCD patients with a history of Tourette syndrome may represent a subtype of the disorder in which two neurotransmitters and the balance between them are involved in the pathophysiology of their symptoms.

Consistent with the role of both serotonin and dopamine in OCD, some OCD patients benefit from treatment with the new serotonin-dopamine antagonists (also known as atypical antipsychotics), especially when there is inadequate response to an SSRI. On the other hand, other patients have no therapeutic response to these new agents, and the condition of still others is even worsened by these drugs. The atypical antipsychotics and serotonin dopamine antagonism are discussed in Chapter 11.

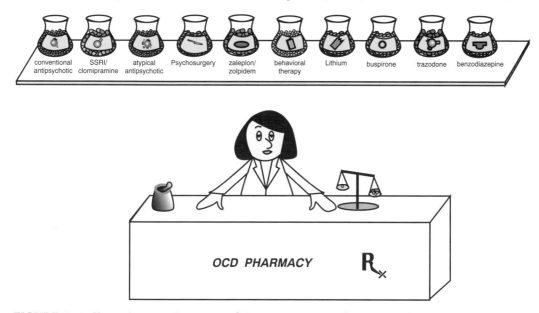

FIGURE 9–1. Shown here are the variety of therapeutic options for treating *obsessive-compulsive disorder* (OCD).

In summary, the hypothesis that an abnormality in neurotransmitter functioning might underlie OCD has generated numerous studies of 5HT and DA neuronal systems. To date, no compelling or consistent neurotransmitter dysfunction has been described that can adequately explain the neurobiological basis for OCD. However, it seems clear that changes in 5HT neuronal systems are caused by the known therapeutic agents for OCD, which suggests an important role for 5HT in mediating treatment responses in OCD.

*Neuroanatomy.* Abnormalities on positron emission tomography (PET) scans of neuronal activity of cortical projections to the basal ganglia have been confirmed by a number of investigators in OCD patients. Specifically, projections from the orbitofrontal–medial prefrontal cortex may be implicated in OCD. Such PET-demonstrated abnormalities in cortical projections to the basal ganglia may even be linked to the severity of symptoms in OCD patients, since they diminish as OCD patients improve, whether that improvement occurs after drug treatment or after behavioral therapy (see Fig. 5–53).

## Drug Treatments

A summary of OCD treatments is shown in Figure 9–1, and combination therapies are depicted graphically in Figure 9–2.

*Serotonin reuptake inhibitors.* Clomipramine is a tricyclic antidepressant first recognized more than 30 years ago as an effective treatment for depression. It has only been recognized widely and on a worldwide basis for the treatment of OCD since the

# OCD Combos

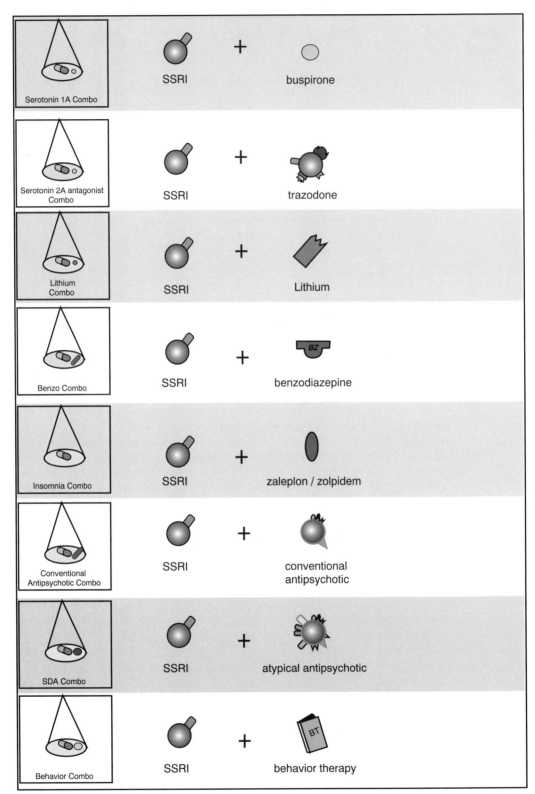

**Serotonin 1A Combo:** SSRI + buspirone

**Serotonin 2A antagonist Combo:** SSRI + trazodone

**Lithium Combo:** SSRI + Lithium

**Benzo Combo:** SSRI + benzodiazepine

**Insomnia Combo:** SSRI + zaleplon / zolpidem

**Conventional Antipsychotic Combo:** SSRI + conventional antipsychotic

**SDA Combo:** SSRI + atypical antipsychotic

**Behavior Combo:** SSRI + behavior therapy

mid-1980s. Originally, the efficacy of clomipramine in OCD was debated because depression is frequently present in OCD patients, leading some researchers to propose that clomipramine was only effective in treating concomitant depressive symptoms and not the obsessions and compulsions in these patients. Others suggested that clomipramine was only effective in treating core OCD symptoms if symptoms of depression were also present. However, it is now clearly recognized that clomipramine has unique anti-OCD effects independent of its antidepressant effects in OCD patients.

Since clomipramine is a potent inhibitor of serotonin reuptake, it is hypothesized that the anti-OCD effects of clomipramine are linked to its serotonin reuptake blocking properties. This is strongly supported by the findings that all five of the SSRIs are also effective in treating OCD. Although clomipramine is also metabolized to a norepinephrine reuptake blocker (i.e., desmethylclomipramine), there does not appear to be a robust role for norepinephrine reuptake blockade in the mechanism of action of clomipramine, since more selective noradrenergic reuptake inhibitors such as desipramine and nortriptyline appear to have little or no anti-OCD actions. Recent findings even suggest that it may be necessary to have serotonin reuptake blockade to treat comorbid depression in OCD. In patients with both OCD and depression, an SSRI was found to improve both, but the norepinephrine reuptake inhibitor desipramine not only failed to improve OCD as expected, but also was less effective that the SSRI in treating the concomitant depression. This suggests that although depression in general may involve serotonin, norepinephrine, or both, the depression that coexists with OCD may be particularly serotonergic.

Although similarities exist between the treatment of OCD with SSRIs and the treatment of depression with SSRIs, there are also some important differences. In general, doses of SSRIs for treating OCD are greater than doses for treating depression. Also, the onset of therapeutic effects may be even more delayed in OCD (6 to 12 weeks or longer) than in depression (4 to 8 weeks) following SSRI administration (Table 9–5).

There are also differences in treatment responses between OCD and depression following SSRI treatment. Whereas many patients with depression recover completely after SSRI treatment, the average response of an OCD patient is about a 35% reduction in symptoms after 12 weeks of treatment (Table 9–5). Relapse rates appear to be higher and to occur sooner after drug discontinuation in OCD than in depression.

One other important difference in the mechanism of SSRIs in OCD versus depression is that the therapeutic response in OCD may be less dependent on the immediate availability of 5HT than is the therapeutic response in depression. Thus, when tryptophan is depleted from depressed patients and 5HT synthesis is suddenly diminished, patients who have responded to SSRIs transiently deteriorate until 5HT

---

FIGURE 9–2. Various treatments can be given in combination for obsessive-compulsive disorder (OCD) (i.e., **OCD combos**). The basis of all combination treatments is a serotonin selective reuptake inhibitor (SSRI) or clomipramine. Added to this basis may be a serotonin 1A partial agonist, a serotonin 2A antagonist, lithium, a benzodiazepine or a sedative-hypnotic, a conventional antipsychotic or an atypical antipsychotic, or behavioral psychotherapy.

Table 9–5. *Profile of serotonin selective reuptake inhibitors (SSRIs) in obsessive-compulsive disorder (OCD)*

The starting dose for OCD is the same as the starting dose for depression

The maintenance dose for OCD may be higher than the maintenance dose for depression because therapeutic effects are not as robust for SSRIs in OCD.

Usual clinical response is less robust in OCD than in depression, usually with less than 50% reduction of symptoms, although this can range from complete reduction to no reduction for individual patients.

The onset of response is slower in OCD than in depression, about 12 to 26 weeks being required to determine whether a response will be seen.

Target symptoms do not worsen before they improve once treatment with an SSRI is initiated.

Some patients respond much better to one SSRI than to another.

synthesis is restored. By contrast, when tryptophan is depleted from OCD patients who have responded to SSRI treatment, their OCD symptoms are not worsened. This may suggest that SSRIs work via a different mechanism in OCD than they do in depression. They certainly appear to be working on serotonin in different pathways in OCD (Fig. 5–53) than they do in depression (Fig. 5–52).

In summary, SSRIs undoubtedly improve symptoms in OCD, just as they improve symptoms in depression. However, as compared to the use of SSRIs in depression, OCD responses to SSRIs specifically require 5HT and not norepinephrine reuptake inhibition, the OCD responses are generally slower, less robust, more likely to relapse after SSRI discontinuation, and not as immediately dependent on synaptic 5HT availability.

*Adjunctive treatments.* Although SSRIs are the foundation of treatment for OCD, many patients are refractory to SSRI treatment, or their responses are incomplete and unsatisfactory. This has led to a variety of strategies to augment SSRIs to attain a more satisfactory therapeutic response (Fig. 9–2). Augmentation strategies include those that are directed at serotonergic functioning, those that are pharmacological but directed at other neurotransmitter systems, and those that are nonpharmacological.

SEROTONERGIC AUGMENTATION STRATEGIES    Since SSRIs do not work well for all OCD patients and do not work at all as monotherapies for some OCD patients, psychopharmacologists have attempted to boost the effectiveness of SSRIs with various agents capable of augmenting serotonergic action. These have been previously discussed in the treatment of depression in Chapter 7, and several are outlined in Figures 7–31 to 7–33 and in Figure 7–37. Such serotonin 1A, serotonin 2A, and lithium augmentation strategies can also be effective in OCD (see Fig. 9–2).

NEUROTRANSMITTER COMBINATION STRATEGIES    Rather than boosting the SSRI with a pharmacologic intervention aimed at helping the SSRI at the serotonergic neuron, it is also possible that adding another neurotransmitter mechanism to the SSRI's action at the serotonin neuron would boost the SSRI's action indirectly. At least two such strategies have proved useful in some OCD patients whose response to SSRIs is unsatisfactory.

For example, one possibility for boosting the SSRI is to add a benzodiazepine, especially clonazepam (Fig. 9–2). The SSRI boosting effect of clonazepam may be mediated partially by allowing a high dose of SSRI to be tolerated, partially by reducing nonspecific anxiety symptoms associated with OCD, and partially by a direct serotonin-enhancing action of clonazepam itself. Other benzodiazepines can be added for treatment of concomitant generalized anxiety. Sedative-hypnotic non-benzodiazepines such as zaleplon or zolpidem or sedative-hypnotic benzodiazepines may also have to be added for short-term reduction of associated insomnia, particularly when initiating treatment with an SSRI (Fig. 9–2).

As discussed earlier, the addition of a conventional antipsychotic that blocks DA receptors can be useful in some patients with OCD, particularly those with concomitant Tourette syndrome. Other OCD patients, including those who have associated schizophreniform symptoms or whose obsessions border on delusions without any insight, may also respond to the boosting effect of a conventional antipsychotic agent (Fig. 9–2). As also mentioned above, augmenting the treatment of some patients with an atypical antipsychotic may be helpful, but this can be tricky, because other patients may be made worse (Fig. 9–2).

BEHAVIORAL THERAPY   The most common concomitant therapy to use with SSRIs is behavioral psychotherapy (Fig. 9–2). Used by itself in selected cases, behavioral therapy can be as effective as SSRIs, and its therapeutic effects may last longer after discontinuance of treatment than the therapeutic effects of SSRIs after they are stopped. Little is known from formal studies combining SSRIs with behavioral therapy, but it is well known from anecdotal clinical experience that this combination can be much more powerful than SSRIs or behavioral therapy alone. Although behavioral therapy may have enduring effects that carry over after the sessions are finished, SSRIs apparently have to be given indefinitely in OCD.

PSYCHOSURGERY   For extremely severe cases refractory to all these treatments alone and in combination, there is the possibility to gain some relief from a neurosurgical procedure cutting the neuronal loop connecting the cortex with the basal ganglia. Few centers have any experience with this procedure in OCD, and long-term outcomes are as yet unknown. However, early results in some patients with very severe, very refractory OCD cases are encouraging, but this is not an option for most patients with refractory OCD.

*New prospects.* Given that there are at least five serotonin reuptake blockers available to treat OCD, and that each is roughly comparable the other in efficacy, it does not seem likely that much more therapeutic ground will be gained merely by developing yet another SSRI for OCD. On the other hand, it is not clear what pharmacological mechanism to target other than serotonin reuptake blockade in order to devise an effective anti-OCD therapy.

It is theoretically possible that novel agents combining the actions of single agents might be more powerful than a drug that is merely an SSRI. However, this is purely hypothetical at the moment because the mechanisms of action of the combinations described above are not proved. It is also possible that certain novel agents acting

Table 9–6. *Symptoms of a panic attack*

| |
|---|
| Palpitations, pounding heart, or accelerated heart rate |
| Sweating |
| Trembling or shaking |
| Sensations of shortness of breath or smothering |
| Feeling of choking |
| Chest pain or discomfort |
| Nausea or abdominal distress |
| Feeling dizzy, unsteady, lightheaded, or faint |
| Derealization (feelings of unreality) or depersonalization (being detached from oneself) |
| Fear of losing control or going crazy |
| Fear of dying |
| Paresthesias |
| Chills or hot flushes |

uniquely on serotonin and other neurotransmitter systems and being tested as antidepressants or antipsychotics will also prove to be anti-OCD agents, such as substance P and neurokinin antagonists. If the past is any indication of the future, new treatments of OCD may arise from agents being tested for depression.

## Panic Attacks and Panic Disorder

### Clinical Description

A panic attack is a discrete episode of unexpected terror accompanied by a variety of physical symptoms. Associated symptoms include fear and anxiety, as well as catastrophic thinking with a sense of impending doom or the belief that loss of control, death, or insanity is imminent. Physical symptoms can be neurologic, gastrointestinal, cardiac, or pulmonary and therefore may mimic many different types of medical illnesses. Panic attacks have therefore sometimes been called the "great medical imposters." Behaviors associated with panic attacks typically include an attempt to flee the situation and eventually to avoid anxiety-producing situations or any situation that has previously been associated with a panic attack.

A panic attack usually lasts from 5 to 30 minutes, with the symptoms peaking at about 10 minutes, but attacks have been reported to last for hours. A person must have at least 4 of the 13 symptoms listed in Table 9–6 for an episode to be classified as a panic attack. Panic attacks may occur during sleep, in which case they are known as nocturnal panic attacks. These attacks may wake the person from sleep but are otherwise similar in symptoms to daytime panic attacks. A majority of patients with panic disorder will experience nocturnal panic, but only a few patients describe having the majority of their panic attacks at night.

It is common to confuse panic attacks with panic disorder. Many psychiatric disorders can have panic attacks associated with them (Table 9–7). However, to qualify for the diagnosis of panic disorder itself, patients must have some panic attacks that are entirely *unexpected* (Table 9–7). Panic attacks can also be reproducibly triggered by certain specific situations for various individuals, and therefore can be

Table 9–7. *Not all panic attacks are panic disorder*

| Diagnosis | Spontaneous Panic Attacks | Situational Panic Attacks | Anticipatory Anxiety | Symptoms of Autonomic Arousal | Phobic Avoidance |
|---|---|---|---|---|---|
| Panic disorder | +++ | +/− | +++ | +++ | + |
| Agoraphobia | +/− | +/− | +++ | ++ | +++ |
| Social phobia | − | ++ | ++ | ++ | +++ |
| Specific phobia | +/− | +++ | ++ | ++ | +++ |
| PTSD | +/− | + | +/− | +++ | + |
| GAD | +/− | +/− | +/− | + | +/− |

+ to +++, present; −, not usually present; +/−, frequently present but not needed for diagnosis.

*expected* (Table 9–7). Situations that frequently act as triggers for panic attacks include driving or riding in a vehicle, especially in heavy rain or over bridges, shopping in crowded stores, and waiting in lines. The perception of lack of control or feeling "trapped" is a common theme in situational triggers.

As already emphasized, not all who have panic attacks have panic disorder (Table 9–7), and the distinguishing factor is the type of panic attacks. Patients with social phobia, posttraumatic stress disorder, or specified phobias will frequently experience panic attacks that are *expected*, since they are in response to specific situations or stimuli. However, such patients do not experience *unexpected* panic attacks. Unexpected panic attacks are thus uniquely characteristic of panic disorder. The DSM-IV diagnostic criteria for panic disorder are given in Table 9–8. Panic disorder can occur with or without a type of phobic avoidance behavior called *agoraphobia*. The diagnostic criteria for agoraphobia are also listed in Table 9–8, and the clinical characteristics of agoraphobia are discussed below in the section on phobic disorders.

Panic disorder, therefore, is the presence of recurrent unexpected panic attacks followed by at least a 1-month period of persistent anxiety or concern about recurrent attacks or consequences of attacks, or by significant behavioral changes related to the attacks. The presence of persistent anxiety or behavioral changes is important, because approximately 10% of the normal population report having had panic attacks at some time in their lives; however, since they do not develop persistent anxiety and do not modify their behavior, they do not develop panic disorder.

Panic disorder affects up to 2% of the population, but less than one-third receive treatment. Panic disorder typically begins in late adolescence or early adulthood but can present in childhood. Onset is rare after age 45. Panic disorder is more prevalent in women, who have perhaps twice the rate in men. Genetic studies demonstrate a 15 to 20% rate of panic disorder in relatives of patients with panic disorder, including a 40% concordance rate for panic disorder in monozygotic twins.

Although not generally recognized by medical or mental health practitioners, panic disorder patients have a suicide rate comparable with that of patients with major depression; 20 to 40% of panic disorder patients report having made suicide attempts, and about half admit to having had suicidal ideation. This high rate of suicide attempts does not appear to be caused by the presence of depression in panic disorder patients.

Table 9–8. *DSM-IV diagnostic criteria for panic disorder*

1. Recurrent unexpected panic attacks
2. At least one of the attacks has been followed by one month or more of the following:
   a. Persistent concern about having additional attacks
   b. Worry about the implications of the attack or its consequences (losing control, having a heart attack, "going crazy")
   c. A significant change in behavior related to the attacks
3. May or may not meet the diagnostic criteria for agoraphobia. The diagnostic criteria for concomitant agoraphobia include:
   a. Anxiety about being in places or situations from which escape is difficult or in which help may not be available in the event of an unexpected or situationally predisposed panic attack or panic-like symptoms. Agoraphobic fears typically involve characteristic clusters of situations, which include being outside the home alone, standing in a line or being in a crowd, being on a bridge, and traveling in a bus, train, or automobile.
   b. The situations are avoided, are endured with marked distress or with anxiety about having a panic attack or panic-like symptoms, or require the presence of a companion.
   c. The anxiety or phobic avoidance is not better accounted for by another mental disorder, such as social phobia (e.g., avoidance limited to social situations because of fear of embarrassment), specific phobia (e.g., avoidance limited to a single situation such as elevators), obsessive-compulsive disorder (e.g., avoidance of dirt on someone for fear of contamination), posttraumatic stress disorder (e.g., avoidance of stimuli associated with a severe stressor), or separation anxiety disorder (e.g., avoidance of leaving home or relatives).
4. The panic attacks are not due to the direct physiological effects of a substance or a general medical condition.
5. The panic attacks are not better accounted for by another mental disorder such as those listed above under diagnostic criteria for concomitant agoraphobia.

Panic disorder patients report a subjective feeling of poor physical and emotional health, impaired social and marital functioning, and increased financial dependency. Because of this disorder, 70% of patients lose or quit their jobs, with an average length of work disability of more than $2^{1}/_{2}$ years, and 50% are unable to drive more than 3 miles from their home. Panic disorder patients also have the highest use of emergency rooms of any psychiatric population.

## Biological Basis of Panic Disorder

### Neurotransmitter dysregulation

NOREPINEPHRINE   One theory about the biological basis of panic disorder is that there is an initial excess of norepinephrine (Fig. 9–3). This theory is supported by evidence that panic disorder patients are hypersensitive to alpha-2 antagonists and hyposensitive to alpha-2 agonists. Thus, yohimbine, an alpha-2 antagonist, acts as a promoter of norepinephrine release by "cutting the brake cable" of the presynaptic norepinephrine autoreceptor, as shown earlier in Figure 7–6. The consequence

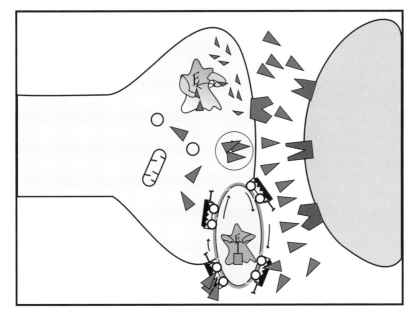

FIGURE 9–3. One theory about the *biological basis of panic disorder* is that there is an excess of norepinephrine, causing intermittent and chaotic discharge of noradrenergic neurons from the locus coeruleus.

of yohimbine administration is an exaggerated response in panic disorder patients, including the precipitation of overt panic attacks. Caffeine is also panicogenic. That is, caffeine is an adenosine antagonist and can be synergistic with norepinephrine. When panic patients are given the caffeine equivalent of four to six cups of coffee, many experience a panic attack, whereas most normal subjects do not panic. On the other hand, panic patients have a blunted physiological response to postsynaptic adrenergic agonists, perhaps as a consequence of an overactive noradrenergic system. Thus, there may be a dysregulation in the noradrenergic system, with changes in the sensitivity of noradrenergic neurons and their receptors altering their physiological functioning and contributing to the pathophysiology of panic attacks.

GAMMA AMINOBUTYRIC ACID (GABA)    The neurotransmitter GABA and its allosteric modulation by benzodiazepines have also been implicated in the biological basis of panic disorder. That is, it appears that the ability of benzodiazepines to modulate GABA is out of balance. This may be due to changes in the amounts of endogenous benzodiazepines (i.e., "the brain's own Xanax" or "Valium-like compound"), or to alterations in the sensitivity of the benzodiazepine receptor itself.

Very little is known about endogenous benzodiazepine ligands, so most of the emphasis has been placed on investigating the responsivity of the benzodiazepine receptor in panic disorder patients. Nevertheless, it is possible that the brain makes less than the necessary amount of an endogenous full agonist and thus has less ability to decrease anxiety on its own owing to a postulated deficiency in a naturally occurring benzodiazepine full agonist. Alternatively, it is possible that the brain is producing an excess in anxiogenic inverse agonists, causing the panic disorder patient to have more anxiety and panic attacks due to such a postulated and unwanted increase in a naturally occurring benzodiazepine inverse agonist.

These are just theoretical possibilities, but some data do actually suggest an abnormality in the benzodiazepine receptor in panic disorder patients, in which the "set point" is shifted toward the inverse agonist conformation (Fig. 9–4). Conceptually, the resting state of the GABA-A–benzodiazepine–chloride channel receptor complex is shifted to the left in the agonist spectrum already discussed (see Fig. 7–25). Thus, chloride channel conductance is already too diminished due to an altered sensitivity of the benzodiazepine receptor site (Fig. 9–4). Evidence for this comes from the fact that such patients require administration of exogenous benzodiazepine ligands (i.e., real Xanax [alprazolam] or real clonazepam) to reset the receptor complex's set point back to normal. Also, flumazenil, which is neutral and without behavioral effects in normal subjects because it acts as a relatively pure antagonist, can act differently in panic disorder patients. In these patients, some but not all studies suggest that flumazenil acts as an inverse agonist, perhaps via an abnormal shift of the set point to the right, toward an inverse agonist conformation. Thus, whereas flumazenil acts as an antagonist with no behavioral effects in normal subjects, it acts as a partial inverse agonist in panic patients and provokes panic attacks in these patients.

CHOLECYSTOKININ (CCK)    The tetrapeptide CCK causes more panic attacks when infused into patients with panic disorder than it does in normal volunteers, which suggests increased sensitivity of the brain type of CCK receptor, known as CCK-B. Unfortunately, in early investigations CCK-B antagonists did not appear to be effective for panic disorder. Nevertheless, agents with novel pharmacological mechanisms of action are sometimes evaluated for their potential antipanic actions by testing whether they can block CCK-induced panic attacks.

*Respiratory hypotheses*

CARBON DIOXIDE AND LACTATE HYPERSENSITIVITY    Another theory regarding the biological substrate for panic disorder proposes that panic attacks are a result of abnormalities in respiratory function. This theory is based on observations that panic disorder patients experience panic attacks more readily than normal control subjects after exercising, when breathing carbon dioxide, or when given lactate. This has generated a theory of carbon dioxide hypersensitivity or lactate hypersensitivity in panic disorder patients, with a corollary hypothesis that panic patients demonstrate these findings because they are chronic hyperventilators. Lactate may induce panic because it is a potent respiratory stimulant, and panic disorder patients may be more sensitive to agents that promote respiratory drive.

FALSE SUFFOCATION ALARM THEORY    This theory proposes that panic disorder patients have a suffocation monitor located in the brainstem, which misinterprets signals and misfires, triggering a "false suffocation alarm" (panic attack). Many factors are consistent with this hypothesis, including the above-mentioned theory of chronic hyperventilation and carbon dioxide hypersensitivity. The disorder of Ondine's curse (congenital central hypoventilation syndrome) appears to be virtually the opposite of panic disorder and is characterized by a diminished sensitivity of the

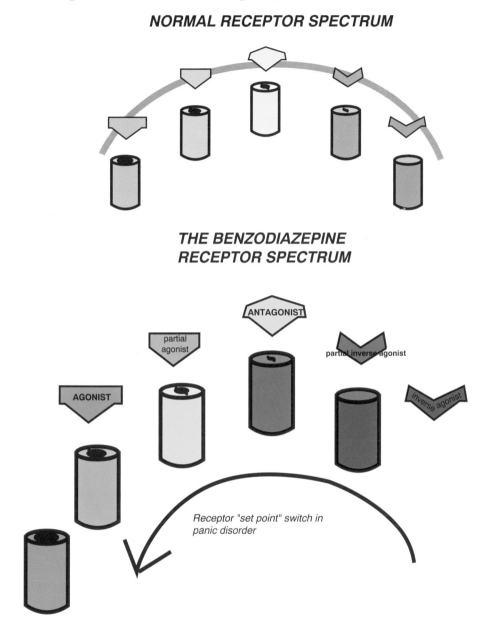

## NORMAL RECEPTOR SPECTRUM

## THE BENZODIAZEPINE
## RECEPTOR SPECTRUM

FIGURE 9–4. Another theory about the *biological basis of panic disorder* is an abnormality in the set point for benzodiazepine receptors. Perhaps the sensitivity of these receptors is switched to the left in this spectrum, rendering the receptors less sensitive to full agonists and experiencing antagonists as inverse agonists.

suffocation alarm, causing sufferers from this disorder to lack adequate breathing, especially when asleep. These various observations support the existence of a distinct suffocation monitor, which is overly sensitive in panic disorder and not sensitive enough in Ondine's curse. According to this theory, spontaneous (i.e., unexpected) panic attacks are thought to be mediated by this mechanism whereas chronic anxiety or fear is not.

*Neuroanatomic findings.* Positron emission tomography (PET) scans of patients experiencing a panic attack suggest abnormalities of neuronal activity projections to the hippocampus, possibly causing asymmetry of metabolic activity. Animal studies suggest that the locus coeruleus appears central to modulation of vigilance, attention, and anxiety or fear. Thus, hypersensitivity of the limbic system has been considered a possible etiology or mechanism mediating panic disorder. Few human studies have been conducted, but lactate-sensitive patients with panic disorder have been found to have abnormal hemispheric asymmetry of parahippocampal blood flow on PET scans. Also, patients with temporal lobe epileptic foci frequently experience panic-like symptoms; however, only an extremely small minority of panic disorder patients have been found to have abnormal electroencephalograms. Nevertheless, the ictal seizure-like analogy may be useful, for panic may be tantamount to seizure-like neuronal activation in parts of the brain that mediate emotions, whereas true epilepsy may involve locations in the brain mediating movement and consciousness rather than emotions of anxiety and panic (see Figs. 4–19 and 4–20).

Since there are both noradrenergic projections to the hippocampus from the locus coeruleus and serotonergic projections to the hippocampus from the raphe, it is possible that dysregulation of these projections may account for neurophysiological abnormalities hypothesized to occur in panic attacks. Changing the outputs of these monoamine neurotransmitter systems to the hippocampus may also explain the therapeutic actions of various antidepressants that reduce panic attacks (see Figs. 5–26 and 5–54).

## Treatments

Figure 9–5 shows the variety of options for treating panic disorders.

*Serotonin selective reuptake inhibitors.* Many medications originally developed or used in treatment of depression have been found to be effective in treating panic disorder, especially the SSRIs. The documentation of efficacy for panic disorder and of the safety of these agents has now made them first-line treatments for this condition. Since many patients have coexisting depression and panic disorder, SSRIs can treat both conditions in the same patient at the same time. Each of the five SSRIs (fluoxetine, paroxetine, sertraline, fluvoxamine, and citalopram) has advantages and disadvantages for individual patients with panic disorder. However, all SSRIs have been shown to be about equally effective in large-scale studies and to take on average 3 to 8 weeks before benefit may be noticed (about the same time as it takes antidepressants to work). Patients with panic disorder tend to be more sensitive to SSRIs (and indeed to all antidepressants) than are depressed patients, since they can easily develop jitteriness or even short-term worsening of their panic when treatment is initiated. Thus, panic patients usually start at a lower dose than depressed patients. Doses must generally be increased to the same or greater levels as antidepressants over time and as tolerated (see Table 9–9). The five SSRIs are all discussed in detail in Chapter 6.

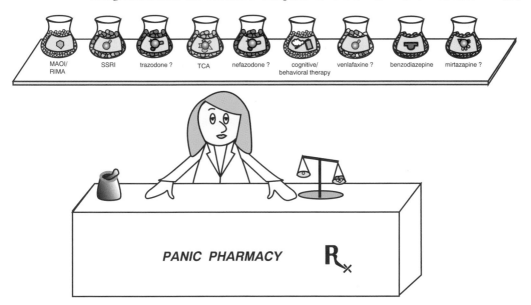

| MAOI/<br>RIMA | SSRI | trazodone ? | TCA | nefazodone ? | cognitive/<br>behavioral therapy | venlafaxine ? | benzodiazepine | mirtazapine ? |

PANIC PHARMACY     R$_x$

FIGURE 9–5. Shown here are the variety of therapeutic options for treating **panic disorder**.

Table 9–9. *SSRI profile for panic/social phobia and PTSD*

Usual starting dose is lower than the starting dose for depression due to activating
  symptoms
Panic and other target symptoms may therefore get worse before they get better
Maintenance doses will be higher than starting doses, and may need to be higher than
  usual antidepressant doses, particularly for paroxetine.
Onset of action is usually 2 to 8 weeks.
Usual response is more than 50% reduction of symptoms, especially in combination with
  other treatments such as benzodiazepines, trazodone, or cognitive behavioral
  psychotherapy.

*Newer antidepressants.* Although the SSRIs are the only antidepressants formally approved for the treatment of panic disorder, recent evidence suggests that several
other antidepressants are promising treatments for panic disorder as well. These
include nefazodone, venlafaxine XR, mirtazapine, and reboxetine. Bupropion, however, does not seem to have apparent antipanic actions. Since the documentation of
efficacy of these newer antidepressants in panic disorder is still emerging, they tend
to be used as second-line therapy after SSRIs fail to improve panic or in patients
who cannot tolerate them.

*Tricyclic antidepressants.* Imipramine and clomipramine have been the most extensively
studied of the tricyclic antidepressants and both have demonstrated efficacy in treating panic disorder. Other tricyclic antidepressants that have shown some evidence
of efficacy include desipramine, doxepin, amitriptyline, and nortriptyline.

The tricyclics have few or no overall advantages compared with SSRIs, although occasionally a patient will respond to a tricyclic and not to an SSRI. The tricyclics have disadvantages that make them second- or third-line treatments for panic disorder, including anticholinergic side effects, orthostatic hypotension, and weight gain (due to actions at receptors discussed in Chapter 6).

*Monoamine Oxidase (MAO) Inhibitors.* The classical irreversible MAO inhibitors are effective in treating panic disorder, with anecdotal observations suggesting that they may be even more effective than imipramine. Clinical experience with reversible inhibitors of MAO A (RIMAs) (see Chapter 6) is also favorable for the treatment of panic disorder. However, the RIMAs may be somewhat less effective than the irreversible MAO inhibitors, but this is not well established. The disadvantages of the MAO inhibitors make them second- or third-line treatments for panic disorder; these include orthostatic hypotension, weight gain, sexual dysfunction, and dietary restrictions (low tyramine diet), with the potential for a tyramine-induced hypertensive crisis. The RIMAs appear safer, with lessened potential for side effects, as discussed in Chapter 6, but also possibly with less efficacy.

*Benzodiazepines.* Benzodiazepines have become adjunctive treatment to antidepressants (particularly SSRIs), especially for long-term treatment when dependence on benzodiazepines can become problematic. The primary advantage to using benzodiazepines is rapid relief from anxiety and panic attacks. As already mentioned, antidepressants have a delayed therapeutic onset. The disadvantages of benzodiazepines include sedation, cognitive clouding, interaction with alcohol, physiological dependence, and the potential for a withdrawal syndrome. Misinformation and stigma about the benzodiazepines can prevent patients from accepting appropriate treatment with these agents and can prevent clinicians from prescribing them.

High-potency benzodiazepines (alprazolam, clonazepam) generally are more effective in panic disorder than low-potency benzodiazepines (diazepam, lorazepam, etc.). Although less research has been done on the low-potency benzodiazepines, it is generally accepted that they frequently result in sedation prior to adequately relieving panic attacks. The reader is referred to the discussion of benzodiazepines in Chapter 8 for a detailed overview of mechanism of action. A critique of the issues of benzodiazepine dependence and appropriate use is given in Chapter 13.

Currently, many physicians adopt a "benzodiazepine-sparing strategy" by using benzodiazepines when necessary but conservatively. That is, benzodiazepines can often be helpful when treatment is initiated or when a rapid-onset therapeutic effect is desired. They can also help improve the short-term tolerability of SSRIs by blocking the jitteriness and exacerbation of panic sometimes observed when initiating treatment with an SSRI or other antidepressant. Benzodiazepines can also be useful to "top up" the patient's treatment on an as-needed basis for sudden and unexpected decompensation or short-term psychosocial stressors. Finally, if a patient is not fully responsive to an antidepressant or combinations of antidepressants, long-term treatment with concomitant benzodiazepines and antidepressants may become necessary to effect full or adequate control of symptoms. Sometimes, once symptoms are suppressed for several months to a year, the benzodiazepine can be slowly discontinued and the patient maintained long-term on the antidepressant alone. The consequences of inadequate treatment of panic disorder can be very severe loss of social and occupational functioning, as well as suicide, and must be weighed as the risk/benefit ratio for benzodiazepine treatment is calculated for each patient individually.

Alprazolam has been researched more extensively than any other benzodiazepine in panic disorder, and is very effective. Because of its short duration of action, it generally must be administered in three to five daily doses. Clonazepam, which has a longer duration of action than alprazolam, has also been investigated in panic disorder. It can generally be administered twice a day. Clonazepam is reported to have less abuse potential than alprazolam and to be easier to taper during discontinuation owing to its longer half-life.

*Cognitive and behavioral psychotherapies.* Cognitive and behavioral psychotherapies are commonly combined in the treatment of panic disorder with or without agoraphobia. Cognitive therapy focuses on identifying the cognitive distortions and modifying them, whereas behavioral therapy specifically attempts to modify a patient's responses, often through exposure to situations or physiologic stimuli that are associated with panic attacks. Behavioral therapy appears to be most effective in treating the phobic avoidance aspect of panic disorder and agoraphobia and does not appear as effective in treating the panic attacks. These treatments have had as high a rate of effectiveness as have the antipanic drugs. Furthermore, for those who are able to complete an adequate period of behavioral treatment, their improvements are perhaps more likely to be sustained after discontinuing treatment than are drug-induced improvements after discontinuation of antipanic drugs.

*Combination therapies.* The term combination therapy can refer either to combinations of two drugs or to combinations of antipanic drugs with cognitive-behavioral psychotherapy (Fig. 9–6). Combining two drugs for the treatment of panic disorder remains an underdeveloped approach, since few studies have been made comparing single-mode and combination therapy. However, as in the treatment of depression (discussed extensively in Chapter 7), common clinical practice for treating many panic disorder patients is indeed the artful choosing of combinations of available treatments. Tailoring a treatment program to the individual patient is becoming the state of the art, although such combinations are generally inadequately investigated in controlled clinical trials. Figure 9–6 summarizes various options for combination treatments of panic disorder.

DRUG COMBINATIONS    Probably the most common combination treatment is concomitant use of an SSRI and a benzodiazepine, especially on initiation of treatment (Fig. 9–6). The benzodiazepines (especially alprazolam and clonazepam) not only appear to act synergistically to increase the onset of therapeutic action and perhaps even boost the efficacy of SSRIs, but they also appear to block the anxiogenic actions of the SSRIs and lead to better tolerability as well as the ability to attain therapeutic dosing levels for the SSRIs. Sometimes sedative-hypnotics such as zaleplon or zolpidem are required in addition to an SSRI, especially on initiation of SSRI treatment.

Some of the same augmentation strategies discussed in detail in Chapter 7 for the treatment of depression, mentioned above for the treatment of OCD, can also be applied to the treatment of panic disorder. Thus, adding the 5HT2A antagonist trazodone to an SSRI can boost the actions of an SSRI, as possibly also could the

# Panic Combos

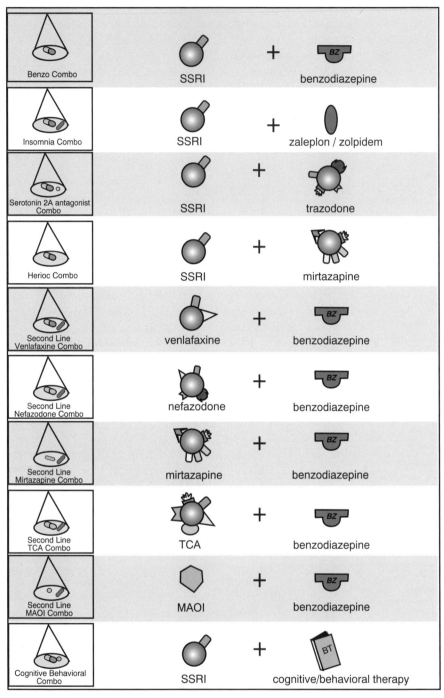

FIGURE 9–6. Various treatments can be given in combination for panic disorder (i.e., **panic combos**). The basis of all many combination treatments is a serotonin selective reuptake inhibitor (SSRI). Other antidepressants such as venlafaxine, nefazodone, mirtazapine, tricyclic antidepressants, and monoamine oxidase inhibitors can all have antipanic actions, although they are second-line treatments, as are the benzodiazepines. On the other hand, benzodiazepines are often added to SSRIs, particularly at the initiation of an SSRI and intermittently when there is breakthrough panic. Cognitive and behavioral psychotherapies can also be added to any of these drug treatments.

combination of mirtazapine with an SSRI (heroic combo in Fig. 9–6). Other medication combinations include some of the newer antidepressants whose efficacy in panic is being documented now (including venlafaxine, nefazodone, and mirtazapine) with a benzodiazepine (Fig. 9–6). Even tricyclic antidepressants and MAO inhibitors have a role in treating panic disorder, especially when other antidepressants or combination fail and possibly in combination with a benzodiazepine (Fig. 9–6).

COGNITIVE-BEHAVIORAL PSYCHOTHERAPY COMBINATIONS WITH ANTIPANIC DRUGS    Virtually any antipanic agent can be combined with cognitive-behavioral therapy in well selected patients. Many clinicians consider some patients to be so anxious or depressed or disabled initially that they are unable to participate in or receive much benefit from psychotherapy, so these patients are sometimes excluded from psychotherapy until their symptoms improve somewhat on medication. Other therapists may believe that benzodiazepines interfere significantly in cognitive-behavioral therapy, since a certain amount of anxiety must be present for behavioral therapy to be effective. Until conclusive data are reported, there is no contraindication for using combination therapy, and there may be additional benefit. Nevertheless, the combination of drugs and behavioral therapy must be individualized for the case at hand.

*Relapse after medication discontinuation.* Relapse rates after discontinuation of antidepressants in the treatment of major depressive disorder have been much more thoroughly studied than have relapse rates of panic disorder in patients discontinued from antipanic agents. Although panic disorder can frequently be in remission within 6 months of beginning treatment, on the basis of existing studies, the relapse rate is apparently very high once treatment is stopped, even for patients who have had complete resolution of symptoms. When a patient has been asymptomatic on medication for 6 to 12 months, it may be reasonable to have a trial off medication. If medication is discontinued, this should be done slowly, and the benzodiazepines in particular should be tapered over a period of at least 2 months and possibly as long as 6 months. More commonly now, panic disorder is considered a chronic illness, which requires maintenance therapy. Investigations are underway to provide much clearer guidelines for chronic therapy in panic disorder, but they tend to mirror the guidelines developed for the long-term maintenance treatment of depression, discussed in Chapter 5.

*New prospects*

NOVEL ANTIDEPRESSANTS    Given the importance of SSRIs in the treatment of panic disorder, other, newer antidepressants are developing an efficacy portfolio for panic disorder (and other anxiety disorders) as well. Thus, venlafaxine XR, nefazodone, and mirtazapine hold promise for the treatment of panic disorder. One early study also suggests that the new antidepressant reboxetine may be effective in panic disorder.

NOVEL SEROTONERGIC AGENTS    The same agents in testing as antidepressants and discussed in the section "Other antidepressants in clinical trials," in Chapter 7, may also be promising antipanic agents. Such compounds tend to be tested first as antidepressants and then for anxiety disorders such as panic disorder. This includes agents that are 5HT1A antagonists, 5HT1D antagonists, neurokinin antagonists, and other neuropeptide antagonists.

PARTIAL AGONISTS AT BENZODIAZEPINE RECEPTORS  As discussed for general anxiolytic agents in Chapter 8, the partial benzodiazepine agonists could be a theoretical advance over the marketed benzodiazepines. Partial agonists should have the same efficacy as full agonists but less potential for sedation, dependence, and withdrawal effects.

NONBENZODIAZEPINE LIGANDS AT BENZODIAZEPINE SITES  This is a variation on the theme of partial benzodiazepine agonists, as these agents act at the same or similar site as benzodiazepines but are not structurally related to them. Thus, the pharmacology of nonbenzodiazepines is that of a partial agonist, but their chemistry is different from that of a benzodiazepine. This is similar to the approach that novel sedative-hypnotics such as zaleplon and zolpidem have taken, and perhaps a less sedating nonbenzodiazepine partial agonist could hold promise for the treatment of panic disorder.

REVERSIBLE INHIBITORS OF MONOAMINE OXIDASE A  Clinical experience with RIMAs in those countries where these agents are approved for marketing or testing suggests potential utility as antipanic agents. Further research is required to determine the relative advantages and relative efficacy of these compounds as compared with available antipanic agents.

## Phobic Disorders: Specific Phobias, Social Phobia, and Agoraphobia

### Clinical Description of Phobias and Phobic Disorders

Phobia is fear, and there are several disorders that are classified as phobias. Here we will briefly discuss agoraphobia, specific phobias, and social phobia, also known as social anxiety disorder.

*Agoraphobia* literally translated means "fear of the marketplace," or essentially fear of going out from one's home. However, the diagnosis of agoraphobia more precisely refers to anxiety about being in all the different situations from which escape might be difficult or in which help may not be available in the event of having a panic attack. This anxiety leads to avoidance of such situations (called phobic avoidance), often to the extent that the patient becomes housebound. Agoraphobia is usually seen in conjunction with panic disorder, but it can be a separate disorder when it is diagnosed as "agoraphobia without history of panic disorder." About one-third of panic disorder patients also have agoraphobia. Patients who have panic disorder accompanied by agoraphobia appear to have a more severe and complicated course than patients with panic disorder alone.

*Specific phobias* used to be called "simple phobias." They are excessive and unreasonable fears of specific objects or situations, such as flying in an airplane, heights, animals, seeing an injection, or seeing blood. In specific phobias, exposure to the feared situation or object causes an immediate anxiety response or even a full-blown panic attack. In *social phobia*, on the other hand, there is an intense, irrational fear of social or performance situations in which the patient is exposed to unfamiliar people or to possible scrutiny by others and anticipates humiliation or embarrassment. Some investigators consider social phobia to be at one end of a spectrum ranging from shyness to avoidant personality disorder to generalized social phobia.

There is both a generalized and a more discrete type of social phobia. In the generalized type, the patient fears practically all social situations in which evaluation and scrutiny are possible. It is significantly more common than the discrete type, in which the individual fears a very specific social situation, usually of public speaking or public performance. Generalized social phobia is also more severe and disabling than discrete social phobia.

Estimates of the incidence of social phobia range from 1.3% to more than 10% of the population, and twice as many women as men are affected. First-degree relatives of social phobics have a greater prevalence of social phobia than the general population. Social phobia usually has an early onset, between 11 and 15 years of age, and has a chronic, unremitting course, with significant lifelong disability. Children as young as 21 months who exhibit behavioral inhibition (intense anxiety and fear when faced with new social situations) have an increased prevalence of childhood anxiety phenomena, including social phobia-like symptoms as well as agoraphobia-like symptoms by the time they are 8 years old.

Two-thirds of social phobics are single, divorced, or widowed. More than half of all patients with social phobia never completed high school. In fact, one-fifth of social phobics are unable to work and must therefore collect welfare or disability benefits.

The most common fears among social phobics are speaking in front of a small group of people, speaking to strangers, meeting new people, eating in public, or being stared at. These fears are different from the fears of people with panic disorder, who mostly wish to avoid driving, shopping, being in crowds, or using elevators. More than half of social phobics will suffer at some point in their lifetime from a specific phobia as well.

*Social phobia* and *specific phobia* can be distinguished from panic disorder by the fact that panic attacks, if present, are in response to specific situations and do not occur unexpectedly. Also, the fear in social phobia is a fear of humiliation, shame, or embarrassment instead of a fear of having a panic attack. Somatic symptoms differ between panic disorder patients with agoraphobia and with social phobia, with blushing more common among social phobics. Difficulty in breathing, dizziness, and syncope occur more frequently among the agoraphobics. The DSM-IV diagnostic criteria for social phobia are given in Table 9–10.

## Biological Basis of Social Phobia

The neurobiology of social phobia remains obscure. A state of noradrenergic over-activity in social phobia is suggested by the symptoms of tremor, tachycardia, and blushing (see Fig. 9–3). Because of these observations, in fact, the first somewhat effective treatments for social phobia were beta adrenergic blockers. Studies of neurotransmitters and neuroimaging are still not able to suggest a biological basis for social phobia, but numerous such studies are in progress.

Table 9–10. *DSM IV diagnostic criteria for social phobia*

A.  Social phobia is characterized by a marked and persistent fear of one or more social or performance situations in which the person is exposed to unfamiliar people or to possible scrutiny by others. The individual fears that he or she will act in a way (or show anxiety symptoms) that will be humiliating or embarrassing. *Note*: In children there must be evidence of the capacity for age-appropriate social relationships with familiar people, and the anxiety must occur in peer settings, not just in interactions with adults.

B.  Exposure to the feared social situation almost invariably provokes anxiety, which may take the form of a situationally bound or situationally predisposed panic attack. *Note*: In children the anxiety may be expressed by crying, tantrums, freezing, or shrinking from social situations with unfamiliar people.

C.  The person recognizes that the fear is excessive or unreasonable. *Note*: In children this feature may be absent.

D.  The feared social or performance situations are voided or else are endured with intense anxiety or distress.

E   The avoidance, anxious anticipation, or distress in the feared social or performance situation interferes significantly with the person's normal routine, with occupational or academic functioning, or with social activities or relationships, or there is marked distress about having the phobia.

F.  In individuals under age 18, the duration is at least 6 months.

G.  The fear of avoidance is not due to the direct physiological effects of a substance or a general medical condition and is not better accounted for by another mental disorder (panic disorder with or without agoraphobia, separation anxiety disorder, body dysmorphic disorder, a pervasive developmental disorder, or schizoid personality disorder).

H.  If a general medical condition or another mental disorder is present, the fear in criterion A is unrelated to it, that is, the fear is not of stuttering, trembling in Parkinson's disease, or exhibiting abnormal eating behavior in anorexia or bulimia nervosa.

## Drug Treatments for Social Phobia

The earliest and unfortunately still one of the commonest treatments of social phobia is self-medication with alcohol. The behaviorally disinhibiting actions of alcohol allow many social phobics to engage in social contacts that would otherwise be impossible. Legitimate therapeutic drugs for social phobia are now being discovered at a fast pace (Fig. 9–7). In fact, one of the SSRIs (paroxetine) already has been formally approved for use in the treatment of social phobia, and several other SSRIs and antidepressants are rapidly accumulating evidence of their efficacies in this condition as well. Specifically, studies of all five SSRIs (paroxetine, fluvoxamine, fluoxetine, sertraline, and citalopram) have indicated their efficacy in social phobia. Currently, SSRIs are considered first-line treatments for social phobia.

In addition, several of the newer antidepressants also appear to be effective in social phobia, including venlafaxine, nefazodone, and perhaps others. Although there

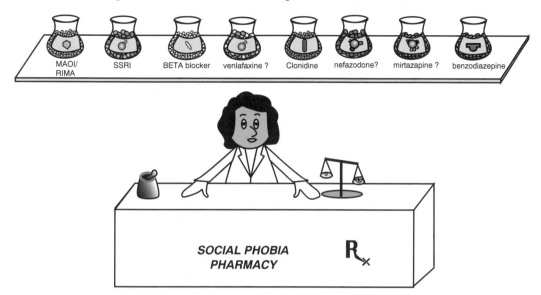

FIGURE 9–7. Shown here are the variety of therapeutic options for treating **social phobia**. Combination treatments are similar to those for panic disorder, but there is less experience with them and less documentation of how they work uniquely for patients with social phobia.

is evidence of efficacy for both the irreversible and the reversible MAO inhibitors in social phobia, there is far less evidence for the usefulness of tricyclic antidepressants. Today, MAO inhibitors are second- or third-line treatments for patients resistant to treatment with SSRIs or other newer antidepressants.

Benzodiazepines, especially clonazepam, appear efficacious in social phobia, although there have been relatively few trials and small numbers of patients studied. Beta blockers may work in patients with discrete phobias, such as fear of public speaking, but are rather underwhelming as treatments for the generalized type of social phobia. Buspirone monotherapy and clonidine monotherapy have also been investigated, with no clear consensus on their therapeutic usefulness in social phobia. Augmentation strategies for the treatment of social phobia resistant to the various monotherapies mentioned here are also in their infancy and tend to follow the strategies used for severe cases of treatment-resistant depression when monotherapies are ineffective.

### Psychotherapeutic Treatments

Psychotherapeutic treatments for social phobia are also in their relative infancy. Relaxation techniques, while sometimes advocated as part of anxiety management, are difficult to apply to patients with social phobia. Exposure therapy, on the other hand, can be successfully implemented if the anxiety-provoking stimuli are categorized into common themes and if the patient practices increasing the frequency of exposure to these stimuli throughout the day. Major cognitive distortions are maintained by social phobics during social situations. For example, they overestimate the scrutiny of others, attribute critical thoughts to others, underestimate their own social skills, and fear the responses of others to their anxiety. For such patients, cognitive restructuring can be helpful. The task is to challenge and reorganize unrealistic, emotional, and catastrophic thoughts. Cognitive and behavioral techniques in a group setting may be the best psychosocial interventions for social phobic patients, especially when combined with drug therapy.

### New prospects

As social phobia is only recently becoming better recognized and researched, better documentation for the various treatments mentioned above is now evolving. This applies especially to the five SSRIs and to some of the newer antidepressants such as venlafaxine XR. Guidelines are emerging for the use of high-potency benzodiazepines, MAO inhibitors, RIMAs, beta blockers, and various drugs in combination as second- or third-line treatments for social phobia.

Under investigation at the present time is virtually every compound being studied in depression and in panic disorder. Perhaps new and effective treatments for social phobia will arise from this same pool of compounds.

## Posttraumatic Stress Disorder

### Clinical Description

Posttraumatic stress disorder (PTSD) is another anxiety disorder that can be characterized by attacks of anxiety or panic, but it is notably different from panic disorder or social phobia in that the initial anxiety or panic attack is in response to a real threat (being raped, for example) and subsequent attacks are usually linked to memories, thoughts, or flashbacks of the original trauma. The lifetime incidence of PTSD is about 1%. Patients have disturbed sleep and frequent sleep complaints. Comorbidities with other psychiatric disorders, especially depression and drug and alcohol abuse, are the rule rather than the exception. The DSM-IV diagnostic criteria are given in Table 9–11.

### Biological Basis

The biology of PTSD is only now beginning to be investigated. Some evidence suggests an overactive noradrenergic nervous system, with an exaggerated startle response and autonomic hyperarousal. Because of associated memory problems, some investigators are focusing on the potential role of the hippocampus. Early findings suggest that there may be a reduction in hippocampal volume, perhaps due to an abnormal stress response similar to that hypothesized for depression (see Figures 5–63 and 5–64 and discussion on brain derived neurotrophic factor (BDNF)).

### Treatments

Drug treatments for PTSD (Fig. 9–8) have until recently focused upon treating the associated comorbidities, especially depression. Because of the high degree of concomitant drug and alcohol abuse, benzodiazepines are usually best avoided.

Just as has been the case for every other anxiety disorder subtype, the SSRIs appear to be the treatment of choice for PTSD (Fig. 9–8). Numerous trials are in

Table 9–11. *DSM IV diagnostic criteria for posttraumatic stress disorder*

A. The person has been exposed to a traumatic event in which both of the following were present:
  1. The person experienced, witnessed, or was confronted with an event or events that involved actual or threatened death or serious injury or a threat to the physical integrity of others.
  2. The person's response involved intense fear, helplessness, or horror. *Note*: In children this may be expressed instead by disorganized or agitated behavior.

B. The traumatic event is persistently reexperienced in one or more of the following ways:
  1. Recurrent and intrusive distressing recollections of the event including images, thoughts, or perceptions. *Note*: In young children, repetitive play may occur in which themes or aspects of the trauma are expressed.
  2. Recurrent distressing dreams of the event. *Note*: In children there may be frightening dreams without recognizing conflict.
  3. Acting or feeling as if the traumatic event were recurring (includes a sense of reliving the experience, illusions, hallucinations, and dissociative flashback episodes, including those that occur on awakening or when intoxicated). *Note*: In children trauma-specific reenactment may occur.
  4. Intense psychological distress at exposure to internal or external cues that symbolize or resemble an aspect of the traumatic event.

C. Persistent avoidance of stimuli associated with the trauma and numbing of general responsiveness (not present before the trauma), as indicated by three or more of the following:
  1. Efforts to avoid thoughts, feelings, or conversations associated with the trauma
  2. Efforts to avoid activities, places, or people that arouse recollection of the trauma
  3. Inability to recall an important aspect of the trauma
  4. Markedly diminished interest or participation in significant activities
  5. Feeling of detachment or estrangement from others
  6. Restricted range of effect (e.g., unable to have loving feelings)
  7. Sense of a foreshortened future (e.g., does not expect to have a career, marriage, children, or normal life span)

D. Persistent symptoms of increased arousal, not present before the trauma, as indicated by two or more of the following:
  1. Difficulty in falling or staying asleep
  2. Irritability or outbursts of anger
  3. Difficulty in concentrating
  4. Hypervigilance
  5. Exaggerated startle response

E. Duration of the disturbance (symptoms in B, C, D) is more than 1 month.

F. The disturbance causes clinically significant distress or impairment in social, occupational, or other important areas of functioning.

progress with these agents and with several of the newer antidepressants as well, including nefazodone. Although there is some evidence that tricyclic antidepressants and MAO inhibitors may have some efficacy in PTSD, they are relegated to second- or third-line use. Anecdotes suggest that beta blockers and mood stabilizers may be useful for some patients. In the future, as investigations proceed at a fast pace, several antidepressants are likely to emerge as first-line treatments for PTSD.

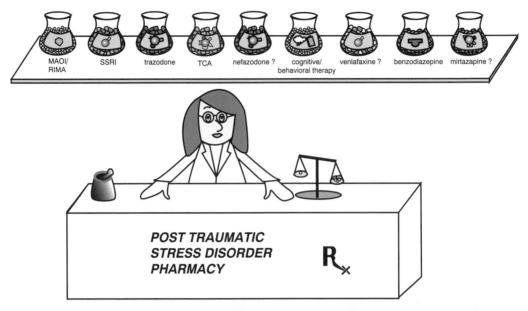

FIGURE 9–8. Shown here are the variety of therapeutic options for treating **posttraumatic stress disorder** (PTSD). Combination treatments for PTSD are very poorly documented but very frequently used. The PTSD combinations are similar to those for depression and for panic disorder.

## Summary

In this chapter we have given clinical descriptions and have also explored the biological basis and a variety of treatments for numerous anxiety disorder subtypes, including obsessive-compulsive disorder, panic disorder, social phobia, and posttraumatic stress disorder.

*Obsessive-compulsive disorder* may be linked to abnormalities of the neurotransmitters serotonin and dopamine. The neuroanatomical basis of OCD may be related to dysfunction in the basal ganglia. The hallmark of treatment for OCD is use of SSRIs plus the tricyclic antidepressant clomipramine. *Panic disorder* is characterized by unexpected panic attacks, possibly linked to abnormalities in the neurotransmitters norepinephrine and GABA, in the sensitivity of benzodiazepine receptors, or even in the regulation of respiration. Drug treatments include SSRIs, several of the newer antidepressants, high-potency benzodiazepines, many tricyclic antidepressants, and MAO inhibitors.

*Social phobia* is characterized by expected panic attacks, that is, attacks are expected in situations of public scrutiny because of the fear the patient has of that situation. The biological basis of social phobia is obscure. Treatment is with SSRIs and perhaps other antidepressants, benzodiazepines, and sometimes beta blockers. *Posttraumatic stress disorder* is a reaction to traumatic events, is associated with a hyperaroused autonomic nervous system, and appears to respond to SSRI treatment.

# PSYCHOSIS AND SCHIZOPHRENIA

*Psychosis* is a difficult term to define and is frequently misused, not only in the newspapers and movies and on television, but unfortunately among mental health professionals as well. Stigma and fear surround the concept of psychosis and the

Table 10–1. *Disorders in which psychosis is a defining feature*

| |
| --- |
| Schizophrenia |
| Substance-induced (i.e., drug-induced) psychotic disorders |
| Schizophreniform disorder |
| Schizoaffective disorder |
| Delusional disorder |
| Brief psychotic disorder |
| Shared psychotic disorder |
| Psychotic disorder due to a general medical condition |

average citizen worries about long-standing myths of "mental illness," including "psychotic killers," "psychotic rage," and the equivalence of "psychotic" with the pejorative term "crazy."

We have already discussed public misconceptions about mental illness in Chapter 5 on depression (Table 5–1). There is perhaps no area of psychiatry where misconceptions are greater than in the area of psychotic illnesses. The reader is well served to develop an expertise on the facts about the diagnosis and treatment of psychotic illnesses in order to dispel unwarranted beliefs and to help destigmatize this devastating group of illnesses. This chapter is not intended to list the diagnostic criteria for all the different mental disorders in which psychosis is either a defining feature or an associated feature. The reader is referred to standard reference sources (DSM-IV and ICD-10) for that information. Although schizophrenia will be emphasized here, we will approach psychosis as a syndrome associated with a variety of illnesses which are all targets for antipsychotic drug treatment.

## Clinical Description of Psychosis

Psychosis is a syndrome, which is a mixture of symptoms that can be associated with many different psychiatric disorders but is not a specific disorder itself in diagnostic schemes such as DSM-IV or ICD-10. At a minimum, psychosis means delusions and hallucinations. It generally also includes symptoms such as disorganized speech, disorganized behavior, and gross distortions of reality testing.

Therefore, psychosis can be considered to be a set of symptoms in which a person's mental capacity, affective response, and capacity to recognize reality, communicate, and relate to others are impaired. Psychotic disorders have psychotic symptoms as their defining features, but there are other disorders in which psychotic symptoms may be present but are not necessary for the diagnosis.

Those *disorders that require the presence of psychosis* (Table 10–1) as a *defining* feature of the diagnosis include schizophrenia, substance-induced (i.e., drug-induced) psychotic disorder, schizophreniform disorder, schizoaffective disorder, delusional disorder, brief psychotic disorder, shared psychotic disorder, and psychotic disorder due to a general medical condition. *Disorders that may or may not have psychotic symptoms* (Table 10–2) as an *associated* feature include mania and depression as well as several cognitive disorders such as Alzheimer's dementia.

Psychosis itself can be paranoid, disorganized-excited, or depressive. Perceptual distortions and motor disturbances can be associated with any type of psychosis.

Table 10–2. *Disorders in which*
*psychosis is an associated feature*

Mania
Depression
Cognitive disorders
Alzheimer dementia

*Perceptual distortions* include being distressed by hallucinatory voices; hearing voices that accuse, blame, or threaten punishment; seeing visions; reporting hallucinations of touch, taste, or odor; or reporting that familiar things and people seem changed. *Motor disturbances* are peculiar, rigid postures; overt signs of tension; inappropriate grins or giggles; peculiar repetitive gestures; talking, muttering, or mumbling to oneself; or glancing around as if hearing voices.

## Paranoid Psychosis

In paranoid psychosis, the patient has paranoid projections, hostile belligerence, and grandiose expansiveness. *Paranoid projection* includes preoccupation with delusional beliefs; believing that people are talking about oneself; believing one is being persecuted or conspired against; and believing people or external forces control one's actions. *Hostile belligerence* is verbal expression of feelings of hostility; expressing an attitude of disdain; manifesting a hostile, sullen attitude; manifesting irritability and grouchiness; tending to blame others for problems; expressing feelings of resentment; and complaining and finding fault, as well as expressing suspicion of people. *Grandiose expansiveness* is exhibiting an attitude of superiority; hearing voices that praise and extol; and believing one has unusual powers, is a well-known personality, or has a divine mission.

## Disorganized-Excited Psychosis

In a disorganized-excited psychosis, there is conceptual disorganization, disorientation, and excitement. *Conceptual disorganization* can be characterized by giving answers that are irrelevant or incoherent; drifting off the subject; using neologisms; or repeating certain words or phrases. *Disorientation* is not knowing where one is, the season of the year, the calendar year, or one's own age. *Excitement* is expressing feelings without restraint; manifesting hurried speech; exhibiting an elevated mood or an attitude of superiority; dramatizing oneself or one's symptoms; manifesting loud and boisterous speech; exhibiting overactivity or restlessness; and exhibiting excess of speech.

## Depressive Psychosis

Depressive psychosis is characterized by retardation, apathy, and anxious self-punishment and blame. *Retardation and apathy* are manifested by slowed speech; indifference to one's future; fixed facial expression; slowed movements; deficiencies in recent memory; blocking in speech; apathy toward oneself or one's problems; slovenly appearance; low or whispered speech; and failure to answer questions. *Anxious self-punishment and blame* involve the tendency to blame or condemn oneself; anxiety about specific matters; apprehensiveness regarding vague future events; an attitude of self-deprecation; manifesting a depressed mood; expressing feelings of guilt and remorse; preoccupation with suicidal thoughts, unwanted ideas, and specific fears; and feeling unworthy or sinful.

This discussion of clusters of psychotic symptoms does not constitute diagnostic criteria for any psychotic disorder. It is given merely as a description of several types of symptoms in psychosis to give the reader an overview of the nature of behavioral disturbances associated with the various psychotic illnesses.

## Five Symptom Dimensions in Schizophrenia

Although schizophrenia is the commonest and best known psychotic illness, it is not synonymous with psychosis but is just one of many causes of psychosis. Schizophrenia affects 1% of the population, and in the United States there are over 300,000 acute schizophrenic episodes annually. Between 25 and 50% of schizophrenia patients attempt suicide, and 10% eventually succeed, contributing to a mortality rate eight times as high as that of the general population. In the United States over 20% of all Social Security benefit days are used for the care of schizophrenic patients. The direct and indirect costs of schizophrenia in the United States alone are estimated to be in the tens of billions of dollars every year.

Schizophrenia by definition is a disturbance that must last for six months or longer, including at least one month of delusions, hallucinations, disorganized speech, grossly disorganized or catatonic behavior, or negative symptoms. *Delusions* usually involve a misinterpretation of perceptions or experiences. The most common type of delusion in schizophrenia is persecutory, but the delusions may include a variety of other themes, including referential (i.e., erroneously thinking that something refers to oneself), somatic, religious, or grandiose. *Hallucinations* may occur in any sensory modality (e.g., auditory, visual, olfactory, gustatory, and tactile), but auditory hallucinations are by far the most common and characteristic hallucinations in schizophrenia.

Although not recognized formally as part of the diagnostic criteria for schizophrenia, numerous studies subcategorize the symptoms of this illness (as well as symptoms of some other disorders) into five dimensions: positive symptoms, negative symptoms, cognitive symptoms, aggressive/hostile symptoms, and depressive/anxious symptoms (Fig. 10–1). Several illnesses other than schizophrenia share these symptoms dimensions as well (Figs. 10–2 to 10–6).

### Positive Symptoms

Positive symptoms seem to reflect an *excess* of normal functions (Table 10–3) and typically include delusions and hallucinations; they may also include distortions or exaggerations in language and communication (disorganized speech), as well as in behavioral monitoring (grossly disorganized or catatonic or agitated behavior).

Disorders in addition to schizophrenia that can have positive symptoms include bipolar disorder, schizoaffective disorder, psychotic depression, Alzheimer's disease

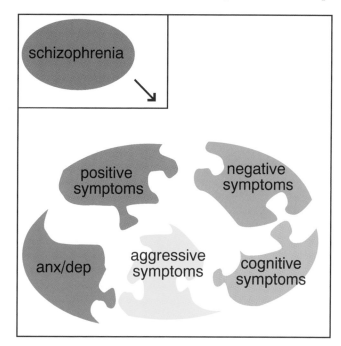

FIGURE 10–1. The **five symptom dimensions** of schizophrenia include not only positive and negative symptoms but also cognitive symptoms, aggressive/hostile symptoms, and depressive and anxious symptoms (anx/dep).

and other organic dementias, childhood psychotic illnesses, drug induced psychoses, and others (Fig. 10–2).

## Negative Symptoms

Negative symptoms (Table 10–4) include at least five types of symptoms (all starting with the letter *a*): (1) *affective flattening*, consisting of restrictions in the range and intensity of emotional expression; (2) *alogia*, consisting of restrictions in the fluency and productivity of thought and speech; (3) *avolition*, consisting of restrictions in the initiation of goal-directed behavior; (4) *anhedonia*, that is, lack of pleasure; and (5) *attentional impairment*.

Negative symptoms commonly are considered a *reduction* in normal functions in schizophrenia, such as blunted affect, emotional withdrawal, poor rapport, passivity, and apathetic social withdrawal. Difficulty in abstract thinking, stereotyped thinking, and lack of spontaneity are associated with long periods of hospitalization and poor social functioning.

Negative symptoms in schizophrenia can be either primary or secondary (Fig. 10–3). Primary negative symptoms are considered to be those that are core to primary deficits of schizophrenia itself. Other core deficits of schizophrenia that may manifest themselves as negative symptoms may be those associated with or thought to be secondary to the positive symptoms of psychosis. Other negative symptoms are considered to be secondary to extrapyramidal symptoms (EPS), especially those

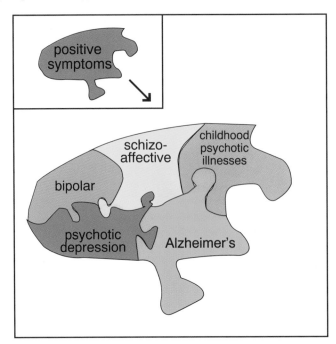

FIGURE 10–2. **Positive symptoms** are associated not just with schizophrenia, but also with bipolar disorder, schizoaffective disorder, childhood psychotic illnesses, psychotic depression, Alzheimer's disease, and other disorders as well.

caused by antipsychotic drugs. Negative symptoms can also be secondary to depressive symptoms or to environmental deprivation.

### Cognitive Symptoms

Cognitive symptoms of schizophrenia and other illnesses of which psychosis may be an associated feature can overlap with negative symptoms. They include specifically the thought disorder of schizophrenia and the sometimes odd use of language, including incoherence, loose associations, and neologisms. Impaired attention and impaired information processing are other specific cognitive impairments associated with schizophrenia. In fact, the most common and the most severe of the cognitive impairments in schizophrenia can include impaired verbal fluency (ability to produce spontaneous speech), problems with serial learning (of a list of items or a sequence of events), and impairment in vigilance for executive functioning (problems with sustaining and focusing attention, concentrating, prioritizing, and modulating behavior based on social cues).

Schizophrenia is certainly not the only disorder with such impairments in cognition. Autism, poststroke dementia, Alzheimer's disease, and many other organic dementias (parkinsonian/Lewy body dementia, frontotemporal/Pick's dementia, etc.) are also associated with some cognitive dysfunctions similar to those seen in schizophrenia (Fig. 10–4).

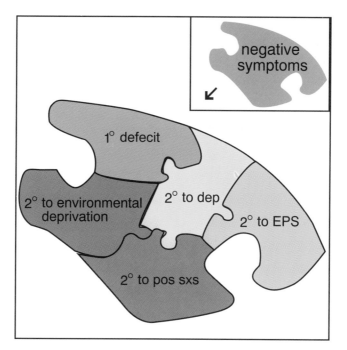

FIGURE 10–3. **Negative symptoms** in schizophrenia can either be a primary deficit of the illness (1° deficit) or secondary to depression (2° to dep), secondary to extrapyramidal symptoms (2° to EPS), secondary to environmental deprivation, or even secondary to positive symptoms (2° to pos sxs) in schizophrenia.

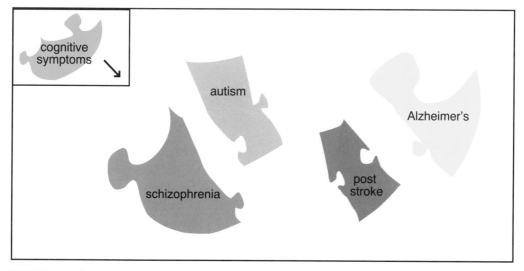

FIGURE 10–4. **Cognitive symptoms** are not just associated with schizophrenia, but also with several other disorders, including autism, Alzheimer's disease, and conditions following cerebrovascular accidents (poststroke).

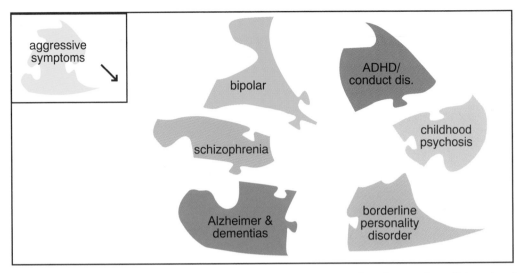

FIGURE 10–5. **Aggressive symptoms and hostility** are associated with several conditions in addition to schizophrenia, including bipolar disorder, attention deficit hyperactivity disorder (ADHD) and conduct disorder (conduct dis.), childhood psychosis, Alzheimer's and other dementias, and borderline personality disorder, among others.

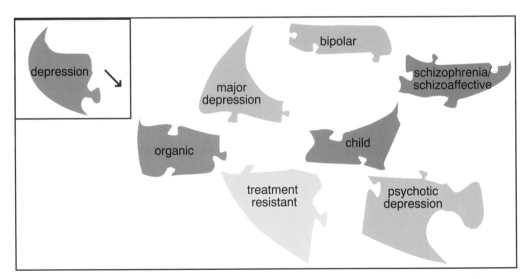

FIGURE 10–6. **Depressive and anxious symptoms** are not only a hallmark of major depressive disorder but are frequently associated with other psychiatric disorders, including bipolar disorder, schizophrenia, and schizoaffective disorder; with organic causes of depression, such as substance abuse; with childhood mood disorders (child); with psychotic forms of depression; and with mood and psychotic disorders resistant to treatment with drugs (treatment-resistant), among others.

372

Table 10–3. *Positive symptoms of psychosis*

Delusions
Hallucinations
Distortions or exaggerations in language and communication
Disorganized speech
Disorganized behavior
Catatonic behavior
Agitation

Table 10–4. *Negative symptoms of psychosis*

Blunted affect
Emotional withdrawal
Poor rapport
Passivity
Apathetic social withdrawal
Difficulty in abstract thinking
Lack of spontaneity
Stereotyped thinking
Alogia: restrictions in fluency and productivity of thought and speech
Avolition: restrictions in initiation of goal-directed behavior
Anhedonia: lack of pleasure
Attentional impairment

### Aggressive and Hostile Symptoms

Aggressive and hostile symptoms can overlap with positive symptoms but specifically emphasize problems in impulse control. They include overt hostility, such as verbal or physical abusiveness or even assault. Such symptoms also include self-injurious behaviors, including suicide and arson or other property damage. Other types of impulsiveness, such as sexual acting out, are also in this category of aggressive and hostile symptoms.

Although aggressive symptoms are common in schizophrenia, they are far from unique to this condition. Thus, these same symptoms are frequently associated with bipolar disorder, childhood psychosis, borderline personality disorder, drug abuse, Alzheimer and other dementias, attention deficit hyperactivity disorder, conduct disorders in children, and many others (Fig. 10–5).

### Depressive and Anxious Symptoms

Depressive and anxious symptoms are frequently associated with schizophrenia, but this does not necessarily mean that they fulfill the diagnostic criteria for a comorbid anxiety or affective disorder. Nevertheless, depressed mood, anxious mood, guilt, tension, irritability, and worry frequently accompany schizophrenia. These various symptoms are also prominent features of major depressive disorder, psychotic depression, bipolar disorder, schizoaffective disorder, organic dementias, and childhood psychotic disorders, among others, and particularly of treatment-resistant cases of depression, bipolar disorder, and schizophrenia (Fig. 10–6).

## Four Key Dopamine Pathways and the Biological Basis of Schizophrenia

The biological basis of schizophrenia remains unknown. However, the monoamine neurotransmitter dopamine has played a key role in hypotheses about certain aspects of the five dimensions of symptoms in schizophrenia, discussed above.

Four well-defined dopamine pathways in the brain are shown in Figure 10–7. They include the mesolimbic dopamine pathway, the mesocortical dopamine pathway, the nigrostriatal dopamine pathway, and the tuberoinfundibular dopamine pathway.

### Mesolimbic Dopamine Pathway and the Dopamine Hypothesis of the Positive Symptoms of Psychosis

The *mesolimbic dopamine pathway* projects from dopaminergic cell bodies in the ventral tegmental area of the brainstem to axon terminals in limbic areas of the brain, such as the nucleus accumbens (Fig. 10–8). This pathway is thought to have an important role in emotional behaviors, especially auditory hallucinations but also delusions and thought disorder (Fig. 10–9).

For more than 25 years, it has been observed that diseases or drugs that increase dopamine will enhance or produce positive psychotic symptoms, whereas drugs that decrease dopamine will decrease or stop positive symptoms. For example, stimulant drugs such as amphetamine and cocaine release dopamine and if given repetitively, can cause a paranoid psychosis virtually indistinguishable from schizophrenia. Stimulant drugs are discussed in Chapters 12 (cognitive enhancers) and 13 (drug abuse). Also, all known antipsychotic drugs capable of treating positive psychotic symptoms are blockers of dopamine receptors, particularly D2 dopamine receptors. Antipsychotic drugs are discussed in Chapter 11. These observations have been formulated into a theory of psychosis sometimes referred to as the dopamine hypothesis of schizophrenia. Perhaps a more precise modern designation is the *mesolimbic dopamine hypothesis of positive psychotic symptoms*, since it is believed that it is hyperactivity specifically in this particular dopamine pathway that mediates the positive symptoms of psychosis (Fig. 10–9). Hyperactivity of the mesolimbic dopamine pathway hypothetically accounts for positive psychotic symptoms whether those symptoms are part of the illness of schizophrenia or of drug-induced psychosis, or whether positive psychotic symptoms accompany mania, depression, or dementia. Hyperactivity of mesolimbic dopamine neurons may also play a role in aggressive and hostile symptoms in schizophrenia and related illnesses, especially if serotonergic control of dopamine is aberrant in patients who lack impulse control.

### Mesocortical Dopamine Pathway

A pathway related to the mesolimbic dopamine pathway is the *mesocortical dopamine pathway* (Fig. 10–10). Its cell bodies arise in the ventral tegmental area of the brainstem, near the cell bodies for the dopamine neurons of the mesolimbic dopa-

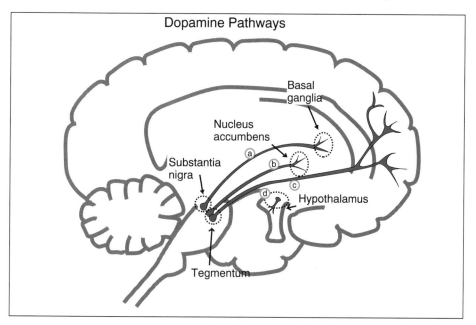

FIGURE 10–7. **Four dopamine pathways in the brain.** The neuroanatomy of dopamine neuronal pathways in the brain can explain both the therapeutic effects and the side effects of the known antipsychotic agents. (a) The **nigrostrial dopamine pathway** projects from the substantia nigra to the basal ganglia, is part of the extrapyramidal nervous system, and controls movements. (b) The **mesolimbic dopamine pathway** projects from the midbrain ventral tegmental area to the nucleus accumbens, a part of the limbic system of the brain thought to be involved in many behaviors, such as pleasurable sensations, the powerful euphoria of drugs of abuse, as well as delusions and hallucinations of psychosis. (c) A pathway related to the mesolimbic dopamine pathway is the **mesocortical dopamine pathway.** It also projects from the midbrain ventral tegmental area, but sends its axons to the limbic cortex, where they may have a role in mediating negative and cognitive symptoms of schizophrenia. (d) The fourth dopamine pathway of interest controls prolactin secretion and is called the **tuberoinfundibular dopamine pathway.** It projects from the hypothalamus to the anterior pituitary gland.

mine pathway. However, the mesocortical dopamine pathway projects to areas of the cerebral cortex, especially the limbic cortex. The role of the mesocortical dopamine pathway in mediating negative and/or cognitive symptoms of schizophrenia is still a matter of debate. Some researchers believe that negative symptoms and possibly certain cognitive symptoms of schizophrenia may be due to a deficit of dopamine in mesocortical projection areas, such as the *dorsolateral prefrontal cortex* (Figs. 10–10 and 10–11). The behavioral deficit state suggested by negative symptoms certainly implies underactivity or even "burnout" of neuronal systems. This may be related to excitotoxic overactivity of *glutamate systems,* discussed earlier in Chapter 4 and shown in Figure 4–9 (see also the discussion of neurodegenerative hypotheses of schizophrenia below). An ongoing degenerative process in the mesocortical dopamine pathway could explain a progressive worsening of symptoms and an ever-increasing deficit state in some schizophrenic patients.

In this formulation of negative and cognitive symptoms of schizophrenia as a dopamine deficiency state of mesocortical dopamine neurons, the deficiency could

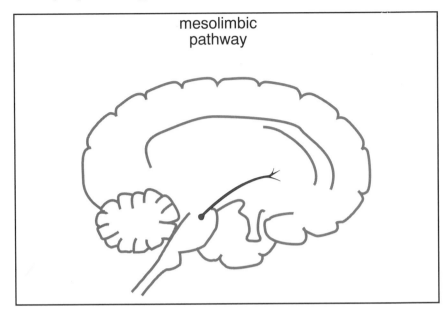

FIGURE 10–8. This diagram shows the **mesolimbic dopamine pathway,** which is thought to be hyperactive in schizophrenia and to mediate the **positive symptoms** of psychosis.

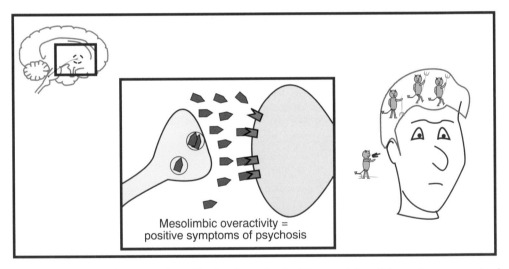

FIGURE 10–9. **The dopamine hypothesis of psychosis.** Hyperactivity of dopamine neurons in the mesolimbic dopamine pathway theoretically mediates the positive symptoms of psychosis, such as delusions and hallucinations. This pathway is also involved in pleasure, reward, and reinforcing behavior, and many drugs of abuse interact here.

hypothetically be either a primary dopamine deficit or a dopamine deficit secondary to inhibition by an excess of serotonin in this pathway (Fig. 10–11). The dopamine deficiency could also be secondary to blockage of dopamine 2 receptors by antipsychotic drugs. This will be discussed in greater detail in Chapter 11. Theoretically,

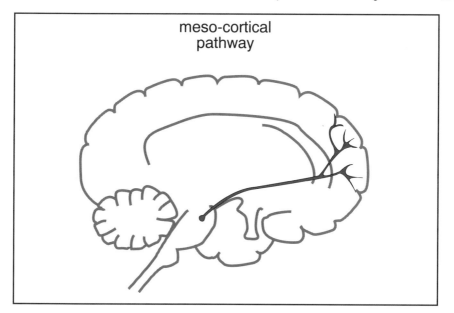

FIGURE 10–10. The **mesocortical dopamine pathway** mediates the negative and cognitive symptoms of psychosis.

increasing dopamine in the mesocortical dopamine pathway might improve negative symptoms or possibly even cognitive symptoms. However, since there is hypothetically already an excess of dopamine in the mesolimbic dopamine pathway, any further increase of dopamine in that pathway would actually worsen positive symptoms. Thus, this poses a therapeutic dilemma: How can one increase dopamine in the mesocortical pathway simultaneously with decreasing dopamine activity in the mesolimbic dopamine pathway? The extent to which atypical antipsychotics have provided a solution to this therapeutic dilemma will be discussed in Chapter 11.

### Nigrostriatal Dopamine Pathway

Another key dopamine pathway in brain is the *nigrostrial dopamine pathway*, which projects from dopaminergic cell bodies in the substantia nigra of the brainstem via axons terminating in the basal ganglia or striatum (Fig. 10–12). The nigrostrial dopamine pathway is a part of the extrapyramidal nervous system and controls motor movements. Deficiencies in dopamine in this pathway cause movement disorders, including Parkinson's disease, which is characterized by rigidity, akinesia or bradykinesia (i.e., lack of movement or slowing of movement), and tremor. Dopamine deficiency in the basal ganglia also can produce akathisia (a type of restlessness) and dystonia (twisting movements, especially of the face and neck). These movement disorders which can be replicated by drugs that block dopamine 2 receptors in this pathway, will be discussed in Chapter 11.

Hyperactivity of dopamine in the nigrostriatal pathway is thought to underlie various hyperkinetic movement disorders, such as chorea, dyskinesias, and tics. Chronic blockade of dopamine 2 receptors in this pathway may result in a hyper-

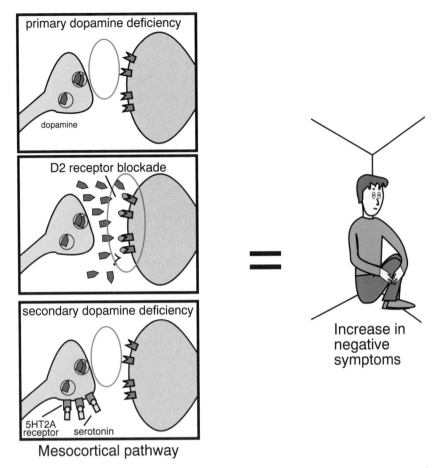

FIGURE 10–11. Several different causes of **dopamine deficiency** may result in **negative and cognitive symptoms**. In schizophrenia itself, there may be a primary dopamine (DA) deficiency or a DA deficiency secondary to blockade of postsynaptic D2 dopamine receptor by an antipsychotic drug. If serotonin is hyperactive, this may also cause a relative DA deficiency by inhibiting DA release. Either primary or secondary DA deficiency in this pathway may cause cognitive blunting, social isolation, indifference, apathy, and anhedonia.

kinetic movement disorder known as *neuroleptic-induced tardive dyskinesia*, which will be discussed further in Chapter 11.

### Tuberoinfundibular Dopamine Pathway

The dopamine neurons that project from the hypothalamus to the anterior pituitary are known as the *tuberoinfundibular dopamine pathway* (Fig. 10–13). Normally, these neurons are active and *inhibit* prolactin release. In the postpartum state, however, their activity is decreased, and therefore prolactin levels can rise during breast-feeding, so that lactation will occur. If the functioning of tuberoinfundibular dopamine neurons is disrupted by lesions or drugs, prolactin levels can also rise. Elevated prolactin levels are associated with galactorrhea (breast secretions), amenorrhea,

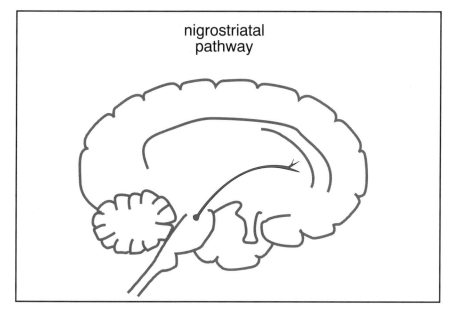

FIGURE 10–12. The **nigrostriatal dopamine pathway** is part of the extrapyramidal nervous system and plays a key role in regulating movements. When dopamine is deficient, it can cause parkinsonism with tremor, rigidity, and akinesia/bradykinesia. When DA is in excess, it can cause hyperkinetic movements such as tics and dyskinesias.

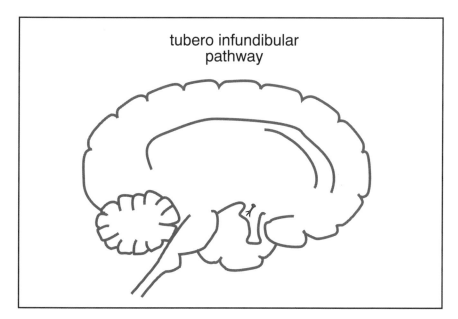

FIGURE 10–13. The **tuberoinfundibular** dopamine pathway from hypothalamus to anterior pituitary regulates prolactin secretion into the circulation. Dopamine inhibits prolactin secretion.

and possibly other problems, such as sexual dysfunction. Such problems can occur after treatment with many antipsychotic drugs that block dopamine 2 receptors, as will be discussed further in Chapter 11.

## Neurodevelopmental Hypotheses of Schizophrenia

One leading hypothesis for the etiology of schizophrenia is that this illness originates from abnormalities in fetal brain development during the early stages of neuronal selection (Fig. 4–6) and migration (Fig. 4–7). Although the symptoms of schizophrenia are usually not evident until the late teens to the twenties it may be that "the die is cast" much earlier. That is, an abnormal degenerative process may be "turned on" genetically very early in fetal brain development. However, symptoms do not occur until the brain extensively revises its synapses in adolescence, and it is hypothetically this normal restructuring process that unmasks the problems of neuronal selection and migration that were previously hidden. Although one idea is that the degenerative process may only do this type of fetal "hit and run" damage, it is also possible that the degenerative process continues during the symptomatic phase of schizophrenia, as discussed below in relation to the neurodegenerative hypothesis and combined neurodevelopmental/neurodegenerative hypothesis of schizophrenia.

Other support for the possibility that schizophrenia could have a neurodevelopmental basis includes observations that schizophrenia is increased in those with a fetal history of obstetric complications ranging from viral infections to starvation to autoimmune processes and other such problems in the pregnant mother. These observations suggest that an insult to the brain early in fetal development could contribute to the cause of schizophrenia. These risk factors may all have the final common pathway of reducing nerve growth factors (see Figs. 1–22 and 5–64), and also stimulating certain noxious processes that kill off critical neurons, such as cytokines, viral infection, hypoxia, trauma, starvation, or stress. This may be mediated either by apoptosis or by necrosis (Fig. 1–18). The result (reviewed in Fig. 10–14) could be either overt structural abnormalities or more subtle problems, including selection of the wrong neurons to survive in the fetal brain (Fig. 4–6), neuron migration to the wrong places (Fig. 4–7), neuron innervation of the wrong targets (Figs. 4–8 and 4–9), and mixup of the nurturing signals so that what innervates these neurons is also mixed up (Figs. 1–19, 1–20, and 1–21). Problems with proteins involved in the structural matrix of synapses (such as synapsins) may occur in schizophrenia, leading to reduced numbers of synaptic vesicles, aberrant synapse formation, and delays or reduction in synapse formation.

If schizophrenia is caused by abnormal early brain development (cf. Figs. 10–15 and 10–16), it may be virtually impossible to reverse such abnormalities in adulthood. On the other hand, some day it may be possible to compensate for such postulated neurodevelopmental difficulties by other mechanisms or to interrupt an ongoing mechanism still present in the symptomatic patient. Therefore, it will be critical to learn what neurodevelopmental abnormalities may exist in schizophrenia in order to devise strategies for reducing their potential impact. It may even be possible to identify such abnormalities in presymptomatic individuals or to exploit the plasticity of adult neurons to compensate for neurodevelopmentally endowed dysfunction. These are bold and unsubstantiated theoretical extrapolations based on

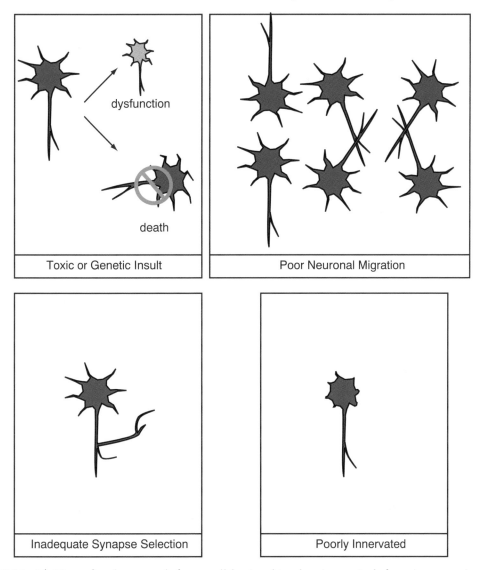

FIGURE 10–14. **Neurodevelopmental abnormalities** in schizophrenia may include toxic or genetic insults to neurons, either killing them or rendering their functioning inadequate; poor neuronal migration during fetal brain development; inadequate and improper selection of synaptic targets during synaptogenesis, especially before the age of 6; and/or inadequate innervation received from inputs of other neurons.

the most optimistic therapeutic visions; current molecular and neurodevelopmental approaches have not yet evolved into successful therapeutic strategies.

Strong evidence for a genetic basis of schizophrenia comes from twin studies, as already discussed in Chapter 4. Scientists have been trying for a long time to identify abnormal genes in schizophrenia (Fig. 10–17) and the consequences that such abnormal genes could have on molecular regulation of neuronal functioning in schizophrenic patients (Fig. 10–18). It is already clear that the causes of psychotic illnesses

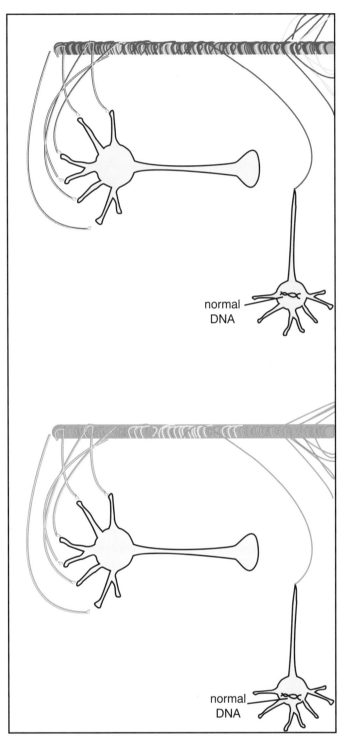

FIGURE 10–15. **Neurodevelopmental theories of schizophrenia** suggest that something goes wrong with the genetic program for the **normal formation of synapses and migration of neurons** in the brain during the prenatal and early childhood formation of the brain and its connections. Depicted here is a concept of how a neuron with normal genetic programming would develop and form synaptic connections.

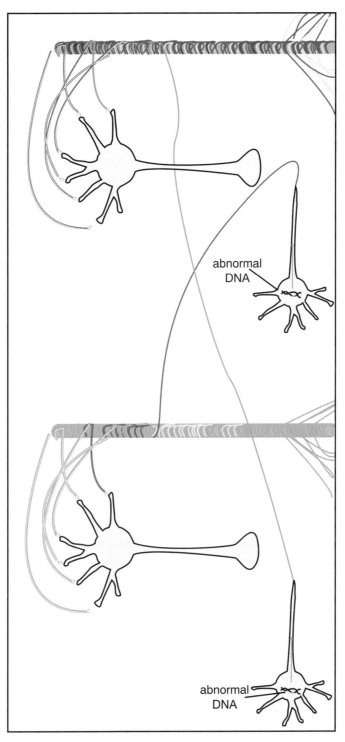

FIGURE 10–16. According to neurodevelopmental theories of schizophrenia, an abnormality in the DNA of a schizophrenic patient may cause the **wrong synaptic connections** to be made during the prenatal and early childhood formation of the brain and its connections. Schizophrenia may be the result of abnormal development of the brain from the beginning of life either because the wrong neurons are selected to survive into adulthood or because those neurons that do survive fail to migrate to the correct parts of the brain, fail to form appropriate connections, and then are subject to breakdown when put to use by the individual in late adolescence and adulthood.

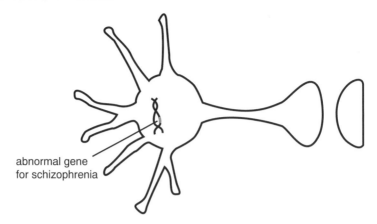

FIGURE 10–17. This figure shows one of the several **postulated abnormal genes** in schizophrenia that may contribute to the risk of this illness. Here it is lying dormant in the cell. In this case, it does not produce abnormal gene products or cause schizophrenia. Thus, it is not contributing to the risk of illness.

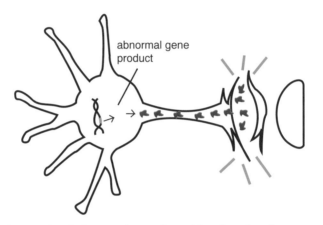

FIGURE 10–18. Here, the postulated **abnormal gene for schizophrenia** is being expressed, leading to an abnormal gene product that contributes to the risk of schizophrenia because it causes disruption in the functioning of the neuron. The manner of the disruption is additive with other risks from other genes and other environmental factors, with just the right timing and in just the right sequence; this, in turn, leads to psychosis and the other symptoms of schizophrenia.

such as schizophrenia and bipolar disorder are not going to be single abnormalities in a major genetic locus of DNA, like those already proven for diseases such as Huntington's disease. Rather, *multiple* genetic abnormalities are likely to *each* contribute in complex ways to a vulnerability to schizophrenia and other psychotic illnesses, perhaps only when other critical environmental inputs are also present. Thus, the genetic basis of schizophrenia is not likely to be as simple as depicted in Figures 10–17 and 10–18; rather, a whole list of abnormally acting genes and their corresponding gene products, triggered from both inherited and acquired risk factors, are hypothesized to act together or in just the right sequence to cause the evolution of the symptom clusters known as schizophrenia. It will be important to

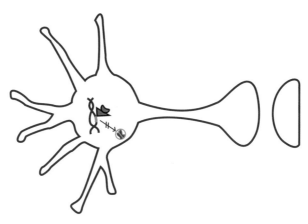

FIGURE 10–19. A highly theoretical direct **genetic approach to therapeutics** in schizophrenia is based on the notion that if dormant risk factors could be identified in the genome, perhaps drugs could prevent the expression of such genes and thus prevent the triggering of the disease process leading to schizophrenia.

determine just how these gene products participate in mediating the symptoms of schizophrenia, because only then could a logical biochemical rationale be found for preventing or interrupting these abnormalities by interfering with gene transcription, for example (Fig. 10–19), by blocking the action of unwanted gene products, or by substituting for the action of missing gene products. This is not likely to be simple, as multiple simultaneous drugs acting to compensate for each genetic abnormality might prove to be necessary, and treatments based on this approach do not appear to be imminent.

## Neurodegenerative Hypotheses of Schizophrenia

The presence of both functional and structural abnormalities demonstrated in neuroimaging studies of the brain of schizophrenics suggests that a neurodegenerative process with progressive loss of neuronal function may be ongoing during the course of the disease. A neurodegenerative condition is also suggested by the progressive nature of the course of illness in schizophrenia (Fig. 10–20). Such a course of illness is not consistent with simply being the result of a static and previously completed pathological process.

Schizophrenia progresses from a largely asymptomatic stage prior to the teen years (phase I in Fig. 10–20), to a prodromal stage of "oddness" and the onset of subtle negative symptoms in the late teens to early twenties (phase II in Fig. 10–20). The active phase of the illness begins and continues throughout the twenties and thirties with destructive positive symptoms, characterized by an up-and-down course with treatment and relapse, with the patient never quite returning to the same level of functioning following acute relapses or exacerbations (phase III in Fig. 10–20). Finally, the disease can reach a largely stable level of poor social functioning and prominent negative and cognitive symptoms, with some ups and downs but at a considerable step-off from baseline functioning, suggesting a more static phase of illness sometimes called "burnout" in the forties or later in life (phase IV in Fig. 10–20).

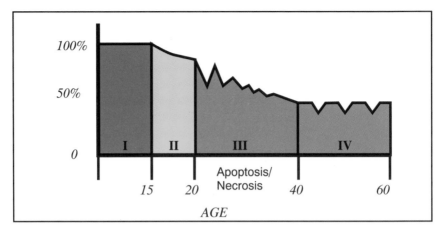

FIGURE 10–20. The **stages of schizophrenia** are shown here over a lifetime. The patient has full functioning (100%) early in life and is virtually asymptomatic (stage I). However, during a prodromal phase (stage II) starting in the teens, there may be odd behaviors and subtle negative symptoms. The acute phase of the illness usually announces itself fairly dramatically in the twenties (stage III), with positive symptoms, remissions, and relapses but never a complete return to previous levels of functioning. This is often a chaotic stage of the illness, with a progressive downhill course. The final phase of the illness (stage IV) may begin in the forties or later, with prominent negative and cognitive symptoms and some waxing and waning during its course, but often more of a burnout stage of continuing disability. There may not necessarily be a continuing and relentless downhill course, but the patient may become progressively resistant to treatment with antipsychotic medications during this stage.

The fact that a schizophrenic patient's responsiveness to antipsychotic treatment can change (and lessen) over the course of illness also suggests an ongoing neurodegenerative process of some kind. For example, the time it takes for a schizophrenic patient to go into remission increases in each successive psychotic relapse. A patient may be less responsive to antipsychotic treatment during successive episodes or exacerbations, so that residual symptoms remain as well as decrements in the patient's functional capacities. This development of treatment resistance during successive episodes of the illness suggests that "psychosis is hazardous to the brain." It thus seems possible that patients who receive early and effective continuous treatment may prevent disease progression or at least the development of treatment resistance.

*Excitotoxicity*

One major idea proposed to explain the downhill course of schizophrenia and the development of treatment resistance is that neurodegenerative events in schizophrenia may be mediated by a type of excessive action of the neurotransmitter glutamate that has come to be known as *excitotoxicity*. The excitotoxic hypothesis of schizophrenia proposes that neurons degenerate because of excessive excitatory neurotransmission at glutamate neurons. This process of excitotoxicity, already discussed in Chapter 4, not only is a hypothesis to explain neurodegeneration in schizophrenia but also has been invoked as an explanation for neurodegeneration in any number of neurological and psychiatric conditions, including Alzheimer's disease and other degenerative dementias, Parkinson's disease, amytrophic lateral sclerosis (Lou Gehrig's disease), and even stroke.

In order to understand the hypothesis of excessive excitation of neurons by glutamate, it is necessary to understand glutamatergic neurotransmission.

## Glutamatergic Neurotransmission

*Glutamate synthesis.* The amino acid glutamate or glutamic acid is a neurotransmitter, but its predominant use is as an amino acid building block for protein biosynthesis. When used as a neurotransmitter, it is synthesized from glutamine (Fig. 10–21), which is converted to glutamate by an enzyme in mitochondria called *glutaminase*. It is then stored in synaptic vesicles for subsequent release during neurotransmission. Glutamine itself can be obtained from glial cells adjacent to neurons. The glial cells help to support neurons both structurally and metabolically. In the case of glutamate neurons, nearby glia can provide glutamine for neurotransmitter glutamate synthesis. In this case, glutamate from metabolic pools in the glia is converted into glutamate for use as a neurotransmitter. This is accomplished by first converting glutamate into glutamine in the glial cell via the enzyme glutamine synthetase. Glutamine is then transported into the neuron for conversion into glutamate for use as a neurotransmitter (Fig. 10–21).

*Glutamate removal.* Glutamate's actions are stopped not by enzymatic breakdown, as in other neurotransmitter systems, but by removal by two transport pumps. The first of these pumps is a presynaptic glutamate transporter, which works as do all the other neurotransmitter transporters already discussed for monoamine neurotransmitter systems such as dopamine, norepinephrine, and serotonin. The second transport pump, located on nearby glia, removes glutamate from the synapse and terminates its actions there. Glutamate removal is summarized in Figure 10–22.

*Glutamate receptors.* There are several types of glutamate receptors (Fig. 10–23), including N-methyl-*d*-asparate (NMDA), alpha-amino-3-hydroxy-5-methyl-4-isoxazole-propionic acid (AMPA), and kainate, all named after the agonists that selectively bind to them. Another type of glutamate receptor is the metabotropic glutamate receptor, which may mediate long-lasting electrical signals in the brain by a process called *long-term potentiation* which appears to have a key role in memory functions.

The NMDA, AMPA, and kainate subtypes of glutamate receptors are probably all linked to an ion channel. The metabotropic glutamate receptor subtype, however, belongs to the G protein–linked superfamily of receptors. The specific functioning of the various subtypes of glutamate receptors is the focus of intense debate. The actions at NMDA receptors will be emphasized here in our discussions on excitotoxicity.

Just as does the GABA-benzodiazepine receptor complex discussed in Chapter 8 (see Figs. 8–18 to 8–20), the NMDA glutamate–calcium channel complex also has multiple receptors surrounding the ion channel, which act in concert as *allosteric modulators* (Fig. 10–24). One modulatory site is for the neurotransmitter *glycine*; another is for *polyamines*, and yet another is for *zinc* (Fig. 10–24). The *magnesium* ion can block the calcium channel at yet another modulatory site, which is presumably inside the ion channel or closely related to it. Another inhibitory modulatory site,

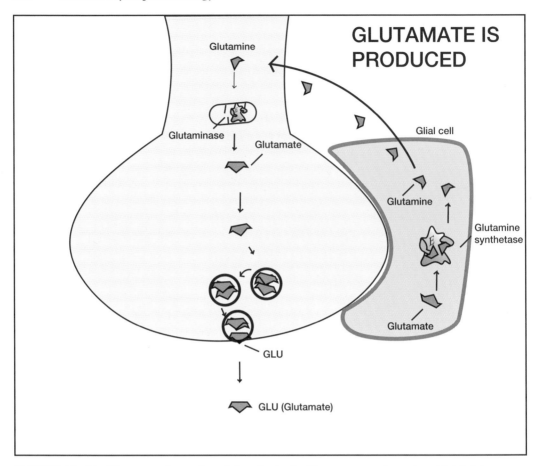

FIGURE 10–21. **Glutamate is produced** (synthesized). Glutamate or glutamic acid (**glu**) is a neurotransmitter that is an amino acid. Its predominant use is not as a neurotransmitter but as an amino acid building block of protein synthesis. When used as a neurotransmitter, it is synthesized from **glutamine**. Glutamine is turned into glutamate by an enzyme present in mitochondria called **glutaminase**. It is then stored in synaptic vesicles for subsequent release during neurotransmission. Glutamine itself can be obtained from glial cells adjacent to neurons. Glial cells have a supportive role to neurons, helping to support them both structurally and metabolically. In the case of glutamate neurons, nearby glia can provide glutamine for neurotransmitter glutamate synthesis. In this case, glutamate from metabolic pools in the glia is converted into glutamate for use as a neurotransmitter. This is accomplished by first converting glutamate into glutamine in the glial cell via the enzyme **glutamine synthetase**. Glutamine is then transported into the neuron for conversion into glutamate for use as a neurotransmitter.

located inside the ion channel, is sometimes called the *PCP site* since the psychotomimic agent phencylclidine (PCP) binds to this site (Fig. 10–24). Since PCP induces a psychotic state with some similarities to schizophrenia (see Chapter 13 on drug abuse), it is possible that such psychotic symptoms in schizophrenia may be modulated by dysfunction in the NMDA subtype of glutamate receptor.

Antagonists for any of the various modulatory sites around the NMDA–calcium channel complex would possibly restrict the flow of calcium and close the channel and therefore be candidates for neuroprotective agents. Such antagonists are being

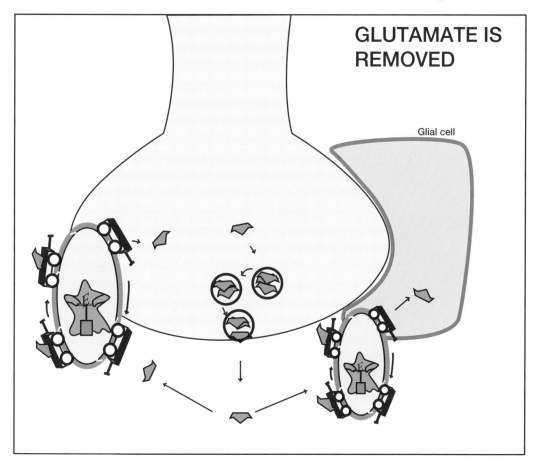

**GLUTAMATE IS REMOVED**

Glial cell

FIGURE 10–22. **Glutamate removal**. Glutamate's actions are stopped, not by enzymatic breakdown as in other neurotransmitter systems, but by removal by two transport pumps. The first of these pumps is a presynaptic glutamate transporter, which works in the same way as all the other neurotransmitter transporters already discussed for monoamine neurotransmitter systems such as dopamine, norepinephrine, and serotonin. The second transport pump, located on nearby glia, removes glutamate from the synapse and terminates its actions there.

developed and tested in various disorders hypothesized to be mediated by an excitotoxic mechanism, such as schizophrenia and Alzheimer's disease.

*Excitotoxicity and the glutamate system in neurodegenerative disorders such as schizophrenia.* The NMDA subtype of glutamate receptor is thought to mediate normal excitatory neurotransmission (Fig. 10–25) as well as neurodegenerative excitotoxicity in the glutamate excitation spectrum shown in Figure 10–26. Excitotoxicity could mediate the final common pathway of any number of neurological and psychiatric disorders characterized by a neurodegenerative course. The basic idea is that the normal process of excitatory neurotransmission runs amok. Instead of normal excitatory neurotransmission, things get out of hand, and the neuron is literally excited to death (Fig. 10–26). The excitotoxic mechanism is thought to begin with a pathological process which eventually triggers reckless glutamate activity (starting with Fig. 10–27).

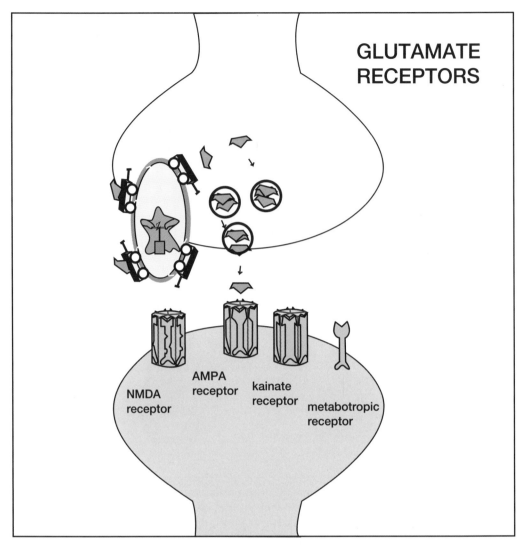

**GLUTAMATE RECEPTORS**

FIGURE 10–23. **Glutamate receptors.** There are several types of glutamate receptors, including three that are linked to ion channels: N-methyl-*d*-aspartate (NMDA), alpha-amino-3-hydroxy-5-methyl-4-isoxazolepropionic acid (AMPA), and **kainate**, all named after the agonists that selectively bind to them. Another type of glutamate receptor is the **metabotropic** glutamate receptor, which is a G protein–linked receptor and which may mediate long-lasting electrical signals in the brain by a process called long-term potentiation, which appears to have a key role in memory functions.

FIGURE 10–24. **Five modulatory sites on the N-methyl-*d*-aspartate (NMDA) receptor.** The NMDA glutamate–calcium channel complex has multiple receptors in and around it, which act in concert as **allosteric modulators.** Three of these modulatory sites are located around the NMDA receptor. One of these modulatory sites is for the neurotransmitter **glycine,** another is for **polyamines,** and yet another is for **zinc.** Two of the modulatory sites are located inside or near the ion channel itself. The **magnesium** ion can block the calcium channel at one of these modulatory site, which is presumably inside the ion channel or close to it. The other inhibitory modulatory site, located inside the ion channel, is sometimes called the **PCP site,** since the psychotomimic agent phencylclidine (PCP) binds to this site.

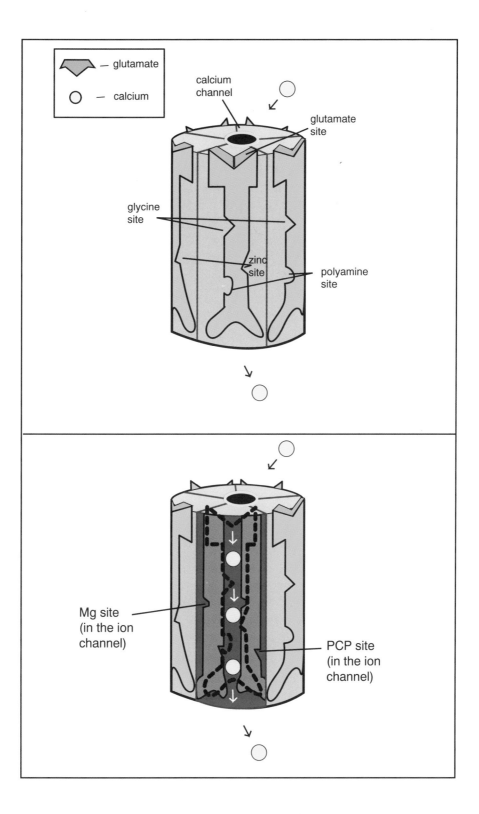

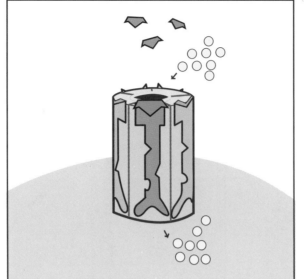

Normal excitatory
neurotransmission

FIGURE 10–25. Shown here is **normal excitatory neurotransmission** at the N-methyl-*d*-aspartate (NMDA) type of glutamate receptor. The NMDA receptor is a **ligand-gated ion channel**. This rapidly transmitting ion channel is an **excitatory** calcium channel. Occupancy of NMDA glutamate receptors by glutamate causes calcium channels to open and the neuron to be excited for neurotransmission.

This could cause dangerous opening of the calcium channel, because if too much calcium enters the cell through open channels, it would poison the cell by activating intracellular enzymes (Fig. 10–28) that form potentially dangerous free radicals (Fig. 10–29). Too many free radicals would eventually overwhelm the cell with toxic actions on cellular membranes and organelles (Fig. 10–30), ultimately killing the cell (Fig. 10–31).

A limited form of excitotoxicity may be useful as a "pruning" mechanism for normal maintenance of the dendritic tree (see Fig. 1–23), getting rid of cerebral "dead wood" like a good gardener; however, excitotoxicity to an excess is hypothesized to cause various forms of neurodegeneration, ranging from slow, relentless neurodegenerative conditions such as schizophrenia and Alzheimer's disease to sudden, catastrophic neuronal death such as stroke (Fig. 10–26).

## Experimental Therapeutic Approaches

### *Blocking Neurodegeneration and Apoptosis: Glutamate Antagonists, Free-Radical Scavengers, and Caspase Inhibitors*

Various experimental therapeutics based on glutamate, excitotoxicity, and free radicals are being developed. It is possible that glutamate antagonists, especially NMDA antagonists, as well as various antagonists of other allosteric sites at the NMDA receptor, such as the glycine site, may be neuroprotective (Fig. 10–32). Such compounds have been tested in animal models and are in development for human conditions ranging from stroke to schizophrenia to Alzheimer's disease. Some drugs are

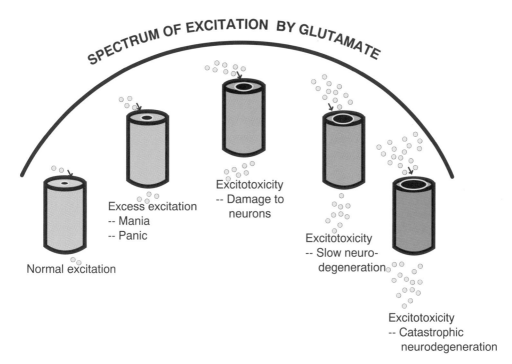

SPECTRUM OF EXCITATION BY GLUTAMATE

Excitotoxicity
-- Damage to
neurons

Excess excitation
-- Mania
-- Panic

Excitotoxicity
-- Slow neuro-
degeneration

Normal excitation

Excitotoxicity
-- Catastrophic
neurodegeneration

FIGURE 10–26. **Neuroprotection, excitotoxicity, and the glutamate system in degenerative disorders**. A major research strategy for the discovery of novel therapeutics in Alzheimer's disease is to target the glutamate system, which might mediate progressive neurodegeneration by an excitotoxic mechanism. Such an excitotoxic mechanism may play a role in various other neurodegenerative diseases such as schizophrenia, Parkinson's disease, Huntington's disease, amyotrophic lateral sclerosis, and even stroke. The **spectrum of excitation by glutamate** ranges from **normal neurotransmission**; to excess neurotransmission, causing pathological symptoms such as **mania** or **panic**; to excitotoxicity, resulting in **minor damage to dendrites**; to **slow progressive excitotoxicity**, resulting in neuronal degeneration such as occurs in Alzheimer's disease; to **sudden and catastrophic excitotoxicity** causing neurodegeneration, as in stroke.

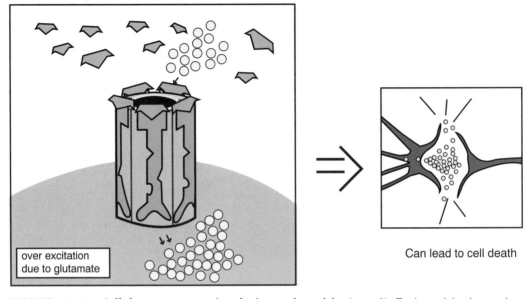

over excitation
due to glutamate

Can lead to cell death

FIGURE 10–27. *Cellular events occurring during excitotoxicity* (**part 1**). Excitotoxicity is a major current hypothesis for explaining a neuropathological mechanism that could mediate the final common pathway of any number of neurological and psychiatric disorders characterized by a neurodegenerative course. The basic idea is that the normal process of excitatory neurotransmission runs amok, and instead of normal excitatory neurotransmission, things get out of hand and the neuron is literally excited to death. The excitotoxic mechanism is thought to begin with a pathological process that triggers excessive glutamate activity. This causes excessive opening of the calcium channel, shown here, beginning the process of poisoning of the cell by allowing too much calcium to enter it.

under development as free-radical scavengers, which have the chemical property of being able to soak up and neutralize toxic free radicals like a chemical sponge and remove them (Fig. 10–33). A weak scavenger that has been tested in Parkinson's disease and tardive dyskinesia is vitamin E. A more powerful set of agents are the lazaroids (so named because of their putative actions of raising degenerating neurons, like Lazarus, from the dead). Another therapeutic approach has to do with blocking the enzyme system that may be necessary for apoptosis to occur, namely the caspase enzymes.

### Presymptomatic Treatment

One idea that is gaining interest and generating debate is the possibility of intervening early in the course of schizophrenia by treating with atypical antipsychotic agents during the prodromal phase prior to the onset of active psychotic symptoms (see Fig. 10–20, stage II). This strategy is causing debate, and even controversy, for there is no assurance that early intervention will lead to improved outcomes, especially since diagnosis of schizophrenia is not very accurate at this point in the illness. Nevertheless, since it is theoretically possible that psychosis itself could be damaging to the brain as a result of excitotoxic neuronal destruction during acute psychosis, there is the provocative possibility that one might be able to abort the illness and modify its natural history by early intervention. It seems obvious that psychosis is

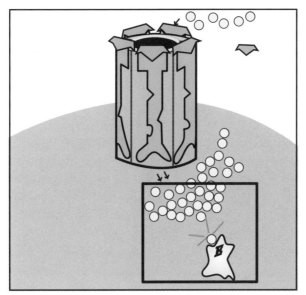

Excess calcium
activates enzyme

FIGURE 10–28. *Cellular events occurring during excitotoxicity* (**part 2**). The internal milieu of a neuron is very sensitive to calcium, as a small increase in calcium concentration will alter all sorts of enzyme activity, as well as neuronal membrane excitability. If calcium levels rise too much, they will begin to activate enzymes that can be dangerous for the cell owing to their ability to trigger a destructive chemical cascade.

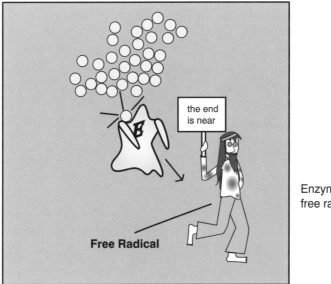

Enzyme produces
free radical

FIGURE 10–29. **Cellular events occurring during excitotoxicity** (**part 3**). Once excessive gluta-mate causes too much calcium to enter the neuron and calcium **activates dangerous enzymes, these enzymes go on to produce troublesome free radicals.** Free radicals are chemicals that are capable of destroying other cellular components, such as organelles and membranes, by destructive chemical reactions.

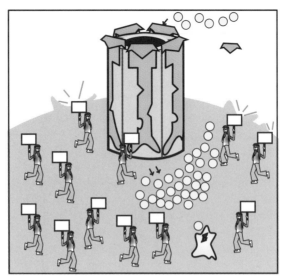

Free radicals begin destroying the cell

FIGURE 10–30. **Cellular events occurring during excitotoxicity (part 4).** As the calcium accumulates in the cell, and the enzymes produce more and more free radicals, they begin to indiscriminately destroy parts of the cell, especially its neuronal and nuclear membranes and critical organelles such as energy-producing mitochondria.

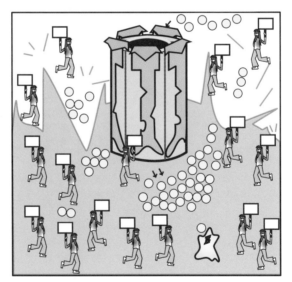

Finally, free radicals destroy the cell

FIGURE 10–31. **Cellular events occurring during excitotoxicity (part 5).** Eventually, the damage is so great that the free radicals essentially destroy the whole neuron.

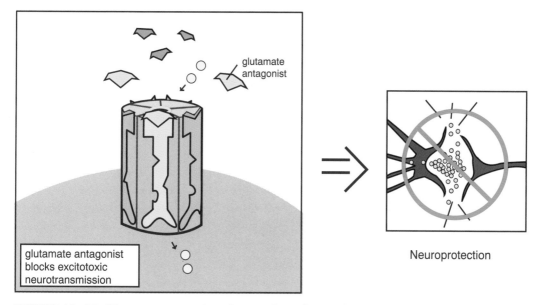

FIGURE 10–32. Glutamate antagonists. **Antagonists of glutamate** at the NMDA agonist site can block excitotoxic neurotransmission and exert neuroprotective actions. Such drugs stop excessive calcium entry and its consequences. These agents are in experimental testing for various neurodegenerative disorders and stroke.

not good for the brain, as exemplified by data from studies showing that patients who are ill for a shorter time prior to initiating treatment with antipsychotic drugs are more likely to respond to them than are those with longer duration of symptoms before treatment is begun. This suggests that an active phase of schizophrenia may reflect a morbid process that begins as early as the prodromal/presymptomatic stage, and which if allowed to persist, can impair the patient's ability to respond to treatment when finally instituted. Some investigators are even extending these ideas to interventions aimed at relatively asymptomatic first-degree relatives of persons with many schizophrenic patients in the family. Whether it will ever be possible to modify or abort the course of schizophrenia is an exciting if perplexing methodological issue for future research.

## Combined Neurodevelopmental/Neurodegenerative Hypothesis

It may be difficult to conceive of a purely neurodevelopmental process that would be completed early in life, that would be entirely asymptomatic until the disease process begins, and that would generate a downhill course and waxing and waning symptomatology. Thus, schizophrenia may be a neurodegenerative process superimposed on a neurodevelopmental abnormality (Fig. 10–34). Candidate neurons for the site of neurodegeneration include dopamine projections to the cortex and glutamate projections back from the cortex to subcortical structures. It is even possible that excitotoxicity occurs in these structures when positive symptoms are produced during psychotic relapses.

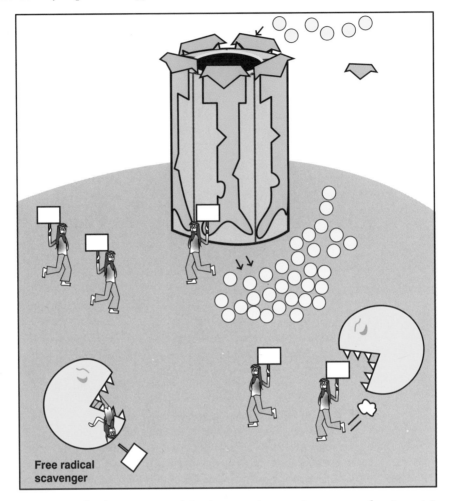

FIGURE 10–33. **Free radicals** are generated in the neurodegenerative process of excitotoxicity. A drug acting as a **free-radical scavenger**, which acts as a chemical sponge by soaking up toxic free radicals and removing them, would be neuroprotective. Vitamin E is a weak scavenger. Other free-radical scavengers, such as the lazaroids (so named because of their putative properties of raising degenerating neurons, like Lazarus, from the dead) are also being tested.

## Summary

This chapter has provided a clinical description of psychosis, with special emphasis on the psychotic illness schizophrenia. We have explained the dopamine hypothesis of schizophrenia, which is the major hypothesis for explaining the mechanism for the positive symptoms of psychosis (delusions and hallucinations).

The four major dopamine pathways in the brain have been described. The mesolimbic dopamine system, which may mediate the positive symptoms of psychosis; the mesocortical system, which may mediate the negative symptoms and cognitive symptoms of psychosis; the nigrostriatal system, which mediates extrapyramidal

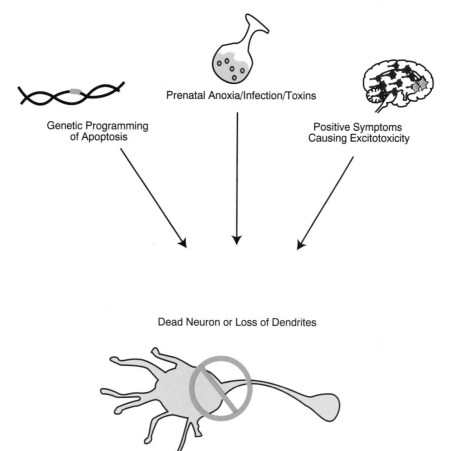

Genetic Programming
of Apoptosis

Prenatal Anoxia/Infection/Toxins

Positive Symptoms
Causing Excitotoxicity

Dead Neuron or Loss of Dendrites

FIGURE 10–34. **Neurodegenerative causes of schizophrenia** may lead to a final common pathway either of neuronal death or possibly of destruction of synapses and the axons and dendrites of such synapses. The causes can range from predetermined genetic programming of neuronal or synaptic destruction; to fetal insults such as anoxia, infection, toxins, or maternal starvation; to perhaps a destructive effect of the positive symptoms themselves on synapses and neurons via glutamate-mediated excitotoxicity.

movement disorders such as Parkinson's disease and tardive dyskinesia; and the tuberoinfundibular system, which controls plasma prolactin levels.

We have also developed the major neurodevelopmental and neurodegenerative hypotheses for schizophrenia and have explained glutamate neurotransmission and the phenomenon of excitotoxicity.

# CHAPTER 11

# ANTIPSYCHOTIC AGENTS

This chapter will explore the various drug treatments for psychotic disorders, with special emphasis on schizophrenia. Such treatments include not only conventional antipsychotic drugs but also the newer atypical antipsychotic drugs, which are rapidly replacing the older conventional agents. We will also take a look into the future at the drugs under development for psychosis, especially schizophrenia. Mood stabilizers for bipolar disorders were covered in Chapter 7.

The specifics of antipsychotic drug treatments will differ, of course, depending on the psychotic disorder (i.e., schizophrenia or other), as well as on how the patient has responded to treatments in the past. Economic considerations are unfortunately also a factor, as the newer drugs are quite expensive; fortunately, they may reduce the overall cost of treatment. Also, antipsychotic treatments can vary, notably in terms of how individual patients respond to specific antipsychotic drugs, doses, durations of treatment, and combinations with additional psychotropic medications. The reader is referred to standard reference manuals and textbooks for practical prescribing information, such as drug doses, because as in past chapters, this chapter will emphasize basic pharmacologic concepts of mechanisms of action and not practical issues such as to how to prescribe these drugs. The pharmacological concepts developed here should, however, help the reader understand the rationale for how to use antipsychotic agents based on their interactions with different neurotransmitter systems in the central nervous system. Such interactions can often explain both the therapeutic actions and side effects of antipsychotic medications and are thus very helpful background information for prescribers.

## Conventional Antipsychotic Drugs

The earliest effective treatments for schizophrenia and other psychotic illnesses arose from serendipitous clinical observations rather than from scientific knowledge of the neurobiological basis of psychosis or the mechanism of action of effective antipsychotic agents. Thus, the first antipsychotic drugs were discovered by accident in the 1950s when a putative antihistamine (chlorpromazine) was serendipitously observed to have antipsychotic effects when tested in schizophrenic patients. Chlorpromazine indeed has antihistaminic activity, but its therapeutic actions in schizophrenia are not mediated by this property. Once chlorpromazine was observed to be an effective antipsychotic agent, it was tested experimentally to uncover its mechanism of antipsychotic action.

Early in the testing process, chlorpromazine and other antipsychotic agents were all found to cause *neurolepsis*, known as an extreme slowness or absence of motor movements as well as behavioral indifference in experimental animals. The original antipsychotics were first discovered largely by their ability to produce this effect in experimental animals and are thus sometimes called neuroleptics. A human counterpart of neurolepsis is also caused by these original (i.e., conventional) antipsychotic drugs and is characterized by psychomotor slowing, emotional quieting, and affective indifference.

### Blockade of Dopamine 2 Receptors as the Mechanism of Action of Conventional Antipsychotics

By the late 1960s and 1970s it was widely recognized that the key pharmacologic property of all neuroleptics with antipsychotic properties was their ability to block dopamine 2 receptors (Fig. 11–1). This action has proved to be responsible not only for the antipsychotic efficacy of conventional antipsychotic drugs but also for most of their undesirable side effects, including neurolepsis.

The therapeutic actions of conventional antipsychotic drugs is due to blockade of D2 receptors specifically in the mesolimbic dopamine pathway (Fig. 11–2). This has the effect of reducing the hyperactivity in this pathway that is postulated to cause the positive symptoms of psychosis, as discussed in Chapter 10 (see Figs. 10–8 and 10–9). All conventional antipsychotics reduced positive psychotic symptoms about equally in schizophrenic patients who were studied in large multicenter trials. That is not to say that one individual patient might not occasionally respond better to one conventional antipsychotic agent than to another, but there is no consistent difference in antipsychotic efficacy among the conventional antipsychotic agents. A list of many conventional antipsychotic drugs is given in Table 11–1.

Unfortunately, it is not possible to block just these D2 receptors in the mesolimbic dopamine (DA) pathway with conventional antipsychotics because these drugs are delivered throughout the entire brain after oral ingestion. Thus, conventional antipsychotics will seek out every D2 receptor throughout the brain and block them

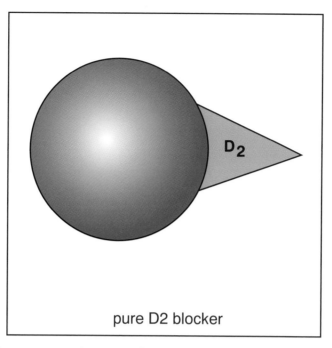

pure D2 blocker

FIGURE 11−1. This icon represents the notion of a single pharmacologic action, namely *dopamine 2 (D2) receptor antagonism*. Although actual drugs have multiple pharmacologic action, this single action idea will be applied conceptually in several of the following figures.

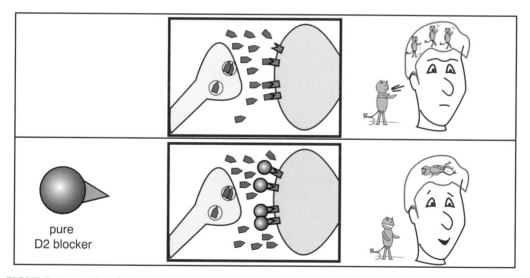

pure
D2 blocker

FIGURE 11−2. The *dopamine receptor antagonist hypothesis* of antipsychotic drug action for *positive symptoms* of psychosis in the *mesolimbic* dopamine pathway is shown here. Blockade of postsynaptic dopamine 2 receptors by a dopamine 2 antagonist acting in the mesolimbic dopamine pathway is hypothesized to mediate the antipsychotic efficacy of the antipsychotic drugs and their ability to diminish or block positive symptoms.

403

Table 11–1. *Conventional antipsychotic agents used to treat psychosis and schizophrenia in the United States*

| Generic Name | Trade Name |
| --- | --- |
| Acetophenazine | Tindal |
| Carphenazine | Proketazine |
| Chlorpromazine | Thorazine |
| Chlorprothixene | Taractan |
| Clozapine | Clozaril |
| Fluphenazine | Prolixin; Permitil |
| Haloperidol | Haldol |
| Loxapine | Loxitane |
| Mesoridazine | Serentil |
| Molindone | Moban; Lidone |
| Perphenazine | Trilafon |
| Pimozide | Orap[a] |
| Piperacetazine | Quide |
| Prochlorperazine | Compazine[b] |
| Thioridazine | Mellaril |
| Thiothixene | Navane |
| Trifluoperazine | Stelazine |
| Triflupromazine | Vesprin |

[a]Approved in the United States for Tourette syndrome.
[b]Approved in the United States for nausea and vomiting as well as psychosis.

all (see Fig. 10–7). This leads to a high "cost of doing business" in order to get the mesolimbic D2 receptors blocked.

Specifically, the D2 receptors will also be blocked in the mesocortical DA pathway (Fig. 11–3), where DA may already be deficient in schizophrenia (see Figs. 10–10 and 10–11). When this happens, it can cause or worsen negative and cognitive symptoms. This is sometimes called the *neuroleptic-induced deficit syndrome* because it looks so much like the negative symptoms produced by schizophrenia itself and is reminiscent of neurolepsis in animals.

When D2 receptors are blocked in the nigrostriatal DA pathway, it produces disorders of movement that can appear very much like those in Parkinson's disease; this is why these movements are sometimes called drug-induced parkinsonism (Fig. 11–4). Since the nigrostriatal pathway is part of the extrapyramidal nervous system, these motor side effects associated with blocking of D2 receptors in this part of the brain are sometimes also called extrapyramidal symptoms, or EPS.

Worse yet, if these D2 receptors in the nigrostriatal DA pathway are blocked chronically (Fig. 11–5), they can produce a hyperkinetic movement disorder known as *tardive dyskinesia*. This movement disorder causes facial and tongue movements such as constant chewing, tongue protrusions, and facial grimacing, as well as limb movements, which can be quick, jerky or choreiform (dancing). Tardive dyskinesia is thus caused by long-term administration of conventional antipsychotics and is

Mesocortical pathway

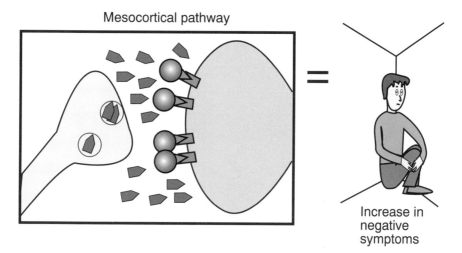

Increase in
negative
symptoms

FIGURE 11–3. When **postsynaptic dopamine** *2 receptors* are blocked by dopamine 2 antagonist acting in the **mesocortical** dopamine pathway, this can cause emotional blunting and cognitive problems that mimic the **negative symptoms** of schizophrenia. Sometimes these cognitive side effects of antipsychotics are called the "neuroleptic induced deficit syndrome." If a patient already has these symptoms before treatment, medication with drugs that block these receptors can make their negative symptoms worse.

Nigrostriatal pathway

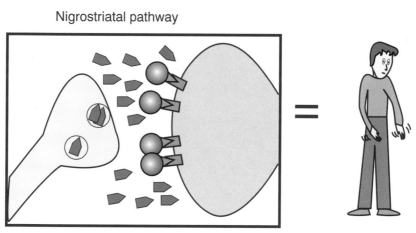

EPSs

FIGURE 11–4. When dopamine 2 receptors are blocked by dopamine 2 antagonists in the postsynaptic projections of the *nigrostriatal* pathway, it produces disorders of movement, which can appear very much like those in Parkinson's disease. That is why these movements are sometimes called drug-induced parkinsonism. Since the nigrostriatal pathway projects to the basal ganglia, a part of the so-called extrapyramidal nervous system, side effects associated with blockade of dopamine 2 receptors there are sometimes also called extrapyramidal symptoms (EPS).

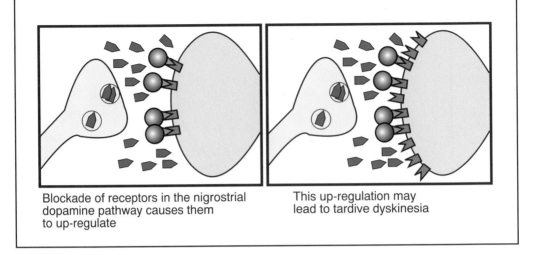

Blockade of receptors in the nigrostrial
dopamine pathway causes them
to up-regulate

This up-regulation may
lead to tardive dyskinesia

FIGURE 11–5. **Long-term** blockade of dopamine 2 receptors by dopamine 2 antagonists in the **nigrostriatal** dopamine pathway may cause these receptors to up-regulate. A clinical consequence of this may be the hyperkinetic movement disorder known as **tardive dyskinesia**. This up regulation may be the consequence of the neuron's futile attempt to overcome drug-induced blockade of its dopamine receptors.

thought to be mediated by changes, sometimes irreversible, in the D2 receptors of the nigrostriatal DA pathway. Specifically, these receptors are hypothesized to become supersensitive or to up-regulate (i.e., increase in number), perhaps in a futile attempt to overcome drug-induced blockade of these receptors (Fig. 11–5).

About 5% of patients maintained on conventional antipsychotics will develop tardive dyskinesia every year (i.e., 20% by 4 years), which is not a very encouraging prospect for a lifelong illness starting in the early twenties. If the D2 receptor blockade is removed early enough, tardive dyskinesia may reverse. This reversal is theoretically due to resetting of these receptors by an appropriate decrease in the number or sensitivity of D2 receptors in the nigrostrial pathway once the antipsychotic drugs that had been blocking these receptors are removed. However, after long-term treatment, the D2 receptors apparently cannot or do not reset back to normal, even when conventional antipsychotic drugs are discontinued. This leads to irreversible tardive dyskinesia, which continues whether conventional antipsychotic drugs are administered or not.

Dopamine 2 receptors in the fourth DA pathway, namely the tuberoinfundibular DA pathway, are also blocked by conventional antipsychotics, and this causes plasma prolactin concentrations to rise, a condition called *hyperprolactinemia* (Fig. 11–6). This is associated with conditions called galactorrhea (breast secretions) and amenorrhea (irregular menstrual periods). Hyperprolactinemia may thus interfere with fertility, especially in women. Hyperprolactinema might lead to more rapid demineralization of bones in postmenopausal women who are not receiving estrogen replacement therapy. Other possible problems associated with elevated prolactin levels include sexual dysfunction and weight gain, although the role of prolactin in causing such problems is not clear.

Tuberoinfundibular pathway

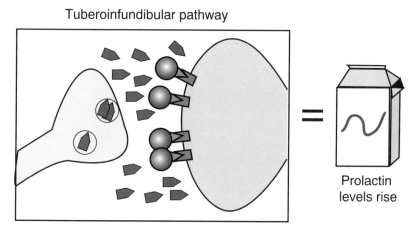

Prolactin
levels rise

FIGURE 11–6. The **tuberoinfundibular** dopamine pathway controls **prolactin** secretion. When dopamine 2 receptors in this pathway are blocked by dopamine 2 antagonists, prolactin levels rise, sometimes so much so that women may begin lactating inappropriately, a condition known as galactorrhea.

### *The Dilemma of Blocking D2 Dopamine Receptors in All Four Dopamine Pathways*

It should now be obvious that the use of conventional antipsychotic drugs presents a powerful dilemma. That is, there is no doubt that conventional antipsychotic medications have dramatic therapeutic actions on positive symptoms of psychosis by blocking hyperactive dopamine neurons in the mesolimbic dopamine pathway. However, there are four dopamine pathways in the brain, and it appears that blocking dopamine receptors in only one of them is useful, whereas blocking dopamine receptors in the remaining three pathways may be harmful.

Specifically, while delusions and hallucinations are reduced when mesolimbic D2 receptors are blocked, negative and cognitive symptoms of psychosis may be worsened when mesocortical D2 receptors are blocked; EPS and tardive dyskinesia may be produced when nigrostriatal D2 receptors are blocked; and hyperprolactinemia and its complications may be produced when tuberoinfundibular D2 receptors are blocked. The pharmacologic quandary here is: What should one do if one wishes to decrease dopamine in the mesolimbic dopamine pathway in order to treat positive psychotic symptoms, which are theoretically mediated by hyperactive mesolimbic dopamine neurons, and yet simultaneously increase dopamine in the mesocortical dopamine pathway to treat negative and cognitive symptoms, while leaving dopaminergic tone unchanged in both the nigrostriatal and tuberoinfundibular dopamine pathways to avoid side effects?

This dilemma may have been solved in part by the atypical antipsychotic drugs described in the following section and is one of the reasons why the atypical antipsychotic agents are rapidly replacing the conventional ones in the treatment of schizophrenia and other psychotic disorders throughout the world.

## Risks and Benefits of Long-Term Treatment with Conventional Antipsychotics

Although the conventional antipsychotics reduce positive psychotic symptoms in most patients after several weeks of treatment, discontinuing these drugs causes relapse of psychosis in schizophrenic patients at the rate of approximately 10% per month, so that 50% or more have relapsed by 6 months after medication is discontinued. Despite this powerful incentive for patients to continue long-term treatment with conventional antipsychotics to prevent relapse, the unfortunate fact that all four dopamine pathways are blocked by these drugs means that the trade-off for many patients is that the benefits of long-term treatment are not considered worth the problems they cause. This leads many patients to discontinue treatment, become noncompliant, and relapse, with a "revolving door" life-style in and out of the hospital. Patients too commonly select the risk of relapse over subjectively unacceptable side effects of the conventional antipsychotics. Especially unacceptable to patients are motor restlessness and EPS such as akathisia, rigidity, and tremor, as well as cognitive blunting and social withdrawal, anhedonia, and apathy. There is even the possibility of a rare but potentially fatal complication called the *neuroleptic malignant syndrome*, which is associated with extreme muscular rigidity, high fever, coma, and even death. Fortunately, the burden of side effects with treatment by atypical antipsychotics appears to be much less than that with conventional antipsychotics and can lead to better compliance and long-term outcomes, as discussed in the next section on atypical antipsychotic drugs.

## Muscarinic Cholinergic Blocking Properties of Conventional Antipsychotics

In addition to blocking D2 receptors in all four dopamine pathways, conventional antipsychotics have other important pharmacologic properties (Fig. 11–7). One particularly important pharmacologic action of some conventional antipsychotics is their ability to block muscarinic cholinergic receptors. This can cause undesirable side effects, such as dry mouth, blurred vision, constipation, and cognitive blunting (Fig. 11–8). Differing degrees of muscarinic cholinergic blockade may also explain why some conventional antipsychotics have a greater propensity to produce extrapyramidal side effects than others. That is, those conventional antipsychotics that cause more EPS are the agents that have only weak anticholinergic properties, whereas those conventional antipsychotics that cause fewer EPS are the agents that have stronger anticholinergic properties.

How does muscarinic cholinergic receptor blockade reduce the EPS caused by dopamine D2 receptor blockade in the nigrostriatal pathway? The reason seems to be that dopamine and acetylcholine have a reciprocal relationship in the nigrostriatal pathway (see Figs. 11–9 to 11–11). Dopamine neurons in the nigrostriatal dopamine pathway make postsynaptic connections with cholinergic neurons (Fig. 11–9). Dopamine normally inhibits acetylcholine release from postsynaptic nigrostriatal cholinergic neurons, thus suppressing acetylcholine activity there (Fig. 11–9). If dopamine can no longer suppress acetylcholine release because dopamine receptors are being blocked by a conventional antipsychotic drug, then acetylcholine becomes overly active (Fig. 11–10).

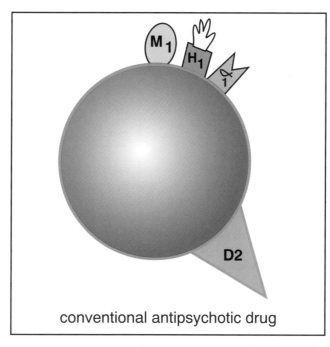

conventional antipsychotic drug

FIGURE 11–7. This figure represents an icon of a **conventional antipsychotic drug**. Such drugs generally have at least four actions: blockade of dopamine 2 receptors (D2); blockade of muscarinic-cholinergic receptors (M1); blockade of alpha 1 adrenergic receptors (alpha 1); and blockade of histamine receptors (antihistaminic actions; [H1]).

One way to compensate for this overactivity of acetylcholine is to block it with an anticholinergic agent (Fig. 11–11). Thus, drugs with anticholinergic actions will diminish the excess acetylcholine activity caused by removal of dopamine inhibition when dopamine receptors are blocked (Fig. 11–11). If anticholinergic properties are present in the same drug with D2 blocking properties, they will tend to mitigate the effects of D2 blockade in the nigrostriatal dopamine pathway. Thus, conventional antipsychotics with potent anticholinergic properties have lower EPS than conventional antipsychotics with weak anticholinergic properties. Furthermore, the effects of D2 blockade in the nigrostriatal system can be mitigated by coadministering an agent with anticholinergic properties. This has led to the common strategy of giving anticholinergic agents along with conventional antipsychotics in order to reduce EPS. Unfortunately, this concomitant use of anticholinergic agents does not lessen the ability of the conventional antipsychotics to cause tardive dyskinesia. It also causes the well-known side effects associated with anticholinergic agents, such as dry mouth, blurred vision, constipation, urinary retention, and cognitive dysfunction.

## Other Pharmacologic Properties of Conventional Antipsychotic Drugs

Still other pharmacologic actions are associated with the conventional antipsychotic drugs. These include generally undesired activity at alpha 1 adrenergic receptors as well as at histamine 1 receptors, as already discussed (Fig. 11–7). Thus, conventional antipsychotic drugs have activities at three of the same neurotransmitter receptors

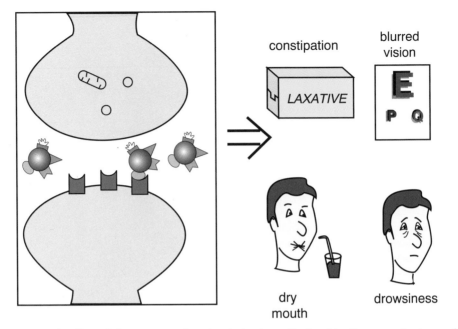

FIGURE 11–8. *Side effects of the conventional antipsychotics* (part 1). In this diagram, the icon of a conventional antipsychotic drug is shown with its M1 anticholinergic-antimuscarinic portion inserted into acetylcholine receptors, causing the side effects of constipation, blurred mouth, dry mouth, and drowsiness.

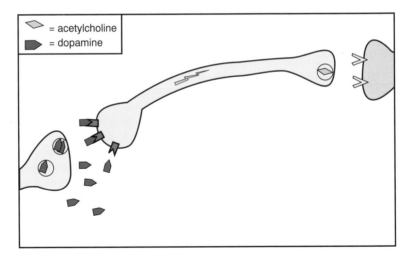

FIGURE 11–9. **Dopamine and acetylcholine** have a reciprocal relationship in the nigrostriatal dopamine pathway. Dopamine neurons here make postsynaptic connections with cholinergic neurons. Normally, **dopamine suppresses acetylcholine** activity.

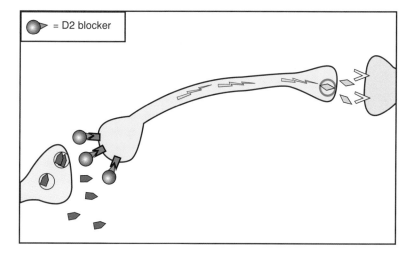

FIGURE 11–10. This figure shows what happens to acetylcholine activity when **dopamine receptors are blocked**. As dopamine normally suppresses acetylcholine activity, removal of dopamine inhibition causes an **increase in acetylcholine** activity. Thus, if dopamine receptors are blocked, acetylcholine becomes overly active. This is associated with the production of extrapyramidal symptoms (EPS). The pharmacological mechanism of EPS therefore seems to be a relative dopamine deficiency and an acetylcholine excess.

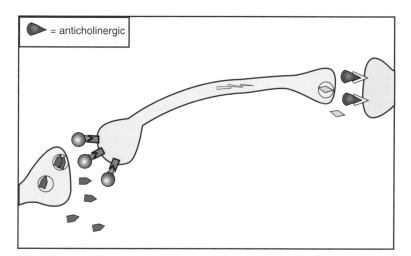

FIGURE 11–11. One **compensation** for the overactivity of acetylcholine that occurs when dopamine receptors are blocked is to block the acetylcholine receptors with an **anticholinergic agent**. Thus, anticholinergics overcome excess acetylcholine activity caused by removal of dopamine inhibition when dopamine receptors are blocked by conventional antipsychotics. This also means that extrapyramidal symptoms (EPS) are reduced.

that mediate the well characterized side effects of the tricyclic antidepressants, which were discussed in Chapter 6 (see Figs. 6–27 and 6–30 to 6–32). That is, these drugs have antihistaminic properties (causing weight gain and drowsiness) (Fig. 11–12), alpha 1 adrenergic blocking properties (causing cardiovascular side effects such

## H1 INSERTED

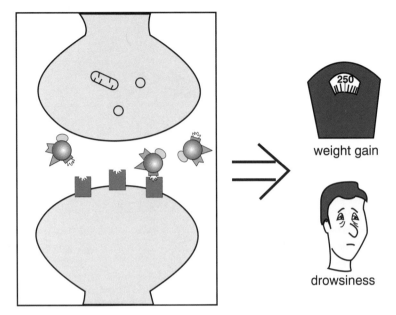

FIGURE 11–12. *Side effects of conventional antipsychotics*, part 2. In this diagram, the icon of a conventional antipsychotic drug is shown with its H1 (antihistamine) portion inserted into histamine receptors, causing the side effects of weight gain and drowsiness.

## $\alpha_1$ INSERTED

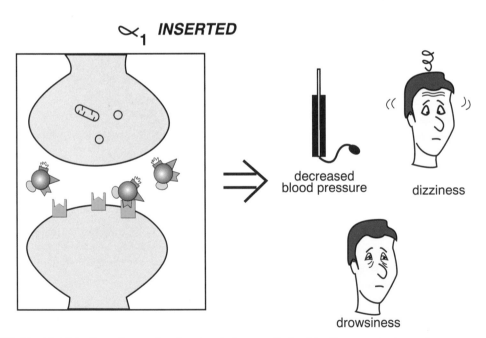

FIGURE 11–13. *Side effects of conventional antipsychotics*, part 3. In this diagram, the icon of a conventional antipsychotic drug is shown with its alpha 1 (alpha 1 antagonist) portion inserted into alpha 1 adrenergic receptors, causing the side effects of dizziness, decreased blood pressure, and drowsiness.

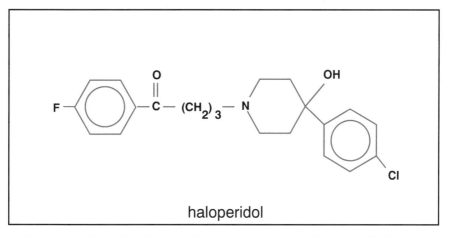

FIGURE 11–14. Structural **formula** of **haloperidol**, one of the most widely prescribed conventional antipsychotic drugs during the height of the conventional antipsychotic era, prior to the mid-1990s.

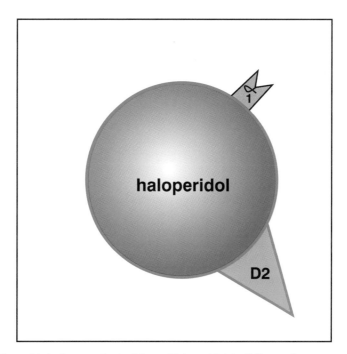

FIGURE 11–15. **Haloperidol** pharmacological icon. Haloperidol is different from many of the other conventional antipsychotic drugs in that it is more potent; it also lacks potent antimuscarinic and antihistaminic binding activities. Otherwise, its clinical profile is highly conventional.

as orthostatic hypotension and drowsiness) (Fig. 11–13), and muscarinic cholinergic blocking properties (causing dry mouth, blurred vision, constipation, urinary retention, and cognitive dysfunction) (Fig. 11–8). Conventional antipsychotic agents differ in terms of their ability to block the various receptors represented in Figure 11–7. For example, the popular conventional antipsychotic haloperidol (Figs. 11–14

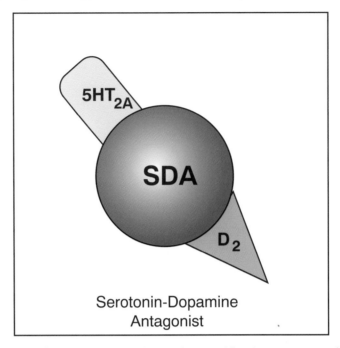

FIGURE 11–16. **Serotonin-dopamine antagonist** (SDA) icon. This icon represents the dual pharmacologic actions that define SDAs, namely blockade of serotonin 2A (5HT2A) receptors, as well as blockade of dopamine 2 (D2) receptors.

and 11–15) has relatively little anticholinergic or antihistaminic binding activity (Fig. 11–15). Because of this, conventional antipsychotics may differ somewhat in their side effect profiles, even if they do not differ overall in their therapeutic profiles. That is, some conventional antipsychotics are more sedating than others; some have more ability to cause cardiovascular side effects than others; and some are more potent than others.

## Atypical Antipsychotic Drugs: Serotonin-Dopamine Antagonism and What Several Antipsychotic Drugs Have in Common

What is an atypical antipsychotic? From a pharmacological perspective, the atypical antipsychotics as a class may be defined in part as serotonin-dopamine antagonists (SDAs) (Fig. 11–16). Several other distinguishing pharmacological characteristics will be discussed in the following section. In this section, we will first discuss how the atypical antipsychotics all derive some of their "atypical" clinical properties from exploiting the different ways that serotonin and dopamine interact within the four key dopamine pathways in the brain. Thus, it is very important to understand serotonin-dopamine interactions in each of the four dopamine pathways.

From a clinical perspective, an atypical antipsychotic, however, is defined in part by the clinical properties that distinguish such drugs from conventional antipsychotics, namely, low extrapyramidal symptoms and efficacy for negative symptoms. By understanding the difference between blocking dopamine D2 receptors alone with a conventional antipsychotic versus blocking serotonin 2A receptors and D2 receptors simultaneously with an atypical antipsychotic in the various dopamine pathways (described below), it should be clear why the atypical antipsychotics have several distinct and atypical clinical properties in common. In this section, we will discuss those features shared by the atypical antipsychotics. Later, we will show that atypical antipsychotics also have features that distinguish one from another. Both the overlapping and the distinguishing features are based on pharmacological mechanisms and clinical observations. Here we will start with the rules (i.e., similarities among the five atypical antipsychotics clozapine, risperidone, olanzapine, quetiapine, and ziprasidone) before discussing the exceptions (i.e., differences among them). Currently, these are the five drugs in psychiatric practice throughout the world that are considered to be atypical antipsychotics by the following three pharmacologic and clinical criteria: (1) atypical antipsychotics have serotonin 2A–dopamine 2 antagonist pharmacological properties, whereas conventional antipsychotics are only dopamine 2 antagonists; (2) atypical antipsychotics cause fewer EPS than conventional antipsychotics; and (3) atypical antipsychotics improve positive symptoms as well as do conventional antipsychotics. Some may argue that zotepine should be included in this group, as should sertindole, recently withdrawn from marketing with the possibility of returning in the future. These are included in the section on potential new drugs of the future.

## Serotonin-Dopamine Antagonism and Serotonergic Control of Dopamine Release in the Four Key Dopamine Pathways

Serotonin has important influences on dopamine, but that influence is quite different in each of the four dopamine pathways. Understanding the differential serotonergic control of dopamine release in each of these four pathways is critical to understanding the differential actions of antipsychotic drugs that block only dopamine 2 receptors (i.e., the conventional antipsychotics) versus antipsychotic drugs that block both serotonin 2A and dopamine 2 receptors (i.e., the atypical antipsychotics). That is, serotonin inhibits dopamine release from dopaminergic axon terminals in the various dopamine pathways, but the degree of control differs from one dopamine pathway to another.

## Serotonin-Dopamine Interactions in the Nigrostriatal Pathway

Serotonin inhibits dopamine release, both at the level of dopamine cell bodies and at the level of dopaminergic axon terminals (Fig. 11–17). Serotonin neurons from the brainstem raphe innervate the dopamine cell bodies in the substantia nigra and also project to the basal ganglia, where serotonin axon terminals are in close proximity to dopamine axon terminals (Figs. 11–17 to 11–20). In both areas, serotonin interacts with postsynaptic serotonin 2A receptors on the dopamine neuron, and this inhibits dopamine release. Thus, in the nigrostriatal dopamine pathway, serotonin exerts powerful control over dopamine release because it occurs at two levels. At the level of serotonergic innervation of the substantia nigra, axon terminals arriving from the raphe synapse on cell bodies and dendrites of dopaminergic cells (Figs. 11–18 to 11–20). At the level of the axon terminals, however, serotonergic interaction with dopamine neurons may be via axoaxonal synapses or via volume (nonsynaptic) neu-

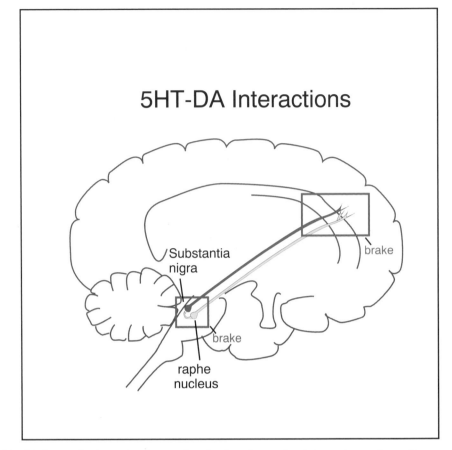

FIGURE 11–17. Serotonin-dopamine interactions in the **nigrostriatal** dopamine pathway. **Serotonin inhibits dopamine release**, both at the level of dopamine cell bodies in the brainstem substantia nigra and at the level of the axon terminals in the basal ganglia–neostriatum (see also Figs. 11–18 through 11–20). In both cases, the release of serotonin acts as a "**brake**" on dopamine release.

rotransmission from serotonin that diffuses to dopamine axon terminals from nearby serotonin axon terminals but without a synapse (Figs. 11–18 to 11–20). In both cases, however, serotonin interacts via serotonin 2A receptors on the dopamine neuron, which inhibit dopamine release. A close-up of the action of serotonin's inhibitory actions on dopamine release from nigrostriatal dopamine axon terminals is shown in Figs. 11–21 and 11–22.

### The Nigrostriatal Pathway and the Pharmacology of Low Extrapyramidal Symptoms

Serotonin 2A antagonism fortunately reverses dopamine 2 antagonism in the nigrostriatal dopamine pathway. Since stimulating 5HT2A receptors inhibits dopamine release (e.g., Fig. 11–22), it would make sense that the opposite would also hold true: in other words, blocking 5HT2A receptors should promote dopamine release. Indeed, this is the case (see Figs. 11–23 and 11–24). When dopamine release

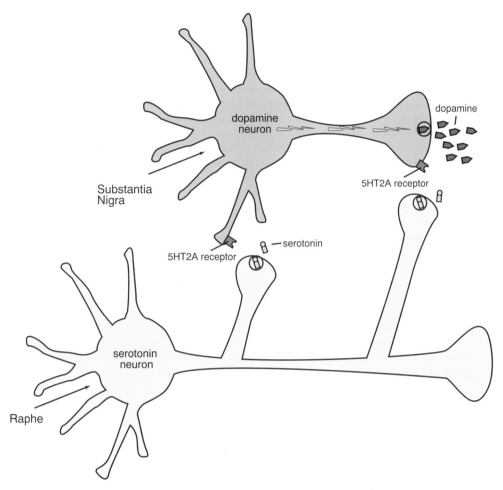

FIGURE 11–18. *Serotonin regulation of dopamine release from nigrostriatal dopamine neurons*, part 1. Here, dopamine is being freely released from its axon terminal in the striatum because there is no serotonin causing any inhibition of dopamine release.

is enhanced by an atypical antipsychotic via blockade of 5HT2A receptors, this allows the extra dopamine to compete with the atypical antipsychotic to reverse the blockade of D2 receptors (Fig. 11–24). Thus, 5HT2A antagonism reverses D2 antagonism in the nigrostriatal dopamine pathway. Not surprisingly, this leads to a reduction or even an absence of EPS and tardive dyskinesia, because there is a reduction of D2 receptor blockade in this pathway.

The serotonin-dopamine antagonism (SDA) properties of the atypical antipsychotics all exploit this ability of serotonin 2A antagonism to play a sort of indirect "tug-of-war" with dopamine 2 antagonism by causing dopamine release, which in turn mitigates or reverses dopamine 2 antagonism. Which one wins—D2 antagonism, or dopamine stimulation—depends on the drug (for conventional antipsychotics, D2 antagonism always wins), the dose (D2 antagonism is more likely to win at higher doses of atypical antipsychotics), and the pathway in the brain, as explained below.

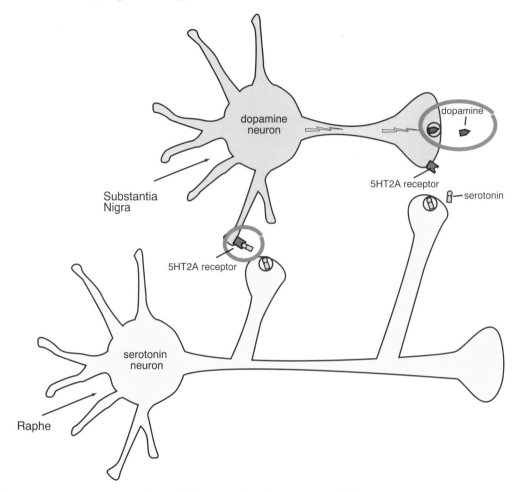

FIGURE 11–19. *Serotonin regulation of dopamine release from nigrostriatal dopamine neurons,* part 2. Now, serotonin is being released from a synaptic connection projecting from the raphe to the substantia nigra and terminating on a postsynaptic serotonin 2A (5HT2A) receptor (*bottom red circle*). Because of this, dopamine release from its axonal terminal is now inhibited (*top red circle*).

In the nigrostriatal dopamine pathway, positron emission tomography (PET) scans document that atypical antipsychotics bind to fewer D2 receptors in the basal ganglia in schizophrenic patients than do conventional antipsychotics at matched antipsychotic efficacies (Figs. 11–25 and 11–26). Thus, about 90% of D2 receptors are blocked when a patient takes an antipsychotic dose of a conventional antipsychotic (Fig. 11–25), but less than 70 to 80% are blocked with an atypical antipsychotic (Fig. 11–26). This puts the threshold of D2 blockade below the level necessary to produce EPS in many patients. Thus, in the SDA tug-of-war in the nigrostriatal pathway, dopamine release is sufficient to reduce D2 antagonist binding just enough to create the best known atypical clinical feature of these agents, namely, reduced EPS without loss of antipsychotic efficacy. Thus, this is a win for dopamine release over dopamine blockade in the nigrostriatal tug-of-war.

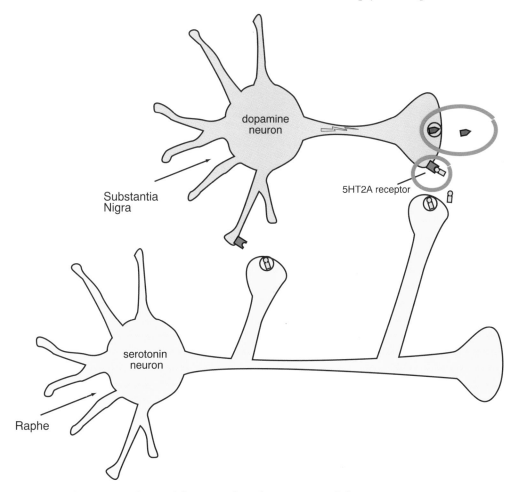

FIGURE 11–20. *Serotonin regulation of dopamine release from nigrostriatal dopamine neurons*, part 3. Here, serotonin is being released from a synaptic connection projection from axoaxonal contacts or by volume neurotransmission between serotoninergic axon terminals and dopamine axon terminals, resulting in serotonin occupying a postsynaptic serotonin 2A (5HT2A) receptor (*bottom red circle*). Because of this, dopamine release from its axonal terminal is now inhibited (*top red circle*).

### The Mesocortical Pathway and the Pharmacology of Improved Negative Symptoms

Serotonin 2A antagonism not only reverses dopamine 2 antagonism but causes a net increase in dopamine activity in the mesocortical dopamine pathway, where the balance between serotonin and dopamine is different from that in the nigrostriatal dopamine pathway. That is, unlike the nigrostriatal dopamine pathway, in which dopamine 2 receptors predominate, there is a preponderance of serotonin 2A receptors over dopamine 2 receptors in many parts of the cerebral cortex. Thus, in the mesocortical dopamine pathway, atypical antipsychotics with SDA properties have a more profound effect in blocking densely populated cortical serotonin 2A receptors, thereby increasing DA release, than in blocking thinly populated cortical D2 recep-

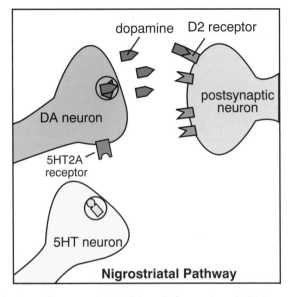

FIGURE 11–21. Enlarged view of **serotonin** (5HT) and **dopamine** (DA) interactions in the **nigrostriatal** dopamine pathway. Normally, serotonin inhibits dopamine release. In this figure, dopamine is being released because no serotonin is stopping it. Specifically, no serotonin is present at its 5HT2A receptor on the nigrostriatal dopaminergic neuron (but see Fig. 11–22).

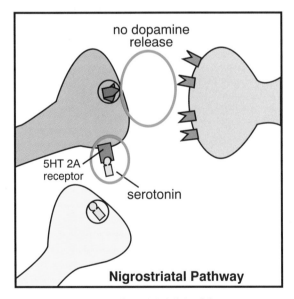

FIGURE 11–22. Now dopamine (DA) release is being **inhibited** by serotonin (5HT) in the nigrostriatal dopamine pathway. When serotonin occupies its 5HT2A receptor on the dopamine neuron (*lower red circle*), this inhibits dopamine release, so there is no dopamine in the synapse (*upper red circle*). Compare this with Figure 11–21.

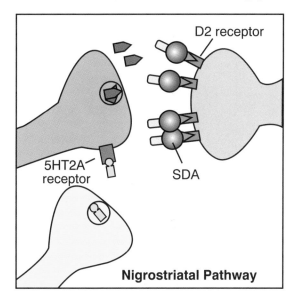

**Nigrostriatal Pathway**

FIGURE 11–23. Here postsynaptic dopamine 2 receptors are being blocked by a serotonin-dopamine antagonist (SDA) atypical antipsychotic in the **nigrostriatal** dopamine pathway. This shows what would happen if only the dopamine 2 blocking action of an atypical antipsychotic were active— namely, the drug would only bind to postsynaptic D2 receptors and block them. However, see Figure 11–24.

tors. This results in considerable amounts of serotonin 2A antagonist binding and also of dopamine release, but not much dopamine 2 antagonism in this part of the brain. Bottom line? Dopamine release wins again over dopamine blockade in the mesocortical tug-of-war. Dopamine release in this part of the brain should be theoretically favorable for ameliorating negative symptoms of schizophrenia, and clinical trials show that atypical antipsychotics improve negative symptoms better than either placebo or conventional antipsychotics. Recall that dopamine deficiency in the mesocortical dopamine pathway is hypothesized to be one of the contributing causes of the negative symptoms of schizophrenia (Fig. 11–27). Thus, the nature of serotonin-dopamine antagonism in the mesocortical dopamine pathway has helped atypical antipsychotics to resolve the dilemma of how to increase theoretically deficient dopamine in the mesocortical dopamine pathway to treat negative symptoms and yet simultaneously to reduce theoretically hyperactive dopamine in the mesolimbic dopamine pathway to treat positive symptoms.

Positron emission tomography scans reveal that an antipsychotic dose of a conventional antipsychotic drug does not block serotonin 2A receptors in the cortex as expected, because these drugs lack such binding properties (Fig. 11–28), but that an antipsychotic dose of an atypical antipsychotic causes a nearly complete blockade of the serotonin 2A receptors there (Fig. 11–29). Where serotonin 2A receptors are blocked, dopamine is being released (see Fig. 11–27), which explains in part why atypical antipsychotics improve negative symptoms better than do conventional antipsychotics. Clearly, other neurochemical mechanisms are operative in the pathophysiology of negative symptoms, but serotonin and dopamine may make an important contribution, as explained by these actions in the mesolimbic pathway.

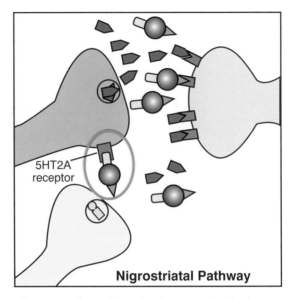

**Nigrostriatal Pathway**

FIGURE 11–24. This figure shows how dopamine 2 (D2) receptor blockade is **reversed** by serotonin 2A receptor blockade in the **nigrostriatal** pathway. In contrast to Figure 11–23, this figure shows the dual action of the serotonin-dopamine antagonists (SDAs). Only the first action was shown in Figure 11–23, namely, binding to D2 receptors. The second action is shown here, namely, binding to serotonin 2A (5HT2A) receptors). The interesting thing is that this second action actually reverses the first. That is, blocking a 5HT2A receptor reverses the blockade of a D2 receptor. This happens because dopamine is released when serotonin can no longer inhibit its release. Another term for this is disinhibition. Thus, blocking a 5HT2A receptor disinhibits the dopamine neuron, causing dopamine to pour out of it. The consequence of this disinhibition is that the dopamine can then compete with the SDA for the D2 receptor and reverse the inhibition there. That is why **5HT2A blockers reverse D2 blockers in the striatum**. As D2 blockade is thereby reversed, SDAs cause little or no EPS or tardive dyskinesia.

## The Tuberoinfundibular Pathway and the Pharmacology of Reduced Hyperprolactinemia

Serotonin 2A antagonism may reverse dopamine 2 antagonism in the tuberoinfundibular pathway. There is an antagonistic and reciprocal relationship between serotonin and dopamine in the control of prolactin secretion from the pituitary lactoroph cells. That is, dopamine inhibits prolactin release by stimulating D2 receptors (Fig. 11–30), whereas serotonin promotes prolactin release by stimulating 5HT2A receptors (Fig. 11–31).

Thus, when D2 receptors are blocked by a conventional antipsychotic, dopamine can no longer inhibit prolactin release, so prolactin levels rise (Fig. 11–32). However, in the case of an atypical antipsychotic, there is simultaneous inhibition of 5HT2A receptors, so serotonin can no longer stimulate prolactin release (Fig. 11–33). This tends to mitigate the hyperprolactinemia of D2 receptor blockade. Although this is interesting theoretical pharmacology, in practice not all serotonin-dopamine antagonists reduce prolactin secretion to the same extent, and some do not reduce it at all.

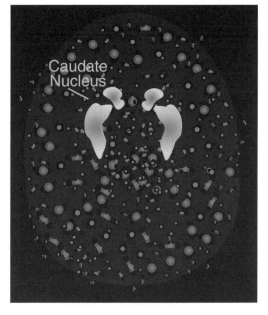

conventional antipsychotic

FIGURE 11–25. Artist's concept of a **conventional antipsychotic** drug binding to postsynaptic **dopamine 2 receptors** in the **nigrostriatal** pathway. Autoradiographic and radioreceptor labeling studies in experimental animals as well as positron emission tomography (PET) scans in schizophrenic patients have established that antipsychotic doses of conventional antipsychotic drugs essentially saturate the binding capacity of these receptors. Bright colors indicate binding to D2 receptors and show here that about 90% of dopamine receptors are being blocked at an antipsychotic dose of a conventional antipsychotic in a schizophrenic patient, which explains why such doses also cause EPS.

### The Mesolimbic Pathway and the Pharmacology of Improved Positive Symptoms

Serotonin 2A antagonism fortunately fails to reverse D2 antagonism in the mesolimbic system. If serotonin 2A antagonism reverses, at least in part, the effects of D2 antagonism in several dopamine pathways, then why does it not reverse the antipsychotic actions of D2 blockade in the mesolimbic dopamine pathway? Evidently, the antagonism by serotonin of the effects of dopamine in this pathway is not robust enough to cause the reversal of D2 receptors by atypical antipsychotics or to mitigate the actions of atypical antipsychotics on positive symptoms of psychosis.

### Summary of Actions of Atypical Antipsychotics as a Class

In summary, for conventional antipsychotics dopamine blockade wins the tug-of-war in every dopamine pathway, resulting in antipsychotic actions for positive symptoms, but at a cost of worsened, or at least not improved, negative symptoms, production of EPS, tardive dyskinesia, and hyperprolactinemia. On the other hand, it appears that atypical antipsychotics let you "have your cake and eat it too," that is, dopamine blockade wins the all important tug of war over dopamine release where it must win to treat disruptive positive symptoms, namely, in the mesolimbic dopamine

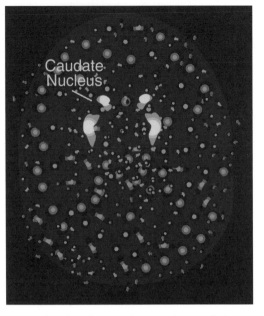

serotonin-dopamine antagonist

FIGURE 11–26. Artist's concept of an **atypical antipsychotic** drug binding to postsynaptic **dopamine 2 receptors** in the **nigrostriatal** pathway. Although this patient is receiving as much antipsychotic benefit as the patient in the previous scan (Fig. 11–25), the binding of drug to D2 receptors in the striatum is less intense in color, indicating only about 70 to 80% blockade of receptors. This reduction is sufficient to put the patient below the threshold for EPS. Thus, this patient has the benefit of the drug's antipsychotic actions, but no EPS. Presumably, blockade of D2 receptors in the mesolimbic dopamine pathway (not shown), which is the target for reducing positive symptoms of psychosis, is matched for both patients in Figures 11–25 and 11–26, which is why they both have relief of psychosis.

pathway. However, the very opposite is occurring simultaneously in the mesocortical dopamine pathway when an atypical antipsychotic is administered, since dopamine release wins the tug of war over dopamine blockade in that area of the brain, and negative symptoms are consequently improved, not worsened as they often are with conventional antipsychotics. The "icing" on the cake is that during atypical antipsychotic drug administration, dopamine release wins the tug-of-war over dopamine blockade both in the nigrostriatal and tuberoinfundibular dopamine pathways to an extent sufficient to reduce EPS and hyperprolactinemia as well, leading largely to elimination of these disabling side effects for many patients as compared with taking conventional antipsychotic drugs. This mix of favorable outcomes appears to be due largely to the differences between serotonin-dopamine antagonism in different parts of the brain, so that simultaneous blockade of D2 receptors and 5HT2A receptors can do nearly the opposite things in the same brain at the same time with the same drug!

Although there are obviously many other factors at play here and this is an overly simplistic explanation, it is a useful starting point for beginning to appreciate the pharmacological actions of atypical antipsychotics as a class of drugs.

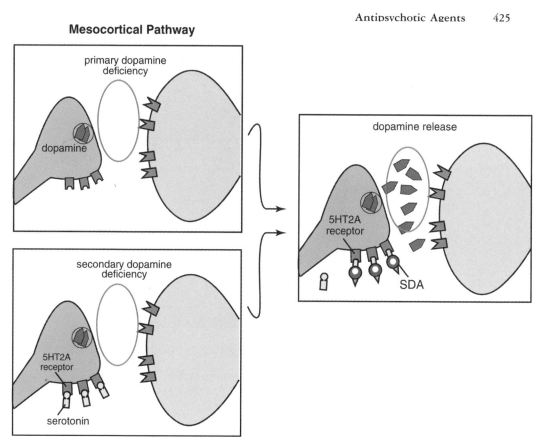

**Mesocortical Pathway**

FIGURE 11–27. The **mesocortical** dopamine pathway may mediate deficits in **cognitive functioning** and **negative symptoms** in schizophrenia because of a relative deficiency in dopamine, due either to a primary deficiency or to various secondary causes, such as serotonin excess. In either case, blockade of 5HT2A receptors with an atypical antipsychotic should lead to dopamine release, which could compensate for the dopamine deficiency and improve negative and cognitive symptoms.

## Atypical Antipsychotics: Several Unique Drugs or One Class of Several Drugs?

Serotonin-dopamine antagonism is a key concept for explaining some of the atypical clinical actions of several atypical antipsychotics, but it is not a sufficient explanation for all the properties of these unique therapeutic agents. Some serotonin-dopamine antagonists do not have the atypical clinical properties of the five well-established atypical antipsychotics cited above (e.g., loxapine is a serotonin-dopamine antagonist but considered to be a conventional antipsychotic, especially at high doses). Also, some drugs (e.g., amisulpride) with low EPS are not necessarily serotonin-dopamine antagonists. Furthermore, some serotonin-dopamine antagonists at high doses begin to lose their atypical properties (e.g., risperidone). Thus, other pharmacologic and clinical factors must be considered to gain a full understanding of the several antipsychotics currently considered atypical. Here, we will consider five agents on an ever-expanding list of atypical antipsychotics: clozapine, risperidone, olanzapine,

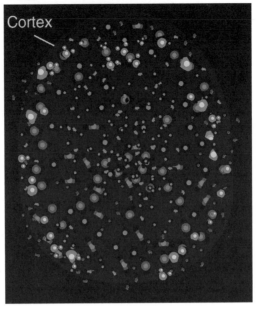

conventional antipsychotic

FIGURE 11–28. Artist's concept of a **conventional antipsychotic drug** binding to postsynaptic **serotonin 2A receptors** in the **cerebral cortex**, including mesocortical dopaminergic projections and dorsolateral prefrontal cortex. Autoradiographic and radioreceptor labeling studies in experimental animals as well as positron emission tomography (PET) scans in schizophrenic patients have established that antipsychotic doses of conventional antipsychotic drugs essentially bind to none of these receptors. Bright colors indicate binding to 5HT2A receptors, and the lack of any receptors lighting up here confirms the lack of binding to cortical 5HT2A receptors. Where cortical 5HT2A receptors are blocked, dopamine is being released. This patient is receiving an antipsychotic dose of a conventional antipsychotic, but there is no effect on 5HT2A receptors in the cortex because these drugs do not interact with 5HT2A receptors. See the contrast with Figure 11–29.

quetiapine, and ziprasidone. Several other candidates are considered in later sections as well.

In addition to the earlier limited definition of an atypical antipsychotic as an agent with serotonin 2A and dopamine 2 antagonist properties associated with decreased EPS, there are other pharmacologic properties associated with the five currently marketed atypical antipsychotics. Furthermore, no two agents have exactly identical properties, including multiple pharmacologic actions at serotonin and dopamine receptor subtypes in addition to SDA actions (e.g., D1, D3, and D4 as well as 5HT1A, 5HT1D, 5HT2C, 5HT3, 5HT6, and 5HT7) (Fig. 11–33) and multiple pharmacologic actions at other neurotransmitter receptors (such as alpha 1 and alpha 2 noradrenergic, muscarinic cholinergic, and histamine 1 receptors, as well as both the serotonin and norepinephrine reuptake pumps) (Fig. 11–34).

Not only do the atypical antipsychotics have incremental pharmacological actions beyond SDA actions, but they also have additional favorable and unfavorable clinical properties beyond the limited clinical definition of reduced EPS and actions on positive symptoms of psychosis. These additional favorable properties include the ability to improve negative symptoms in schizophrenic patients better than do con-

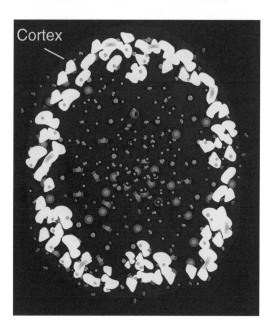

serotonin-dopamine antagonist

FIGURE 11–29. Artist's concept of an **atypical antipsychotic drug** binding to postsynaptic **serotonin 2A (5HT2A) receptors** in **cerebral cortex**, including mesocortical dopamine projections and dorsolateral prefrontal cortex. Autoradiographic and radioreceptor studies in animals as well as positron emission tomography (PET) scans in schizophrenic patients have established that 5HT2A receptors in the cortex are essentially saturated by antipsychotic doses of atypical antipsychotic drugs. Presumably, dopamine release occurs at the sites where there is 5HT2A binding, and that could lead to improvement in cognitive functioning and negative symptoms by a mechanism not possible for conventional antipsychotic agents (cf. Fig. 11–28).

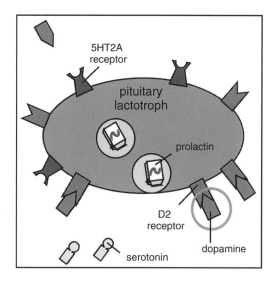

FIGURE 11–30. **Dopamine inhibits prolactin** release from pituitary lactotroph cells in the pituitary gland (*red circle*).

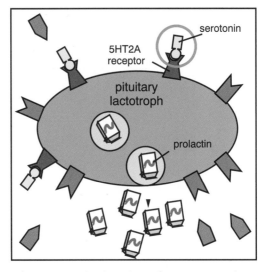

FIGURE 11–31. **Serotonin stimulates prolactin** release from pituitary lactotroph cells in the pituitary gland (*red circle*). Thus, serotonin and dopamine have a reciprocal regulatory action on prolactin release, and oppose each other's actions.

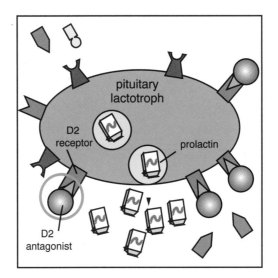

FIGURE 11–32. **Conventional antipsychotic drugs** are D2 antagonists and thus oppose dopamine's inhibitory role on prolactin secretion from pituitary lactotrophs. Therefore, drugs that block D2 receptors **increase prolactin** levels (*red circle*).

ventional antipsychotics; the ability to cause little or no elevation of prolactin levels; the ability to improve positive symptoms in schizophrenic patients resistant to conventional antipsychotics; the ability to improve mood and reduce suicide not only in patients with schizophrenia but also in bipolar patients in manic, mixed, and depressed phases of their illnesses. Additional unfavorable clinical properties of atypical antipsychotics can include weight gain, sedation, seizures, or agranulocytosis.

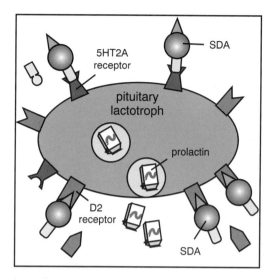

FIGURE 11–33. This figure shows how serotonin 2A antagonism **reverses** the ability of dopamine 2 (D2) antagonism to increase prolactin secretion. As **dopamine and serotonin have reciprocal regulatory roles** in the control of **prolactin** secretion, one cancels the other. Thus, stimulating 5HT2A receptors reverses the effects of stimulating D2 receptors (cf. Figs. 11–30 and 11–31). The same thing works in reverse, namely, blockade of 5HT2A receptors (shown here) reverses the effects of blocking D2 receptors (shown in Fig. 11–32).

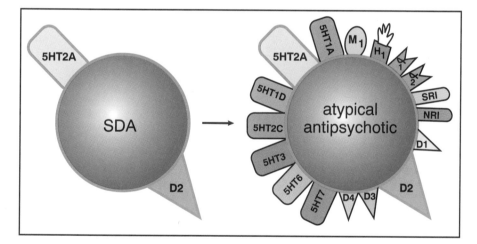

FIGURE 11–34. **Beyond the SDA concept.** Atypical antipsychotics are not merely simple serotonin-dopamine antagonists (SDAs). In truth, they have some of the most complex mixtures of pharmacologic properties in psychopharmacology. Shown here is an icon with all these properties. Beyond antagonism of serotonin 2A and dopamine 2 receptors, some agents in this class interact with multiple other receptor subtypes for both dopamine and serotonin, including 5HT1A, 5HT1D, 5HT2C, 5HT3, 5HT6, 5HT7, and D1, D3, and D4. Other neurotransmitter systems are involved as well, including both norepinephrine and serotonin reuptake blockade, as well as antimuscarinic, antihistaminic, and alpha 1 adrenergic plus alpha 2 adrenergic blockade. No two atypical antipsychotics, however, have identical binding properties, which probably helps to explain why they all have distinctive clinical properties.

429

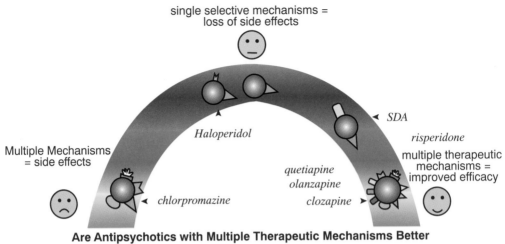

single selective mechanisms =
loss of side effects

◀ SDA

*Haloperidol*

*risperidone*

Multiple Mechanisms
= side effects

multiple therapeutic
mechanisms =
improved efficacy

*quetiapine*
*olanzapine*

◀ *chlorpromazine*

*clozapine* ▶

**Are Antipsychotics with Multiple Therapeutic Mechanisms Better
than Selective Dopamine 2 Antagonists?**

FIGURE 11–35. Are antipsychotics with **multiple therapeutic mechanisms** better than selective D2 antagonists or selective SDAs? The original phenothiazine antipsychotics are conceptualized as conventional antipsychotics with the desirable pharmacologic property of D2 antagonism, whereas their other pharmacologic properties are considered unwanted, and the cause of side effects (see left hand of spectrum). Thus, when higher-potency D2 antagonists with lesser secondary pharmacologic properties were introduced, such as haloperidol, this was considered an advance (see middle of spectrum). During this era, the idea was that the most desirable agents were those with the greatest selectivity and with only one primary action, namely D2 antagonism. Next, in the SDA era, the concept was developed that, at a minimum, 5HT2A antagonism (SDA) should be combined with D2 antagonism to make a more efficacious, better tolerated antipsychotic, namely an atypical antipsychotic. Taking things a step further is the proposition that even greater efficacy can be attained with a further mix of pharmacologic properties, especially for treatment-refractory schizophrenia and for treating additional dimensions of symptoms in schizophrenia beyond positive and negative symptoms, such as mood and cognition symptoms.

Each of the major atypical antipsychotics differs on how well these various favorable and unfavorable clinical features have been established in large clinical trials. Furthermore, individual patients can have responses very different from the median response predicted from group outcomes of clinical trials, as well as very different responses to one of these agents as compared with another. In practice, therefore, the currently marketed agents in the atypical antipsychotic class can each be appreciated as much for the differences they have from one another as for the pharmacological and clinical actions they share.

Although it is not yet clear why the various atypical antipsychotics differ from each other, the answer is most likely to be found in the pharmacologic properties, other than serotonin 2A dopamine–2 antagonism, that they do *not* share in common. Although some of these properties are still unknown, many of them are known (and are shown in Figure 11–34 and in the individual icons for the various atypical antipsychotics discussed later in this chapter). Of the 17 pharmacologic properties detailed in these icons, some undoubtedly mediate side effects, and others may mediate additional therapeutic actions mentioned here. This raises the question: Are atypical antipsychotics with multiple therapeutic mechanisms better than those with fewer therapeutic mechanisms (see Fig. 11–35)? This theme of multiple pharmacologic mechanisms possibly having synergistic actions has already been discussed extensively in Chapter 7 for antidepressants (see Fig. 7–3).

The idea of synergy among multiple pharmacologic mechanisms also forms the rationale for combining drugs of differing therapeutic actions in patients who do not respond to various antidepressants with single pharmacologic mechanisms, as discussed extensively in Chapter 7. Could such a rationale also explain why one schizophrenic patient may sometimes respond to an atypical antipsychotic with one specific blend of multiple pharmacologic mechanisms better than to another atypical antipsychotic with a different mixture of such mechanisms? Head-to-head comparisons of atypical antipsychotics are only beginning to help develop a rational basis for choosing one atypical antipsychotic over another now that the superiority of this class of agents over conventional antipsychotics seems well established. Currently, the best atypical antipsychotic for an individual patient is often discovered by trial and error. Because differences among the drugs in this class can be important, a brief discussion of each of the five agents currently in clinical use is included here. Other specific agents will be discussed in later sections of this chapter.

## Clozapine

Clozapine is considered to be the prototype of the atypical antipsychotics, as it was the first to be recognized as having few if any extrapyramidal side effects, not causing tardive dyskinesia, and not elevating prolactin. Clozapine is one of five antipsychotics with somewhat related chemical structures (Fig. 11–36). Although certainly a serotonin 2A–dopamine 2 antagonist, clozapine also has one of the most complex

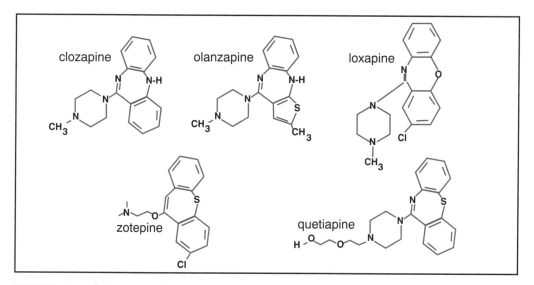

FIGURE 11–36. Structural formulas for clozapine and four other antipsychotics, namely, olanzapine, quetiapine, loxapine, and zotepine. Interestingly, all five of these are also SDAs, but not all of them appear to be atypical antipsychotics (e.g., loxapine is conventional, and zotepine is still being characterized). Also, clinical properties and pharmacological characteristics vary considerably among those that are clearly atypical (i.e., clozapine, olanzapine, and quetiapine).

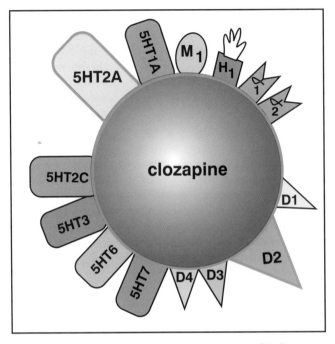

FIGURE 11–37. **Clozapine's** pharmacologic icon. The most prominent binding properties of cloza-pine are represented here; it has perhaps one of the most complex binding portfolios in psychophar-macology. Its binding properties vary greatly with technique and species and from one laboratory to another. This icon portrays a qualitative consensus of current thinking about the binding properties of clozapine, which are constantly being revised and updated.

pharmacologic profiles in psychopharmacology, let alone among the atypical anti-psychotics (Fig. 11–37).

Clozapine is the one atypical antipsychotic recognized as particularly effective when conventional antipsychotic agents have failed. Although patients may occa-sionally experience an "awakening" (in the Oliver Sachs sense), characterized by return to a near normal level of cognitive, interpersonal, and vocational functioning and not just significant improvement in positive symptoms of psychosis, this is unfortunately quite rare. The fact that it can be observed at all, however, gives hope to the possibility that a state of wellness might some day be achieved in schizo-phrenia by the right mix of pharmacologic mechanisms. Such awakenings have been observed on rare occasions in association with treatment with other atypical anti-psychotics as well, but rarely if ever in association with conventional antipsychotic treatment.

Clozapine is also the only antipsychotic drug associated with the risk of a life-threatening and occasionally fatal complication called *agranulocytosis* which occurs in 0.5 to 2% of patients. Because of this, patients must have their blood counts mon-itored weekly for the first 6 months of treatment and then every 2 weeks for as long as they are treated. Clozapine also entails an increased risk of seizures, especially at high doses. It can be very sedating and is associated with the greatest degree of weight gain among the antipsychotics. Thus, clozapine may have the greatest efficacy but the most side effects among the atypical antipsychotics.

Pharmacologists have been attempting to define what it is about clozapine's biochemical mechanism of action that accounts for its special efficacy as well as its side effects. As discussed extensively in this chapter, SDA properties may account in part for reducing EPS, for reducing tardive dyskinesia, and perhaps even for lack of prolactin elevation; SDA properties may even help explain improvement in negative symptoms of schizophrenia. However, the concept of SDA does not appear to explain the therapeutic actions of clozapine in treatment-resistant cases because clozapine is superior to other agents that share this property.

Serotonin-dopamine antagonist properties also do not explain clozapine's side effects of weight gain, sedation, seizures, and agranulocytosis. The mechanism of clozapine's induction of agranulocytosis remains unclear, but fortunately no other atypical antipsychotic drug appears to share this problem. Seizures are also poorly understood but are not a serious problem for any other atypical antipsychotic. Weight gain, most notorious for clozapine among all of the atypical antipsychotics, appears to correlate best with its antihistaminic binding properties, perhaps made worst by concomitant serotonin 2C antagonist actions. Sedation may be linked to antihistaminic and anticholinergic actions.

In view of the risk/benefit ratio for clozapine, this agent is not generally considered a first-line agent for the treatment of psychosis but one to consider when several other agents have failed. It is especially useful in quelling violence and aggression in difficult patients, may reduce suicide rates in schizophrenia, and may reduce tardive dyskinesia severity, especially over long treatment intervals.

### Risperidone

This agent has a different chemical structure (Fig. 11–38) and a considerably simpler pharmacologic profile than clozapine (Fig. 11–39). Risperidone is especially atypical at lower doses but can become more "conventional" at high doses in that EPS can occur if the dose is too high. Risperidone thus has favored uses, not only in schizophrenia at moderate doses but also for conditions in which low doses of conventional antipsychotics have been used in the past, for example, for elderly patients with

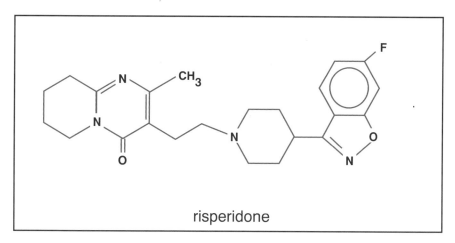

risperidone

FIGURE 11–38. Structural formula of risperidone.

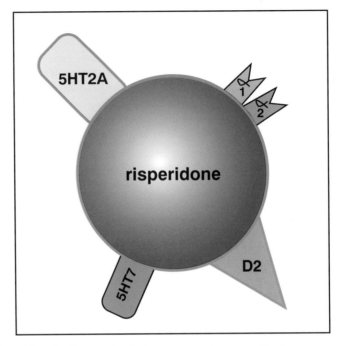

FIGURE 11–39. **Risperidone**'s pharmacologic icon, portraying a qualitative consensus of current thinking about the binding properties of this drug. Among the atypical antipsychotics, it has one of the simplest pharmacologic profiles and comes closest to an SDA. As with all atypical antipsychotics discussed in this chapter, binding properties vary greatly with technique and species and from one laboratory to another; they are constantly being revised and updated.

psychosis, agitation, and behavioral disturbances associated with dementia (see also Chapter 12) and for children and adolescents with psychotic disorders. Although risperidone is an SDA, for reasons that are not clear it elevates prolactin to the same degree as conventional antipsychotics, even at low doses.

Many studies show that risperidone is a highly effective agent for positive symptoms of schizophrenia and also improves negative symptoms of schizophrenia better than do conventional antipsychotics. Early studies show a very low incidence of tardive dyskinesia with long-term use and also show that some patients improve on risperidone when conventional antipsychotics fail, although probably not as well as they would on clozapine. Ongoing studies suggest that risperidone may improve cognitive functioning not only in schizophrenia, but also in dementias, such as Alzheimer's disease. Risperidone may also improve mood in schizophrenia and in both the manic and depressed phases of bipolar disorder. There is less weight gain with risperidone than with some other atypical antipsychotic agents, perhaps because risperidone does not block histamine 1 receptors, but weight gain is still a problem for some patients.

## Olanzapine

Although olanzapine has a chemical structure related to that of clozapine (Fig. 11–36), it is more potent than clozapine and has several differentiating pharmacologic

(Fig. 11–40) and clinical features, not only as compared with clozapine (Fig. 11–37) but also as compared with risperidone (Fig. 11–39). Olanzapine is atypical in that it generally lacks EPS, not only at moderate doses but usually even at high doses. Thus, olanzapine tends to be used for some of the most difficult cases of schizophrenia, bipolar disorder, and other types of psychosis in which good control of psychosis without EPS is still desired, yet aggressive treatment is required. On the other hand, this approach can be very expensive.

Olanzapine lacks the extreme sedating properties of clozapine but can be somewhat sedating. Olanzapine is associated with weight gain, perhaps because of its antihistaminic and serotonin 2C antagonist properties (Fig. 11–40). Olanzapine does not often raise prolactin. Early studies suggest a very low incidence of tardive dyskinesia with long-term use and also suggest that some patients improve with olanzapine when conventional antipsychotics fail, although probably not as much as they would with clozapine. Many studies demonstrate that olanzapine is highly effective for positive symptoms of schizophrenia and also improves negative symptoms of schizophrenia better than do conventional antipsychotics. Ongoing studies also show that olanzapine improves mood, not only in schizophrenia but also in the manic and depressed phases of bipolar disorder, suggesting that it may be a first-line treatment for bipolar disorder, as discussed in Chapter 7. Some studies suggest that olanzapine may improve cognitive functioning in schizophrenia and in dementia.

## Quetiapine

Quetiapine also has a chemical structure related to that of clozapine (Fig. 11–36), but it has several differentiating pharmacologic (Fig. 11–41) and clinical features, not only as compared with clozapine (Fig. 11–37) but also as compared with risperidone (Fig. 11–39) and olanzapine (Fig. 11–40). Quetiapine is very atypical in that it causes virtually no EPS at any dose and no prolactin elevations. Thus, quetiapine tends to be the preferred atypical antipsychotic for patients with Parkinson's disease and psychosis. It is also useful in schizophrenia, bipolar disorder, and other types of psychosis, in which it has few extrapyramidal side effects.

Quetiapine can cause some weight gain, as it blocks histamine 1 receptors. It has shown species-specific inhibition of cholesterol biosynthesis in the lens of some animals, where it can cause cataracts, but is not documented to do this in humans. Some patients improve on quetiapine when conventional antipsychotics fail, although probably not as well as on clozapine. Studies demonstrate that quetiapine is highly effective for the positive symptoms and also improves the negative symptoms of schizophrenia. Ongoing studies are beginning to show that quetiapine may improve mood in schizophrenia and in the manic and depressed phases of bipolar disorder. Some studies suggest that quetiapine may improve cognitive functioning in schizophrenia and also in dementia.

## Ziprasidone

Ziprasidone has a novel chemical structure (Fig. 11–42) and a quite novel pharmacological profile as compared with the other atypical antipsychotics (Fig. 11–43). Ziprasidone appears to be atypical, like the other agents in this class, in that it has low EPS and causes little or no prolactin elevation. Its major differentiating feature

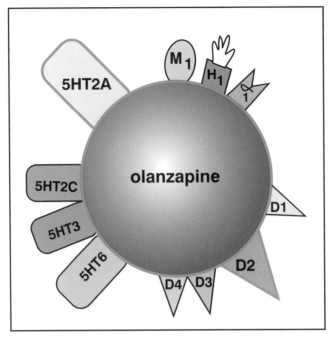

FIGURE 11–40. **Olanzapine**'s pharmacologic icon, portraying a qualitative consensus of current thinking about the binding properties of this drug. It has a complex pharmacology overlapping, yet different from, that of clozapine. As with all atypical antipsychotics discussed in this chapter, binding properties vary greatly with technique and species and from one laboratory to another; they are constantly being revised and updated.

within this class may be that it seems to have little or no propensity to cause weight gain, perhaps because it has no antihistaminic properties, although it does have serotonin 2C antagonist actions. Also, ziprasidone is the only atypical antipsychotic that is a serotonin 1D antagonist, a serotonin 1A agonist, and also inhibits both serotonin and norepinephrine reuptake. These latter pharmacologic actions would be expected to be both proserotonergic and pronoradrenergic, which might contribute to ziprasidone's favorable behavior as concerns weight but would predict antidepressant and anxiolytic actions as well. Antidepressant actions are being actively tested in schizophrenia and bipolar disorder to determine whether ziprasidone's theoretically advantageous pharmacological features will be demonstrable in head-to-head comparisons with other atypical antipsychotic agents.

Some patients improve with ziprasidone when conventional antipsychotics fail, although probably not as much as with clozapine. Studies demonstrate that ziprasidone is highly effective for the positive symptoms and also improves the negative symptoms of schizophrenia. Some studies suggest that ziprasidone may improve cognitive functioning in schizophrenia and also in dementia.

## Pharmacokinetic Considerations for the Atypical Antipsychotic Drugs

Many of the general principles of pharmacokinetics were introduced in Chapter 6 on antidepressants (see also Figs. 6–8 through 6–20). Here we will discuss some specific pharmacokinetic issues relating to antipsychotic drugs.

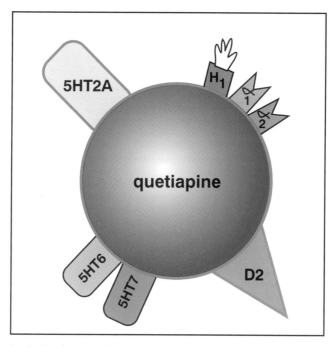

FIGURE 11–41. **Quetiapine**'s pharmacologic icon, portraying a qualitative consensus of current thinking about the binding properties of this drug. It has a unique pharmacological profile, different from those of all other atypical antipsychotics. As with all atypical antipsychotics discussed in this chapter, binding properties vary greatly with technique and species and from one laboratory to another; they are constantly being revised and updated.

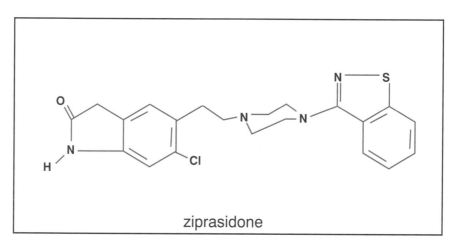

FIGURE 11–42. Structural **formula** of **ziprasidone**.

## Cytochrome P450 1A2

Recall that one of the key drug-metabolizing enzymes is the cytochrome P450 (CYP450) enzyme called 1A2. Two atypical antipsychotic drugs are substrates of 1A2, namely olanzapine and clozapine. That means that when they are given con-

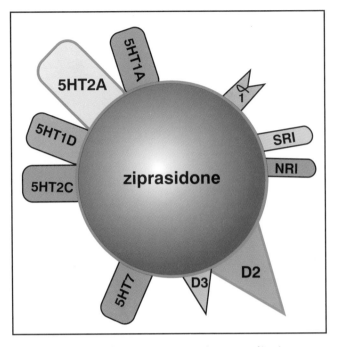

FIGURE 11–43. **Ziprasidone**'s pharmacologic icon, portraying a qualitative consensus of current thinking about the binding properties of this drug. It is the only atypical antipsychotic with 5HT1D antagonist and serotonin-norepinephrine reuptake blocking properties. As with all atypical antipsychotics discussed in this chapter, binding properties vary greatly with technique and species and from one laboratory to another; they are constantly being revised and updated.

comitantly with an inhibitor of this enzyme, such as the antidepressant fluvoxamine, their levels could rise (Fig. 11–44). Although this may not be particularly clinically important for olanzapine (other than causing slightly increased sedation), it could potentially raise plasma levels sufficiently in the case of clozapine to increase the risk of seizures. Thus, the dose of clozapine may need to be lowered when administering it with fluvoxamine, or another antidepressant may need to be chosen.

On the other hand, when an inducer of 1A2 is given concomitantly with either of the two antipsychotic substrates of 1A2, the level of the antipsychotic may fall. This happens when a patient begins to smoke, because smoking induces 1A2, and this would cause levels of olanzapine and clozapine to fall (Fig. 11–45). Theoretically this might cause patients stabilized on an antipsychotic dose to relapse if the levels fell too low. Also, cigarette smokers may require higher doses of these atypical antipsychotics than nonsmokers.

### Cytochrome P450 2D6

Another cytochrome P450 enzyme of importance to atypical antipsychotic drugs is 2D6. Risperidone, clozapine, and olanzapine are all substrates for this enzyme (Fig. 11–46). Risperidone's metabolite is also an active atypical antipsychotic (Fig. 11–47), but the metabolites of clozapine and olanzapine are not. Recall that some antidepressants are inhibitors of CYP450 2D6 and thus can raise the levels of these

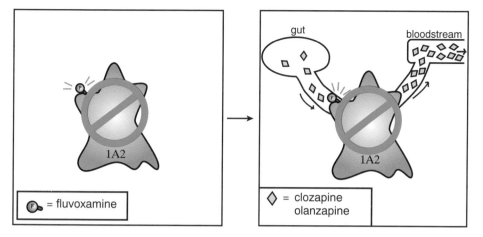

FIGURE 11–44. Clozapine and olanzapine are **substrates** for cytochrome P450 1A2 (CYP450 1A2). When these drugs are given with an inhibitor of this enzyme, such as the antidepressant fluvoxamine, plasma levels of olanzapine and clozapine can rise.

three atypical antipsychotics (Fig. 11–48). For risperidone the clinical significance of this is uncertain, since both the parent drug and the metabolite are active. Theoretically, the dose of olanzapine and clozapine may have to be lowered when given with an antidepressant that blocks 2D6, although this is not often necessary in practice.

### Cytochrome P450 3A4

The CYP450 enzyme 3A4 metabolizes several atypical antipsychotics, including clozapine, quetiapine, ziprasidone, and sertindole (Fig. 11–49). Several psychotropic drugs are weak inhibitors of this enzyme, including the antidepressants fluvoxamine, nefazodone, and norfluoxetine, which is an active metabolite of fluoxetine. Several nonpsychotropic drugs are powerful inhibitors of 3A4, including ketoconazole (antifungal), protease inhibitors (for human immunodeficiency virus (HIV) infections) and erythromycin (antibiotic). For the four atypical antipsychotics that are metabolized by 3A4, the clinical implication is that concomitant administration with a 3A4 inhibitor may require dosage reduction of the atypical antipsychotic (Fig. 11–50).

Drugs can not only be substrates for a cytochrome P450 enzyme or an inhibitor of a P450 enzyme, they can also be inducers of a cytochrome P450 enzyme and thereby increase the activity of that enzyme. This was discussed in Chapter 6 for CYP450 3A4, and the induction of 3A4 activity by the anticonvulsant and mood stabilizer carbamazepine was given as an example (Fig. 6–19). Since mood stabilizers may be frequently mixed with atypical antipsychotics, it is possible that carbamazepine may be added to the regimen of a patient previously stabilized on clozapine, quetiapine, ziprasidone, or sertindole. If so, the doses of these atypical antipsychotics may need to be increased over time to compensate for the induction of 3A4 by carbamazepine.

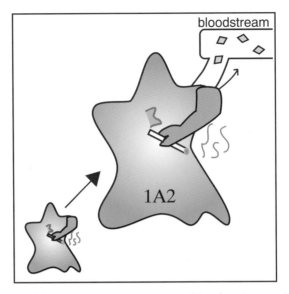

FIGURE 11–45. **Cigarette smoking**, quite common among schizophrenics, can induce the enzyme CYP450 1A2 and lower the concentration of drugs metabolized by this enzyme, such as olanzapine and clozapine. Smokers may also require higher doses of these drugs than nonsmokers.

On the other hand, if carbamazepine is stopped in a patient receiving one of these four atypical antipsychotics, the antipsychotic dose may need to be reduced, because the autoinduction of 3A4 by carbamazepine will reverse over time (Fig. 11–51).

## Atypical Antipsychotics in Clinical Practice

The atypical antipsychotics are still relatively new, particularly some members. Information about new drugs is first available from clinical trials and then modified by observations from clinical practice, and the atypical antipsychotics are no exception to this pattern. Some findings from clinical practice have already confirmed those from clinical trials for the three marketed atypical antipsychotics (i.e., risperidone, olanzapine, and quetiapine) and are generally applicable to choosing an atypical antipsychotic for patients with a wide variety of psychotic disorders, although least is known about ziprasidone, the newest member of this group.

There are four main favorable findings.

First, atypical antipsychotics undoubtedly cause far fewer EPS than do conventional antipsychotics and often cause essentially no EPS (i.e., they really do perform in this respect, as predicted pharmacologically and as advertised). Second, atypical antipsychotics reduce negative symptoms of schizophrenia better than do conventional antipsychotics, but this may be because they do not make things worse as much as because they really reduce negative symptoms. The magnitude of this effect is not as robust as the effects on EPS, and further innovations will be necessary to solve the negative symptom problem in schizophrenia—nevertheless, this is a good start. Third, atypical antipsychotics reduce affective symptoms in schizophrenia and related disorders such as treatment-resistant depression and in bipolar disorder, where treatment effects appear to be quite robust. Fourth, atypical antipsychotics may

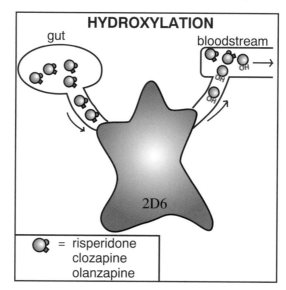

FIGURE 11–46. Several atypical antipsychotics are **substrates** for the enzyme **CYP450 2D6**, including risperidone, clozapine, and olanzapine.

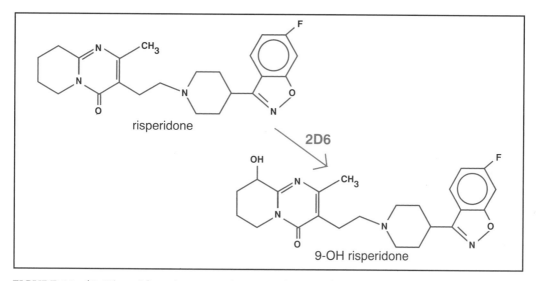

FIGURE 11–47. **Risperidone** is converted to an **active metabolite** by the enzyme CYP450 2D6.

possibly reduce cognitive symptoms in schizophrenia and related disorders such as Alzheimer's disease.

The magnitude of these properties is far from trivial and, in fact, makes the four atypical antipsychotics risperidone, olanzapine, quetiapine, and ziprasidone easily preferable as first-line therapies for psychosis, with conventional antipsychotics and clozapine as second-line therapies.

On the other hand, not everything that is suggested from controlled clinical trials of restricted populations of patients undergoing studies in ideal situations turns out

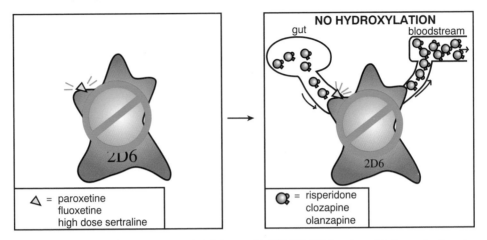

FIGURE 11–48. Several antidepressants are **inhibitors** of **CYP450 2D6** and could theoretically raise the levels of 2D6 substrates such as risperidone, olanzapine, and clozapine. However, this is not usually clinically significant.

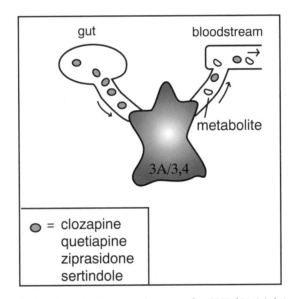

FIGURE 11–49. Several atypical antipsychotics are **substrates** for **CYP450 3A4**, including clozapine, quetiapine, ziprasidone, and sertindole.

to be applicable in the real world of clinical practice. Some of the perceptions from longer-term experience deriving from clinical practice that differ from the early indications arising from clinical trials may be summarized as follows.

First, different atypical antipsychotics can have clinically distinctive effects in different patients, unlike conventional antipsychotics, which mostly have the same clinical effects in different patients. Thus, median clinical effects in clinical trials may not be the best indicator of the range of clinical responses possible for individual patients. Second, optimal doses suggested from clinical trials often do not match

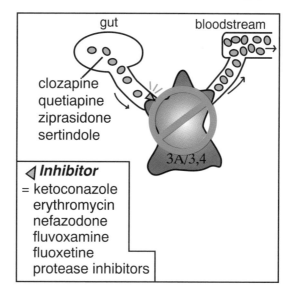

FIGURE 11–50. There are several **inhibitors** of **CYP450 3A4** that may increase levels of some atypical antipsychotics. The inhibitors are shown here, and the atypical antipsychotics including clozapine, quetiapine, ziprasidone, and sertindole, are shown as well.

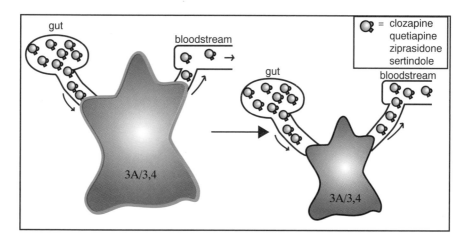

FIGURE 11–51. The enzyme **CYP450 3A4** can be **induced** by the anticonvulsant and mood stabilizer carbamazepine. If this agent is stopped in a patient who is receiving an atypical antipsychotic that is a substrate for this same enzyme (i.e., clozapine, quetiapine, ziprasidone, or sertindole), the doses of these antipsychotics may need to be reduced because the autoinduction of 3A4 by carbamazepine will reverse over time once it is discontinued.

optimal doses used in clinical practice, being too high for some drugs and too low for others. Third, atypical antipsychotics may not work as fast as conventional antipsychotics for acutely psychotic, aggressive, agitated patients requiring sedation and onset of action within minutes; for such patients, conventional antipsychotics or sedating benzodiazepines may be useful as adjuncts or as substitutes. Finally, although virtually all studies are head-to-head comparisons of monotherapies and/or placebo, many patients receive two antipsychotic drugs in clinical settings. Sometimes this is rational and justified, but often it is not.

## Use of Atypical Antipsychotics for Positive Symptoms of Schizophrenia and Related Disorders

Although the usefulness of the atypical antipsychotics is best documented for the positive symptoms of schizophrenia, numerous studies are documenting the utility of these agents for the treatment of positive symptoms associated with several other disorders (discussed in Chapter 10; see Fig. 10–2). Atypical antipsychotics have become first-line acute and maintenance treatments for positive symptoms of psychosis, not only in schizophrenia but also in the acute manic and mixed manic-depressed phases of bipolar disorder; in depressive psychosis and schizoaffective disorder; in psychosis associated with behavioral disturbances in cognitive disorders such as Alzheimer's disease, Parkinson's disease, and other organic psychoses; and in psychotic disorders in children and adolescents (Fig. 11–52, first-line treatments). In fact, current treatment standards have evolved in many countries so that atypical antipsychotics have largely replaced conventional antipsychotics for the treatment of positive psychotic symptoms except in a few specific clinical situations.

One area of continuing use for conventional antipsychotics is in an especially acute setting with an uncooperative patient, where a drug with not only a rapid onset of action but also an intramuscular dosage formulation may be preferred (Fig. 11–52, in case of emergency). In practice, this can mean using sedating benzodiazepines as well as a few of the old-fashioned conventional antipsychotics available for intramuscular administration, such as haloperidol and loxapine. Several atypical antipsychotics are in the late testing stages for acute and chronic intramuscular administration.

Another area of continuing use of conventional antipsychotics is for the noncompliant patient who may require monthly injections of a depot antipsychotic. No atypical antipsychotic is yet available for depot administration, although such formulations are under development. Otherwise, most clinicians generally try several different atypical antipsychotics before resorting to a trial of clozapine (with its encumbrance of weekly or biweekly blood counts), conventional antipsychotics, or various combination therapies of atypical antipsychotics with other agents (Fig. 11–52 second- and third-line treatments).

## Use of Atypical Antipsychotics to Treat Disorders of Mood in Schizophrenia and Related Disorders

Profound mood-stabilizing effects of the atypical antipsychotic drugs were observed once their antipsychotic effects were documented. These effects on mood appear to be quite independent of their effects on positive symptoms of psychosis. The most dramatic story may be how impressive the atypical antipsychotics are turning out to be for the treatment of bipolar disorder (Fig. 11–53). Although the best documented effect of these drugs is to reduce psychotic symptoms in the acute manic phase of bipolar disorder, it is clear that these agents also stabilize mood and can help in some of the most difficult cases, such as those marked by rapid cycling and mixed simultaneous manic-depressed states that are often nonresponsive to mood

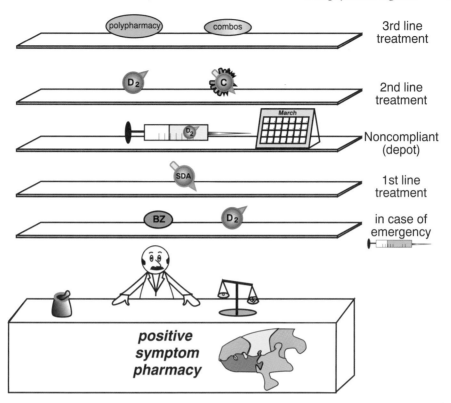

FIGURE 11–52. **Positive symptom pharmacy.** First-line treatment of positive symptoms is now atypical antipsychotics (SDA), not only for schizophrenia but also for positive symptoms associated with bipolar disorder, Alzheimer's disease, childhood psychoses, and other psychotic disorders. However, conventional antipsychotics (D2) and benzodiazepines (BZ) are still useful for acute intramuscular administration (in case of emergency), and D2 for monthly depot injections for noncompliant patients, as well as for second-line use after several atypical agents fail. Clozapine (C), polypharmacy, and combinations (combos) are relegated to second- and third-line treatment for positive symptoms of psychosis.

stabilizers and worsened by antidepressants. The atypical antipsychotics can help stabilize such patients for maintenance treatment, reduce the need for destabilizing antidepressants, and help boost the efficacy of concomitantly administered mood stabilizers.

Mood symptoms of depression are associated with many conditions in addition to major depressive disorder, including mood and anxiety symptoms in schizophrenia, schizoaffective disorder, bipolar manic/depressed/mixed/rapid cycling states, organic mood disorders, psychotic depression, childhood and adolescent mood disorders, treatment-resistant mood disorders, and many more (see Chapter 10, Fig. 10–6). Atypical antipsychotics are enjoying expanded use for the treatment of symptoms of depression and anxiety in schizophrenia that are troublesome but not severe enough to reach the diagnostic threshold for a major depressive episode or anxiety disorder; in these cases the antipsychotics are used not only to reduce such symptoms but hopefully also to reduce suicide rates, which are so high in schizophrenia (Fig. 11–53). Atypical antipsychotics may also be useful adjunctive treatments to anti-

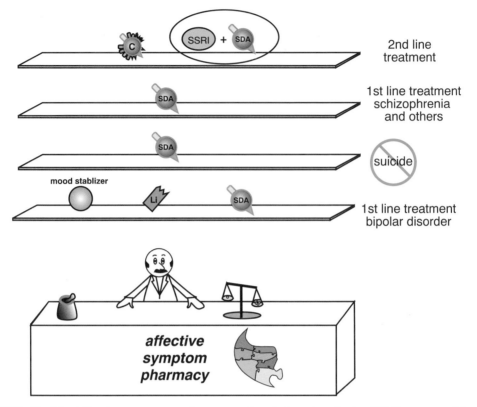

FIGURE 11–53. **Affective symptom pharmacy.** Atypical antipsychotics (SDA) are surprisingly effective in stabilizing mood in a number of disorders and are now becoming first-line treatments not only for psychotic symptoms of bipolar disorder (see positive symptom pharmacy in Fig. 11–52), but also for stabilizing manic, mixed, rapid cycling, and treatment-resistant mood states in bipolar patients (first-line treatment). Atypical agents may even reduce suicide rates among schizophrenic patients as well as bipolar disorder patients and improve mood and anxiety, even depression, in a number of disorders other than major depression. Atypical antipsychotics are also employed as adjuncts to anti-depressants in treatment-resistant cases of nonpsychotic unipolar depression (second-line treatment). (Li is lithuim; C is clozapine; SSRI is serotonin selective reuptake inhibitor.)

depressants for unipolar depressed, nonpsychotic patients when several other anti-depressants have failed.

## Use of Atypical Antipsychotics for Cognitive Symptoms of Schizophrenia and Related Disorders

The severity of cognitive symptoms correlates with the long-term prognosis of schizophrenia. Cognitive symptoms clearly are a dimension of psychopathology that cuts across many disorders in psychiatry and neurology (see Chapter 10; Fig. 10–4). The atypical antipsychotics may improve cognition in several of these disorders and do this independently of their ability to reduce positive symptoms of psychosis (Fig. 11–54). In schizophrenia, there may be improvements in verbal fluency, serial learning, and executive functioning. In Alzheimer's disease, there may be improve-

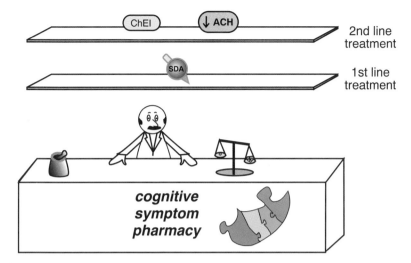

FIGURE 11–54. **Cognitive symptom pharmacy**. Atypical antipsychotic drugs (SDA) may improve cognitive functions in both schizophrenic and Alzheimer patients (first-line treatment). They may boost the actions of cholinesterase inhibitors (ChEIs) in Alzheimer's disease. It may also be useful to discontinue any anticholinergic medication that you can, a welcome bonus when switching from conventional antipsychotics to atypical antipsychotics (decreased A Ch).

ments in memory and behavior, which could be additive or even synergistic with the improvement attained with concomitant treatment with other types of cognitive enhancers, such as the cholinesterase inhibitors (see Chapter 12). Much work is ongoing to see how treatment with atypical antipsychotics can optimize cognitive function in schizophrenia and related disorders.

## Use of Atypical Antipsychotics for Negative Symptoms of Schizophrenia

The negative symptoms of schizophrenia are thought to constitute a particularly unique feature, although certain aspects of these symptoms can overlap with symptoms that are not unique to schizophrenia itself (see Chapter 10 and Fig. 10–3). Any improvement in negative symptoms that can be gained from treatment with atypical antipsychotics is very important because the long-term outcome of schizophrenia is more closely correlated with severity of negative symptoms than it is with the severity of positive symptoms. However, it is already clear that significantly more robust treatment effects will be necessary than those offered by atypical antipsychotics if such symptoms are to be eliminated in the vast majority of schizophrenic patients. Nevertheless, there are two approaches to improving negative symptoms in the short run. First, negative symptoms secondary to conventional antipsychotics can be readily reduced by substituting an atypical antipsychotic (Fig. 11–55). Second, atypical antipsychotics actually improve negative symptoms. Olanzapine and risperidone have already documented better negative symptom improvement than conventional antipsychotics (Fig. 11–55, first-line treatment); quetiapine and ziprasidone have so far documented better negative symptom improvement than placebo (Fig. 11–55, second-line treatment).

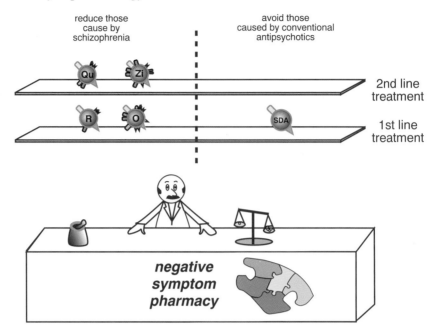

FIGURE 11–55. **Negative symptom pharmacy**. Negative symptoms can be improved in schizophrenia, both by switching from conventional antipsychotics, that make these symptoms worse to atypical antipsychotics (SDA) that do not (right-hand side of pharmacy) or by the direct effects of atypical antipsychotics that boost negative symptoms. Olanzapine (O) and risperidone (R) both improve negative symptoms in schizophrenics better than do haloperidol or placebo in head-to-trials (first line treatments). Ziprasidone (Zi) and quetiapine (Qu) so far both improve negative symptoms in schizophrenics as well as haloperidol and better than placebo in head-to-head trials (second-line treatments).

## Use of Atypical Antipsychotics for Treating Hostility, Aggression, and Poor Impulse Control in Schizophrenia and Related Disorders

Patients with schizophrenia can obviously be hostile and aggressive, toward self, staff, family, and property. This may take the form of suicide attempts, self-mutilation, poor impulse control, drug abuse, verbal abuse, physical abuse, and/or threatening behavior and may not directly correlate with positive symptoms. It can be a particular problem in a forensic setting. Such problems are commonly a symptom dimension in many psychiatric disorders other than schizophrenia, including many childhood and adolescent disorders such as conduct disorder, oppositional defiant disorder, autism, mental retardation, and attention deficit hyperactivity disorder, as well as borderline personality disorder, bipolar disorders, and various types of organic disorders and brain damage, including head injury, stroke, and Alzheimer's disease (see Chapter 10 and Fig. 10–5). This dimension of psychopathology obvious cuts a wide swath across psychiatric disorders and is not necessarily associated with psychosis. Both conventional and atypical antipsychotics reduce such symptoms (Fig. 11–56), but there are far more studies of hostility and aggression in psychotic illnesses than in nonpsychotic illnesses.

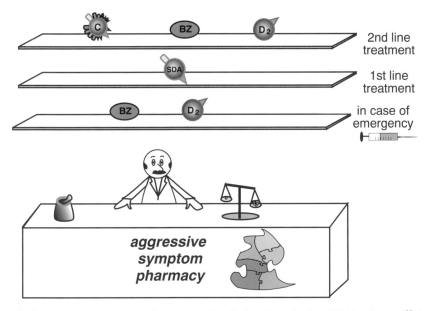

FIGURE 11–56. **Aggressive symptom pharmacy**. Atypical antipsychotics (SDA), when sufficiently effective, are preferable (first line) to conventional antipsychotics (D2) for the management of aggression, hostility, and impulse control because of their more favorable side effect profiles. However, in an acute situation, intramuscular conventional antipsychotics or benzodiazepines (BZ) may be useful, and conventional antipsychotics or clozapine (C) may be required when atypical antipsychotics are not effective (second-line).

### *Antipsychotic Polypharmacy and Managing Treatment Resistance in Schizophrenia*

Schizophrenic patients usually respond to treatment with any single antipsychotic drug, whether conventional or atypical, by improving their positive symptoms at least 30 or 40% on standardized rating scales after a month or two of treatment. However, if a treatment effect of this order of magnitude is not observed after an adequate trial with the first antipsychotic agent (usually an atypical antipsychotic agent according to current treatment guidelines), most clinicians switch to another atypical antipsychotic drug. When switching from one atypical antipsychotic to another, it is frequently prudent to cross-titrate, that is, build down the dose of the first drug while building up the dose of the other (Fig. 11–57). This leads to transient administration of two drugs, but is justified in order to reduce side effects and the risks of rebound symptoms as well as to accelerate the administration of the second drug. However, it is also possible to become trapped in cross-titration (Fig. 11–58). That is, when switching, the patient may improve in the middle of cross-titration, and the clinician may decide to continue both drugs rather than to complete the switch. This type of polypharmacy is not justified, since current treatment guidelines (e.g., those of the American Psychiatric Association) recommend that only after several failures with sequential monotherapies, including consideration of clozapine and conventional antipsychotics, should long-term polypharmacy with two antipsychotics be given.

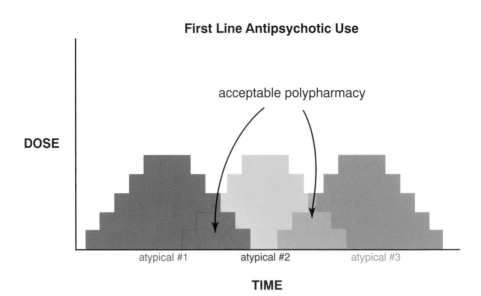

**First Line Antipsychotic Use**

DOSE

acceptable polypharmacy

atypical #1    atypical #2    atypical #3

**TIME**

FIGURE 11–57. When **switching** from one atypical antipsychotic to another, it is frequently prudent to **cross-titrate**, that is, to build down the dose of the first drug while building up the dose of the other. This leads to transient administration of two drugs but is justified in order to reduce side effects and the risk of rebound symptoms and to accelerate the administration of the second drug.

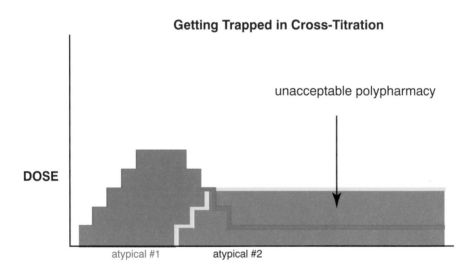

**Getting Trapped in Cross-Titration**

unacceptable polypharmacy

DOSE

atypical #1    atypical #2

**TIME**

FIGURE 11–58. **Getting trapped in cross-titration.** When switching from one atypical antipsychotic to another, the patient may improve in the middle of cross-titration. The polypharmacy that results if cross-titration is stopped and the patient continues both drugs indefinitely without a monotherapy trial of the second drug is not currently justified.

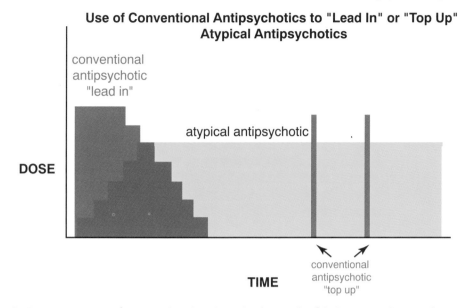

## Use of Conventional Antipsychotics to "Lead In" or "Top Up" Atypical Antipsychotics

conventional
antipsychotic
"lead in"

atypical antipsychotic

**DOSE**

**TIME**

conventional
antipsychotic
"top up"

FIGURE 11–59. Use of **conventional antipsychotics** to "**lead in**" or "*top up*" atypical antipsychotics. One of the most important and justified uses of antipsychotic polypharmacy is to lead in to treatment with a conventional antipsychotic when an unmedicated patient is acutely psychotic, combative, or out of control. Such patients may also require periodic top-up for bouts of aggressiveness, which allows more rapid and robust relief of symptoms than an additional dose of the maintenance atypical antipsychotic can provide.

However, conventional antipsychotics may be added to atypical antipsychotics to "lead in" the initiation of atypical antipsychotic administration for the treatment of positive symptoms, when the more rapid onset of action of the conventional antipsychotics is necessary; the conventional antipsychotics then can be phased out while the atypical antipsychotics are phased in for maintenance in a less acute situation (Fig. 11–59). Conventional antipsychotics may also be useful to periodically "top up" patients receiving atypical antipsychotic maintenance treatment who are experiencing bouts of aggressiveness, thereby also allowing for more rapid and more robust relief of symptoms than an additional dose of the maintenance atypical antipsychotic (Fig. 11–59).

One might expect that with several atypical antipsychotics, plus clozapine, and several conventional antipsychotics, if one follows treatment guidelines, the odds of using long-term maintenance polypharmacy might be relatively low and something reserved as a last resort and for the sickest of the sick. However, audits of antipsychotic use in clinical practice suggest that up to a fourth of outpatients and up to half of inpatients take two antipsychotic drugs for long-term maintenance treatment. Is this a viable therapeutic option for treatment-resistant patients or a dirty little secret of irrational drug use? Whatever it is, the use of two antipsychotic drugs seems to be one of the most practiced and least investigated phenomena in clinical psychopharmacology. It may occasionally be useful to combine two agents when no single agent is effective. On the other hand, it has not proved useful to combine two antipsychotics to get supra-additive antipsychotic effects, such as "wellness" or "awakenings." Although depressed patients frequently recover (see Chapter 5, Fig.

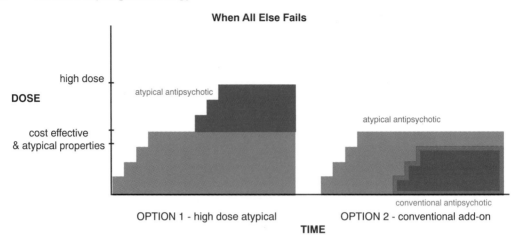

FIGURE 11–60. **When all else fails**, if all of the atypical antipsychotics show insufficient efficacy, it may be necessary to use **high doses**. This is quite costly and leads to loss of the atypical therapeutic advantages of such drugs. Another option is to give a second antipsychotic from the conventional class to **augment** an inadequately efficacious atypical antipsychotic.

5–3), schizophrenic patients rarely achieve wellness, no matter what drug or drug combination is given. Thus, current treatment guidelines suggest that maintenance of patients on two antipsychotics or even very high doses of atypical antipsychotics should be done sparingly when all else fails (Fig. 11–60), and only when clearly demonstrated to be beneficial.

## Other Antipsychotics and Future Antipsychotics

Innovation in the area of schizophrenia is one of the most active research areas in psychopharmacology. Although this is a most exciting topic, it may not be of interest to every reader, and especially not to the beginner or to the generalist. These readers may wish to skip to the summary at the end of the chapter.

### Past as Prologue for Future Antipsychotics

Perhaps the first antipsychotics to have the atypical clinical property of low EPS were thioridazine and mesoridazine, which achieve their clinical effect by potent anticholinergic binding rather than highly potent SDA pharmacology. Sulpiride and amisulpiride are benzamide antipsychotics with low EPS but are neither highly anticholinergic nor serotonin-dopamine antagonists (SDAs). Their exact mechanism of low EPS is not clear but is hypothesized to be related to a preference for meso-limbic over nigrostriatal dopamine receptors in animal models. It is not clear, however, whether they share any of the other features characteristic of SDA atypical antipsychotics, such as improvement in negative symptoms.

Zotepine is an SDA available in several countries, including Japan and some European countries, and has a chemical structure related to that of clozapine (Fig. 11–36) but with distinguishing pharmacologic (Fig. 11–61) and clinical properties. Although an SDA, some EPS have nevertheless been observed, as have prolactin

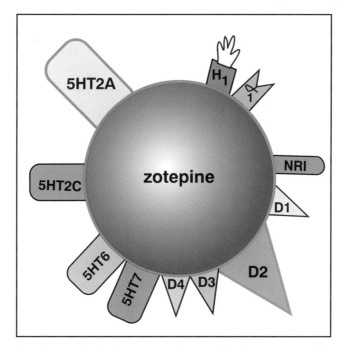

FIGURE 11–61. **Zotepine** pharmacologic icon, portraying a qualitative consensus of current thinking about the binding properties of this drug. As with all atypical antipsychotics discussed in this chapter, binding properties vary greatly with technique and species and from one laboratory to another; they are constantly being revised and updated.

elevations. As with clozapine, there is an increased risk of seizures, especially at high doses, as well as weight gain and sedation. However, there is no clear evidence yet that zotepine is as effective as clozapine for patients who fail to respond to conventional antipsychotics. It is interesting, however that zotepine inhibits norepinephrine reuptake, which suggests potential antidepressant actions. More clinical research is in progress to determine whether zotepine is superior to conventional antipsychotics or to atypical antipsychotics for the treatment of positive symptoms or negative symptoms.

Loxapine is another SDA with a structure related to that of clozapine (Fig. 11–36) but with unique pharmacological properties (Fig. 11–62). As usually dosed, it has an entirely conventional antipsychotic profile, including EPS and elevations in prolactin. There are hints, however, that it may be somewhat atypical at doses much lower than those usually administered, and this has been confirmed by human positron emission tomography (PET) scans. It is one of the few agents available for intramuscular administration and usually causes no weight gain, or it may even cause weight loss. A principal metabolite has noradrenergic reuptake blocking properties, suggesting possible antidepressant actions.

Sertindole is another SDA. It has a structural formula based on serotonin (Fig. 11–63) and also a unique pharmacological profile (Fig. 11–64). It was originally approved in several European countries and then withdrawn from marketing for further investigation of its cardiac properties. It may become available in the future if these issues are satisfactorily resolved. Sertindole causes virtually no EPS at any

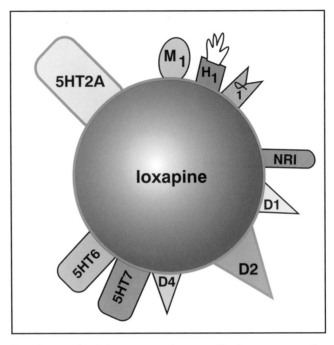

FIGURE 11–62. **Loxapine** pharmacologic icon, portraying a qualitative consensus of current thinking about binding properties of this drug. As with all atypical antipsychotics discussed in this chapter, binding properties vary greatly with technique and species and from one laboratory to another; they are constantly being revised and updated.

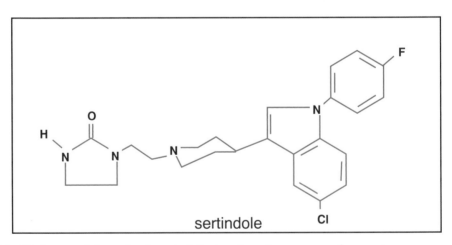

FIGURE 11–63. Structural **formula** of **sertindole**, based on the structure of serotonin.

dose and only rare prolactin elevations. It also causes less weight gain than most other antipsychotics, and like ziprasidone, it does not block histamine receptors, although it does block 5HT2C receptors (Fig. 11–64). It has proved useful in schizophrenia, bipolar disorder, and other types of psychosis, where it has few EPS side effects. Some patients improve with sertindole when conventional antipsychotics

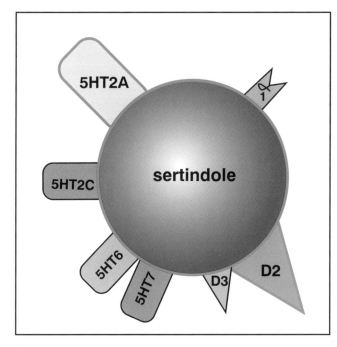

FIGURE 11–64. **Sertindole** pharmacologic icon, portraying a qualitative consensus of current thinking about binding properties of this drug. As with all atypical antipsychotics discussed in this chapter, binding properties vary greatly with technique and species and from one laboratory to another; they are constantly being revised and updated.

fail, although probably not as much as with clozapine. Studies demonstrate that sertindole is highly effective for positive symptoms of schizophrenia and also improves negative symptoms of this disorder.

## Novel Serotonergic and Dopaminergic Mechanisms

Iloperidone is a compound in clinical development with SDA properties, but it has even more potent alpha 1 antagonist properties. Mazapertine is a D2 antagonist, but rather than 5HT2A antagonist properties, it has 5HT1A agonist actions. Nemonapride is a D2 (D3, D4) antagonist and 5HT1A agonist as well. The selective 5HT2A antagonist MDL-100,907 was recently dropped from clinical development, as was the 5HT2A/2C antagonist ritanserin in prior years, both for lack of robust efficacy in schizophrenia. However, there remains some continuing interest in both 5HT2C selective agonists and antagonists, several of which are in early development. There are even novel and selective 5HT6 and 5HT7 antagonists in development as well.

On the dopamine side of the equation, one of the most promising agents in late clinical development is aripiprazole, theoretically a presynaptic D2 autoreceptor agonist. This compound is postulated to exert its antipsychotic actions in a manner far different from serotonin-dopamine antagonism: that is, it may shut off the presynaptic dopamine terminal and stop dopamine release in the mesolimbic dopamine pathway by stimulating presynaptic D2 receptors. The agents CI-1007 and DAB-

452 may have a similar mechanism of action. Several selective D4 antagonists have been tested in schizophrenia, with generally disappointing results, although some trials are continuing. Such compounds, some more selective for D4 receptors than others, include YM-43611, nemonapride, fananserin, L-745,870, PNU-101,387G, NGD-94-4, LU-111,995, and others. Several selective D3 antagonists are being developed, because most known D2 antagonists block D3 receptors as well. It is theoretically possible that pure D3 antagonists, which increase psychomotor behavior in rodents, might activate such behaviors in schizophrenia and thus reduce negative symptoms. Other compounds in testing for schizophrenia include D2 modulators-"normalizers" and D2 partial agonists (e.g., terguride, CI-1007, PNU 9639) and D1-like selective antagonists.

## Novel Neurotransmitter Mechanisms Other Than Serotonin and Dopamine for Therapeutic Strategies in Schizophrenia

*Sigma antagonists.* The physiological functions of the sigma receptors remain poorly characterized; thus, these receptors remain in many ways the "sigma enigma." Originally categorized as one type of opiate receptor, they are now associated with the actions of the psychotomimetic agent phencyclidine (PCP) (see Fig. 10−20 and also Chapter 13 on drug abuse) and the activity of the N-methyl-*d*-aspartate (NMDA) subtype of glutamate receptors (see Figs. 10−18 and 10−19). Theoretically, a sigma antagonist could block any PCP-like actions occurring in schizophrenia. Although early testing of the sigma antagonist BMY-14,802 in schizophrenia was not impressive, other antagonists with greater selectivity, especially SR31742A, have been developed and have entered testing. A combined sigma/5HT1A agonist/5HT reuptake inhibitor, OPC14523, is being tested in depression.

*Cannabinoid antagonists.* Cannabinoid receptors are discussed in further detail in Chapter 13 on drug abuse. An antagonist to cannabinoid 1 (CB1) receptors, SR141716A, reduces the activity of mesolimbic dopamine neurons in animal models, suggesting possible antipsychotic actions in schizophrenia and leading to testing in schizophrenic patients.

*Neurotensin antagonists.* Neurotensin is a peptide neurotransmitter, which is colocalized with dopamine in the mesolimbic dopamine pathway, but is much lower in concentration in the nigrostriatal and mesocortical dopaminergic pathways. A nonpeptide antagonist SR-142948 is in clinical testing in schizophrenia as a theoretical agent that could reduce positive symptoms without producing EPS by exploiting differential actions on the mesolimbic rather than nigrostriatal dopamine system.

*Cholecystokinin.* Cholecystokinin (CCK) is also colocalized with dopaminergic neurons and has two receptor subtypes, CCK-A being predominantly outside of and CCK-B within the central nervous system. Studies of CCK agonists and antagonists to date have not given clear clues as to their potential for therapeutic actions in schizophrenia.

*Substance P and the neurokinins.* The substance P and neurokinin family of peptide neurotransmitters was extensively discussed in Chapter 5 (see Figs. 5−69 through

5–73). Antagonists to all three neurokinin receptors (i.e., NK-1, NK-2, and NK-3) are now in clinical testing for a variety of indications, predominantly depression. Several are being tested in schizophrenia as well.

*Alpha-7-nicotinic cholinergic agonists.* Although the role of therapeutics for cognition will be more extensively discussed in the chapter on cognitive enhancers (Chapter 12), it is appropriate to consider the role of cognitive enhancers in schizophrenia as well, for this too is a disorder characterized in part by cognitive dysfunction. Furthermore, cholinergic deficiency may not be exclusively associated with Alzheimer's disease, since the alpha 7 nicotinic cholinergic receptor has been implicated in the familial transmission of sensory gating deficits in families with schizophrenia. Deficits in activity at this receptor could theoretically predispose patients to problems with learning efficiency and accuracy and underlie delusional thinking and social dysfunction. In addition, heavy smoking in many schizophrenics (about two-thirds of a North American population of schizophrenics are smokers compared with about one-fourth of nonschizophrenics) is consistent with the high concentration of nicotine necessary to activate the receptor and with the receptor's rapid desensitization. Thus, there are numerous theoretically appealing hypotheses on why to target this receptor to improve particularly cognitive functioning in schizophrenia and in Alzheimer's disease as well.

## Future Combination Chemotherapies for Schizophrenia and Other Psychotic Disorders

Given the economic incentives for providing the "cure" and treatment of choice for psychotic disorders, it is not difficult to understand why most drug development activities for the psychoses target a single disease mechanism, with the goal of discovering the principal therapy for that disorder. In reality, it is probably overly simplistic to conceptualize disorders with psychotic features as products of single disease mechanisms. Diseases such as schizophrenia, bipolar disorder, and Alzheimer's disease not only have psychotic features, but a behavioral dimension, a mood dimension, a cognitive dimension, and in some cases a neurodegenerative dimension. It is difficult to conceptualize how such complex disorders could ever be satisfactorily treated with a single entity acting by a single pharmacologic mechanism. For instance, how could a single therapeutic agent for schizophrenia simultaneously treat the positive symptoms of psychosis, the negative symptoms of psychosis, the cognitive symptoms, and the mood symptoms, prevent further neurodegeneration, and repair neurodevelopmental abnormalities?

Perhaps psychopharmacological treatments for psychotic disorders in the future will need to borrow a chapter out of the book of cancer chemotherapy and HIV/AIDS therapy, in which the standard of treatment is to use multiple drugs simultaneously to attain therapeutic synergy. Combination chemotherapy for malignancy uses the approach of adding together several independent therapeutic mechanisms. When successful, this results in a total therapeutic response that is greater than the sum of its parts.

This approach often has the favorable consequence of simultaneously diminishing total side effects, since adverse experiences of multiple drugs are mediated by different pharmacological mechanisms and therefore should not be additive. Clinical trials with multiple therapeutic agents working by several mechanisms can be quite difficult to undertake, but as there is a clinical trials methodology that exists in the cancer chemotherapy and HIV/AIDS literature, it may be an approach that should be applied to complex neurodegenerative disorders with multiple underlying disease mechanisms, such as schizophrenia. Thus, schizophrenia treatments of the future will almost undoubtedly combine an atypical antipsychotic for positive and negative symptoms and for mood, cognition, and hostility, without causing EPS, tardive dyskinesia, or hyperprolactinemia, with some sort of booster treatment to attain even better relief of negative symptoms (more dopamine?) and cognitive symptoms (alpha 7 nicotinic cholinergic agonist?). Possibly an additional neuroprotective agent (perhaps a glutamate antagonist) will be helpful if stopping future psychotic episodes alone is not sufficient to arrest the downhill course of illness. In the long run, some sort of molecular-based therapy to prevent genetically programmed disease progression or to reverse the consequences of aberrant neurodevelopment may also form part of the portfolio of treatments for schizophrenia.

## Summary

This chapter has reviewed the pharmacology of conventional dopamine 2 antagonist antipsychotic drugs, as well as the new atypical antipsychotic agents that are largely replacing them in clinical practice. The overlapping features of serotonin 2A–dopamine 2 antagonism of the atypical antipsychotics were discussed, as well as multiple unique features that differentiate each of these agents from each other. Pharmacokinetic considerations for the atypical antipsychotic drugs were reviewed, as were various issues important in the use of these agents in clinical practice. Finally, a wide-ranging view of future therapies for schizophrenia was discussed.

# CHAPTER 12

# COGNITIVE ENHANCERS

Pharmacological agents are increasingly being used to enhance cognition. Some agents that enhance cognition, such as antidepressants and atypical antipsychotics, are believed to act in part by improving syndromes that are not categorized primarily as cognitive disorders. These drugs were discussed in previous chapters (see Chapters 6 and 7 on antidepressants and Chapter 11 on antipsychotics). Here we will review pharmacological agents that enhance cognition in disorders with prominent and primary cognitive features. We will discuss the use of such cognitive enhancers from a psychopharmacological perspective rather than from a disease perspective by considering cognitive enhancement in two broad categories, namely, the enhancement of attention with stimulants and the enhancement of memory with cholinesterase inhibitors. This chapter emphasizes concepts about the mechanism of action of psychopharmacological agents rather than specific dosing or prescribing tips, which the reader should obtain by consulting standard prescribing guides. Other important management issues for patients with cognitive disturbances also are not covered here, including diagnostic issues and nonpharmacological management, which can be critical to the outcome for a patient. However, a solid concept of how drugs act on the brain's psychopharmacological mechanisms is an important foundation for understanding how to use these agents and why they work.

## Enhancement of Attention

### Dopamine, Norepinephrine, and the Neuropharmacology of Attention

The catecholamine neurotransmitters dopamine and norepinephrine have the best documented roles in attention, concentration, and associated cognitive functions such as motivation, interest, and learning tasks dependent on being adequately aroused, yet focused. In our earlier discussion of norepinephrine, we emphasized the role of prefrontal noradrenergic pathways in sustaining and focusing attention, as well as in mediating energy, fatigue, motivation, and interest (Chapter 5, Fig. 5–25). In Chapter 10, we emphasized the role of the mesocortical dopamine projection in mediating cognitive functions such as verbal fluency, serial learning, vigilance for executive functioning, sustaining and focusing attention, prioritizing behavior, and modulating behavior based upon social cues (Fig. 10–10). Those discussions were related to how attention is altered in depression (Chapter 5) and schizophrenia (Chapter 10). It should not be surprising if these same pathways and neurotransmitters are implicated in "primary" disorders of attention, such as attention deficit disorder, or in other cognitive disorders such as Alzheimer's disease and various dementias.

Although arousal is usually considered to be a state of increased dopamine and norepinephrine and inattentiveness is considered to reflect deficiencies in these neurotransmitters in these pathways, this is only somewhat true even in persons without a cognitive disorder. Thus, more of these neurotransmitters will enhance attention, but only to a certain extent. Too much of a good thing, like dopamine or norepinephrine, will actually lead to deterioration in cognitive performance. Thus, "hyperarousal" is more likely to be associated with *inability* to concentrate than with heightened attention span.

### Attention Deficit Disorder

Although there are many disorders of attention, ranging from lack of appropriate sleep or motivation in a normal person, to medication side effects to any number of psychiatric and cognitive disorders, here we will only discuss attention deficit disorder, the disorder of attention for which there is the greatest use of stimulant medications as therapeutic agents.

Diagnostic criteria for an "inattentive" type of attention deficit disorder in adults or children must include at least six symptoms of inattention, lasting for at least 6 months. Such symptoms include

1. Often failing to give close attention to details or making careless mistakes in schoolwork, work, or other activities

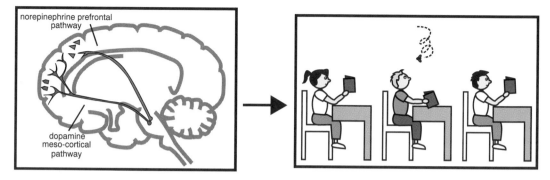

FIGURE 12–1. Noradrenergic and dopaminergic pathways of **attention**. The **noradrenergic** pathway projecting from the locus coeruleus in the brainstem to the frontal cortex and the **dopaminergic** pathway projecting from the ventral tegmental area in the brainstem to mesocortical and dorsolateral prefrontal cortical areas may be the hypothetical mediators of attention, arousal, concentration, and other related cognitive functions. If they fail to function, inattentiveness and attention deficit may result.

2. Often having difficulty sustaining attention in tasks or play activities
3. Often not seeming to listen when spoken to directly
4. Often not following through on instructions and failing to finish school-work, chores, or duties in the workplace (not due to oppositional behavior or failure to understand instructions)
5. Often having difficulty organizing tasks and activities
6. Often avoiding, disliking, or being reluctant to engage in tasks that require sustained mental effort (such as schoolwork or homework)
7. Often losing things necessary for tasks or activities (e.g., toys, school as-signments, pencils, books, or tools)
8. Being often easily distracted by extraneous stimuli
9. Being often forgetful in daily activities
10. Some symptoms of impairment present before age 7

Full diagnostic criteria may be found in DSM IV.

Such symptoms of inattention may map to dopamine and/or norepinephrine dys-function in critical areas of the cerebral cortex controlling cognition (Fig. 12–1). It seems as though patients with such symptoms need a boost in their dopamine/norepinephrine actions, and indeed when they are given agents that boost these systems, their symptoms of inattentiveness can improve.

### Stimulants and Prodopaminergic/Pronoradrenergic Agents as Enhancers of Attention

The most commonly used agents to enhance attention in attention deficit disorder are the stimulants methylphenidate and *d*-amphetamine. Other effective stimulants are not as widely used, pemoline because of liver toxicity and methamphetamine because of its greater abuse potential. Methylphenidate and *d*-amphetamine act pre-dominantly by releasing dopamine from presynaptic dopamine terminals (Figs. 12–2 and 12–3). These agents not only block the dopamine transporter but may actually

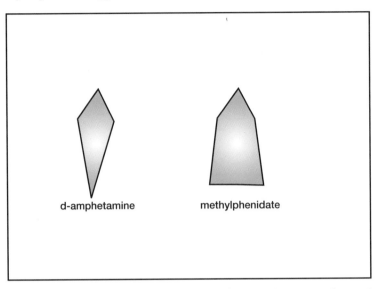

FIGURE 12–2. Icons for *d*-amphetamine and methylphenidate. Both compounds are classified as stimulants, as they both promote the availability of dopamine, thereby enhancing ("stimulating") attention (see also Fig. 12–3).

reverse its direction and make dopamine reverse out of the nerve terminal. Methylphenidate seems to act less quickly but is longer-acting than *d*-amphetamine.

Another form of amphetamine, called *l*-amphetamine, actually releases norepinephrine (Figs. 12–4 and 12–5) as well as dopamine (Fig. 12–3) by a similar mechanism. Some patients respond better to a mixture of *d,l*-amphetamine salts than to pure *d*-amphetamine, perhaps because of the beneficial action of norepinephrine. Other compounds acting on the noradrenergic system that can be beneficial for symptoms of inattentiveness in attention deficit disorder include alpha 2 agonists such as clonidine and guanfacine (Fig. 12–6). Recall that the cognitive effects of norepinephrine in the prefrontal cortex are hypothesized to be mediated in part by postsynaptic alpha 2 adrenergic receptors, as was discussed in Chapter 5 (see Fig. 5–25). Both clonidine and guanfacine are direct-acting alpha 2 adrenergic agonists, which may enhance cognition and attention by this mechanism in attention deficit disorder. It is theoretically possibly that the noradrenergic selective reuptake inhibitor reboxetine could have helpful effects in attention deficit disorder. The prodopaminergic and pronoradrenergic antidepressant bupropion, discussed in Chapter 6 (see Figs. 6–48 and 6–49) can be useful in improving attention in some cases of attention deficit disorder.

## Hyperactivity and Impulsivity Associated with Inattentiveness

No discussion of attention deficit disorder would be complete without mentioning that these patients frequently also have problems with hyperactivity and impulse control, characterized by at least six of the following symptoms for at least 6 months.

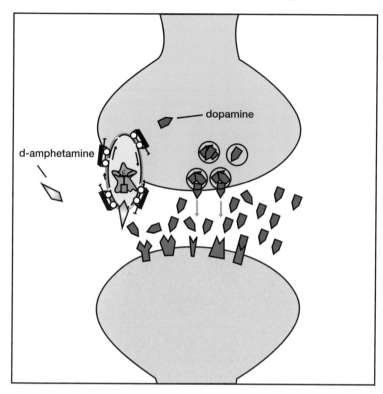

FIGURE 12–3. When *d*-**amphetamine** binds to the presynaptic dopamine transporter on the do-pamine neuron, it not only blocks dopamine reuptake but actually causes dopamine release. There may be a preference or selectivity for cortical over striatal dopamine presynaptic terminals by *d*-amphetamine, so lower doses may have preferential effects on attention rather than on motor activity. Methylphenidate has a similar action, which is not quite as rapid but longer-lasting in many patients.

*Hyperactivity symptoms*

1. Frequent fidgeting with hands or feet or squirming in seat
2. Often leaving seat in classroom or in other situations in which remaining seated is expected
3. Frequent running about or climbing excessively in situations in which it is inappropriate (in adolescents or adults, may be limited to subjective feelings of restlessness)
4. Frequent difficulty playing or engaging in leisure activities quietly
5. Often "on the go" or acting as if "driven by a motor"
6. Frequent excessive talking

*Impulsivity symptoms*

1. Often blurting out answers before questions have been completed
2. Frequent difficulty awaiting turn
3. Frequent interruption of or intruding on others (e.g., butting into conversations or games)

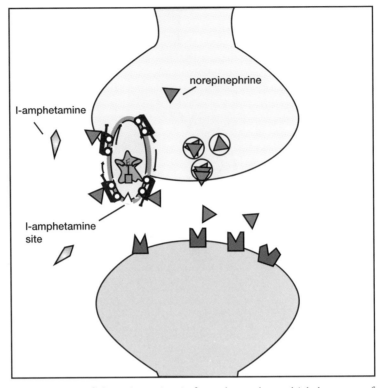

FIGURE 12–4. The enantiomer of *d*-amphetamine is ***l*-amphetamine**, which has no preference between the norepinephrine and the dopamine transporters. Thus, it will target both the **norepinephrine** reuptake site (shown here), as well as the dopamine reuptake site (shown in Fig. 12–2). *d*-Amphetamine is selective for the dopamine transporter.

The symptoms of hyperactivity and impulsivity in this disorder to not appear to be mediated by the same dopaminergic and noradrenergic pathways that mediate the inattentiveness of attention deficit disorder. The most likely candidate to mediate both the hyperactivity and the impulsivity in this condition is the nigrostriatal dopamine pathway (Fig. 12–7). Motor activity is controlled by this pathway. Glutamatergic input from the cortex theoretically also acts as an inhibitory input to the striatum to suppress unwanted obsessions, compulsions, and impulses from other parts of the brain. Although both motor hyperactivity and/or impulsivity and inattentiveness in attention deficit disorder are controlled by dopamine, different pathways are involved (cf. Figs. 12–1 and 12–7). Furthermore, clinical experience suggests that when patients with both sets of clinical symptoms are treated with stimulants (not all patients have both types of problems), low doses seem to prefer the cortex, so there are effects on attention that can appear before effects on motor behaviors. This may be due to greater sensitivity to stimulants of mesocortical dopamine terminals as compared with nigrostriatal dopamine terminals in many patients with attention deficit disorder.

Some unexpected clinical observations have become apparent after several decades of treating attention deficit disorder patients with potentially abusable stimulants (the psychopharmacology of stimulant abuse is discussed in Chapter 13). That is,

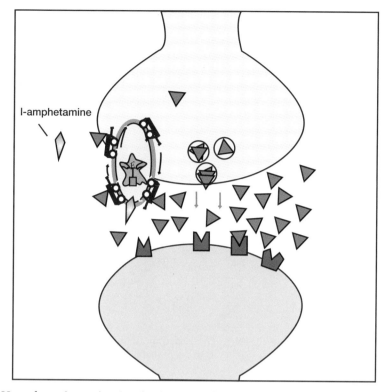

FIGURE 12–5. Here, *l*-amphetamine is releasing **norepinephrine** from presynaptic noradrenergic neurons. It also does this from dopamine neurons, just as shown for *d*-amphetamine in Figure 12–3. When *l*-amphetamine binds to the presynaptic norepinephrine transporter on the norepinephrine presynaptic nerve terminal, it not only blocks norepinephrine reuptake but actually causes norepinephrine release. Thus, *l*-amphetamine releases both norepinephrine and dopamine, whereas *d*-amphetamine is selective for dopamine. Since norepinephrine and dopamine can have different if related cognitive functions in different patients, then *d*- and *l*-amphetamine can have different cognitive effects as well.

the dopamine systems of these patients do not necessarily behave as do those of other individuals when exposed to chronic treatment with stimulants.

Specifically, in attention deficit disorder patients, there is "paradoxical" calming and mental focusing at low doses as well as *reduction* of hyperactive motor movements at higher stimulant doses, whereas many "normal" subjects who take stimulants can become overstimulated and "wired" mentally, and hyperactive with fidgety, excessive motor movements. Furthermore, attention deficit disorder patients show little or no evidence of tolerance or the need for escalating doses over time, whereas others who use stimulants often need higher and higher doses to achieve an enhancement of attention. Still another difference is that in attention deficit disorder patients, there is surprisingly little or no evidence of the phenomenon of "reverse tolerance" or sensitization seen in amphetamine and cocaine abusers, causing psychosis and stimulant abuse (see Chapter 13 on drug abuse for discussion of this phenomenon).

On the other hand, there is also the sense among many clinicians that attention deficit disorder is overdiagnosed and stimulants overprescribed and that these observations do not hold when stimulants are too freely prescribed. Nevertheless, there

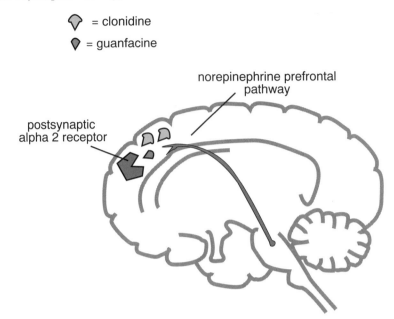

$\mathsf{Q}$ = clonidine

$\mathsf{\Phi}$ = guanfacine

FIGURE 12–6. Postsynaptic **alpha 2** adrenergic receptors are postulated to mediate **cognitive** effects of **norepinephrine** in the frontal cortex. Direct-acting alpha 2 agonists such as clonidine and guanfacine can be helpful in attention deficit disorder, perhaps because of actions at this site.

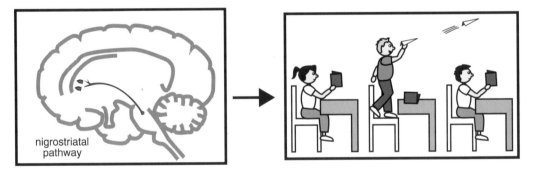

FIGURE 12–7. **Motor hyperactivity** is mediated by **dopaminergic** activity in the **nigrostriatal** pathway. Impulsivity may be inhibited by cortical inhibitory glutamatergic inputs passing through the striatum. Although increasing dopamine in this pathway with stimulants can lead to increased motor behavior and increased impulsivity in normal subjects, it can have a paradoxical motor calming effect and a reduction in behavior impulsivity in patients with attention deficit disorder.

remains a core of individuals with inattentiveness who undoubtedly benefit from stimulant treatment by experiencing a significant enhancement of their attention span and ability to focus and concentrate.

### New Developments for Enhancing Attention

Mood stabilizers and atypical antipsychotics may be helpful in patients who fail to have adequate responses to stimulants, alpha 2 adrenergic agonists, or bupropion, especially if they are misdiagnosed bipolar disorder patients or have comorbid bipolar disorder. Other antidepressants such as venlafaxine may be useful in some cases, and as mentioned earlier, it may be prudent to try reboxetine, although there is little experience with this approach yet.

A new stimulant, modafinil, has been marketed for the treatment of narcolepsy. It has a vague mechanism of action, but may be prodopaminergic, not so much by releasing dopamine as by blocking dopamine reuptake. It may also work through other neurotransmitter systems. There are thus theoretical reasons for considering this agent in disorders of attention. Perceptin (GT2331) is a centrally acting H3 antihistamine, an autoreceptor antagonist whose blockade causes a reduction of histamine release and enhancement of cognitive arousal.

## Enhancement of Memory

### Acetylcholine and the Neuropharmacology of Memory

Memory is obviously one of the most complex functions of the brain and ultimately involves many neuronal pathways and many neurotransmitter systems. However, we currently know that certain disorders disrupt cholinergic neurotransmission specifically and that new therapeutic agents that boost cholinergic neurotransmission can enhance memory in patients with such disorders. Thus, the modern psychopharmacologist requires a working knowledge of cholinergic pharmacology, the disorders that disrupt it, and the therapeutic agents currently available that can improve memory function by acting upon it.

*Acetylcholine synthesis.* Acetylcholine (ACh) is a prominent neurotransmitter, which is formed in cholinergic neurons from two precursors, choline and acetyl coenzyme A (AcCoA) (Fig. 12–8). Choline is derived from dietary and intraneuronal sources, and AcCoA is synthesized from glucose in the mitochondria of the neuron. These two substrates interact with the synthetic enzyme choline acetyltransferase to produce the neurotransmitter ACh.

*Acetylcholine destruction and removal.* Acetylcholine is destroyed by an enzyme called acetylcholinesterase (AChE), which turns ACh into inactive products (Fig. 12–9) and is one of two cholinesterase enzymes capable of breaking down ACh. The other is butyrylcholinesterase (BuChE), also known as pseudocholinesterase and nonspecific cholinesterase. Although both AChE and BuChE can metabolize ACh, they are quite different in that they are encoded by separate genes and have different tissue distributions and substrate patterns. There may be different clinical effects of inhibiting these two enzymes as well. High levels of AChE are present in brain, especially in neurons that receive ACh input; BuChE is also present in brain, especially in glial cells. As discussed below, some of the new drugs for Alzheimer's disease specifically inhibit AChE, whereas others inhibit both enzymes. It is AChE that is the key enzyme for inactivating ACh at cholinergic synapses (Fig. 12–9), although BuChE can take on this activity if ACh diffuses to nearly glia. Acetylcholinesterase is also present in skeletal muscle, red blood cells, lymphocytes, and platelets, and butyrylcholinesterase is also present in plasma, skeletal muscle, placenta, and liver.

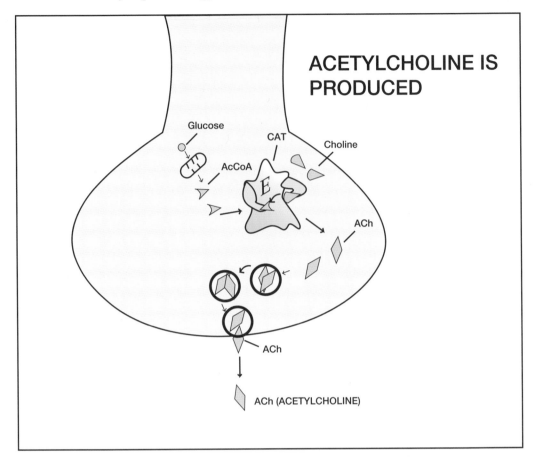

FIGURE 12–8. *Acetylcholine (ACh) is synthesized.* Acetylcholine is a prominent neurotransmitter, which is formed in cholinergic neurons from two precursors, choline and acetyl coenzyme A (AcCoA). Choline is derived from dietary and intraneuronal sources, and AcCoA is made from glucose in the mitochondria of the neuron. These two substrates interact with the synthetic enzyme choline acetyltransferase (CAT) to produce the neurotransmitter acetylcholine (ACh).

Acetylcholine is destroyed too quickly and completely by AChE to be available for transport back into the presynaptic neuron, but the choline that is formed by its breakdown can be transported back into the presynaptic cholinergic nerve terminal by a transporter similar to the transporters for other neurotransmitters discussed earlier in relation to norepinephrine, dopamine, and serotonin neurons. Once back in the presynaptic nerve terminal, this choline can be recycled into acetylcholine synthesis (Fig. 12–8).

*Acetylcholine receptors.* There are numerous receptors for ACh (Fig. 12–10), of which the major subtypes are nicotinic and muscarinic subtypes of cholinergic receptors. Classically, muscarinic receptors are simulated by the mushroom alkaloid muscarine and nicotinic receptors by the tobacco alkaloid nicotine. Nictotinic receptors are all ligand-gated, rapid-onset, and excitatory ion channels, which are blocked by curare. Muscarinic receptors, by contrast, are G protein–linked, can be excitatory or inhib-

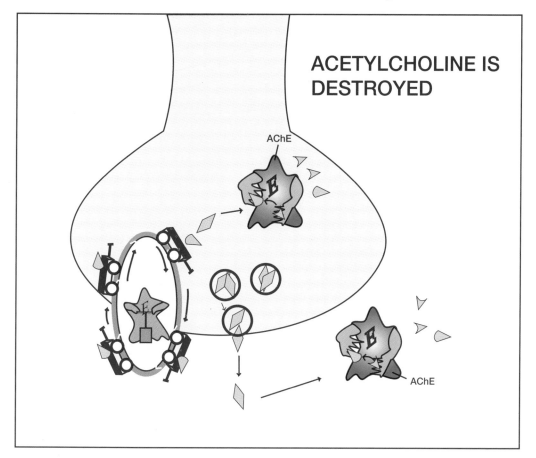

FIGURE 12–9. *Acetylcholine (ACh) destruction and removal.* Acetylcholine is destroyed by an enzyme called acetylcholinesterase (AChE), which turns ACh into inactive products. The actions of ACh can also be terminated by a presynaptic ACh transporter, which is similar to the transporters for other neurotransmitters already discussed earlier in relation to norepinephrine, dopamine, and serotonin neurons.

itory, and are blocked by atropine, scopolamine, and other well-known so-called anticholinergics discussed throughout this text (see, for example Fig. 11–11). Both nicotinic and muscarinic receptors have been further subdivided into numerous receptor subtypes, those for the muscarinic receptors being best known. Perhaps the M1 postsynaptic subtype of muscarinic receptor is the key receptor that mediates memory functions in cholinergic neurotransmission in cerebral cortical sites; however, a role for other cholinergic receptor subtypes has not been ruled out.

*Cholinergic deficiency hypothesis of amnesia.* Numerous investigators have shown that a deficiency in cholinergic functioning is linked to a disruption in memory, particularly short-term memory. For example, blockers of muscarinic cholinergic receptors (such as scolopamine) can produce a memory disturbance in normal human volunteers that has similarities to the memory disturbance in Alzheimer's disease. Boosting cholinergic neurotransmission with cholinesterase inhibitors not only reverses

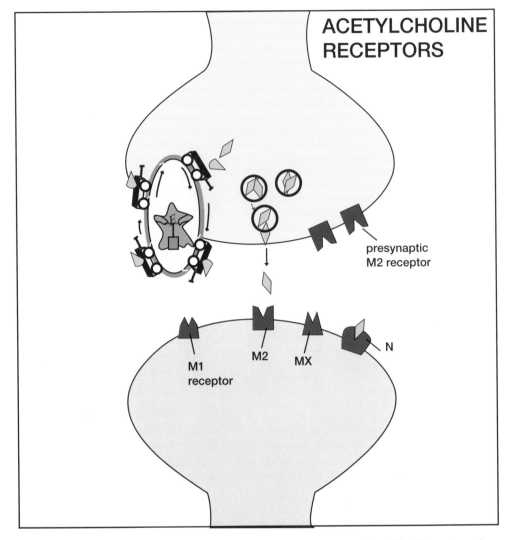

FIGURE 12–10. *Acetylcholine (ACh) receptors.* There are numerous receptors for ACh. The major subdivision is between *nicotinic* (N) and *muscarinic* (M) cholinergic receptors. There are also numerous subtypes of these receptors, best characterized for muscarinic receptor subtypes (M1, M2, Mx). Perhaps the M1 postsynaptic receptor is key to mediating the memory functions linked to cholinergic neurotransmission, but a role for other cholinergic receptor subtypes has not been ruled out.

scopolamine-induced memory impairments in normal human volunteers but also enhances memory functioning in patients with Alzheimer's disease. Both animal and human studies have demonstrated that the nucleus basalis of Meynert is the major brain center for cholinergic neurons that project throughout the cortex. These neurons have the principal role in mediating memory formation (Fig. 12–11). It is suspected that the short-term memory disturbance of Alzheimer patients is due to degeneration of these particular cholinergic neurons. Other cholinergic neurons, such those in the striatum and those projecting from the lateral tegmental area (Fig. 12–12), are not involved in the memory disorder of Alzheimer's disease.

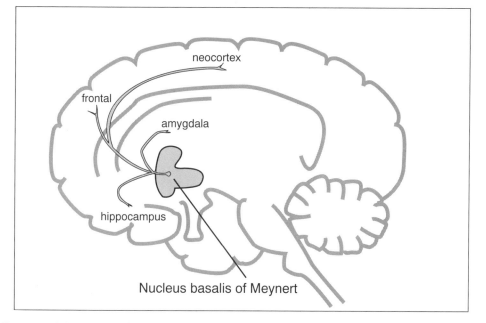

FIGURE 12–11. The **nucleus basalis of Meynert**, located in the basal forebrain, is the principal site of *cholinergic cell bodies* for axons that project to the hippocampus and amygdala and throughout the neocortex. These particular cholinergic neurons are thought to mediate memory and "higher" cortical functions, such as learning, problem solving, and judgment. They degenerate early and progressively throughout the course of Alzheimer's disease.

A "cholinergic deficiency syndrome" due to a limited degeneration of the nucleus basalis could theoretically also be responsible for the more limited short-term memory problems associated with "normal" aging (if there is such a thing), sometimes called mild cognitive impairment. Although Alzheimer's disease may start with a profound cholinergic deficiency, and this is the likely cause of memory disturbances early in its course, the illness is progressive, and many other symptoms develop, such as difficulties in problem solving, judgment, language, and behavior. Thus, it appears that degeneration begins at the nucleus basalis at the time of vague and undiagnosed memory symptoms (Fig. 12–13), spreading to closer projection areas such as the hippocampus, amygdala, and entorhinal cortex by the time of early diagnosis, then spreading diffusely throughout the neocortex by the time of nursing home placement and loss of functional independence, and eventually involving many neurons and neurotransmitters systems by the time of death (Fig. 12–13). Here we will focus just on the cholinergic component of memory and just the memory component of Alzheimer's disease, recognizing that the whole picture is much more complex.

## Impact of Memory Disorders on Cholinergic Neurotransmission

*How Alzheimer's disease kills cholinergic and other neurons leading to memory loss.* Alzheimer's disease is still a pathological, not a clinical diagnosis. It is thus defined by the presence of abnormal degenerative structures seen postmortem in the neocortex,

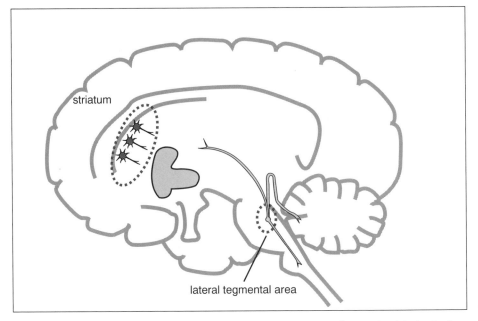

FIGURE 12–12. Other **cholinergic neurons** in the brain are thought to be involved in brain functions other than memory. They include interneurons in the striatum, which are involved in regulating motor movements, and those arising in the lateral tegmental area and projecting rostrally, caudally, and to the cerebellum with a wide variety of functions.

called *neuritic plaques* with *beta-amyloid cores* but also including other proteins such as apolipoprotein A (apo A) (Fig. 12–14) and *neurofibrillary tangles* of abnormally phosphorylated tau proteins (Fig. 12–15). *Neuritic plaques* are extracellular lesions, and their number correlate strongly with cognitive function. Presumably many are formed progressively in the cholinergic neurons of the nucleus basalis of Meynert (Fig. 12–13). *Neurofibrillary tangles* consist largely of a type of protein wrapped into bundles. These proteins are called *tau proteins*, which are chemically altered by being abnormally phosphorylated and then twisted together. The primary element of the neurofibrillary tangle is a paired helical filament, consisting of a ropelike section comprising two fibers wrapped around each other. It is hypothesized that these proteins interfere with nerve functioning in Alzheimer's disease, particularly in cholinergic neurons early in the course of illness, by impairing transport of molecules in the axon of these neurons. As time progresses, the tangles spread, and the consequences of deranged axoplasmic transport appear as a disorder of memory function as well as a disorder of other functions mediated by the cortex (Fig. 12–13).

*Amyloid cascade hypothesis of Alzheimer's disease.* A leading contemporary theory for the biological basis of Alzheimer's disease centers around the formation of beta amyloid. Certainly much of this amyloid destroys cholinergic neurons in the nucleus basalis of Meynert (Fig. 12–11), although the damage becomes more widespread as the disease progresses (Fig. 12–13). Hypothetically, Alzheimer's disease is a disorder in which beta amyloid deposition destroys neurons, in a manner somewhat analogous to that in which the abnormal deposition of cholesterol causes atherosclerosis. Thus,

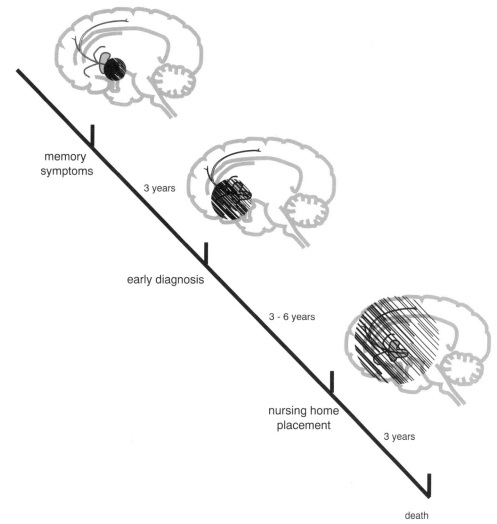

memory
symptoms

3 years

early diagnosis

3 - 6 years

nursing home
placement

3 years

death

**Untreated Course of Alzheimer's Disease**

FIGURE 12–13. The **untreated course of Alzheimer's disease** is progressive and downhill, beginning with very mild and nondiagnostic memory symptoms, probably signaling the beginning of a
process in the nucleus basalis of Meynert. After about 3 years of nonspecific symptoms, a diagnosis of
Alzheimer's disease is made, at which time damage to the cholinergic system has spread at least to
the near projections from the nucleus basalis (i.e.., to the amygdala, hippocampus, and entorhinal
cortex) and the person is losing a great deal of functional independence. In another 3 to 6 years,
neurodegenerative progress now includes the neocortex diffusely; at this stage, the patient is in nursing
home placement, and in a further 3 years is dead.

Alzheimer's disease may be essentially a problem of too much formation of beta
amyloid, or too little removal of it.

One idea is that neurons in some patients destined to have Alzheimer's disease
have an abnormality in the DNA that codes for a protein called *amyloid precursor
protein* (APP) (Fig. 12–16). The abnormal DNA starts a lethal chemical cascade in
neurons (Figs. 12–17 and 12–18), ultimately resulting in Alzheimer's disease (Figs.

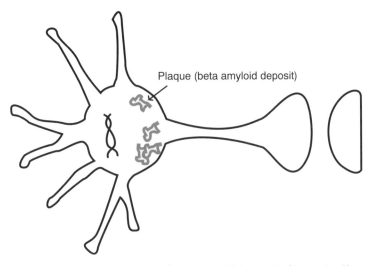

FIGURE 12–14. Postmortem brain pathology defines what Alzheimer's disease is. Shown here are abnormal degenerative structures called **neuritic plaques** with **amyloid cores**.

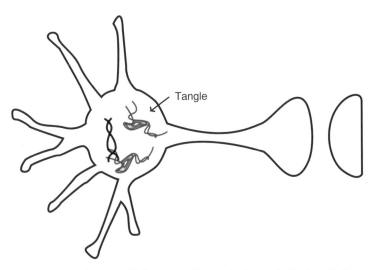

FIGURE 12–15. Another key finding in Alzheimer's disease is the pathological finding of another degenerative structure called **neurofibrillary tangles** made up of abnormally phosphorylated tau proteins.

12–19 and 12–20). Specifically, the abnormal DNA causes the formation of an altered APP (Fig. 12–16), which instead of being removed from the neuron causes formation of beta amyloid deposits (Fig. 12–17). These deposits and fragments go on to form plaques and tangles (Fig. 12–18), the presence of which signals cell damage and cell death (Figs. 12–19 and 12–20). Sufficient cell damage and cell death give rise to the formation of the symptoms in Alzheimer's disease.

Another version of the amyloid cascade hypothesis is the possibility that something is wrong with a protein that binds to amyloid and removes it (Figs. 12–21

# AMYLOID CASCADE HYPOTHESIS

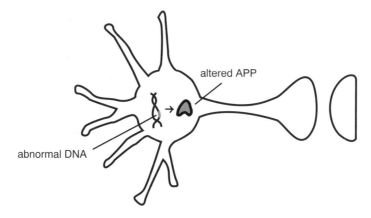

FIGURE 12–16. *The amyloid cascade hypothesis of Alzheimer's disease* (part 1). A leading contemporary theory for the biological basis of Alzheimer's disease centers around the formation of beta amyloid. Perhaps Alzheimer's disease is essentially a disease in which the abnormal deposition of beta amyloid reaches the point of destroying neurons. Thus, Alzheimer's disease may be essentially a problem of too much formation of beta amyloid, or too little removal of it. One idea is that neurons in some patients destined to have Alzheimer's disease have an **abnormality in the DNA** that codes for a protein called amyloid precursor protein (APP). The abnormal DNA starts a lethal chemical cascade in neurons, beginning with the formation of an **altered APP**.

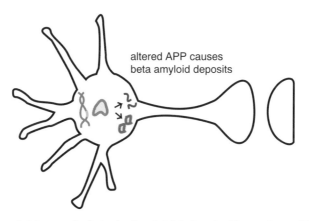

FIGURE 12–17. *The amyloid cascade hypothesis of Alzheimer's disease* (part 2). Once altered amyloid precursor protein (APP) is formed (Fig. 12–16), it leads to the formation of **beta amyloid deposits**.

and 12–22). This protein is called *APO-E*. "Good" APO-E binds to beta amyloid and removes it, preventing the development of Alzheimer's disease and dementia (Fig. 12–21). In the case of "bad" APO-E, a genetic abnormality in APO-E formation causes it to be ineffective in binding beta amyloid. This results in beta amyloid deposition in neurons, which goes on to damage the neurons and cause Alzheimer's disease (Fig. 12–22).

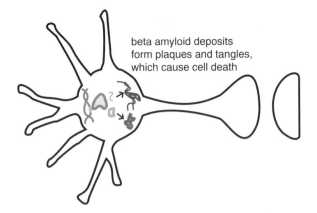

FIGURE 12–18. *The amyloid cascade hypothesis of Alzheimer's disease* (**part 3**). Once beta amyloid deposits are formed from abnormal APP (amyloid precursor protein), the next step is that beta amyloid deposits form plaques and tangles in the neuron.

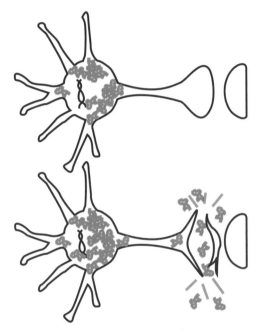

FIGURE 12–19. *The amyloid cascade hypothesis of Alzheimer's disease* (**part 4**). Formation of numerous neuritic plaques eventually causes the neuron to stop functioning and even to die.

Genes coding for APO-E are associated with different risks for Alzheimer's disease. There are three alleles (or copies) of the gene coding for this apolipoprotein which are called E2, E3, and E4. For example, a gene on chromosome 19 that codes for APO-E is linked to many cases of late-onset Alzheimer's disease. Moreover, APO-E is associated with cholesterol transport and involved with other neuronal functions, including repair, growth, and maintenance of myelin sheaths and cell membranes.

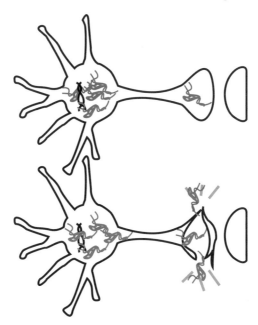

FIGURE 12–20. *The amyloid cascade hypothesis of Alzheimer's disease* (part 5). Formation of numerous neurofibrillary tangles also will eventually cause the neuron to cease to function and even to die.

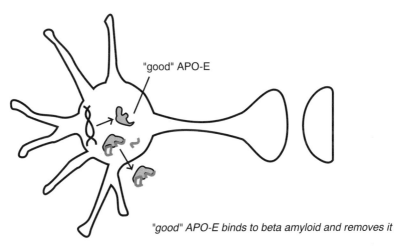

FIGURE 12–21. Another version of the amyloid cascade hypothesis is the possibility that something is wrong with a protein that binds to amyloid and removes it. This protein is called APO-E. In the case of *"good"* APO-E, it binds to beta amyloid and removes it, preventing the development of Alzheimer's disease and dementia.

Having one or two copies of E4 increases the risk of getting Alzheimer's disease, and Alzheimer patients with E4 have more amyloid deposits.

Sporadic cases (i.e., noninherited cases) account for the vast majority of Alzheimer's disease cases, but about 10% of cases are inherited in an autosomal dominant

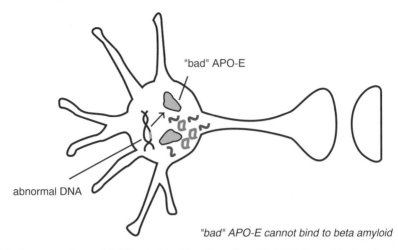

FIGURE 12–22. In comparison with Figure 12–21, where "good" APO-E can bind to beta amyloid and remove it, it is possible that patients with Alzheimer's disease have an **abnormality in their DNA**, which causes the formation of a **defective or "bad" version of the APO-E protein**. In this case, the bad APO-E cannot bind to beta amyloid, so the **amyloid is not removed from the neuron**. Consequently, beta amyloid accumulates, forms plaques and tangles, and the neuron loses its function and dies.

fashion, and they have been intensely investigated for clues to the sporadic disorder. Such rare familial cases are also unusually early in their onset, and, unlike the common sporadic cases, have been linked to mutations in three different chromosomes, namely, 21, 14, and 1. The *first mutation* is on chromosome 21, where there is a defect in the gene for APP, leading to increased deposition of beta amyloid because a longer form of APP is formed. Recall that Down syndrome is a disorder of this same chromosome (i.e., trisomy 21), and virtually all persons with Down syndrome develop Alzheimer's disease if they live past age 50. The *second mutation* known to be associated with a familial form of early-onset Alzheimer's disease is on chromosome 14 in a gene called presenilin 1, which has no known relation to APP. The abnormal protein made by this gene mutation may have effects on membrane ion channels, intracellular protein transport, and cellular differentiation, all of which can affect the rate of neuronal degeneration. The *third mutation* known to be associated with a familial form of early-onset Alzheimer's disease is on chromosome 1, in a similar gene called presenilin 2, also unrelated to APP. It is not clear yet what, if anything, these three mutations in the rare familial cases tell us about the pathophysiology of the usual sporadic, nonfamilial late-onset cases of Alzheimer's disease or, about how cholinergic neurons are damaged in them.

*Other disorders that may kill cholinergic and other neurons, thus leading to memory loss.* Vascular dementia, formerly multi-infarct dementia, is characterized by dementia that classically has a more stepwise downhill course as compared with Alzheimer's disease, which has a more smoothly progressive downhill course. Multi-infact dementia is caused by multiple strokes, which damage the brain sufficiently to cause dementia and often cause focal neurological signs and symptoms as well. *Normal pressure hydrocephalus* can cause dementia from dilated cerebral ventricles. *Creutzfeldt-*

*Jakob disease* can cause dementia from a "slow" viral infection of the brain. *Depression* can cause a false dementia or pseudodementia, which can be reversed by antidepressants in many cases. In *Huntington's disease*, *Parkinson's disease*, and many other neurological disorders, dementia, such as Lewy body dementia, can be associated with various neurological signs and symptoms. These latter dementias are part of a neurodegenerative disorder that destroys various neurons in the brain, including those areas responsible for memory and cognition. Patients with acquired immunodeficiency syndrome (AIDS), often have dementia resulting from a human immunodeficiency virus (HIV) infection of the brain. Frontotemporal dementia, also called Pick's disease, can involve more frontal lobe degeneration and personality changes. There has been little systematic investigation in these various dementias of cholinergic neuronal damage or of the therapeutic benefit of cholinesterase inhibitors, although numerous anecdotal reports suggest that some patients may benefit.

## Cholinesterase Inhibitors as Treatments for Enhancing Memory or Slowing the Pace of Memory Loss in Alzheimer's Disease

No matter how it happens, cholinergic neuronal functioning is one of the earliest neurotransmitters to change in Alzheimer's disease, and it changes dramatically in the first year of symptoms, since the synthetic enzyme for acetylcholine, choline acetyltransferase (Fig. 12–7), may already be decreased by 40 to 90% in the cortex and hippocampus (Fig. 12–13). The nucleus basalis of Meynert also shows progressive neuronal loss in Alzheimer's disease, which correlates with the progressive loss of memory function in this disease (Fig. 12–13). The most successful approach to boosting cholinergic functioning in Alzheimer's patients and improving their memory has been to inhibit acetylcholine destruction by inhibiting the enzyme acetylcholinesterase (Fig. 12–23). This causes the buildup of acetylcholine because it can no longer be destroyed by acetylcholinesterase.

This pharmacologic approach has already led to the approval of two drugs for treatment of memory disorders of Alzheimer's disease in the United States, with several others in the late stages of clinical testing and approval. These drugs enhance memory and are sometimes called *cognitive enhancers* and sometimes *promnestic* (as opposed to an amnestic) *agents*. They are specifically approved to treat Alzheimer's disease. Since these agents appear to depend on the presence of intact postsynaptic cholinergic receptors to receive the benefits of the enhanced cholinergic input, they may be most effective in the early stages of Alzheimer's disease, while postsynaptic cholinergic targets are still present. There is some evidence that cholinesterase inhibitors may even slow the course of the underlying degenerative process in some patients, and thus may have three possible pharmacological benefits mediated by diffuse stimulation of nicotinic and muscarinic cholinergic receptors. These possible benefits are (1) functional improvement of central cholinergic neurotransmission at cholinergic synapses (especially relevant in the neocortex), mediated through muscarinic and nicotinic mechanisms; (2) protection against neuronal degeneration, mediated through nicotine receptor activation; and (3) modification of amyloid precursor protein processing, mediated through M1 receptor activation.

*Donepezil* is currently approved worldwide as a first-line treatment for improving memory or at least slowing the rate of memory loss in Alzheimer's disease. It is a reversible, long-acting, selective piperidine inhibitor of acetylcholinesterase (AchE)

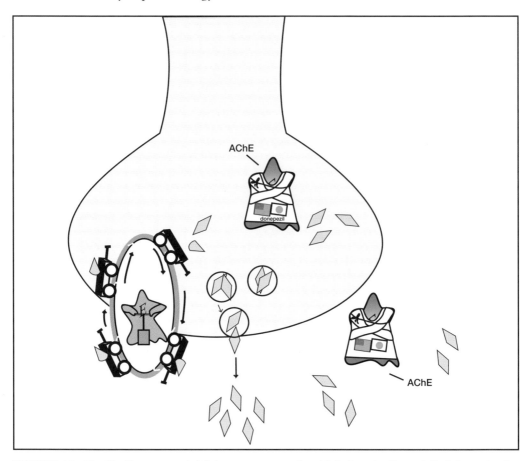

FIGURE 12–23. **Cholinesterase inhibitor treatment for Alzheimer's disease.** Deficiency in cholinergic functioning, due to degeneration in cholinergic projections from the nucleus basalis of Meynert, may be linked to the memory disturbance of Alzheimer's disease. Levels of acetylcholine (ACh) and its synthetic enzyme choline acetyltransferase are greatly reduced in brains of Alzheimer's patients. A powerful and successful mechanism of boosting ACh in the brain is to inhibit ACh destruction by *inhibiting the enzyme acetylcholinesterase* (AChE). This causes the buildup of ACh, which is no longer destroyed by acetylcholinesterase. This approach has led to the only truly effective therapies for the treatment of Alzheimer's disease. Shown here is the current first-line **cholinesterase treatment** in clinical practice, **donepezil**, which inhibits acetylcholinesterase in the cholinergic neuron and its surroundings. Other similar agents are in late clinical testing. Since these agents appear to depend on the presence of intact targets for acetylcholine for maximum effectiveness, they may be most effective in the early stages of Alzheimer's disease, before these targets degenerate. However, the cholinesterase inhibitors may actually slow the degeneration itself by releasing growth factors or by interfering with amyloid deposition.

without inhibition of butyrylcholinesterase (BuChE) (Fig. 12–24). It is easy to dose, and has mostly gastrointestinal side effects, which are mostly transient.

*Tacrine* was the first cholinesterase inhibitor approved for the enhancement of memory associated with Alzheimer's disease in the United States. Because of its short half-life, drug interactions, and hepatic toxicity, it is currently considered second-line therapy for patients who fail to respond to donepezil. Its psychophar-

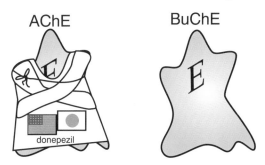

FIGURE 12–24. Icon for the cholinesterase inhibitor **donepezil**. This is the current first-line treatment for Alzheimer's disease, since it is a once daily agent without significant hepatotoxicity. It is a reversible agent, selective for acetylcholinesterase (AChE) over butyrylcholinesterase (BuChE), developed by American and Japanese companies.

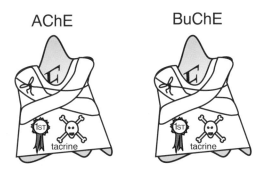

FIGURE 12–25. Icon for the cholinesterase inhibitor **tacrine**. This was the first cholinesterase inhibitor, but since it is a hepatoxotin, it has been relegated to second-line use. Also, it must be given four times daily, is difficult to dose, and has several drug interactions. It is short-acting, reversible, and nonselective, inhibiting both acetylcholinesterase (AChE) and butyrylcholinesterase (BuChE).

macological mechanism of action is reversible inhibition of both AchE and BuChE (Fig. 12–25). It thus has a short half-life, and must be given four times a day with falloff of enzyme inhibition and sometimes of efficacy as well, between doses. Like all cholinesterase inhibitors, its therapeutic benefits on memory and its side effects are dose-related, but because of its short duration of action, it requires very careful dose titration. Tacrine frequently causes hepatic toxicity and thus requires monitoring of liver function during drug administration. There are also several potential significant pharmacokinetic drug interactions, since tacrine is an inhibitor of CYP450 1A2, and its levels are increased by other drugs such as cimetidine. Thus, tacrine not only is a second-line treatment given the current availability of donepezil, but it will likely fall to a third-line treatment once other agents now in late clinical development are approved for clinical use.

*Rivastigmine* is currently in the late stages of clinical development and awaiting approval for marketing in many countries. It is a carbamate, which is "pseudoirreversible" (meaning that it reverses itself over hours) and intermediate-acting, and is selective not only for AChE over BuChE, but perhaps also for AChE in the cortex and hippocampus over AChE in other areas of brain (Fig. 12–26). It appears to have

AChE                    BuChE

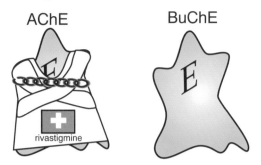

FIGURE 12–26. Icon for the cholinesterase inhibitor **rivastigmine**. This agent is in late development by a Swiss company. It is long-acting, pseudoirreversible, intermediate-acting, and selective for acetylcholinesterase (AChE) over butyrylcholinesterase (BuChE).

AChE                    BuChE

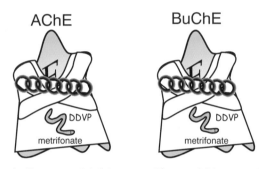

FIGURE 12–27. Icon for the cholinesterase inhibitor **metrifonate**. This agent is in late development for Alzheimer's disease, but is a well-known agent for schistosomiasis. It is a prodrug for 2,2-dichloro-dimethyl-phosphate (DDVP), an irreversible inhibitor of both acetylcholinesterase (AChE) and butyrylcholinesterase (BuChE).

safety and efficacy comparable with those of donepezil, although head-to-head comparisons have not been published.

*Metrifonate* has been used in millions of patients since the 1960s as a treatment for schistosomiasis. More recently, it has been investigated as a cognitive enhancer for Alzheimer's disease patients. Metrifonate itself is not an AChE inhibitor; rather, it is a prodrug, which is gradually converted, nonenzymatically, into another chemical, 2,2-dichlorovinyldimethyl phosphate (DDVP), which is the actual cholinesterase inhibitor. Metrifonate's psychopharmacological mechanism of action is therefore as a prodrug for an organophosphate irreversible, long-acting inhibitor of both AChE and BuChE (Fig. 12–27). Its onset of action is gradual, since it takes some time for DDVP to form with oral administration of metrifonate, and this can improve tolerability as the patient adjusts to cholinesterase inhibition. Some of the best studies linking dose-related AChE inhibition with clinical efficacy in improving memory in Alzheimer's disease have been made with metrifonate. Since inhibition of AChE in red blood cells by metrifonate correlates directly with the agent's inhibition of brain AChE, monitoring of red blood cell AChE has indicated that approximately 50 to 60% enzyme inhibition is sufficient to produce efficacy with acceptable tolerability. Observations of muscular weakness in some patients receiving

AChE

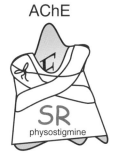

FIGURE 12–28. Icon for the cholinesterase inhibitor **physostigmine**. This agent is used intravenously as a short-acting cholinesterase inhibitor to reverse anticholinergic poisoning and is in testing in an oral sustained-release formulation for Alzheimer's disease.

AChE

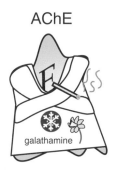

FIGURE 12–29. Icon for the cholinesterase inhibitor **galanthamine**. This agent is naturally present in snowdrops and daffodils and may also have nicotinic agonist or cholinergic-releasing actions as well as cholinesterase actions. It is also in testing for Alzheimer's disease.

long-term treatment with metrifonate in clinical trials have caused reconsideration of dosing and safety issues prior to approval for marketing in some countries.

*Physostigmine* is a very short acting cholinesterase inhibitor normally used intravenously to reverse anticholinergic poisoning. It has been reformulated into an oral sustained-release preparation and successfully tested in Alzheimer's disease (Fig. 12–28), demonstrating efficacy in improving memory and cognition comparable to that of other cholinesterase inhibitors, but it has not yet satisfactorily resolved all safety issues (e.g., nausea and vomiting) that must be resolved for marketing to begin.

*Galanthamine* is a very interesting cholinesterase inhibitor found in snowdrops and daffodils. It may have a dual mechanism of action, matching cholinesterase inhibition with direct nicotinic agonist actions causing acetylcholine release (Fig. 12–29). Early testing in Alzheimer's disease is underway.

*Cholinesterase inhibitors: one class of six drugs or six unique agents?* Soon three to six cholinesterase inhibitors should be available worldwide for the treatment of cholinergic-related memory disturbances in Alzheimer's disease (Fig. 12–30). Use of these agents will likely be expanded to treat cholinergic-related behavioral disturbances in Alzheimer's disease in addition to memory disturbances, since there is evidence that behavioral problems in this disease may also respond to cholinergic

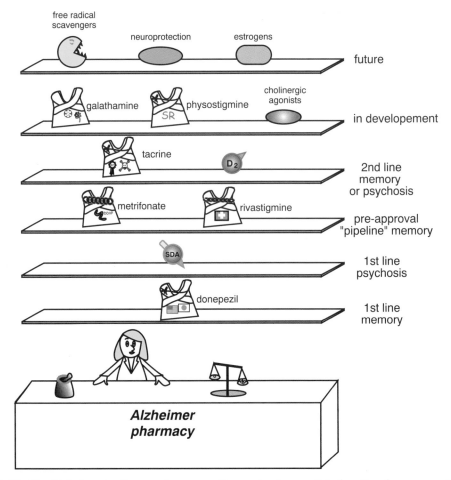

FIGURE 12–30. **Alzheimer's disease pharmacy.** Currently, donepezil is first-line for memory loss, and atypical antipsychotics (SDA) are first-line for positive psychotic symptoms; together they may work synergistically. Soon the cholinesterase inhibitors metrifonate and/or rivastigmine may become available. Second-line treatments are tacrine for memory and conventional antipsychotics (D2) for positive psychotic symptoms. Several other agents are in clinical and preclinical development.

intervention (Fig. 12–31). Even though we have chosen to emphasize the memory impairment of Alzheimer's disease, this disorder obviously has many dimensions of functional impairments, often heralded by mood changes even before cognitive and memory declines, with consequent loss of functional independence, followed by onset of behavioral and finally motor changes (Fig. 12–31). The cholinesterase inhibitors may have synergistic actions with atypical antipsychotics in reducing behavioral disturbances, as discussed in Chapter 11. The cholinesterase inhibitors may also be expanded to uses outside of Alzheimer's disease, for example, to the treatment of memory disorders in other conditions, to the treatment of attention deficit disorder, and to the treatment of bipolar disorder. Thus, a thorough familiarity with these agents will be useful for the informed psychopharmacologist in the coming years, this should including knowing the relative advantages and disadvantages of each of

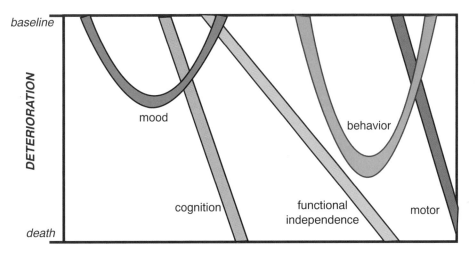

FIGURE 12–31. **Time course of deterioration** of multiple dimensions of symptoms in Alzheimer's disease. Changes in **mood** late in life, particularly if first onset in life and nonresponsive to antidepressants, may be a harbinger for later onset of the memory and **cognitive decline** of Alzheimer's disease. As cognitive decline worsens, **functional impairment** follows shortly thereafter. **Behavioral problems** then begin and become a major management issue in this disorder. Eventually, even **motor** problems develop in the last few years of life. Thus, Alzheimer's disease is certainly not just a disorder of memory, although that has been the dimension emphasized in this chapter.

the various members of this class. Given the advantages of the newer agents, there seems to be little reason to prescribe tacrine any more. Once rivastigmine and metrifonate join donepezil on the market, clinicians will want to know the relative advantages and disadvantages of each of these, however. Unfortunately, direct head-to-head comparisons in Alzheimer's disease are not yet available.

These newer drugs differ mostly in pharmacology and in type and selectivity of enzyme inhibition, which may translate more directly into differences in tolerability and drug interactions than into differences in efficacy. Changes in memory and cognition seem to be about the same for all of the cholinesterase inhibitors when tested against placebo in trials without comparators. Nevertheless, there will undoubtedly be debates on the relative advantages of reversible (short-acting) versus pseudoirreversible (intermediate-acting) versus irreversible (long-acting) enzyme inhibition, as well as on the desirability of selective versus nonselective enzyme inhibition of acetylcholinesterase versus butyrylcholinesterase and of selective versus nonselective inhibition of acetylcholinesterase in various brain regions. Currently, the manner in which these pharmacologic distinctions will translate into clinical advantages or special niche uses for one drug over another is not known and is only likely to be discovered after the compounds have been used extensively in clinical practice. However, it is theoretically possible that drugs that do not inhibit BuChE will have better tolerability, since side effects may be enhanced by the presence of increased ACh in certain tissues. On the other hand, BuChE is present in glia as well as in the plaques, tangles, and amyloid-containing blood vessels in the brains of Alzheimer patients. It is theoretically possible but unproven that inhibiting BuChE at these sites would have a useful boosting function for improving memory.

*The spectrum of potential memory enhancing benefits of the cholinesterase inhibitor class of therapeutic agents.* Cholinergic enhancement compensates for the loss of ACh that occurs as cholinergic neurons degenerate. The cholinergic enhancement strategy has yielded the only successful therapy for improving memory in any cognitive disorder and is specifically approved for treating cognitive symptoms in Alzheimer's disease, but it has obvious limitations. For instance, we have already mentioned that the ideal pharmacologic situation is likely to present itself early in the illness, when postsynaptic neurons and their cholinergic receptors in the cortex are still intact, even though presynaptic cholinergic inputs from the nucleus basalis of Meynert have degenerated. However, not only is it difficult to diagnose patients at this stage of the illness, but it is particularly difficult to monitor the effects of treatment, because the available rating scales are not very sensitive in picking up subtle changes, even in a research setting. Another limitation of the cholinergic approach to enhancing memory in Alzheimer's disease is that as the illness advances, the postsynaptic neurons in the neocortex degenerate, removing the targets for acetylcholine. Furthermore, replacing acetylcholine will not improve functions mediated by the loss of those noncholinergic neurotransmitters.

Studies of the untreated course of Alzheimer's disease (Fig. 12–13), coupled with extensive long-term experience with two cholinesterase inhibitors in clinical practice and several more in clinical trials over the past few years, are helping to set expectations for what these agents can achieve in terms of memory enhancement. As with many psychopharmacological agents, the median response rate of a large group of patients often belies the range of responses exhibited by individuals, and since there is no way of predicting who will experience the more robust clinical responses, only empirical trial and error of individual patients can ultimately tell who will be helped the most by these agents. Nevertheless, the *range* of responses is well known and is summarized in Figures 12–32 to 12–34.

The *best responses* to cholinesterase inhibitors can be substantial improvement, large enough to be noticeable by the patient and his or her caregiver within weeks of initiation of therapy (Fig. 12–32). Some of these patients sustain this robust improvement for many months or have a noticeably slower than expected decline in memory (Fig. 12–32). The *usual (median) response*, however, is for the initial improvement to be statistically detectable on cognitive testing and perhaps to be noticeable by the caregiver, but often not by the patient. Such a response usually lasts about 6 months, and then cognitive functioning, as measured on cognitive testing, is back to where it was before beginning the drug (Fig. 12–33). This response is clearly drug-related, because if the drug is stopped, cognitive function immediately declines back to what would be expected if the patient had never been treated. Thereafter, the decline may be at about the same rate as before taking the drug (Fig. 12–33). Yet another response to cholinesterase inhibition can be to have no immediate improvement but a definite slowing in the expected rate of decline (Fig. 12–34). Of course, some patients do not respond at all, but it is distinctly unusual for a patient to worsen on cholinesterase inhibitor treatment.

As mentioned earlier, all cholinesterase inhibitors seem to have the same ability to improve cognitive function as compared with placebo in large clinical trials, and there are few anecdotes and no head-to-head trials suggesting that patients who do not respond robustly to one cholinesterase agent will respond robustly to another. Substantial improvement in 30-week studies might thus be expected in about one-

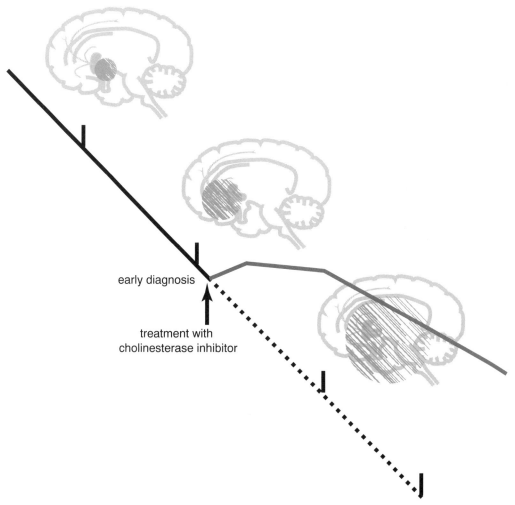

**Best Responders**

FIGURE 12–32. The **best responses** to cholinesterase inhibitor therapy in Alzheimer's disease can be substantial improvement, large enough to be noticeable to the patient and to his or her caregiver within weeks of initiation of therapy. Some of these patients sustain this robust improvement for many months or have a noticeably slower than expected decline in memory.

fourth of patients treated with a cholinesterase inhibitor (and only in 8 to 10% of those given placebo); about 56 to 60% are expected to show either no further deterioration or moderate improvement with the drug (versus 50% or fewer with placebo, this difference being statistically significant).

These findings from the natural history of untreated Alzheimer's disease and how it is modified by cholinesterase inhibitors should help prescribers set realistic expectations for treatment with AChE inhibitors. The hope is that today's improvements from cholinesterase inhibition will be synergistic when combined with agents of differing pharmacologic mechanisms of action in the future and should be considered a very useful first step in treating this devastating illness.

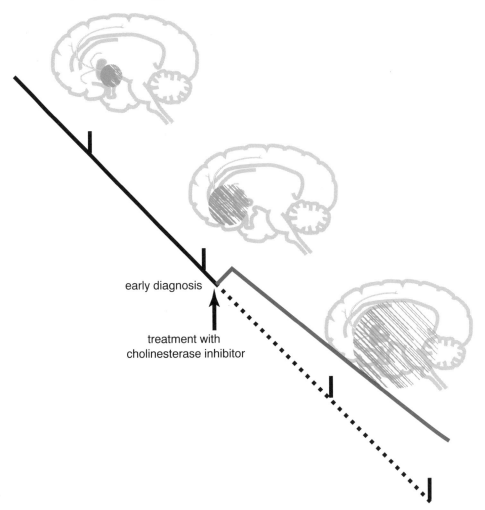

**Usual (Median) Response**

FIGURE 12–33. Usual (median) responders to cholinesterase inhibitor therapy in Alzheimer's disease. The **usual (median) response** to cholinesterase inhibitor therapy is for the initial improvement to be statistically detectable on cognitive testing and perhaps noticeable to the caregiver, but often not to the patient. Such a response usually lasts about 6 months, and then cognitive functioning as measured on cognitive testing is back to where it was before beginning the drug. This response is clearly drug-related, because if the drug is stopped, cognitive function declines back to what would be expected if the patient had never been treated. Thereafter, the decline may be at about the same rate as before taking the drug.

## *Other and Future Memory and Cognitive Enhancers*

Innovation in the area of cognitive enhancers in general and in Alzheimer's disease in particular is one of the most active research areas in psychopharmacology. Although this is a most exciting topic, it may not be of interest to every reader, and especially not to the beginner or to the generalist. These readers may wish to skip to the end of the chapter and to the summary.

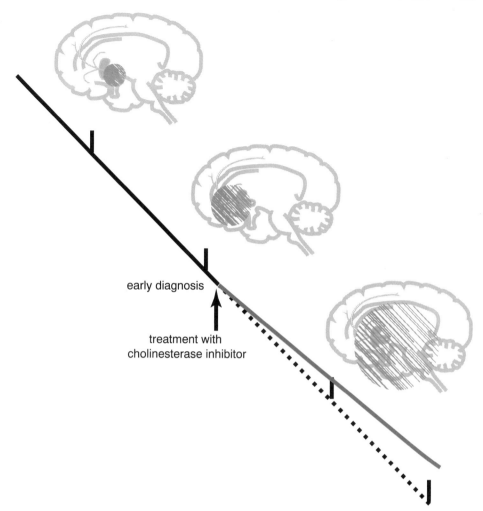

**Palliative Response**

FIGURE 12–34. **Palliative** responders to cholinesterase inhibitor therapy in Alzheimer's disease. Yet another response to cholinesterase inhibition can be no immediate improvement but a definite slowing in the expected rate of decline.

*Agents of unproven or limited efficacy for dementias*

EARLY CHOLINERGIC THERAPIES    The earliest attempts to boost cholinergic functioning in Alzheimer's disease were made with rather rudimentary cholinergic agents, namely, choline and lecithin (phospatidyl choline), the precursors for ACh synthesis. This was based on an analogy with Parkinson's disease, in which neurodegeneration of dopaminergic neurons causes symptoms that can be successfully treated by administering L-DOPA, the precursor of dopamine. Multiple studies of cholinergic precursors have led to essentially negative results, which do not offer meaningful hope for improvement in patients with Alzheimer's disease.

CEREBRAL VASODILATORS    *Cerebral vasodilators* were originally explored as treatments for dementia based on the hypothesis that cognitive loss was caused by atherosclerosis of cerebral vessels. Thus, carbon dioxide, carbonic anhydrase inhibitors, anticoagulants, nicotinic acid (a vitamin B6 derivative), pyritinol, meclofenate, vitamin E, hyperbaric oxygen, papaverine, cyclandelate, isoxuprine, vincamine, and cinnarizine have all been tested to improve oxygen delivery to the brain. However, none of these strategies has proved to be effective, and the hypothesis that faulty circulation is implicated in the dementia process is no longer tenable. Some carryover use of these compounds, which were originally marketed in the era of the "faulty brain circulation hypothesis of dementia," includes use nafridrofuryl in some European countries for elderly confused patients, but improvement is inconsistent. Cinnazine is a vasodilating and calcium antagonist compound prescribed in Europe for vertigo and dementia related to chronic ischemia, with equivocal efficacy. Pentoxifylline is a vasodilator, which may improve memory in animals but has not been conclusively shown to do so in patients with dementia. Nimodipine is a calcium channel blocker marketed for cerebrovascular disease in some countries and specifically for lessening vasospasm in subarachnoid hemorrhage in many countries. It may normalize cellular calcium levels or possibly affect another mechanism, such as calcium-activated enzymes involved in cognition. Nimodipine was therefore tested extensively in Alzheimer's disease, where it failed to show efficacy in improving cognitive functioning. Calcium channel blockers are used as possible neuroprotective and/or cognitive enhancing agents in Japan and in some European countries.

METABOLIC ENHANCERS    So-called metabolic enhancers include Hydergine, the brand name of a mixture of ergot alkaloids, the first FDA-approved drug of this group, which was marketed for a while for the treatment of dementia, although not specifically for memory disturbances in Alzheimer's disease. It also was developed during the era when Alzheimer's disease and dementia in general were believed to result from vascular disease. Hydergine was marketed as a "cerebral vasodilator" owing to its putative but fairly weak alpha adrenergic antagonist actions, which might be expected to cause dilation of blood vessels. Subsequently, the drug was reclassified as a metabolic enhancer because of its ability to change second-messenger cAMP levels, and because of the possibility that it acts as a partial agonist at dopamine, serotonin, and norepinephrine receptors. Several studies of higher doses of Hydergine have shown some beneficial effects in dementia, especially when cognitive impairment is mild. Several reports indicate that improved mood is more pronounced than change in cognitive status. Currently, there is no current acceptance of how Hydergine or other putative metabolic enhancers or cerebral vasodilators might be useful, especially in the United States.

VITAMINS AND HORMONES    Vitamins and hormones such as B12, thiamine, and zinc have been administered since abnormalities have been described in Alzheimer's disease. However, most studies of replacement therapy with these agents have been negative. *Gingko biloba* may improve cognitive functioning according to some reports, although the size of the effect and generalizability of the finding remain uncertain, as do the effects of other herbs. *Chelation* therapy is used by some practitioners to remove aluminum, based on speculation regarding the role of aluminum in Alzheimer's disease. Trials with chelating agents such as desferioxamine, however, have been negative, and the potential efficacy of future chelation therapy is uncertain. Chelation therapy is now largely considered to be an expensive and elaborate placebo for Alzheimer's disease.

NOOTROPIC DRUGS    *Nootropic drugs* are a class of psychotropic drugs that enhance learning acquisition and reverse learning impairments in experimental animals. The term *nootropic* was introduced to describe a group of drugs that have the ability to improve certain brain mechanisms postulated to be associated with mental performance. The hypothesized main features of nootropic agents, in addition to the ability to enhance memory and learning, are the following: (1) facilitation of the flow of information between the cerebral hemispheres; (2) enhancement of the resistance of the brain to physical and chemical assault; and (3) lack of sedative, analgesic, or neuroleptic activity. The naturally occurring agent acetyl-L-carnitine, formed by acetylation of carnitine in mitochondria, has an analogous structure to ACh and is sometimes classified as a nootropic agent or as a weak ACh agonist.

Limited data exist in patients with cerebral ischemia in Japan, some of which suggest improvements in functioning. One idea is that a nootropic drug enhances cellular protection by inhibiting the formation of damaging lipid peroxides in cellular ischemia as well as the increased lactate production that follows interrupted blood flow. The chemical structure of the prototype nootropic, piracetam, is a derivative of gamma aminobutyric acid (GABA). As yet, however, there is no established mechanism of action for nootropics at GABA neurons, GABA receptors, or elsewhere. Some scientists hypothesize that nootropics act as metabolic enhancers by influencing cerebral energy reserves and by increasing energy-containing chemicals such as ATP in the brain. The initial nootropic compound was piracetam, but several more have since been developed, including pramiracetam, oxiracetam, and aniracetam. Limited data suggest that nootropics may be useful in improving memory, mood, or behavioral functioning in patients with mild to moderate senile dementia but not in severely demented patients. These agents are used primarily outside the United States, as no nootropic is approved for any use in the United States.

*Research strategies for age-associated memory impairment, mild cognitive impairment, and presymptomatic or early symptomatic treatment of Alzheimer's disease.* If we live long enough, will we all be demented? Is aging hazardous to our cholinergic neurons? Over half of elderly residents living in the community complain of memory impairment. They have four common complaints; namely, as compared with their functioning of 5 or 10 years ago, they experience a diminished ability (1) to remember names, (2) to find the correct word, (3) to remember where objects are located, and (4) to concentrate. When such complaints occur in the absence of dementia or depression, it is called age-associated memory impairment. Fortunately, it does not appear that the majority of those with such complaints go on to develop Alzheimer's disease, but there is intense interest in early recognition and prevention of progression for those who are destined to have Alzheimer's disease. Thus, we are embarking on an era of extensive presymptomatic and very early symptomatic treatments. This was mentioned briefly as well in Chapter 11 on schizophrenia. The idea here is not to remove current symptoms but to prevent future symptoms and deterioration. There are many methodological and logistical problems with conducting such studies in both schizophrenia and Alzheimer's disease, including the difficulty in deciding which subjects to enter into the study; the expense (because these studies need huge numbers of patients and take a very long time to conduct); the problems in defining satisfactory end points (when does one have early schizophrenia or Alzheimer's disease, etc.?) Assuming that all these methodological points can be addressed, nevertheless a number of novel psychopharmacological agents are being used to test several provocative hypotheses.

First, of course, the cholinesterase inhibitors are being administered to see if they can prevent or delay the onset of dementia. Also, estrogen (in women) and anti-inflammatory agents (in rheumatoid arthritis and in uncontrolled use) have already suggested a lowered incidence of Alzheimer's disease, so these agents are similarly being tested in randomized trials. The idea behind the estrogen trials is that estrogen may be a neurotrophic factor (see Chapter 14 on psychopharmacology of the sexes). The hypothesis behind the anti-inflammatory trials is that amyloid deposition precipitates an inflammatory reaction, which leads to further neuronal damage, but interruption of this reaction, could halt the degenerative process. Thus, a whole host of agents that could theoretically interrupt such an inflammatory cascade are all currently being tested in this manner, including old-fashioned nonsteroidal anti-inflammatory drugs (NSAIDS), the new generation version called cyclooxygenase type 2 (COX-2) inhibitors, the free-radical scavenger vitamin E, and the potential neuroprotective and monoamine oxidase B inhibitor deprenyl.

A theoretical off-shoot of this strategy is to use neuroprotective agents, such as glutamate antagonists, to interrupt a theoretically excitotoxic neurodegenerative process in Alzheimer's disease. This has been discussed extensively in Chapter 10 for schizophrenia (Figs. 10–26 to 10–31), along with potential treatment strategies (Figs. 10–32 and 10–33) that apply to Alzheimer's disease as well. A major research strategy for the discovery of novel therapeutics in Alzheimer's disease is to target the glutamate system, which might mediate progressive neurodegeneration by an excitotoxic mechanism. The therapeutic idea underlying the development of neuroprotective agents is that such drugs could stop inappropriate or excessive excitatory neurotransmission and thereby halt the progressive neurodegenerative course of various neurodegenerative disorders. No such agents are currently available for clinical use. In the long run, it may also be possible to interrupt the loss of degenerating neurons in Alzheimer's disease through apoptotic demise by the administration of caspase inhibitors, as mentioned in Chapter 11 in our discussion of possible novel therapeutics for schizophrenia as well.

*Other research strategies for Alzheimer's disease and other dementias*

CHOLINERGIC STRATEGIES (NONCHOLINESTERASE INHIBITION)   One approach that still has only met with limited success is to target cholinergic receptors selectively with a cholinergic agonist. Various agonists are under investigation, especially agonists for the M1 cholinergic receptor (Fig. 12–35). Nicotinic agonists are also being tested (Fig. 12–36). The possible advantage of stimulating nicotinic cholinergic receptors is suggested by several epidemiological studies finding a lower risk for Alzheimer's disease among smokers. In addition, central nicotinic receptors are reduced in brains of Alzheimer patients. In Chapter 11, we discussed the development of alpha-7-nicotinic cholinergic agonists as a novel therapeutic strategy for schizophrenia. This could be useful for cognitive enhancement in Alzheimer's disease

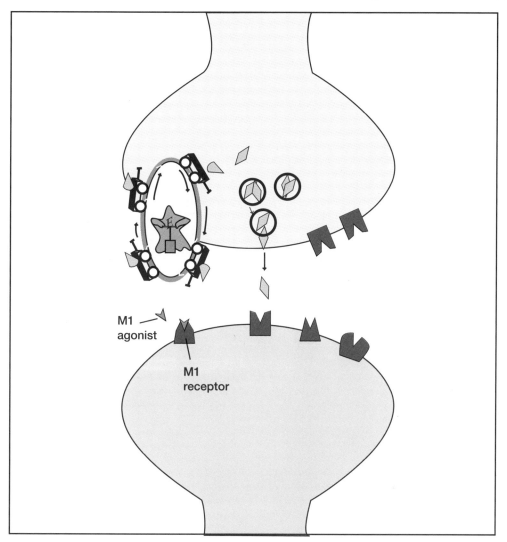

FIGURE 12–35. **Use of agonists for the muscarinic 1 receptor for the treatment of Alzheimer's disease.** Another approach that still has only met with limited success is to target cholinergic receptors selectively with a cholinergic agonist. Various agonists are under investigation, especially agonists for the M1 cholinergic receptor.

as well. Yet another possibility is to develop an agent that can release acetylcholine, perhaps through blocking potassium channels. This approach is heavily dependent, however, on the presence of intact remaining presynaptic cholinergic nerve terminals and may therefore only be effective in the early stages of the disease. Several such agents are under clinical investigation.

ALTERING AMYLOID PRECURSOR PROTEIN OR APO-E BIOSYNTHESIS   Current therapeutics are aimed at the possibility that altering the synthesis of APP (Fig. 12–37) or APO-E (Fig. 12–38) might change the deposition of beta amyloid (see

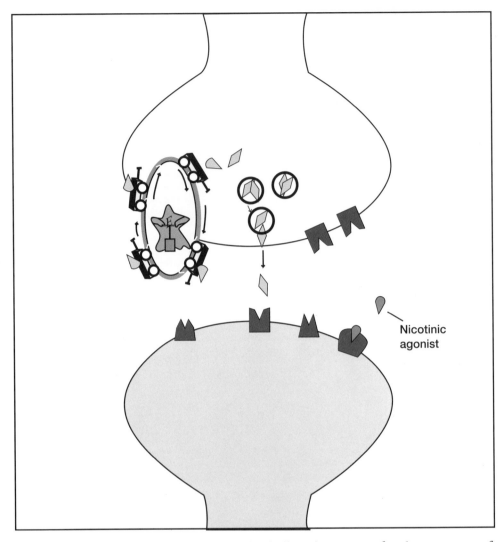

Nicotinic
agonist

FIGURE 12–36. **Use of agonists for the nicotinic cholinergic receptor for the treatment of Alzheimer's disease.** Nicotinic agonists are also being tested in Alzheimer's disease. The possible advantage of stimulating nicotinic cholinergic receptors is suggested by several epidemiological studies finding a lower risk for Alzheimer's disease among smokers. In addition, central nicotinic receptors are reduced in brains of Alzheimer's patients. To date, no such agents have been licensed for the treatment of Alzheimer's disease.

Figs. 12–16 to 12–22) and prevent the progressive course of Alzheimer's disease. Direct inhibition of gene expression for the biosynthesis of these proteins is not currently possible and is currently not a very feasible therapeutic possibility. Perhaps a more realistic therapeutic possibility would be to inhibit the synthesis of beta amyloid, in much the same way that lipid-lowering agents act to inhibit the biosynthesis of cholesterol in order to prevent atherosclerosis. This could be done by means of enzyme inhibitors, such as protease inhibitors, which are at least a theoretical possibility.

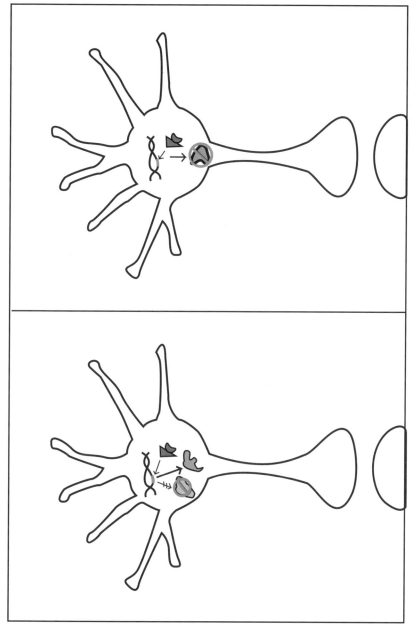

FIGURE 12–37. One current therapeutic approach to preventing the neuronal destruction in Alzheimer's disease is based on the molecular neurobiology of beta amyloid formation and the involvement of amyloid precursor protein (APP) in this process. If the **synthesis of APP could be prevented**, it might change the deposition of beta amyloid and prevent the progressive course of Alzheimer's disease. Another possibility is to inhibit the synthesis of beta amyloid itself, in much the same way that lipid-lowering agents act to inhibit the biosynthesis of cholesterol in order to prevent atherosclerosis.

FIGURE 12–38. Another current therapeutic approach to preventing the neuronal destruction in Alzheimer's disease is also based on the molecular neurobiology of beta amyloid formation but emphasizes the involvement of APO-E binding protein in this process. If the **synthesis of "good" APO-E could be ensured** or the **synthesis of "bad" APO-E prevented**, possibly amyloid would not accumulate in the neuron. Changing the deposition of beta amyloid would hopefully prevent the progressive course of Alzheimer's disease.

NEUROPEPTIDES    Several *neuropeptide* neurotramsitter systems are known to be disturbed in Alzheimer's disease, including somatostatin, corticotropin-releasing factor, neuropeptide Y, and substance P. A somatostatin analogue tested to date has not been effective. Arginine vasopressin and several of its analogues have been extensively studied because of their role in cognition and their demonstrated effects in animal studies of memory. In Alzheimer's disease patients, their use has led to some reports of modest improvements in behavior, with improved energy and mood, but with not much improvement in memory. The same is true of corticotropin agonists, which appear to affect mood and behavior without clear memory or cognitive effects. Studies of thyrotropin-releasing hormone analogues that have procholinergic effects have been largely negative. The opiate antagonist naloxone does not have consistent effects in improving cognition in Alzheimer's disease.

GROWTH FACTORS    Neural regeneration or increased resistance to destructive processes may be achievable with selected neurotrophic factors. Nerve growth factor is the prototype, with particular potential to synergize with cholinergic therapy because its receptors are primarily localized on cholinergic neurons and it is present in relatively high levels in the basal forebrain, where cholinergic neurons degenerate in Alzheimer's disease. There are potential hazards to consider, however, with growth factor treatments. Thus, in addition to cholinergic neural regeneration, there is the possibility of inappropriate "sprouting" and corresponding growth in the wrong fibers. There is also an ominous rise in mRNA for amyloid precursor protein (APP), which may actually cause more formation of unwanted beta amyloid, as well as plaques and tangles. Another growth factor–like substance is GM1 ganglioside. Gangliosides in the brain are complex lipids associated with developing synapses. In several animal models, GM1 has been found capable of preventing neuronal degeneration, and it may also prevent retrograde degeneration of cholinergic neurons in the rat basal forebrain resulting from damage to the cerebral cortex. Although these strategies are in the very earliest stages of development, they represent concrete examples in animal models where endogenous trophic molecules potentially could be used to treat degenerative diseases such as Alzheimer's disease. This has been previously discussed in Chapters 1 and 4 and shown in Figures 1–19, 1–22, and 4–13. It remains a highly theoretical and mostly long-term proposition at this time.

TRANSPLANTATION    The hypothesis that implanting healthy neuronal tissue may promote regeneration and return of function in the diseased brain comes from animal experiments using tissues from fetal central nervous system, peripheral nerve, and cultured cells. When transplanted into the brain, these tissues may exert therapeutic effects via a variety of mechanisms. For example, they may act as a chemical generator (e.g., of growth factors), or as a generator of glial cells, which in turn promote neuronal function. They may also provide the brain with regenerating axons in the transplant material, which may innervate other neurons from the diseased brain. At present, this is a highly theoretical area of research, without current clinical applications and involving many ethical considerations. This has been previously discussed in Chapter 4 and shown in Figure 4–14.

*Future combination chemotherapies for disorders associated with cognitive disturbance and memory loss.* Just as in the case of schizophrenia (as discussed in Chapter 11 on antipsychotics), the future treatment for Alzheimer's disease is not likely to consist of one drug acting by a single pharmacological mechanism. Despite the economic incentives for developing a single treatment of choice and the methodological incentives for studying one drug at a time, it seems likely that a disorder with cognitive and memory disturbance, behavioral disturbance, and a degenerative component will require some kind of combination of drugs, such as a procholinergic agent for memory working with an atypical antipsychotic for behavior and a neuroprotective agent for neurodegeneration, or some such blend. Perhaps psychopharmacological treatments for cognitive disorders in the future will need to borrow a chapter out of the book of cancer chemotherapy and HIV/AIDS therapy, as we have argued as well for new therapies in schizophrenia, where the standard of treatment is to use multiple drugs simultaneously so that several independent therapeutic mechanisms work synergistically to provide a total therapeutic response that is greater than the sum of its parts.

## Summary

In this chapter, we have looked at two topics in cognitive enhancement: attention and memory. We have first reviewed the role of dopamine and norepinephrine/ noradrenaline in the neuropharmacology of attention, and then the syndrome of attention deficit disorder as a common problem associated with a disorder of attention. We then discussed the use of stimulants for improving attention, primarily in attention deficit disorder, and reviewed the pharmacological mechanisms of action of methylphenidate, d and l amphetamine, pemoline, and secondary therapies such as clonidine and guanfacine.

The second major topic of this chapter was the role of acetylcholine in memory, and how cholinergic systems are disrupted in Alzheimer's disease by a number of processes that form plaques and tangles in the cholinergic neurons projecting from the nucleus basalis of Meynert, and more diffusely throughout the brain as well. We then reviewed the major cholinergic strategies for enhancing memory and slowing the rate of memory loss in Alzheimer's disease, namely, cholinesterase inhibition by a number of agents including donepezil and tacrine as well as promising new therapies such as rivastigmine, metrifonate, physostigmine and galanthamine. Finally, numerous strategies for treating Alzheimer's disease based on current understanding of pathophysiologic mechanisms of this disorder were reviewed.

# CHAPTER 13

# PSYCHOPHARMACOLOGY OF REWARD AND DRUGS OF ABUSE

Psychopharmacology is defined in this text as the study of drugs that affect the brain. Until now, all the chapters of this book have addressed how psychotropic drugs affect the brain for therapeutic purposes. Unfortunately, psychotropic drugs can also be abused, and this has caused major public health problems throughout the world. Here we will attempt to explain how abuse of psychotropic agents affects the brain. Our approach to this problem is to discuss how nontherapeutic use, short-term abuse (intoxication), and the complications of long-term abuse affect chemical neurotransmission. We will not discuss the many other important aspects of psychoactive substance abuse, leaving it to other experts to explore such issues as the relationship of drug abuse to economics, criminal behavior, and violence.

## Terminology in Psychoactive Substance Use, Abuse, and Reward

Before exploring the neurochemical mechanisms related to psychoactive substance abuse, it is useful to define several terms as they will be used here (Table 13–1).

Table 13–1. *Nine key terms and their definitions*

Abuse: Self-administration of any drug in a culturally disapproved manner that causes adverse consequences.

Addiction: A behavioral pattern of drug abuse characterized by overwhelming involvement with the use of a drug (compulsive use), the securing of its supply, and a high tendency to relapse after discontinuation.

Dependence: The physiological state of neuroadaptation produced by repeated administration of a drug, necessitating continued administration to prevent the appearance of the withdrawal syndrome.

Reinforcement: The tendency of a pleasure-producing drug to lead to repeated self-administration.

Tolerance: Tolerance has developed when after repeated administration, a given dose of a drug produces a decreased effect, or conversely, when increasingly larger doses must be administered to obtain the effects observed with the original use.

Cross-tolerance and cross-dependence: The ability of one drug to suppress the manifestations of physical dependence produced by another drug and to maintain the physically dependent state.

Withdrawal: The psychologic and physiologic reactions to abrupt cessation of a dependence-producing drug.

Relapse: The reoccurrence on discontinuation of an effective medical treatment of the original condition from which the patient suffered.

Rebound: The exaggerated expression of the original condition sometimes experienced by patients immediately after cessation of an effective treatment.

## Use versus Abuse

Sanctioned uses of drugs have always been defined within a culture and therefore differ across cultures and are prone to change as cultures change over time. When a drug is used in a manner that varies from the use approved by a culture, it is called *abuse*. Therefore, use and abuse of drugs are defined by a culture and not by a psychopharmacological mechanism. *Abuse* is thus defined as the self-administration of any drug in a culturally disapproved manner that causes adverse consequences. It is easier to define and recognize the adverse psychopharmacological consequences of drug self-administration than it is to arrive at a consensus as to what constitutes "cultural disapproval." The purpose of this chapter is not to debate what our culture defines as the line between use and abuse, particularly when that line is blurry. To the brain, it matters little how society defines use versus misuse, and our discussion of the acute actions of psychotropic agents will emphasize how psychopharmacologcal mechanisms are affected in proportion to the *amount* (i.e., dose) of drug being self-administered and the *frequency* of drug self-administration. When the brain's chemical neurotransmission is affected to such a degree that the behavior of individuals takes the form of danger to themselves or others, leading to clinically significant impairment or distress, it is now considered to have passed the threshold of mere use and to qualify for abuse, as defined by the Diagnostic and Statistical Manual of Mental Disorders, 4th Edition (DSM-IV) of the American Psychiatric Association.

*Reinforcement* and reward are the terms that explain in part why individuals repeatedly abuse a drug, namely, the fact that drugs of abuse have various *reinforcing properties*, which cause a pleasure-producing drug to lead to repeated self-administration. The neurochemical basis of reinforcement is thought to depend on the action of drugs on neurotransmission and is related to what happens in the brain when there is *intoxication* with the drug. Intoxication is a reversible drug-specific syndrome characterized by clinically significant maladaptive behavior or psychological changes that are due to the psychopharmacological actions of the drug on neurotransmission. The symptoms of intoxication range from belligerence to changes in mood to cognitive impairment or impaired judgment to impaired social or occupational functioning.

## Addiction, Dependence, Rebound, and Withdrawal

Addiction and dependence are frequently confused. *Addiction* is hard to define, with little consensus on what it means, and in fact is not even defined as a condition in DSM-IV. This term usually refers to a behavioral pattern of drug abuse characterized by overwhelming involvement with use of a drug (compulsive use) and with the securing of its supply and by a high tendency to relapse after discontinuation. *Dependence* is easier to define and will be emphasized in our discussion in this chapter. The term *addiction* is frequently employed by those who are not experts in psychopharmacology when *dependence* is what they mean. *Dependence* is a physiological state of neuroadaptation produced by repeated administration of a drug, necessitating continued administration to prevent the appearance of a withdrawal syndrome. Several things can occur when a drug causes dependence and the individual continues taking it, namely, *cross-dependence, tolerance,* and *cross-tolerance.* Several other things can occur when a drug causes dependence and the individual abruptly stops taking it, namely, *withdrawal* and *rebound,* both defined below. Later, in relationship to specific drugs, the various neuroadaptive mechanisms that mediate each of these effects will also be discussed in terms of the impact that they have on chemical transmission of specific neurotransmitters.

*Tolerance* develops when after repeated administration, a given dose of a drug produces a decreased effect, or conversely, when increasingly larger doses must be administered to obtain the effects observed with the original use. Related to this are *cross-tolerance* and *cross-dependence,* which are the ability of one drug to suppress the manifestations of physical dependence produced by another drug and to maintain the physically dependent state. *Withdrawal* is the term for the adverse psychological and physiological reactions to abrupt cessation of a dependence-producing drug. It is very important to distinguish withdrawal from *rebound,* which are frequently confused, because both are related to the neurochemical changes that mediate dependence. *Rebound* is what happens when tolerance occurs in patients who have taken a drug (usually for a medically sanctioned use), which then is suddenly stopped— their symptoms come back in an exaggerated fashion. *Withdrawal,* on the other hand, is what happens when tolerance occurs in those who have taken a drug (either for abuse or for medically sanctioned use) and then that drug is suddenly stopped— they develop a withdrawal syndrome characterized by craving, dysphoria, and signs of sympathetic nervous system overactivity.

*Dependence* is a term that is not frequently used outside of psychopharmacology but in fact is a key feature of many antihypertensive medications, hormones, and other treatments throughout medicine. Thus, several antihypertensives can produce *rebound* hypertension, worse than the original blood pressure elevation, when sud-

denly discontinued. These patients are not "addicted" to their blood pressure medications although they are dependent on them. Such hypertensive patients who suddenly discontinue these antihypertensive drugs do not experience withdrawal effects,
since their symptoms are an exaggerated manifestation of their original condition,
and not a new set of symptoms such as craving and dysphoria. A panic disorder
patient who suddenly stops a benzodiazepine and then has rebound panic attacks
may be incorrectly accused of being "addicted" to benzodiazepines. As in the case
of the patient discontinuing antihypertensives, this panic patient is dependent on
his or her medication and experiencing rebound, not withdrawal or addiction. These
distinctions among dependence, addiction, rebound, and withdrawal should be kept
in mind when educating patients about their medications associated with these
actions.

## Detoxification

*Detoxification* is the slow tapering of a drug that has caused dependence and would
cause withdrawal if stopped too suddenly. Detoxification can be accomplished either
by slowly withdrawing the dependence-forming drug itself or by substitution of a
cross-dependent drug that has a similar pharmacological mechanism of action. In
either case, detoxification is done by slowly tapering the dependent or cross-
dependent drug so that the neuroadaptational mechanisms of dependence can readapt
during dose tapering and thus prevent withdrawal symptoms. Tapering of a drug
treatment for a medical condition (such as hypertension or panic) that has caused
dependence can also prevent the emergence of rebound. In this case, it is not called
detoxification but tapered discontinuation. Detoxification generally implies a method
to prevent withdrawal, not to prevent rebound.

## Rebound versus Relapse

Another important distinction to make is that between *rebound* and *relapse*, as these
two terms are constantly confused. The term *relapse* was already introduced in our
discussion of depression in Chapter 5. Relapse refers to the reoccurrence of disease
symptoms on discontinuation of an effective medical treatment. Relapse assumes an
underlying medical condition for which the drug was administered and therefore a
medically sanctioned use. Thus, if patients with diabetes mellitus require insulin,
they are generally referred to as insulin-dependent, not addicted to insulin. If such
patients suddenly stop their insulin, glucose will generally return to pretreatment
levels, that is, *relapse* of diabetes, not *rebound* to a worse state of diabetes. Panic
patients who require benzodiazepines to suppress panic attacks can similarly be
referred to a benzodiazepine-dependent, not addicted to benzodiazepines. If such
patients suddenly stop benzodiazepines, they may experience *rebound* panic attacks,
i.e., panic attacks that are more frequent and severe than those of the original panic
disorder. On discontinuation of benzodiazepines, especially if they are tapered over
a long period of time, these patients may very well experience the return of their
usual panic attacks, that is, *relapse* of panic disorder. These patients have not developed withdrawal symptoms just because they experience panic attacks after discontinuing benzodiazepines. However, if they develop insomnia, irritability, seizures,

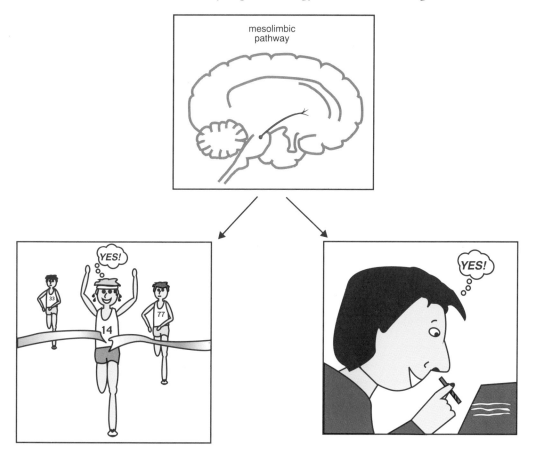

FIGURE 13–1. The **mesolimbic dopamine pathway** mediates the **psychopharmacology of reward**, whether that is a natural high or a drug-induced high.

and agitation, none of which were symptoms of their original panic attacks, they *have* developed symptoms of *withdrawal*.

## Mesolimbic Dopamine Pathway and the Psychopharmacology of Reward

The final common pathway of reinforcement and reward in the brain is hypothesized to be the mesolimbic dopamine pathway (Fig. 13–1). Some even consider this to be the "pleasure center" of the brain and dopamine to be the "pleasure neurotransmitter." There are many natural ways to trigger mesolimbic dopamine neurons to release dopamine, ranging from intellectual accomplishments to athletic accomplishments to enjoying a symphony to experiencing an orgasm. These are sometimes called "natural highs" (Fig. 13–1). The inputs to the mesolimbic pathway that mediate these natural highs include a most incredible "pharmacy" of naturally occurring substances, ranging from the brain's own morphine/heroin (endorphins) to

## drugs affecting the mesolimbic dopaminergic neurons

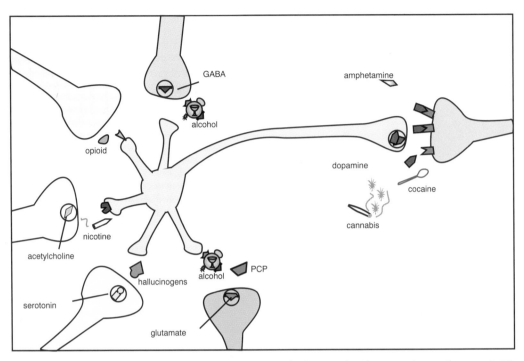

FIGURE 13–2. **Mesolimbic dopamine pathway and the psychopharmacology of reward.** The final common pathway of reward in the brain is hypothesized to be the mesolimbic dopamine pathway. The inputs to this pathway include an incredible "pharmacy" of naturally occurring substances, ranging from the brain's own morphine/heroin (i.e., endorphins) to the brain's own marijuana (i.e., anandamide), to the brain's own cocaine/amphetamine (i.e., dopamine itself). The numerous psychotropic drugs of abuse that occur in nature bypass the brain's own neurotransmitters and directly stimulate the brain's receptors, causing dopamine to be released. Since the brain already uses neurotransmitters that resemble drugs of abuse, it is not necessary to earn the reward naturally, since an artificial "high" can also be obtained on demand. Unfortunately, this can lead to complications. Thus, alcohol, opiates, stimulants, marijuana, benzodiazepines, sedative-hypnotics, hallucinogens, and nicotine all have an impact on this mesolimbic dopaminergic system.

the brain's own marijuana (anandamide), to the brain's own nicotine (acetylcholine), to the brain's own cocaine and amphetamine (dopamine itself) (Fig. 13–2).

The numerous psychotropic drugs of abuse that occur in nature also have a final common pathway of causing the mesolimbic pathway to release dopamine, often in a manner more explosive and pleasurable than that which occurs naturally. These drugs bypass the brain's own neurotransmitters and directly stimulate the brain's own receptors for these drugs, causing dopamine to be released (Fig. 13–2). Since the brain already uses neurotransmitters that resemble drugs of abuse, it is not necessary to earn one's reward naturally, since a much more intense reward can be obtained in the short run and on demand from a drug of abuse than from a natural high with the brain's natural system. However, unlike a natural high, a drug-induced reward causes such wonderful feeding of dopamine to postsynaptic limbic dopamine

2 (D2) sites that they furiously crave even more drug to replenish dopamine once the drug stops working, leading the individual to be preoccupied with finding more drug and thus beginning a vicious circle.

Because there appears to be an optimal range in which D2 receptor stimulation by the mesolimbic dopamine system is reinforcing, the risk of becoming a substance abuser may depend on how many receptors a person has. Thus, in subjects who have only a few receptors for a given substance, taking that substance will not cause much of an effect at first, but the substance will become more and more rewarding as the dose increases. However, in subjects with many receptors for a given substance, taking that substance will be aversive and they will not want to try it again. One might also postulate that in those with few substance receptors, their own internal reward system is not working too well in the first place. This might predispose them to keep trying drugs as a means of compensating for their own naturally decreased activation of reward circuits. In fact, studies in alcoholics, cocaine abusers, and amphetamine abusers show that a low initial response to a drug predicts a high risk for ultimate abuse, whereas a high initial response to a drug predicts a low risk of abuse.

## Stimulants: Cocaine and Amphetamine

Cocaine (Fig. 13–3) has two major properties: it is both a local anesthetic and an inhibitor of monoamine transporters, especially dopamine (Fig. 13–4). Cocaine's local anesthetic properties are still used in medicine, especially by ear, nose, and throat specialists (otolaryngologists). Freud himself exploited this property of cocaine to help dull the pain of his tongue cancer. He may have also exploited the second property of the drug, which is to produce euphoria, reduce fatigue, and create a sense of mental acuity due to inhibition of dopamine reuptake at the dopamine transporter. Cocaine also has similar but less important actions at the norepinephrine and the serotonin transporters (Fig. 13–3). Cocaine may do more than merely block the transporter—it may actually release dopamine (or norepinephrine or serotonin) by reversing neurotransmitter out of the presynaptic neuron via the monoamine transporters (Fig. 13–4).

At higher doses, cocaine can produce undesirable effects, including tremor, emotional lability, restlessness, irritability, paranoia, panic, and repetitive stereotyped behavior. At even higher doses, it can induce intense anxiety, paranoia, and hallucinations, along with hypertension, tachycardia, ventricular irritability, hyperthermia, and respiratory depression. In overdose, cocaine can cause acute heart failure, stroke, and seizures. Acute intoxication with cocaine produces these various clinical effects, depending on the dose; these effects are mediated by inhibition of the dopamine transporter and in turn by the effects of excessive dopamine activity in dopamine synapses, as well as by norepinephrine and serotonin in their respective synapses.

Repeated intoxication with cocaine may produce complex adaptations of the dopamine neuronal system, including both tolerance and, indeed, the opposite phenomenon, called sensitization or *reverse tolerance*. One example of reverse tolerance may be what happens to some abusers on repeated intoxication with cocaine at doses that previously only induced euphoria. In these cases, cocaine causes a behavioral

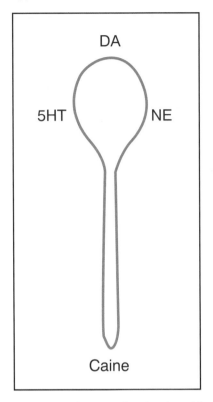

FIGURE 13–3. Icon of **cocaine**. The main mechanism of action is to block reuptake and cause the release of monoamines, principally dopamine (DA), but also norepinephrine (NE) and serotonin (5HT). There is also a local anesthetic action (caine).

reaction that can take the form of an acute paranoid psychosis virtually indistinguishable from paranoid schizophrenia (Fig. 13–5).

This should not be surprising, because the major hypothesis for the etiology of the positive symptoms of psychosis (discussed in Chapter 10 on schizophrenia) is an excess of dopamine activity in this same mesolimbic dopamine pathway (see Fig. 10–9). When the reinforcing properties of cocaine, mediated via mild to moderate stimulation of D2 receptors in this pathway, become "too much of a good thing" (i.e., the compulsive quest for euphoria and pleasure through pleasurable stimulation of these receptors), this eventually results in sensitization of these receptors and induction of *overactivity* in this pathway, reproducing the pathophysiology underlying the positive symptoms of schizophrenia (see Fig. 10–9). This complication of cocaine abuse requires chronic use in order to sensitize the mesolimbic dopamine system, which eventually releases progressively more and more dopamine until repetitive cocaine abuse erupts into frank psychosis. How the dopamine synapse becomes sensitized to cocaine so that this effect can be produced on repeated administration is unknown. Interestingly, treatment with dopamine receptor–blocking atypical antipsychotics or conventional antipsychotics can also relieve the symptoms of cocaine intoxication, as would be expected by analogy with schizophrenia (see Fig. 11–2).

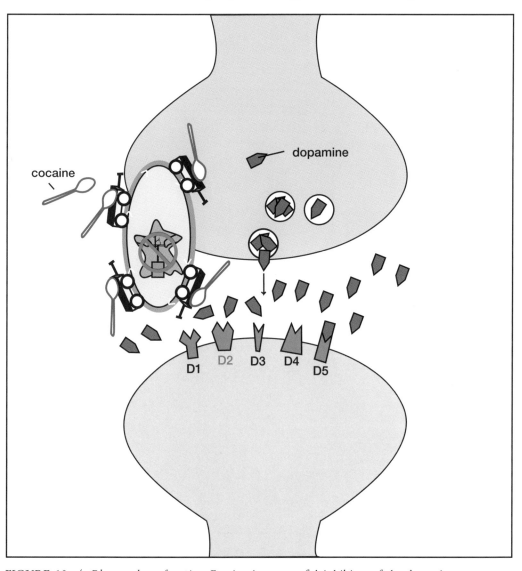

FIGURE 13–4. *Pharmacology of cocaine.* Cocaine is a powerful inhibitor of the dopamine transporter. Blocking this transporter acutely causes dopamine to accumulate, and this produces euphoria, reduces fatigue, and creates a sense of mental acuity. Cocaine has similar but less important actions at the norepinephrine and serotonin transporters.

In addition to the acute intoxicating effects and the chronic reverse tolerance effects of cocaine, all of which are mediated by increasing dopamine levels due to its release from dopamine synapses, there are also longer-term effects of cocaine, possibly due to other, more traditional desensitization types of adaptations of dopamine receptors. As abusers use cocaine for longer and longer periods of time, their dopamine receptors become desensitized (down-regulated) as they adapt to chronic

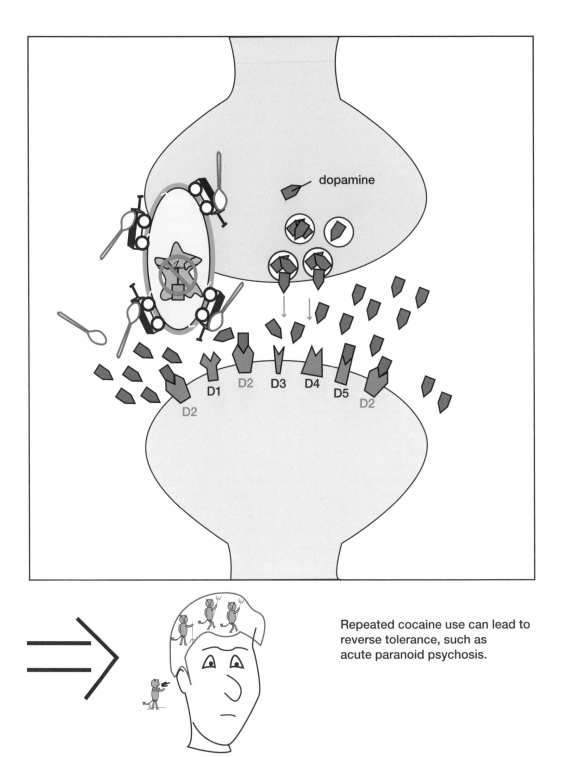

FIGURE 13–5. *Production of reverse tolerance in a cocaine abuser.* Repeated intoxication with cocaine may produce complex adaptations of the dopamine neuronal system, such as sensitization or "reverse tolerance." Thus, in repeat users, cocaine releases more and more dopamine. In such cases doses of cocaine that previously only induced euphoria can create an acute paranoid psychosis virtually indistinguishable from paranoid schizophrenia.

exposure. After consecutive episodes of intoxication followed by abstinence, they mediate an increasingly bothersome withdrawal syndrome.

A subjective experience that may follow the euphoria is a sense of "crashing," characterized by craving more cocaine and accompanied by agitation and anxiety, giving way to fatigue, depression, exhaustion, hypersomnolence, and hyperphagia. After several days, if another dose of cocaine is not taken, the chronic abuser may experience other signs of withdrawal, including anergy, decreased interest, anhedonia, and increased cocaine craving.

Since dopamine neurotransmission via D2 receptors in the mesolimbic dopamine pathway is thought to mediate in large part the psychopharmacology of pleasure and therefore the reinforcing properties of many drugs of abuse, it is not surprising that cocaine abusers describe their highs as more intense and pleasurable than orgasm and their lows as the inability to experience any pleasure whatsoever (anhedonia). These latter complaints are reminiscent of symptoms of depression, and it is not surprising that a condition that acts to mobilize and deplete dopamine and then to desensitize dopamine receptors could create a condition that mimics the signs of major depressive disorder. Interventions aimed at repleting dopamine stores and readapting dopamine receptor sensitivity would be theoretically useful for the cocaine abuser dependent—with both tolerance and reverse tolerance—on cocaine. However, the most useful intervention often is to allow the dopamine system to restore itself with time alone, provided that the abuser can remain abstinent long enough for the system to recover. This, of course is often not feasible or even desired by the abuser. In the future, there may be a "reverse cocaine" available for therapeutic purposes, which would work analogously to the action of a "reverse serotonin selective reuptake inhibitor (SSRI)" or "serotonin reuptake enhancer" tianeptine, as discussed in the section on the mechanism of action of the SSRIs in Chapter 6. This experimental agent for cocaine abuse does not block the reuptake pump for dopamine, nor does it cause a reverse flow of dopamine out of the synapse, as does cocaine; it actually pumps dopamine back into the presynaptic neuron, and is thus a dopamine reuptake enhancer. Another therapeutic possibility for cocaine abusers in the future would be antibodies to cocaine.

*Amphetamines*, especially *d-amphetamine* and *methamphetamine* (Fig. 13–6), also have potent pharmacological effects on the dopamine neuron. Their predominant actions are to release dopamine (Figs. 13–7 and 13–8). Amphetamine and derivatives of amphetamines also have weaker releasing actions at noradrenergic synapses as discussed in Chapter 12 (see Figs. 12–4 and 12–5), and some amphetamine derivatives also release serotonin. Recently, a new neurotransmitter system, called cocaine- and amphetamine-regulated transcript (CART) peptides, has been discovered. This is a peptide neurotransmitter system, identified first as mRNA (i.e., a transcript) that was increased after administration of either cocaine or amphetamine. Now that the peptides for which this RNA codes are being characterized, it appears that these so-called CART peptides probably have a role in drug abuse and in the control of stress and feeding behavior. Their receptors could be a target for future drug abuse therapies.

The clinical effects of amphetamine and its derivatives are very similar to those of cocaine, although the euphoria they produces may be less intense but last longer than that due to cocaine. Signs of amphetamine intoxication, toxicity, overdose, sensitization by production of an acute paranoid psychosis, and withdrawal syndrome are all similar to those described above for cocaine.

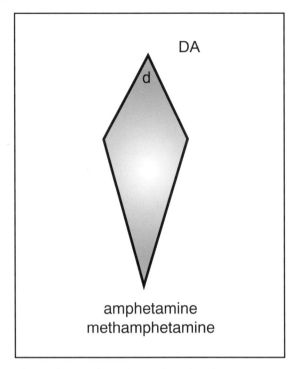

FIGURE 13–6. Icon of **amphetamine/methamphetamine**. Amphetamine (principally *d*-amphetamine) and related derivatives such as methamphetamine are also releasers of dopamine, with a mechanism similar to that described for cocaine.

## Hallucinogens, Designer Drugs, and Phencyclidine

### Hallucinogens

The hallucinogens are a group of agents that produce intoxication, sometimes called a "trip," associated with changes in sensory experiences, including visual illusions and hallucinations, an enhanced awareness of external stimuli, and an enhanced awareness of internal thoughts and stimuli. These hallucinations are produced with a clear level of consciousness and a lack of confusion and may be both psychedelic and psychotomimetic. *Psychedelic* is the term for the subjective experience, due to heightened sensory awareness, that one's mind is being expanded or that one is in unison with mankind or the universe and having some sort of a religious experience. *Psychotomimetic* means that the experience mimics a state of psychosis (see Table 10–3), but the resemblance between a trip and psychosis is superficial at best. As previously discussed, the stimulants cocaine and amphetamine mimic psychosis much more genuinely.

Hallucinogen intoxication includes visual illusions; visual "trails," in which the image smears into streaks as it moves across a trail; macropsia and micropsia; emotional and mood lability; subjective slowing of time; the sense that colors are heard and sounds are seen; intensification of sound perception; depersonalization and derealization. All these effects may be experienced while yet retaining a state of full wakefulness and alertness. Other changes may include impaired judgment, fear of

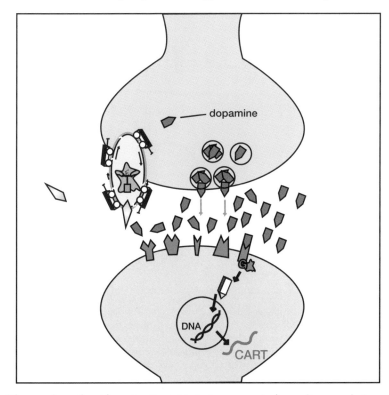

FIGURE 13–7. *Pharmacology of amphetamine (part 1)*. It has recently been discovered that after amphetamine releases dopamine, the postsynaptic targets of amphetamine stimulate the expression of some novel genes, which make messenger RNA for a novel neurotransmitter system. The messenger RNA (or transcript) is called cocaine- and amphetamine-regulated transcript (CART) (see Fig. 13–8). CART is a novel neurotransmitter system, which may be involved in regulating neuronal systems in drug abuse.

losing one's mind, anxiety, nausea, tachycardia, increased blood pressure, and increased body temperature. Not surprisingly, when the list of symptoms above is compared with the list of symptoms for a panic attack in Chapter 9 (Table 9–6), hallucinogen intoxication can cause what is perceived as a panic attack but often called a "bad trip." As intoxication escalates, one can experience an acute confusional state called *delirium*, in which the abuser is disoriented and agitated. This can evolve further into frank psychosis with delusions and paranoia.

Common hallucinogens include two major classes of agents. Agents of the first class (indolealkylamines) resemble serotonin and include the classical hallucinogens *d*-lysergic acid diethylamide (LSD), psilocybin, and dimethyltryptamine (DMT) (Fig. 13–9). Agents of the second class (phenylalkylamines) resemble norepinephrine and dopamine, are also related to amphetamine, and include mescaline, 2,5-dimethoxy-4-methylamphetamine (DOM), and others. More recently, synthetic chemists have come up with some new "designer drugs" such as 3,4-methylenedioxymethamphetamine (MDMA). These are either stimulants or hallucinogens and produce a complex subjective state sometimes referred to as "ecstasy," which is also what abus-

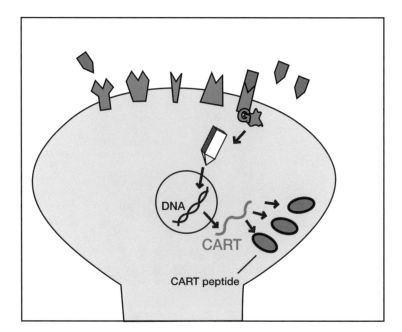

FIGURE 13–8. *Pharmacology of amphetamine (part 2)*. After dopamine is released and the postsynaptic target cells express genes for cocaine- and amphetamine-regulated transcript (CART) as shown in Figure 13–7, the next step is the synthesis of various neurotransmitter CART peptides. These peptides probably have a role not only in drug abuse but also in the control of stress and feeding behavior. Their receptors could be targets for future drug abuse therapies.

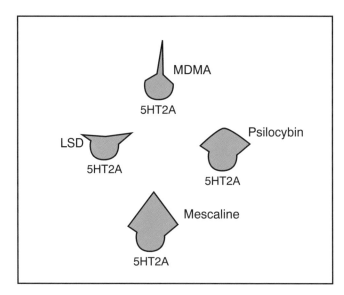

FIGURE 13–9. Icons of **hallucinogens**. Hallucinogens such as lysergic acid diethylamide (LSD), mescaline, psyloscibin, and 3,4-methylenedioxymethamphetamine (MDMA) are partial agonists at 5HT2A receptors.

512

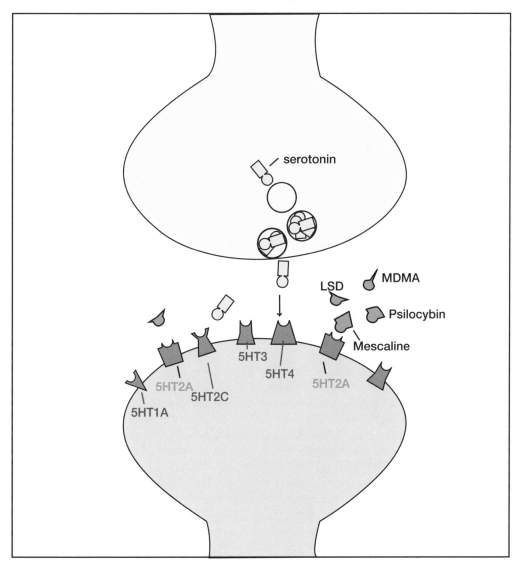

FIGURE 13–10. Here hallucinogenic drugs such as LSD, mescaline, and psilocybin, as well as the "designer drugs" such as MDMA, are interacting as partial agonists at 5HT2A receptors at serotoninergic postsynaptic neuronal sites.

ers call MDMA itself. The effects of MDMA include euphoria, disorientation, confusion, enhanced sociability, and a sense of increased empathy and personal insight.

Hallucinogens have rather complex interactions at neurotransmitter systems, but one of the most prominent is a common action as agonists at serotonin 2A (5HT2A) receptor sites (Fig. 13–10). Hallucinogens certainly have additional effects at other 5HT receptors (especially 5HT1A somatodendritic autoreceptors) and also at other neurotransmitter systems, especially norepinephrine and dopamine, but the relative importance of these other actions are less well known. Also, MDMA appears to be a powerful releaser of serotonin and it and several drugs structurally related to it

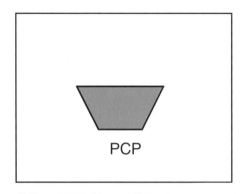

FIGURE 13–11. Icon of **phencyclidine (PCP)**. Phencyclidine is an antagonist of an ion channel site associated with the N-methyl-*d*-aspartate (NMDA) subtype of glutamate receptor.

may even destroy serotonin axon terminals. However, the action that appears to explain a common mechanism for most of the hallucinogens is the stimulation of 5HT2A receptors.

Hallucinogens can produce incredible tolerance, sometimes after a single dose. Desensitization of 5HT2A receptors is hypothesized to underlie this rapid clinical and pharmacological tolerance. Another unique dimension of hallucinogen abuse is the production of "flashbacks," namely the spontaneous recurrence of some of the symptoms of intoxication, which lasts from a few seconds to several hours but in the absence of recent administration of the hallucinogen. This may occur days to months after the last drug experience and can apparently be precipitated by a number of environmental stimuli. The psychopharmacological mechanism underlying flashbacks is unknown, but its phenomenology suggests the possibility of a neurochemical adaptation of the serotonin system and its receptors related to reverse tolerance and incredibly long-lasting. Alternatively, flashbacks could be a form of emotional conditioning triggered when a later emotional experience occurring when one is not taking a hallucinogen nevertheless reminds one of experiences that occurred when intoxicated with a hallucinogen. This could precipitate a whole cascade of feelings that occurred originally while intoxicated with a hallucinogen. This is analogous to the reexperiencing flashbacks that occur without drugs in patients with posttraumatic stress disorder.

### Phencyclidine

Phenylcyclidine (PCP) (Fig. 13–11) was originally developed as an anesthetic but proved to be unacceptable for this use because it induces a unique psychotomimetic-hallucinatory experience. Its structurally related and mechanism-related analogue ketamine is still used as an anesthetic but causes far less of the psychotomimetic-hallucinatory experience. Nevertheless, some people do abuse ketamine, one of the "club drugs," which is sometimes called "special K." Phenylcyclidine causes intense analgesia, amnesia, delirium, stimulant as well as depressant effects, staggering gait, slurred speech, and a unique form of nystagmus (i.e., vertical nystagmus). Higher degrees of intoxication can cause catatonia (excitement alternating with stupor and catalepsy), hallucinations, delusions, paranoia, disorientation, and lack of judgment.

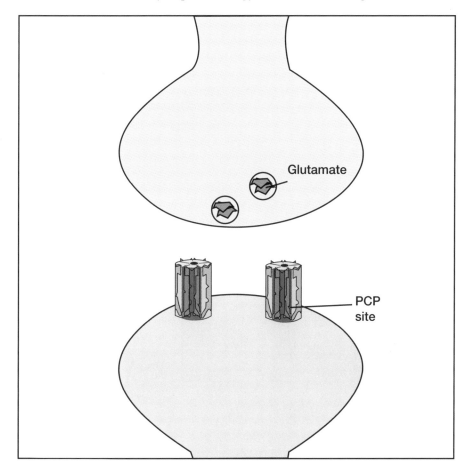

FIGURE 13–12. *Pharmacology of phencyclidine (PCP)*. Phenylcyclidine is an open-channel *antagonist of N-methyl-d-aspartate (NMDA) glutamate receptors* at a site probably closely associated with the calcium ion channel there. This means that its site is probably inside the calcium channel, and it probably works best when the channel is open.

Overdose can include coma, extremely high temperature, seizures, and muscle break-down (rhabdomyolysis).

We have already briefly mentioned the mechanism of action of PCP in Chapter 10 in our discussion on neuroprotective agents (Fig. 10–24). It acts as an allosteric modulator of the NMDA subtype of glutamate receptor (Figs. 13–12 and 13–13). It specifically acts to block this receptor and to decrease the flux of calcium into the cell. Phenylcyclidine itself and other agents that act at the PCP receptor may be neuroprotective, but apparently only at the expense of disrupting memory and causing psychosis (Fig. 13–13).

## Getting Stoned With or Without Inhaling: Marijuana and the Endocannabinoids

Cannabis preparations are smoked in order to deliver their psychoactive substances, cannabinoids, especially THC delta-9-tetrahydrocannabinol (THC) (Fig. 13–14).

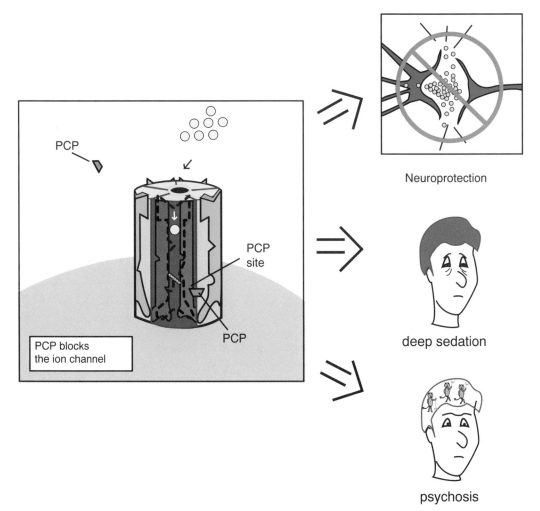

FIGURE 13–13. The PCP site is a modulatory site for the ion channel at the NMDA glutamate receptor–calcium channel complex, which can block this channel and prevent calcium from flowing through it in response to glutamate. This can be neuroprotective at very high doses and sedating or anesthetic at high doses but psychotomimetic at moderate doses.

These smoked substances interact with the brain's own cannabinoid receptors to trigger dopamine release from the mesolimbic reward system. There are two known cannabinoid receptors, CB1 (in the brain, which is coupled via G proteins and modulates adenylate cyclase and ion channels) and CB2 (in the immune system). The CB1 receptors may mediate not only marijuana's reinforcing properties, but also those of alcohol. There is also an endogenous cannabinoid system (the brain's own marijuana) capable of activating these cannabinoid receptors functionally. These *endocannabinoids* are synthesized by neurons and inactivated by reuptake systems and enzymes in both neurons and glia.

Anandamide is one of these endocannabinoids and a member of a new chemical class of neurotransmitters, which is not a monoamine, not an amino acid, and not

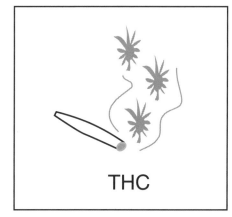

FIGURE 13–14. Icon for **tetrahydrocannabinol (THC)**, the psychoactive ingredient in marijuana.

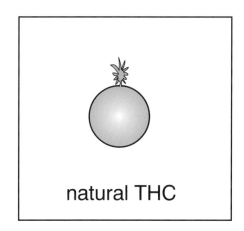

FIGURE 13–15. Icon for **anandamide**, the brain's endocannabinoid (the "brain's own marijuana").

a peptide—it is a lipid, specifically a member of a family of fatty acid ethanolamides (Fig. 13–15). Anandamide shares most but not all of the pharmacologic properties of THC, since its actions at brain cannabinoid receptors are not only mimicked by THC but are antagonized in part by the selective brain cannabinoid antagonist SR141716A (Fig. 13–16). The discovery of this marijuana antagonist (Fig. 13–16) opens the door to using it as a potential therapeutic agent in various types of drug abuse. It is already in clinical testing in schizophrenia (as discussed in Chapter 11), since that disorder is hypothesized to be due to hyperactivity in the same pathway that mediates reward (Fig. 10–9) and is overstimulated by drugs of abuse (Fig. 13–2).

Marijuana can have both stimulant and sedative properties. In usual intoxicating doses, it produces a sense of well-being, relaxation, and friendliness, a loss of temporal awareness, (including confusing the past with the present), slowing of thought processes, impairment of short-term memory, and a feeling of achieving special insights. At high doses, marijuana can induce panic, toxic delirium, and rarely, psy-

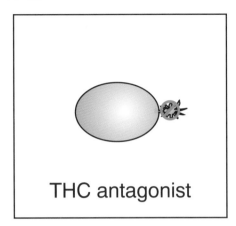

**THC antagonist**

FIGURE 13–16. Icon for **marijuana antagonist**, theoretically a treatment for drug abuse and for use in testing for schizophrenia.

chosis. One complication of long-term use is the so-called amotivational syndrome in frequent users. This syndrome is seen predominantly in heavy daily users and is characterized by the emergence of decreased drive and ambition. It is also associated with other socially and occupationally impairing symptoms, including a shortened attention span, poor judgment, easy distractibility, impaired communication skills, introversion, and diminished effectiveness in interpersonal situations. Personal habits may deteriorate, and there may be a loss of insight and even feelings of deperson-alization. In terms of chronic administration to humans, tolerance to cannabinoids has been well documented, but the question of cannabinoid dependence has always been controversial. The discovery of the brain cannabinoid antagonist SR141716A (Fig. 13–16) has settled this question in experimental animals because it precipitates a withdrawal syndrome in mice chronically exposed to THC. It is therefore highly likely, but not yet proved, that dependence also occurs in humans and is presumably due to the same types of adaptive changes in cannabinoid receptors that occur in other neurotransmitter receptors after chronic administration of other drugs of abuse.

### Nicotine

Cigarette smoking is a nicotine delivery system. Unfortunately, it also delivers car-cinogens and other toxins that damage the heart, lungs, and other tissues as well. In terms of psychopharmacology, nicotine acts directly on nicotinic cholinergic re-ceptors (Fig. 13–17) (see discussion of cholinergic neurons in Chapter 12 and Fig. 12–10). The reinforcing actions of nicotine are very similar to those of cocaine and amphetamine, since dopaminergic cells in the mesolimbic dopamine pathway receive direct nicotinic cholinergic input, which is stimulated by cigarette smoking (Figs. 13–2 and 13–18). This mediates the reward experienced by smokers, including elevation of mood, enhancement of cognition, and decrease of appetite. The psycho-pharmacological and behavioral actions of nicotine, however, appear to be much more subtle than those of cocaine. Whereas cocaine blocks the dopamine transporter and causes a flood of dopamine to act at the dopamine synapse, nicotine may shut down the nicotinic receptor shortly after binding to it (Fig. 13–19), so that neither it nor

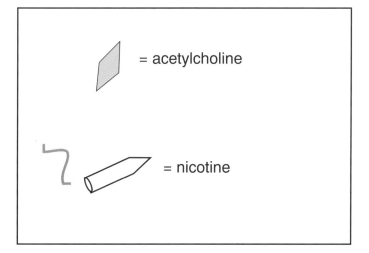

FIGURE 13—17. Icons for **nicotine** and **acetylcholine**.

acetylcholine itself can stimulate the nicotinic receptor any further for a while. Thus, dopaminergic stimulation of mesolimbic dopamine receptors stops after a short period and a small amount of nicotinic stimulation. Instead of the longer and much more intense euphoria of cocaine, the pleasure of nicotine is a desirable but small boost in the sensation of pleasure ("minirush"), followed by a slow decline until the nicotinic receptors switch back on and the smoker takes the next puff or smokes the next cigarette. Nicotine's psychopharmacological effects, therefore, may be somewhat self-regulating, which may explain why its effects on behavior are more limited than the effects of cocaine or amphetamine.

Both stimulant users and smokers may down-regulate their dopamine receptors because of excessive dopamine stimulation. However, nicotine users may up-regulate their nicotinic cholinergic receptors to help compensate for the fact that nicotine keeps turning them off (Fig. 13—20). These possible changes in dopamine and nicotine receptors may be related to the psychopharmacological mechanisms underlying nicotine's profound ability to produce dependence and withdrawal.

Dependence on nicotine causes a withdrawal syndrome characterized by craving and agitation, reminiscent of but less severe than that experienced by a stimulant abuser in withdrawal (Fig. 13—21). The recent availability of a nicotine delivery system through a transdermal patch is popular as a means to assist patients to detoxify from smoking. The pulsatile delivery of nicotine through smoking (Fig. 13—22) can be replaced by continuous delivery through a transdermal skin patch acting similarly to a constant intravenous infusion (Fig. 13—23). The idea is that the nicotine and dopamine receptors are allowed to readapt more gradually toward normal than they would if the smoker suddenly became abstinent. The hope is that the withdrawal syndrome is prevented or blunted when nicotine is delivered transdermally. In addition, the nicotine dose can be progressively decreased, depending on how much dose reduction the abstinent smoker can tolerate. The dose is decreased in a slow, stepwise fashion until the patient is able to tolerate complete abstinence from smoking and complete discontinuation of transdermal nicotine delivery. The success of this approach depends on the motivation of the smoker to quit and the

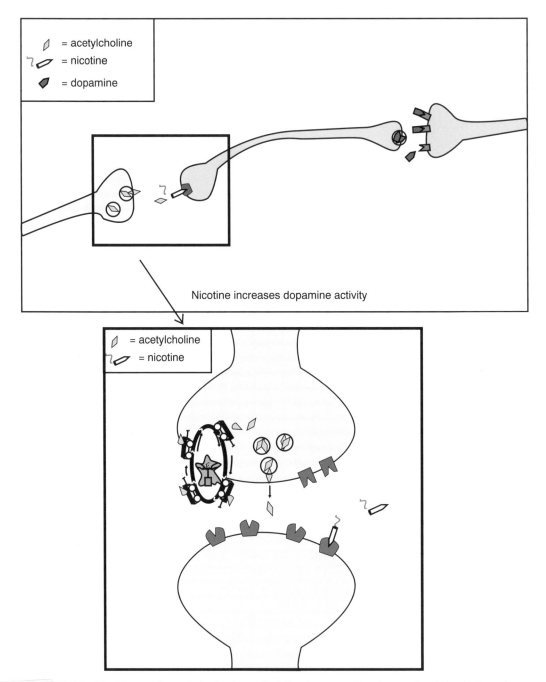

FIGURE 13–18. *Pharmacology of nicotine (part 1)*. Nicotine acts directly on nicotinic cholinergic receptors, which are themselves located in part on mesolimbic dopamine neurons. When nicotine stimulates these receptors (A and B), it causes release of dopamine from the mesolimbic neurons and thereby conveys a sense of reward and pleasure.

use of adjunctive psychological support and information programs to help the smoker cope better with abstinence.

Another approach to facilitating smoking cessation is to reduce the craving that occurs during abstinence (Fig. 13–21) by boosting dopamine with the dopamine and norepinephrine reuptake inhibitor bupropion (see Figs. 6–48 and 6–49). The idea is to give back some of the dopamine downstream to the craving postsynaptic limbic D2 receptors while they are adjusting to the absence of their dopamine "fix" due to the recent withdrawal of nicotine (Fig. 13–24).

## Opiates

Opiates act on a variety of receptors. The three most important subtypes are the mu, delta, and kappa opiate receptors (Fig. 13–25). The brain makes its own endogenous opiate-like substances, sometimes referred to as the "brain's own morphine." They are peptides derived from precursor proteins called pro-opiomelanocortin (POMC), proen-kephalin, and prodynorphin. Parts of these precursor proteins are cleaved off to form endorphins or enkephalins, stored in opiate neurons, and presumably released during neurotransmission to mediate endogenous opiate-like actions (Fig. 13–25). However, the precise number and function of endogenous opiates and their receptors and their role in pain relief and other central nervous system (CNS) actions remain largely unknown.

Exogenous opiates in the form of pain relievers, such as codeine or morphine, or drugs of abuse, such as heroin, are also thought to act as agonists at mu, delta, and kappa opiate receptors (Fig. 13–26), particularly mu receptors. At and above pain-relieving doses, the opiates induce euphoria, which is their main reinforcing property. Opiates can also induce a very intense but brief euphoria, sometimes called a "rush," followed by a profound sense of tranquility, which may last several hours, followed in turn by drowsiness ("nodding"), mood swings, mental clouding, apathy, and slowed motor movements. In overdose, these same agents act as depressants of res-piration and can also induce coma. The acute actions of opiates can be reversed by synthetic opiate antagonists, such as naloxone and naltrexone, which compete as antagonists at opiate receptors.

When given chronically, opiates readily cause both tolerance and dependence. Adaptation of opiate receptors occurs quite readily after chronic opiate administra-tion. The first sign of this is the need of the patient to take a higher and higher dose of opiate in order to relieve pain or to induce the desired euphoria. Eventually, there may be little room between the dose that causes euphoria and that which produces the toxic effects of an overdose. Another sign that dependence has occurred and that opiate receptors have adapted by decreasing their sensitivity to agonist actions is the production of a withdrawal syndrome once the chronically administered opiate wears off. The opiate antagonists such as naloxone can precipitate a withdrawal syndrome in opiate-dependent persons. This withdrawal syndrome is characterized by a feeling of dysphoria, craving for another dose of opiate, irritability, and signs of autonomic hyperactivity, such as tachycardia, tremor, and sweating. Piloerection ("goose bumps") is often associated with opiate withdrawal, especially when the drug is stopped suddenly ("cold turkey"). This is so subjectively horrible that the opiate abuser will often stop at nothing in order to obtain another dose of opiate to relieve symptoms of withdrawal. Thus, what may have begun as a quest for euphoria may end up as a quest to avoid withdrawal. Clonidine, an alpha 2 adrenergic agonist, can reduce signs of autonomic hyperactivity during withdrawal and aid in the detoxification process.

In the early days of opiate use, abuse, and intoxication and prior to completion of the neuroadaptive mechanisms, that mediate opiate receptor desensitization, opiate intoxication alternates with normal functioning. Later, after the opiate receptors adapt and dependency is established, the abuser may experience very little euphoria, but mostly withdrawal-free periods alternating with withdrawal.

Opiate receptors can readapt to normal if given a chance to do so in the absence of additional opiate intake. This may be too difficult for the abuser to tolerate, so reinstitution of another opiate, such as methadone, which can be taken orally and then slowly tapered, may assist in the detoxification process. A partial mu opiate agonist, buprenophine, may also become available in a sublingual dosage formulation to substitute for stronger opiates and then be tapered. It will be combined with the opiate naloxone so that it cannot be abused intravenously. L-Alpha-acetylmethodol acetate (LAAM) is a long-acting orally active opiate with pharmacologic properties similar to those of methadone. Agonist substitution treatments are best used in the setting of a structured maintenance treatment program, which includes random urine drug screening and intensive psychological, medical, and vocational services.

## Alcohol

The pharmacology of alcohol is still relatively poorly characterized, and its mechanism of action is nonspecific since alcohol can have effects on a wide variety of neurotransmitter systems. Neither alcohol's acute intoxicating actions nor its chronic effects of dependence, tolerance, and withdrawal are understood very well. However, various research studies do suggest that alcohol acts not only by enhancing inhibitory neurotransmission at GABA-A receptors (Fig. 13–27), but also by reducing excitatory neurotransmission at the N-methyl-$d$-aspartate (NMDA) subtype of glutamate receptors (Fig. 13–28). That is, alcohol enhances inhibition and reduces excitation, and this may explain its characterization as a "depressant" of CNS neuronal functioning (Fig. 13–29). These effects of alcohol may thus explain some of its in-

---

FIGURE 13–19. *Pharmacology of nicotine (part 2).* Although Figure 13–18 suggests that the pharmacology of nicotine shares similarities with the pharmacology of cocaine, the actions of nicotine appear to be much more subtle than those of cocaine. Whereas cocaine blocks the dopamine transporter and causes a flood of dopamine to act at the dopamine synapse, nicotine stimulation of nicotinic receptors (Fig. 13–19A) may shut down the nicotinic receptor by causing it to withdraw into a membrane pit (Fig. 13–19B) shortly after binding to it, so that it cannot stimulate the nicotinic receptor any further for a time. Thus, dopaminergic stimulation of mesolimbic dopamine receptors stops after a short time and small amount of nicotinic stimulation. Instead of the longer and much more intense euphoria of cocaine, the pleasure of nicotine is a desirable but small boost in the sensation of pleasure (mini-"rush"), followed by a slow decline until the nicotinic receptors switch back on and the smoker takes the next puff or smokes the next cigarette. Nicotine's psychopharmacological effects, therefore, may be somewhat self-regulating, which may explain why its effects on behavior are more limited than the effects of cocaine or amphetamine.

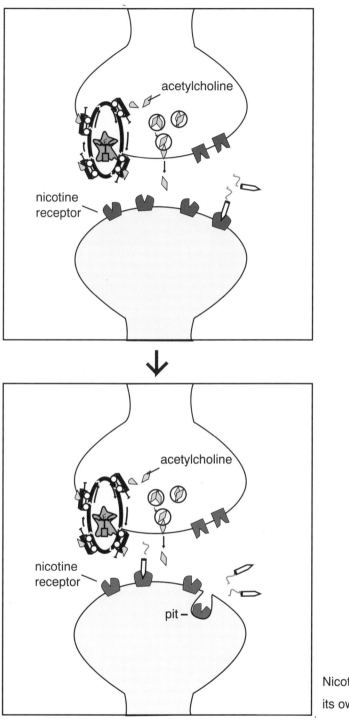

acetylcholine

nicotine
receptor

acetylcholine

nicotine
receptor

pit –

Nicotine will "turn off"

its own receptor for a time

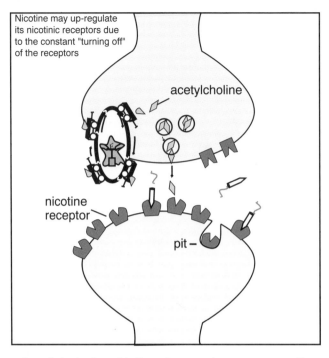

FIGURE 13–20. *Pharmacology of nicotine (part 3).* Over time, smokers may eventually up-regulate their nicotinic cholinergic receptors to help compensate for the fact that nicotine keeps turning them off. These changes in nicotine receptors may be related to the psychopharmacological mechanisms underlying nicotine's profound ability to produce dependence and withdrawal.

toxicating, amnestic, and ataxic effects. However, alcohol's reinforcing effects are theoretically mediated by the effects that its changes in GABA and glutamate have on dopamine release in the mesolimbic dopamine system (Fig. 13–2). Furthermore, it also seems to release both opiates and cannabinoids in the reward system. Blocking cannabinoid receptors in animals reduces craving for alcohol in alcohol dependent animals. Blocking opiate receptors with naltrexone (Fig. 13–29) in alcohol-dependent humans decreases craving and thereby increases abstinence rates. If one drinks when taking naltrexone, the opiates released do not lead to pleasure, so why bother drinking? (Some patients may also say, why bother taking naltrexone, of course, and relapse back into drinking alcohol.) Naltrexone is recommended for use in the first 90 days of abstinence, when the risk of relapse is highest; however, it has been shown to be generally safe and well tolerated by alcoholic patients for up to a year. Nalmefene is a mu opioid antagonist, which is also being tested in alcoholics to determine whether it increases abstinence rates.

Alcamprosate, a derivative of the amino acid taurine, interacts with the NMDA receptor and perhaps can substitute for this effect of alcohol during abstinence (Fig. 13–30). Thus, when alcohol is withdrawn and the mesolimbic D2 receptors are whining for dopamine because of too much glutamate, perhaps alcamprosate substitution will reduce the neuronal hyperexcitability of alcohol withdrawal, resulting

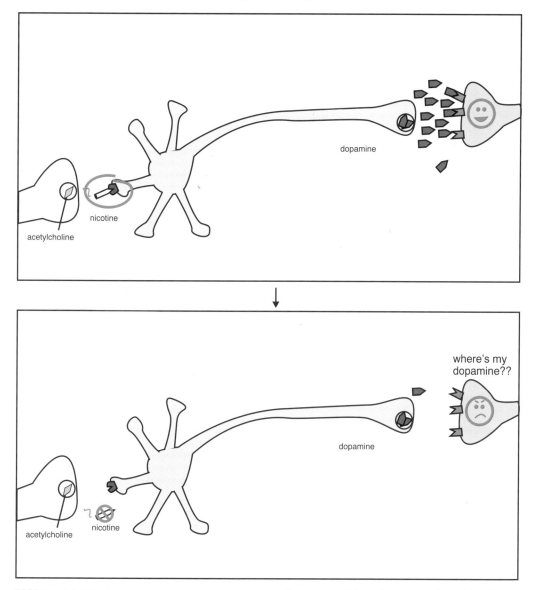

FIGURE 13–21. In the top panel, a regular **smoker delivers reliable nicotine** (red circle), releasing dopamine in the limbic area at frequent intervals, which is very rewarding to the limbic dopamine 2 (D2) receptors on the right. However, during attempts at smoking cessation, dopamine will be cut off when nicotine no longer releases it from the mesolimbic neurons. This upsets the postsynaptic D2 limbic receptors and leads to craving and what some call a "**nicotine fit.**"

in reduced withdrawal distress and craving. Alcamprosate is marketed in Europe and is being tested extensively in the United States.

The subject of how to treat alcohol abuse and dependence is complex, and the most effective treatments are still 12-step programs, which are beyond the scope of this text.

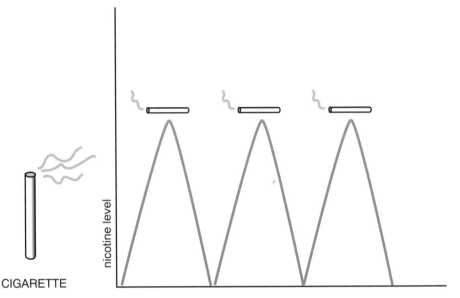

FIGURE 13–22. Cigarette smoking is a *pulsatile nicotine delivery system*. Dependence on nicotine causes a withdrawal syndrome between cigarettes as the nicotine level leaves the blood and the brain. If allowed to progress without another cigarette being smoked, withdrawal from nicotine is characterized by craving and agitation, suggestive of a less severe version of a stimulant abuser in withdrawal.

## Benzodiazepines and Sedative-Hypnotics

### Benzodiazepines

We have already discussed extensively in Chapter 8 the mechanism of the therapeutic actions of benzodiazepines as anxiolytics and sedative-hypnotics and their pharmacologic mechanism as allosteric modulators of GABA-A receptors (Figs. 8–19 to 8–24). This causes a net boosting of chloride conductance through a chloride channel, enhancing inhibitory neurotransmission and causing anxiolytic actions (Fig. 13–31). Such actions are also thought to underlie the production of the reinforcing properties of euphoria and a sedating sort of tranquility, which causes some individuals to abuse these drugs (Fig. 13–2). Excessive actions of benzodiazepines at the same receptors that mediate their therapeutic actions are thought to be the psychopharmacological mechanism of euphoria, drug reinforcement, and at an extreme, overdose.

When benzodiazepines are used or abused chronically, they may cause adaptive changes in benzodiazepine receptors such that their power to modulate GABA-A receptors in response to a benzodiazepine decreases with time (Fig. 13–32). These patients may become irritable or anxious or even experience panic attacks if they suddenly stop taking the drugs (Fig. 13–33). This shift in benzodiazepine abusers to a desensitized receptor (Fig. 13–32) may manifest itself as the need to take higher doses of benzodiazepines to get "high." This receptor desensitization is most likely to be uncovered once chronic abusive benzodiazepine administration is discontinued, particularly if discontinuation is sudden (Fig. 13–33). This desensitized receptor worsens the impact of benzodiazepine discontinuation because the brain, which is

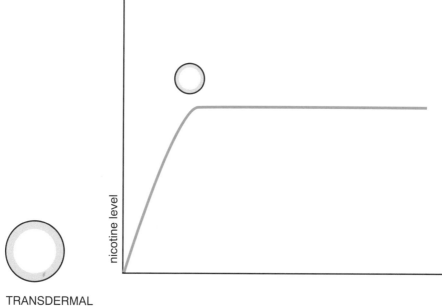

nicotine level

TRANSDERMAL
PATCH

FIGURE 13–23. *Transdermal nicotine administration for the treatment of nicotine withdrawal.* A recently available nicotine delivery system through a transdermal patch is popular as an adjunct in assisting patients to detoxify from smoking. The pulsatile delivery of nicotine through smoking (Fig. 13–22) can be replaced by continuous delivery through a transdermal skin patch, acting similarly to a constant intravenous infusion. The idea is that the nicotine and dopamine receptors are allowed by readapt more gradually to normal than would happen if the smoker suddenly became abstinent. The hope is that the withdrawal syndrome is prevented or blunted when nicotine is delivered transdermally. In addition, the nicotine dose can be progressively decreased depending on how much nicotine dose reduction the abstinent smoker can tolerate. The amount of reduction is increased in a slow, stepwise fashion until the patient is able to tolerate complete abstinence from smoking and complete discontinuation of transdermal nicotine delivery. The success of this approach depends on the motivation of the smoker to quit and the use of adjunctive psychological support and information programs to help the smoker cope better with abstinence.

used to too much benzodiazepine at its receptors, is suddenly starved for benzodiazepine. Therefore, the brain experiences the reverse of benzodiazepine intoxication, namely, dysphoria and depression instead of euphoria, anxiety and agitation instead of tranquility and lack of anxiety, insomnia instead of sedation and sleep, muscle tension instead of muscle relaxation, and at worst, seizures instead of anticonvulsant effects. These actions continue either until benzodiazepine is replaced or until the receptors readapt to the sensitivity they had prior to excessive use of the benzodiazepines. Alternatively, one can reinstitute benzodiazepines but taper them slowly, so that the receptors have time to readapt during dosage reduction and withdrawal symptoms are prevented.

## Sedative-Hypnotics

The pharmacologic mechanisms of drugs are basically the same as those described above for the benzodiazepines. However, these drugs are much less safe in overdose,

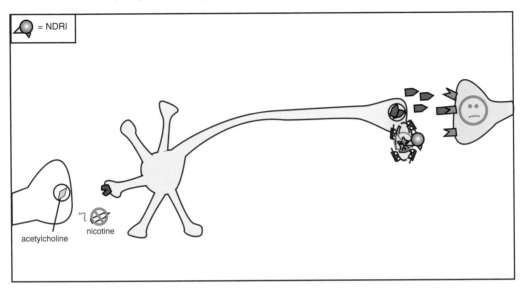

FIGURE 13–24. Rather than substitute a nicotine patch for nicotine cigarettes in **smoking cessation**, another therapeutic approach to diminishing craving during the early stages of smoking cessation is to **deliver a bit of dopamine** itself by blocking dopamine reuptake directly at the nerve terminal with bupropion. Although not as powerful as nicotine, it does take the edge off and makes abstinence more tolerable.

cause dependence more frequently, are abused more frequently, and produce much more dangerous withdrawal reactions. Apparently, the receptor mediating the pharmacologic actions of these agents, presumably an allosteric modulator at GABA-A ligand-gated chloride channels, is even more readily desensitized with even more dangerous consequences than the benzodiazepine receptor (Fig. 13–34). It must also mediate a more intense euphoria and a more desirable sense of tranquility than the benzodiazepine receptor. Since benzodiazepines are frequently an adequate alternative therapy for these drugs, physicians can help minimize abuse of these agents by prescribing them rarely if ever. In the case of withdrawal reactions, reinstituting and then tapering the offending agent under close clinical supervision can assist the detoxification process. These agents include barbiturates and related compounds such as ethclorvynol and ethinamate, chloral hydrate and derivatives; and piperidinedione derivatives such as glutethimide and methyprylon.

## Psychopharmacology of Obesity: My Receptors Made Me Eat It

Metabolism and energy utilization are peripheral endocrine actions. Recent discoveries are lending important insights into how these central and peripheral components of weight control are mediated by receptors for several key neurotransmitters and hormones. Since obesity results from an imbalance between caloric intake and energy expenditure, these new findings suggest that treatment of obesity in the future perhaps will be based both on central mechanisms, which decrease the urge to eat, and on peripheral mechanisms, which increase the mobilization of energy. At present, however, it is useful to be aware that chronic treatment with many psy-

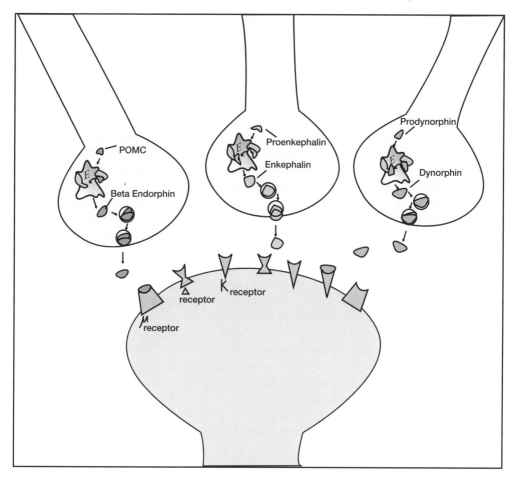

FIGURE 13−25. *Pharmacology of the endogenous opiate systems.* The brain makes its own endogenous opiate-like substances, sometimes referred to as the "brain's own morphine-like molecules." They are peptides derived from a precursor proteins called pro-opiomelanocortin (POMC), proenkephalin, and prodynorphin. Parts of these precursor proteins are cleaved off to form endorphins or enkephalins, stored in opiate neurons, and presumably released during neurotransmission to mediate endogenous opiate-like actions. However, the precise number and function of endogenous opiates and their receptors and their role in pain relief and in other CNS actions remain largely unknown.

chotropic drugs can be associated with changes in weight, particularly weight gain. This is increasingly recognized as a problem for atypical antipsychotics (Table 13−2), although it can also be a problem for many other classes of psychotropic drugs, including antidepressants. Some individuals may abuse stimulants and nicotine for their ability to control weight gain or may struggle with weight gain problems when they try to become abstinent from these agents. Therefore, a brief discussion of the role of receptors and weight is included in this chapter.

## Histamine-1 Receptors

The exact neurotransmitter role of histamine in the CNS remains an enigma. However, regulation of arousal and appetite by histamine has long been suggested by

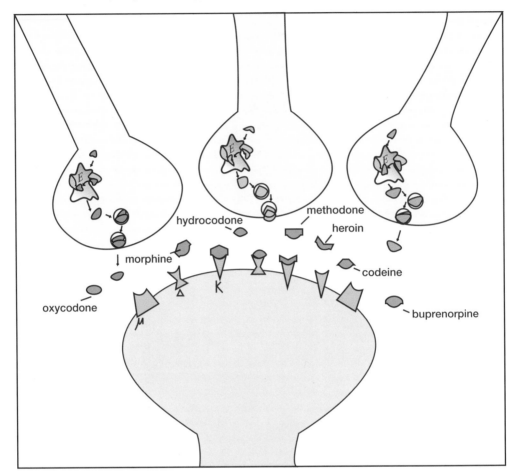

FIGURE 13–26. *Pharmacological actions of opiate drugs.* Opiate drugs act on a variety of receptors, called opiate receptors. Acute actions of opiate drugs cause relief of pain by acting as agonists at opiate receptor subtypes. At and above pain-relieving doses, the opiate drugs induce euphoria, which is the main reinforcing property of the opiates. In sufficient doses, opiates induce a very intense but brief euphoria sometimes called a "rush," followed by a profound sense of tranquility, which may last several hours and is followed in turn by drowsiness ("nodding"), mood swings, mental clouding, apathy, and slowed motor movements. In overdose, these same agents act as depressants of respiration and can also induce coma.

observations that histamine-1 antagonists not only are sedating but also increase appetite and weight in experimental animals and humans. Binding studies of antidepressants and antipsychotics suggest that sedation and weight gain in humans are proportional to their ability to block these histamine receptors. In fact, binding to these receptors correlates best with weight gain among the actions of psychotropic drugs.

## 5-HT2C Receptors

For many years, pharmacologists have known that increasing the availability of serotonin (5-HT) in the synaptic cleft or direct activation of 5-HT receptors reduces

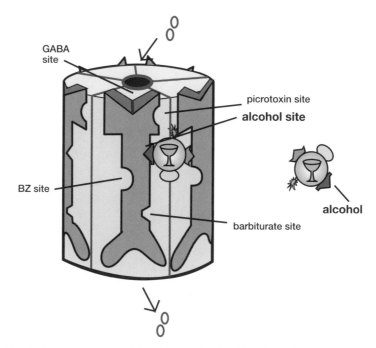

FIGURE 13–27. **Alcohol** mediates some of its pharmacologic effects by enhancing the actions of the **inhibitory GABA A** receptor complex—that is, it enhances inhibition.

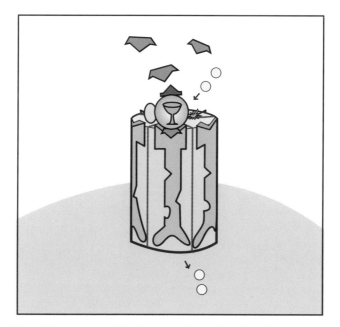

FIGURE 13–28. **Alcohol** mediates some of its pharmacologic effects by decreasing the actions of the **excitatory NMDA** receptor complex—that is, it diminishes excitation.

531

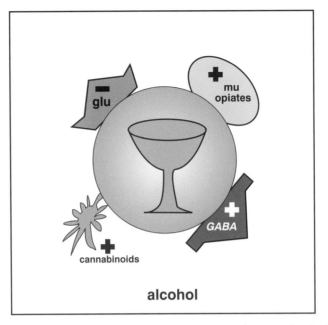

FIGURE 13–29. Icon of **alcohol**. In addition to enhancing GABA inhibition and reducing glutamate excitation, alcohol also enhances euphoric effects by releasing opiates and endocannabinoids, perhaps thereby mediating its "high."

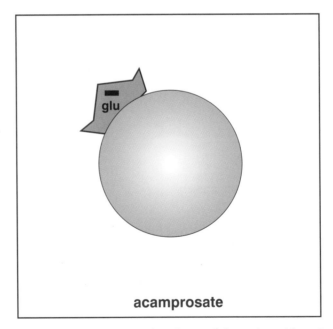

FIGURE 13–30. Icon of **acamprosate**. A structural analogue of the amino acid taurine, acamprosate reduces the excitatory actions of glutamate at the NMDA–calcium channel complex.

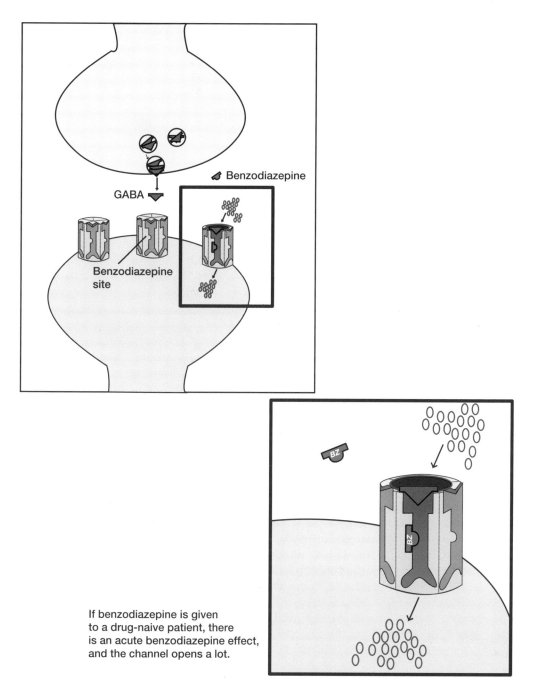

If benzodiazepine is given
to a drug-naive patient, there
is an acute benzodiazepine effect,
and the channel opens a lot.

FIGURE 13–31. *Acute administration of a benzodiazepine to a nondependent individual.* Benzodiazepines act as allosteric modulators of GABA-A receptors. If a benzodiazepine is given to a drug-naive patient, there is an acute benzodiazepine effect, opening the chloride channel maximally. This causes a net boosting of chloride conductance through a chloride channel, enhancing inhibitory neurotransmission and causing anxiolytic actions. Such actions are also thought to underlie production of the reinforcing properties of euphoria or a sedating sort of tranquility, which causes some individuals to abuse these drugs. Excessive actions of benzodiazepines at the same receptors that mediate their therapeutic actions is thought to be the psychopharmacological mechanism of euphoria, drug reinforcement, and at an extreme, overdose.

533

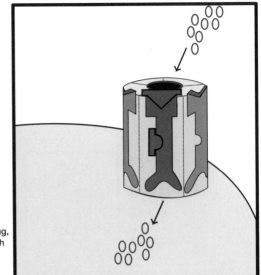

If benzodiazepine is given
to a patient who is tolerant to the drug,
the channel opens a little (still enough
to have an anxiolytic effect)

FIGURE 13–32. *Chronic administration of a benzodiazepine to an individual who has developed tolerance and dependence.* When benzodiazepines are used or abused chronically, they may cause *adaptive changes* in benzodiazepine receptors, such that they become increasingly less powerful in modulating GABA-A receptors in response to a benzodiazepine. Administration of a benzodiazepine to such an individual causes the chloride channel to open less than before but still enough to give an anxiolytic or perhaps a euphoric and drug-reinforcing effect. That effect may be diminished, however, in comparison with acute administration prior to the development of this desensitization and tolerance.

food consumption, while decreasing 5-HT receptor activation brings about the opposite effect. Recent research more specifically implicates the 5-HT2C receptor subtype as playing the key role in regulating appetite. For example, mutant mice that lack the 5-HT2C receptor are obese. Activating 5-HT2C receptors decreases eating behavior in rats. A 5-HT2C mechanism may also underlie weight reduction in humans taking appetite suppressants. Serotonin selective reuptake inhibitors (SSRIs) can also reduce appetite, at least acutely. Fluoxetine, arguably the most anorexigenic of the SSRIs and with a specific indication for bulimia, is also the only SSRI with direct 5-HT2C agonist activity in addition to its 5-HT reuptake blocking properties (see Chapter 6 and Fig. 6–41). The most recently marketed appetite suppressant is sibutramine. Its mechanism works by both 5-HT and norepinephrine reuptake blockade, much like higher doses of venlafaxine (see Chapter 7 and Figs. 7–1 and 7–2). Drugs that block 5HT2C receptors as well as histamine-1 receptors are especially associated with weight gain, although blocking 5HT2C receptors alone is not necessarily associated with weight gain (see Chapter 11 and Table 13–2).

## Beta3-Adrenergic Receptors

The three distinct subtypes of beta receptors are the beta1-adrenergic receptor, which is predominantly a cardiac receptor and the target of beta-blockers; the beta2-

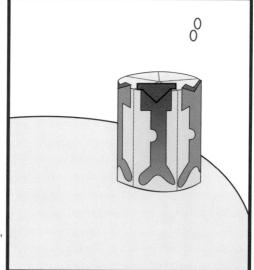

If benzodiazepine is suddenly stopped
for a patient who is tolerant to the drug,
the channel closes, creating anxiety

FIGURE 13–33. *Acute withdrawal of benzodiazepines in a benzodiazepine-dependent individual.* If benzodiazepines are suddenly stopped in a patient who is tolerant to them and dependent on them, benzodiazepine receptors will experience this as an *acute deficiency* at their binding sites. Thus, the presence of desensitized benzodiazepine receptors actually worsens the impact of benzodiazepine discontinuation. The brain, which is used to too much benzodiazepine at its receptors, is suddenly starved for benzodiazepine. Therefore, the brain experiences the reverse of benzodiazepine intoxication, namely, dysphoria and depression instead of euphoria; anxiety and agitation instead of tranquility and lack of anxiety; insomnia instead of sedation and sleep; muscle tension instead of muscle relaxation; and at worst, seizures instead of anticonvulsant effects. These actions continue either until benzodiazepine is replaced or until the receptors readapt to the sensitivity they had prior to excessive benzodiazepine use. Alternatively, one can reinstitute benzodiazepines but taper them slowly, so that the receptors have time to readapt during dosage reduction, and withdrawal symptoms are prevented.

adrenergic receptor, which is in the lungs, where it is the target of bronchodilating agonists, and is also found in the uterus and skeletal muscle; and the beta3-adrenergic receptor, expressed primarily in adipose tissue, where it regulates energy metabolism and thermogenesis (from fat) especially in response to norepinephrine.

Evidence that the beta3-adrenergic receptors play an active role in weight control in humans comes from the finding that a genetic variant of this receptor constitutes a susceptibility factor for the onset of morbid obesity as well as non-insulin-dependent diabetes. Specifically, this variant of the beta3-adrenergic receptor is associated with hereditary obesity in Pima Native Americans from Arizona and has been demonstrated to have an increased incidence in obese patients in Japan. It also exists in nonobese individuals, including one-fourth of African-Americans and about 10% of the general population in Europe and the United States. The various findings suggest a strategy for treating obesity by stimulating metabolism and peripheral burning of fat rather than by acting on central satiety. Sibutramine, for example, increases norepinephrine peripherally at the beta3-adrenergic receptors in adipose tissue, thereby stimulating thermogenesis, increasing oxygen consumption, and thus leading to weight loss.

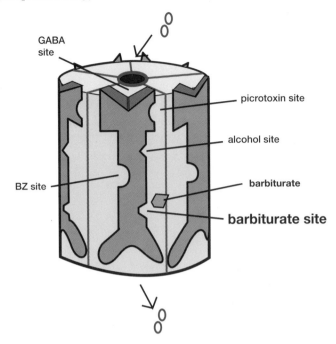

FIGURE 13–34. *Pharmacology of sedative-hypnotic-depressant abuse.* The pharmacologic mechanism of action of these drugs is not yet proven but is thought to be basically the same as that described for the benzodiazepines, namely allosteric modulators at GABA-A ligand-gated chloride channels.

Table 13–2. *Weight gain and antipsychotics (drugs listed in order of increasing weight gain likelihood)*

Loxapine (no weight gain or weight loss)
Molindone
Ziprasidone
Thiothixene
Haloperidol
Risperidone
Chlorpromazine
Sertindole
Quetiapine
Thioridazine
Olanzapine
Zotepine
Clozapine (the most weight gain)

## Neuropeptide Receptors and the Leptin Story

At least three peptides are implicated in the regulation of food intake, energy expenditure, and whole-body energy balance in both rodents and humans and are found both peripherally as hormones and centrally. These are galanin, neuropeptide Y, and leptin. The physiologic roles of these peptides in regulating body weight via their CNS receptors remain somewhat obscure, although the effects of leptin on food intake and energy expenditure are thought to be mediated centrally via neuropeptide Y.

The role of peripheral leptin has been more extensively investigated. Leptin, a member of the interleukin 6 cytokine family, is a peptide found in multiple tissues and secreted by white adipose cells, where it is highly correlated with body fat mass and size of fat cells. The peripheral effects of leptin include regulation of insulin secretion and energy metabolism in fat cells and skeletal muscle, where it seems to play a role in ensuring the maintenance of adequate energy stores, and thereby protects against starvation. It also acts as a metabolic signal that regulates the effect of nutritional status on reproductive function. Cortisol and insulin are potent stimulators of leptin, whereas beta-adrenergic agonists reduce leptin expression.

Administration of leptin to genetically obese mice reduces their food intake and makes them lose weight. Congenital leptin deficiency in humans is associated with severe early-onset obesity. Somewhat paradoxically, however, plasma leptin levels are increased in obese women and decreased in women with anorexia nervosa. Plasma neuropeptide Y and galanin levels are also increased in obese women. Since leptin levels are chronically increased in obese humans, this suggests that obesity may be associated with malfunctioning leptin receptors, a condition called *leptin resistance*, since leptin is unable to generate an adequate response when its receptor is occupied. Improving responsiveness to leptin may be one key to weight loss.

Understanding the neuropharmacology of weight gain will hopefully lead to better management of obesity. In the meantime, prescribers of psychotropic drugs should monitor weight and body mass index and attempt to select drugs that prevent obesity, as well as to manage obesity when it occurs.

## Summary

In this chapter we have attempted to emphasize the psychopharmacological mechanisms of the actions of drugs of abuse and have used these mechanisms to describe drug dependence as well. We have attempted to define the terms frequently used in describing drug abuse and dependence, including abuse, addiction, dependence, reinforcement, tolerance, cross-tolerance and cross-dependence, withdrawal, relapse, and rebound.

We have described the mesolimbic dopamine pathway and the neuropharmacology of reward and have specifically emphasized the mechanism of action of several classes of drugs of abuse, including stimulants (cocaine and amphetamines), hallucinogens, designer drugs and phencyclidine, nicotine, marijuana, opiates, alcohol, benzodiazepines, and sedative-hypnotics. We have even mentioned how receptors and the mesolimbic dopamine pathway could play a role in the psychopharmacology of obesity.

# CHAPTER 14

# SEX-SPECIFIC AND SEXUAL FUNCTION–RELATED PSYCHOPHARMACOLOGY

Psychopharmacology can affect the sexes quite differently. This is just beginning to be recognized and investigated in a systematic manner. This chapter will explore some of the concepts behind treating men and women differently with psychopharmacological agents. One topic that affects both sexes is sexual activity, and this has become of great interest to psychopharmacologists since psychotropic medications are now widely recognized to affect sexual functioning, often negatively. Also, treatments for sexual dysfunction based on altering chemical neurotransmission are becoming available, and therefore the relevant psychopharmacological principles underlying these treatments are reviewed here.

The profound behavioral and neurobiological properties of reproductive hormones, particularly estrogen, are now recognized and are increasingly being exploited for their therapeutic potential in psychopharmacology. These properties will be reviewed in this chapter. Also reviewed here will be the movement to integrate the role of reproductive hormones into psychopharmacology by taking account of a woman's stage in her life cycle (i.e., child, child-bearing potential, pregnant, postpartum, lactating/nursing, perimenopausal, postmenopausal) and whether she is taking estrogens when choosing a psychotropic drug for her.

## Libido

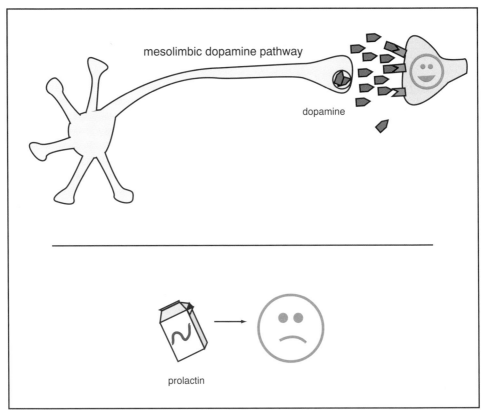

FIGURE 14–1. *Psychopharmacology of the human sexual response*, part 1. **Libido** is the first stage of the human sexual response and is related to desire. It is hypothetically mediated by the mesolimbic dopaminergic reward pathway. This pathway also mediates other "natural highs," as well as the artificial rewards of drug abuse. Prolactin may exert negative influences on sexual functioning by poorly understood mechanisms.

## Neurotransmitters and the Psychopharmacology of the Human Sexual Response

From a simple psychopharmacological perspective, the human sexual response can be divided into three phases, each with distinct and relatively nonoverlapping neurotransmitter functions, namely, libido, arousal, and orgasm.

### Libido

The first stage, libido, is linked to desire for sex, or sex drive, and is hypothetically a dopaminergic phenomenon mediated by the mesolimbic dopaminergic "reward center" (Fig. 14–1). This pathway has already been discussed in Chapter 13 and is well known for being the site of action of drugs of abuse as well as the site of

## Sexual Arousal

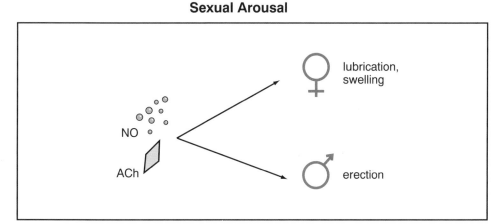

FIGURE 14–2. *Psychopharmacology of the human sexual response*, part 2. Sexual arousal in peripheral genitalia is accompanied by **erections** in men and **lubrication and swelling** in women. Both nitric oxide and acetylcholine mediate these actions.

"natural highs" (see Figs. 13–1 and 13–2). This site may not only mediate orgasm but also libidinous desire prior to the sex act.

Prolactin is hypothesized to have a negative influence on sexual desire, which is interesting because there is a generally reciprocal relationship between dopamine and prolactin (as discussed in Chapter 11; see Fig. 11–30). However, the relationship between prolactin and sexual dysfunction is not well documented and relatively poorly understood.

### Arousal

The second psychopharmacological stage of the sexual response is arousal (Fig. 14–2)—arousal of peripheral genitalia, that is. In men, that means an erection; in women, it means lubrication and swelling. This type of arousal prepares the genitalia for penetration and sexual intercourse. The message of arousal starts in the brain, is relayed down the spinal cord, then into peripheral autonomic nerve fibers that are both sympathetic and parasympathetic, next into vascular tissues, and finally to the genitalia. Along the way, at least two key neurotransmitters are involved, acetylcholine in the autonomic parasympathetic innervation of the genitalia and nitric oxide, which acts on the smooth muscle of the genitalia. Acetylcholine and nitric oxide both promote erections in men and lubrication and swelling in women. Cholinergic psychopharmacology has been extensively discussed in Chapter 12 (see Figs. 12–8 to 12–10). However, nitric oxide is a relatively recently characterized neurotransmitter system in brain and peripheral tissues, and more detailed discussion of this system will help explain its actions in mediating sexual arousal in the human sexual response.

### Nitric Oxide Psychopharmacology

Nitric oxide, a gas, is an improbable compound for a neurotransmitter. It is not an amine, amino acid, or peptide; it is not stored in synaptic vesicles or released by exocytosis; and it does not interact with specific receptor subtypes in neuronal membranes, but it is "NO laughing matter." Specifically, it is not nitrous oxide ($N_2O$) or "laughing gas," one of the earliest known anesthetics. Nitric oxide (NO) is a far different gas, although the two of them are often confused. It is NO that is the neurotransmitter, not $N_2O$. Incredible as it may seem, NO is a poisonous and unstable gas, a component of car fumes, which helps to deplete the ozone layer, yet is also a chemical messenger both in the brain and in blood vessels, including those that control erections in the penis.

Yes, there is NO synthesis by neurons and the penis. Certain neurons and tissues possess the enzyme nitric oxide synthetase (NOS), which forms NO from the amino acid *l*-arginine (Fig. 14–3). Nitric oxide then diffuses to adjacent neurons or smooth muscle and provokes the formation of the second messenger cyclic guanosine monophosphate (cGMP) by activating the enzyme guanylyl cyclase (GC) (Fig. 14–4). Nitric oxide is not made in advance nor is it stored, but it seems to be made on demand and released by simple diffusion. Glutamate and calcium can trigger the formation of NO by activating NOS.

No, there are no NO membrane receptors, in striking contrast to classical neurotransmitters, which have numerous types and subtypes of membrane receptors on neurons. Rather, the target of NO is iron in the active site of GC (Fig. 14–4). Once NO binds to the iron, GC is activated and cGMP is formed. The action of cGMP is terminated by a family of enzymes known as phosphodiesterases (PDEs), of which there are several forms, depending on the tissue (Fig. 14–5).

Yes, there is NO neurotransmitter function. The first known messenger functions for NO were described in blood vessels. By relaxing smooth muscles in blood vessels of the penis, NO can regulate penile erections, allowing blood to flow into the penis. Nitric oxide also can modulate vascular smooth muscle in cardiac blood vessels and mediate the ability of nitroglycerin to treat cardiac angina. Nitric oxide is also a key regulator of blood pressure, platelet aggregation, and peristalsis. Its central nervous system (CNS) neurotransmitter function remains elusive, but it may be a *retrograde neurotransmitter*. That is, since presynaptic neurotransmitters activate postsynaptic receptors, it seems logical that communication in this direction should be accompanied by some form of back talk from the postsynaptic site to the presynaptic neuron. The idea is that NO is prompted to be formed in postsynaptic synapses by some presynaptic neurotransmitters and then diffuses back to the presynaptic neuron, carrying information in reverse. Nitric oxide may also be involved in memory formation, neuronal plasticity, and neurotoxicity.

## Orgasm

The third stage of the human sexual response is orgasm (Fig. 14–6), accompanied by ejaculation in men. Descending spinal serotonergic fibers exert *inhibitory* actions on orgasm via 5HT2A receptors (see Fig. 5–57). Descending spinal noradrenergic fibers (Fig. 5–28) and noradrenergic sympathetic innervation of genitalia *facilitate* ejaculation and orgasm.

In summary, there are three major psychopharmacological stages of the human sexual response (Fig. 14–7). Multiple neurotransmitters mediate these stages, but only some of them are understood. Libido (stage 1) has dopaminergic dimensions to its pharmacology. The mechanism of arousal (stage 2), which is characterized by

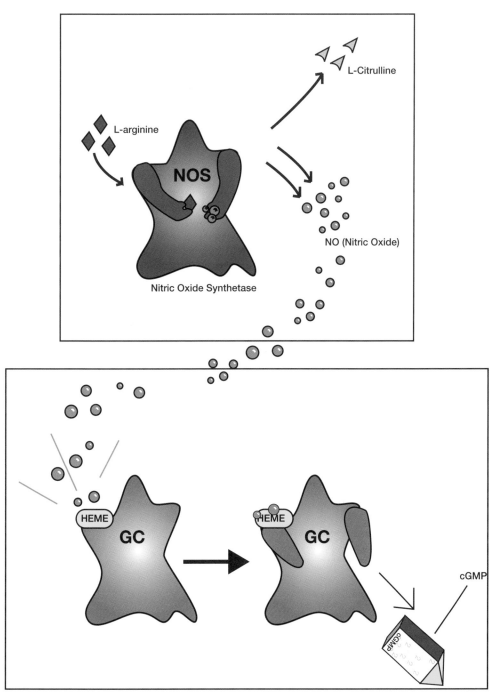

FIGURE 14–3. **Nitric oxide** (NO) is formed by the enzyme nitric oxide synthetase (NOS), which converts the amino acid l-arginine into nitric oxide and l-citrulline.

FIGURE 14–4. Once formed, nitric oxide activates the enzyme **guanylyl cyclase** (GC) by binding to iron (heme) in the active site of this enzyme. When activated, GC makes a messenger, (cyclic guanylate monophosphate (cGMP), which relaxes smooth muscle and performs other physiological functions. In the penis, relaxation of vascular smooth muscle opens blood flow and causes an erection.

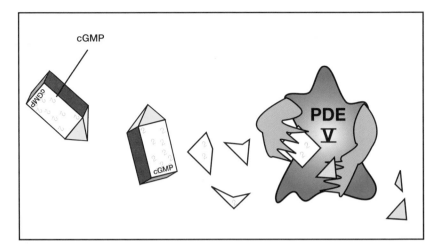

FIGURE 14–5. The action of cGMP is terminated by the enzyme **phosphodiesterase**. In the penis, the type of phosphodiesterase is type V (PDE V).

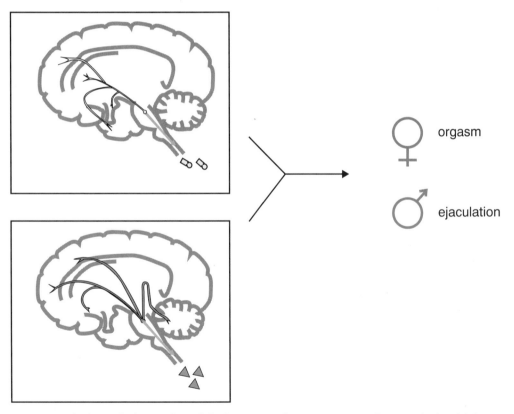

FIGURE 14–6. *Psychopharmacology of the human sexual response*, part 3. **Orgasm** is the third stage of the human sexual response, accompanied by ejaculation in men. Serotonin exerts an inhibitory action on orgasm and norepinephrine an excitatory or facilitatory action.

## Psychopharmacology of Sex

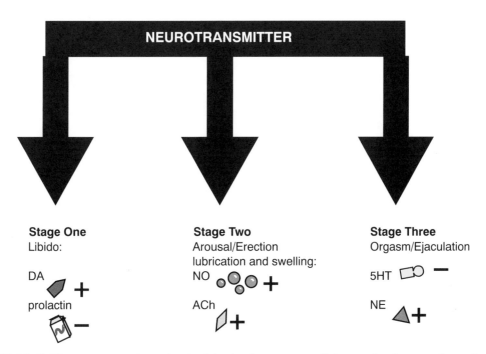

FIGURE 14–7. The neurotransmitters involved in the **three stages of the psychopharmacology of the human sexual response** are summarized here. In stage 1, libido, dopamine exerts a positive influence and prolactin a negative effect. In stage 2, arousal correlates with erections in men and lubrication and swelling in women. Both nitric oxide and acetylcholine facilitate sexual arousal. In stage 3, orgasm, which is associated with ejaculation in men, is inhibited by serotonin and facilitated by norepinephrine.

erection in men and lubrication and swelling in women, involves both cholinergic and nitric oxide pharmacology. Finally, orgasm (stage 3), with ejaculation in men, involves both inhibitory serotonergic input and excitatory noradrenergic input. Although sexual functioning is certainly complex and there are many overlapping functions of these neurotransmitters as well as exceptions to the rules, there are general principles of neurotransmission for each of the various stages of the human sexual response, some of which are reviewed in Figure 14–7.

## Erectile Dysfunction

Impotence, the inability to maintain an erection sufficient for intercourse, is more properly called erectile dysfunction. Up to 20 million men in the United States have this problem to some degree. Another way of stating the problem is that for normal men living in the community who are between 40 and 70 years old, only about half do not have some degree of erectile dysfunction (Fig. 14–8). The problem worsens with age (Fig. 14–9), since 39% of 40-year-olds have some degree of impotence (5% are completely impotent), but by age 70 two-thirds have some degree of impotence (and complete impotence triples to 15%). The multiple causes of erectile

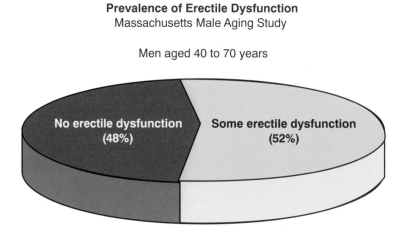

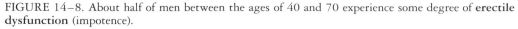

FIGURE 14–8. About half of men between the ages of 40 and 70 experience some degree of **erectile dysfunction** (impotence).

dysfunction include vascular insufficiency, various neurological causes, endocrine pathology (especially diabetes mellitus, but also reproductive hormone and thyroid problems), drugs, local pathology in the penis, and psychological and psychiatric problems.

Until recently, psychopharmacologists were not very useful members of the treatment team for patients with erectile dysfunction, other than to stop the medications they had been prescribing. Effective treatment of "organic" causes of erectile dysfunction until recently was often elusive and usually involved a urological approach, such as prostheses and implants. The old-fashioned surgical strategy bypasses diseased peripheral nerves and inadequate vascular blood supply to the penis to create erections mechanically and on demand, but this approach has serious limitations in terms of patient and partner acceptability. In men who have a "functional" etiology to their erectile dysfunction, the treatment strategy has traditionally taken a psychodynamic and behavioral approach, with attention to partners and functional disorders, psychoeducation, lifestyle changes, and where appropriate, starting (or stopping) psychotropic drugs to treat associated disorders. The typical case of erectile dysfunction, however, has neither a single "organic" cause nor a single "functional" cause but is usually caused by some combination of problems, including use of alcohol, smoking, diabetes, hypertension, antihypertensive drugs, psychotropic drugs, partner problems, performance anxiety, problems with self-esteem, and psychiatric disorders, especially depression.

The topic of erectile dysfunction has become increasingly important in psychopharmacology, not only because there are several psychotropic drugs that cause it but also because of the strikingly high incidence of impotence in several common psychiatric disorders. For example, some studies show that more than 90% of men with severe depression have moderate to severe erectile dysfunction (Fig. 14–10). Another reason for the importance of this topic in psychopharmacology is that effective and simple new psychopharmacological treatment based upon nitric oxide physiology and pharmacology is now available for men with erectile dysfunction.

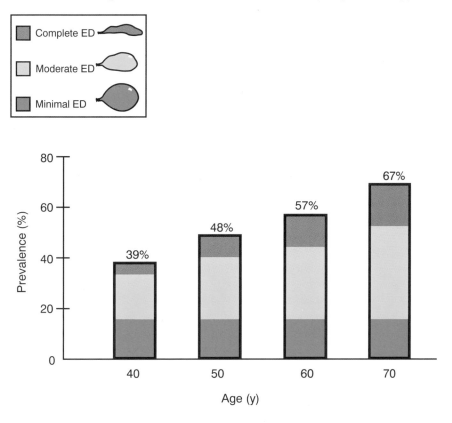

**Association Between Age and Prevalence of Erectile Dysfunction (ED)**
Massachusetts Male Aging Study

FIGURE 14–9. The incidence of erectile dysfunction **increased with age** in this study of normal men between the ages of 40 and 70, from 39% at age 40 to 67% at age 70.

## Psychopharmacology of Erectile Dysfunction

Normally, the desire to have sexual relations is a powerful message sent from the brain down the spinal cord and through peripheral nerves to smooth muscle cells in the penis, triggering them to produce sufficient nitric oxide to form all the cyclic GMP necessary to create an erection (Fig. 14–11). The cyclic GMP lasts long enough for sexual intercourse to occur, but then phosphodiesterase (type V in the penis) eventually breaks down the cGMP (Fig. 14–5), and the erection is lost (called detumescence).

However, if a man smokes, eats to the point of obesity, and has elevated blood glucose and elevated blood pressure, his peripheral nervous system "wires" do not respond adequately to the "let's have intercourse" signal from the brain—in other words, neurological innervation of the penis is rendered faulty, usually by diabetes (Fig. 14–12). Furthermore, there may not be much pressure in the "plumbing"— there may be atherosclerosis of the arterial supply of the penis from hypertension and hypercholesterolemia—when cGMP says "relax the smooth muscle and let the

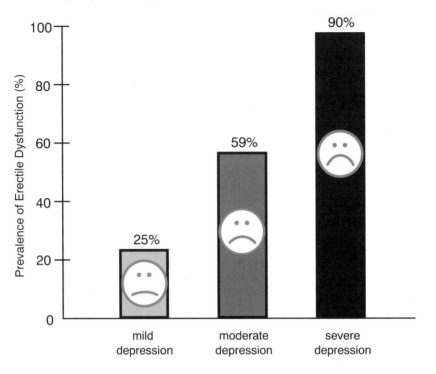

**Association Between Depression and Prevalence of Erectile Dysfunction**
Massachusetts Male Aging Study

FIGURE 14–10. **Erectile dysfunction** is associated with **depression** and increases in frequency as depression worsens. Among severely depressed men, some studies suggest that over 90% are impotent.

blood flow into the penis." In these cases, the desire for intercourse is there, but the signal cannot get through, so insufficient cGMP is formed, and therefore no erection occurs (Fig. 14–12). Similarly, even if a depressed patient experiences sexual desire, there is a general shutdown of neurotransmitter systems centrally and peripherally, resulting in inability to become aroused (Fig. 14–12).

Fortunately, there is a way to compensate for inadequate formation of cGMP. That compensation is a slowing of the rate of destruction of that cGMP that is formed, which is accomplished by inhibiting the enzyme that normally breaks down cGMP in the penis, namely phosphodiesterase type V, with an enzyme inhibitor called sildenafil (Viagra) (Fig. 14–13). Sildenafil will stop cGMP destruction for a few hours and allow the levels of cGMP to build up so that an erection can occur even though the wires and plumbing are still faulty (Fig. 14–13). Interestingly, sildenafil only works if the patient is mentally interested in the sex act and attempts to become aroused, so that at least weak signals are sent to the penis (i.e., it does not work during sleep).

Smooth muscle relaxation is thus the key element in attaining an erection. Administration of prostaglandins can also relax penile smooth muscle and elicit erections in a manner that mimics typical physiological mechanisms. Thus, intrapenile

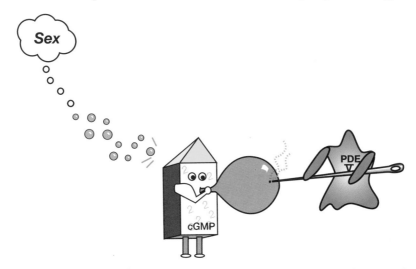

FIGURE 14–11. Under **normal conditions**, when young healthy men are sexually aroused, nitric oxide causes cGMP to accumulate, and cGMP causes smooth muscle relaxation, resulting in a physiological **erection**, indicated here by an inflated balloon. The erection is sustained long enough for sexual intercourse, and then phosphodiesterase V (PDE V) metabolizes cGMP, reversing the erection, indicated here by a pin ready to prick the balloon.

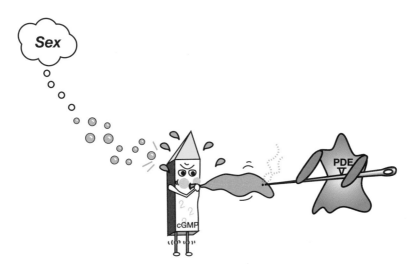

FIGURE 14–12. When a man has diabetes or hypertension, or if he smokes, uses alcohol, takes prescription drugs, or is depressed, there is a good chance that not enough of a signal of sexual desire will be able to get through his peripheral nerves and arteries to produce sufficient amounts of cGMP to cause an erection. This leads to **impotence**.

injection of the prostaglandin alprostadil produces erections not only in men with organic causes of impotence but also in those with functional causes and even in the common situation of multifactorial causes. Limitations of this somewhat masochistic approach include unacceptability of self-injection, lack of spontaneity, and the possibility of "too much of a good thing," namely a prolonged and painful erection,

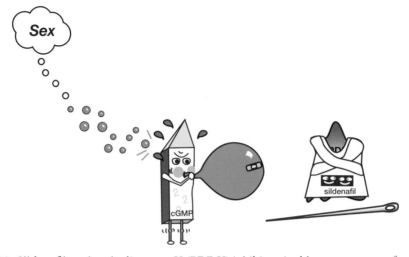

FIGURE 14–13. **Sildenafil**, a phosphodiesterase V (PDE V) inhibitor, is able to compensate for faulty signals through the peripheral nerves and arteries that produce insufficient amounts of cGMP to produce or sustain erections. Sildenafil does this by allowing cGMP to build up, since PDE V can no longer destroy cGMP for a few hours. This is indicated by a patch on the balloon in the figure. The result is that normally inadequate nerves and arteries signaling cGMP formation are now sufficient to inflate the balloon, and therefore an erection can occur and sexual intercourse is now possible, until the sildenafil wears off a few hours later.

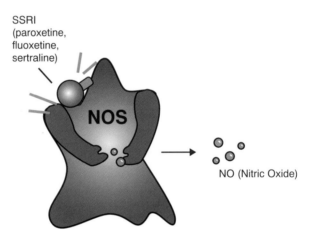

FIGURE 14–14. Some **antidepressants** such as serotonin selective reuptake inhibitors (SSRIs) may inhibit nitric oxide synthetase (NOS) and thereby reduce NO and cause **erectile dysfunction**.

called priapism. Prostaglandin administration *will* cause an erection whether the man is mentally aroused or not.

Other drugs can affect sexual arousal, including some serotonin selective reuptake inhibitors (SSRIs), which may inhibit NOS directly and can thus cause erectile dysfunction (Fig. 14–14), and some dopaminergic agents, which boost NOS and might some day help erectile dysfunction (Fig. 14–15). Anticholinergic agents can interfere directly with arousal and cause erectile dysfunction. Thus, agents such as

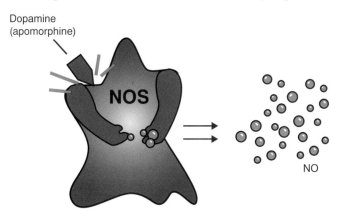

Dopamine
(apomorphine)

NOS

NO

FIGURE 14–15. Some agents that **boost dopamine** (perhaps like apomorphine) are promising experimental drugs for enhancing NOS and may be useful to reverse erectile dysfunction.

antipsychotics and tricyclic antidepressants and others with similar properties can cause erectile dysfunction (Fig. 14–16).

## Psychopharmacology of Sexual Dysfunction

In summary, numerous agents used in psychopharmacology can facilitate or interfere with each of the three stages of the human sexual response (Fig. 14–16). Understanding the basic mechanisms of neurotransmission for each of these stages (Fig. 14–7), as well as the psychopharmacological mechanisms of action of the various psychotropic drugs that impact these neurotransmitter systems, will facilitate the management of psychotropic drugs in patients with sexual dysfunction.

## Estrogen as a Neurotrophic Factor in the Brain

It is well known that ovarian estrogens, especially 17-beta-estradiol, regulate reproductive function and have profound effects on reproductive tissues in women, such as those of the breast and uterus. The long-term positive effects of estrogens outside of the reproductive tissues have also been emphasized, such as estrogen's effects in preserving bone mineralization and in reducing serum cholesterol. Recently there has been growing appreciation for the diversity of effects that estrogen can have on the brain as well, especially in regions of the brain outside of those areas known to be involved in the control of reproductive function and sexual differentiation. These neuronal effects are mediated by the same types of receptors for estrogen that exist in other tissues and have trophic actions on the brain, just as they have on other tissues. Trophic factors have been discussed in Chapter 1 (see Fig. 1–19 and Tables 1–3 and 1–4). In the brain, estrogen's trophic actions trigger the expression of genes that lead to the formation of synapses.

Estradiol modulates gene expression by binding to estrogen receptors (Fig. 14–17). Estrogen receptors differ from tissue to tissue and may differ from brain region to brain region. In addition to various forms of estrogen receptors, there are receptors for progesterone and androgens, as well as for other steroids such as glucocorticoids

## Psychopharmacology of Sex

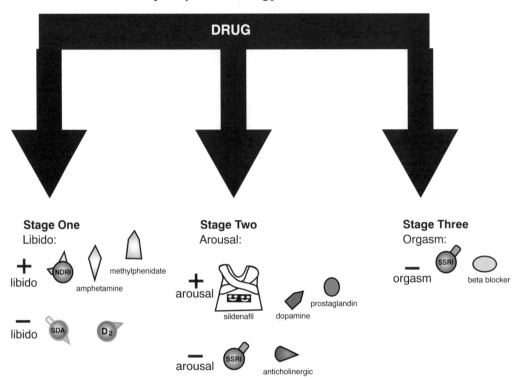

FIGURE 14–16. Psychopharmacological agents can affect **all three stages of the human sexual response**, both positively and negatively, as summarized here. In stage 1, **libido** can be enhanced by the norepinephrine and dopamine reuptake inhibitor (NDRI) bupropion, as well as by the dopamine-releasing stimulants amphetamine and methylphenidate. Libido can also be reduced by the dopamine receptor–blocking antipsychotics, some of which also increase prolactin. Stage 2, **sexual arousal**, can be enhanced by sildenafil, which boosts cGMP action, by prostaglandins, and perhaps by some dopaminergic agents. Sexual arousal can be reduced by some serotonin selective reuptake inhibitors (SSRIs), as well as by agents with anticholinergic properties. Finally, in stage 3, **orgasm** can be inhibited by SSRIs as well as by beta blockers, which block noradrenergic function.

and mineralocorticoids. Unlike neurotransmitter receptors located on neuronal membranes, receptors for estradiol are located in the neuronal nucleus, so estradiol must penetrate the neuronal membrane and the nuclear membrane to find its receptors, which are therefore located near the genes it wishes to influence. These genes are called estrogen response elements (Fig. 14–17).

The expression of these estrogen response elements within the DNA of the neuron progresses generally in the same manner as the expression of other neuronal genes, which has been discussed in Chapter 2 (see Figs. 2–31 to 2–42). The activation of estrogen response elements by estradiol requires "dimerization" (i.e., coupling of two copies of the estrogen receptor) when estrogen binds to the receptor to form an active transcription factor capable of "turning on" the estrogen response element (Fig. 14–18). Formation of transcription factors has also been discussed in Chapter 2 (see Figs. 2–33 and 2–35 to 2–38). Once the estrogen receptors are activated by estradiol into transcription factors, they activate gene expression by the estrogen

cell nucleus

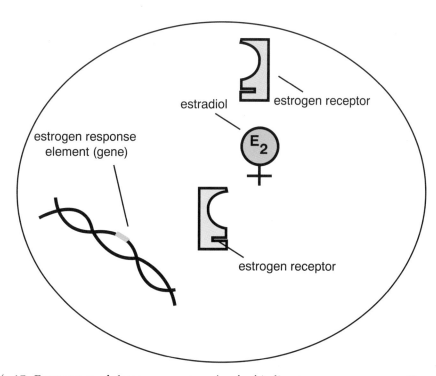

FIGURE 14–17. **Estrogen modulates gene expression** by binding to estrogen receptors. Estrogen receptors differ from tissue to tissue and may differ from brain region to brain region. Unlike neurotransmitter receptors located on neuronal membranes, receptors for estradiol are located in the neuronal cell nucleus, so estradiol must penetrate the neuronal membrane and the nuclear membrane to find its receptors, which are therefore located near the genes that are to be influenced. These genes are called estrogen response elements.

response elements in the neuron's DNA (Fig. 14–19). Gene products that are expressed include direct trophic factors such as nerve growth factor (NGF) and brain-derived neurotrophic factor (BDNF), which can facilitate synaptogenesis and prevent apoptosis and neurodegeneration.

Gene products also include neurotransmitter-synthesizing enzymes for the key monoamine neurotransmitter systems that regulate mood and memory (Figs. 14–20 to 14–22). Thus, the presence of estradiol can be critical to the adequate functioning of the monoamines serotonin (Fig. 14–20) and norepinephrine (Fig. 14–21) in women. Adult men do not respond to estrogen in this manner. The presence of estradiol in aging women but not in aging men can also be critical to the adequate functioning of acetylcholine in the nucleus basalis of Meynert (Fig. 14–22). The role of these key cholinergic neurons in the regulation of memory (see Fig. 12–11) and in the causation of Alzheimer's disease when they degenerate (see Fig. 12–13) have been discussed in Chapter 12. This may explain the emerging role of estrogen in managing memory and Alzheimer's disease in aging women, as discussed below.

Dramatic evidence of estrogen's trophic properties can be observed in hypothalamic and hippocampal neurons in adult female experimental animals within days

cell nucleus

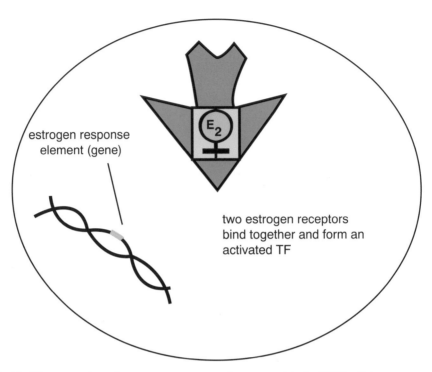

FIGURE 14–18. The expression of **estrogen response elements** with the DNA of the neuron must be initiated by estrogen and its receptor. Activation of these genes by estradiol requires "dimerization" (i.e., coupling of two copies of the estrogen receptor) when estrogen binds to the receptor to form an **active transcription factor** capable of "turning on" the estrogen response element.

and across a single menstrual (estrus) cycle (Figs. 14–23 and 14–24). During the early phase of the cycle, estradiol levels rise, and this trophic influence induces dendritic spine formation, specifically in the ventromedial hypothalamus and on pyramidal neurons in the hippocampus of female rats. Progesterone administration rapidly potentiates this, so spine formation is at its greatest when both estrogen and progesterone peak, just after the first half of the cycle (Fig. 14–23). However, once estrogen levels fall significantly and progesterone levels continue to rise, the presence of progesterone without estrogen triggers down regulation of these spines and removal of the synapses by the end of the estrus cycle (Fig. 14–23). One hypothesis to explain the mechanism of this cyclical formation and removal of synapses is that estrogen may exert its trophic influence through low levels of glutamate activation (Fig. 14–24), leading to spine formation and synaptogenesis: this effect is followed by too much glutamate activation in the absence of estrogen, when progesterone alone leads to excitotoxicity and destruction of these same spines and synapses (Fig. 14–24). The hypothesis of how glutamate might mediate excitotoxic synaptic or neuronal toxicity was introduced in Chapter 4 (see Figs. 4–14 to 4–23) and discussed extensively in Chapter 10 (see Figs. 10–26 to 10–33).

Other evidence for the trophic influences of estrogen comes from what happens when the estrogen's effects are blocked with estrogen receptor antagonists. Tamox-

cell nucleus

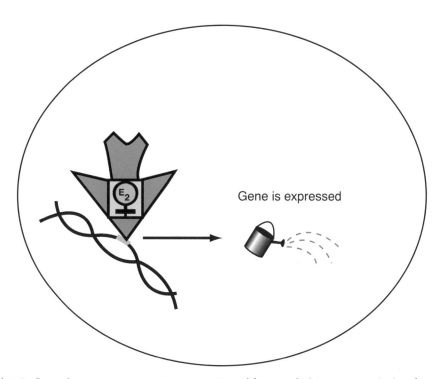

Gene is expressed

FIGURE 14–19. Once the **estrogen receptors** are activated by estradiol into **transcription factors**, they **activate gene expression** by the estrogen response elements in the neuron's DNA. Gene products that are expressed include direct trophic factors such as nerve growth factor (NGF) and brain-derived neurotrophic factor (BDNF), which can facilitate synaptogenesis and prevent apoptosis and neurodegeneration.

ifen is an estrogen receptor antagonist used for the treatment of breast cancer, especially for breast tumors that themselves express estrogen receptors. Blocking estrogen receptors in breast cancer cells with tamoxifen triggers apoptosis (programmed cell death), presumably due to blocking the trophic effect of estrogen in these tumor cells. Interestingly, tamoxifen is an estrogen receptor antagonist in breast and uterus but is actually a partial agonist in preserving bone mineralization and reducing cholesterol. It is also an estrogen receptor antagonist in brain, since it can induce depression that can be difficult to treat with antidepressants. Thus, individual estrogens such as estradiol and tamoxifen all have tissue-selective estrogen agonist, partial agonist, and antagonist activities. This also extends to the new class of estrogens known as selective estrogen receptor modulators (SERMs), of which raloxifene is the newest available member. Such observations may also explain why some women respond differently to one estrogen preparation than to another, and from a behavioral perspective, why they may have different mood and cognitive responses to one estrogen preparation versus another. Unfortunately, very little work has been done to distinguish the pharmacologic effects of the different available estrogen preparations on estrogen receptor binding in the brain, and the only way

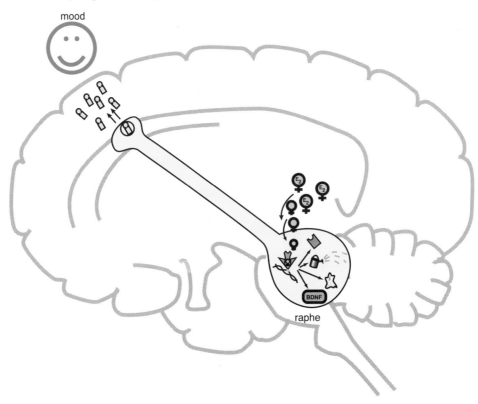

FIGURE 14–20. **Gene products** activated by estradiol interacting with **estrogen response elements** in the serotoninergic neurons of the midbrain raphe include not only **trophic factors,** which nourish the growth and synapses of these neurons with nerve growth factor (NGF) and brain-derived neurotrophic factor (BDNF), but also the **enzymes and receptors** that facilitate **serotonergic** neurotransmission. These receptors may also allow the neuron to have normal mood functions and to be more responsive to antidepressant medications in case of a depressive episode.

to detect these differences at the present time is through trial and error. Nevertheless, the differences in tissue-selective, brain region–selective, or individual-selective estrogen agonist, partial agonist, or antagonist activities can be explained by the fact that there are many different DNA response elements to estrogens, and these may be expressed differently in various tissues, brain regions, and individuals. There may even be state-dependent differences in expression of DNA response elements to estrogens, which vary across the female life cycle or vary depending on the presence or absence of a mood or cognitive disorder. This is the subject of intense current research interest.

## Estrogen and Mood Across the Female Life Cycle

Estrogen levels shift rather dramatically across the female life cycle, all in relationship to various types of reproductive events (Fig. 14–25). Thus, levels begin to rise and then cycle during puberty (see also Fig. 14–23). This cycling persists during the childbearing years, except during pregnancy, when a woman's estrogen levels

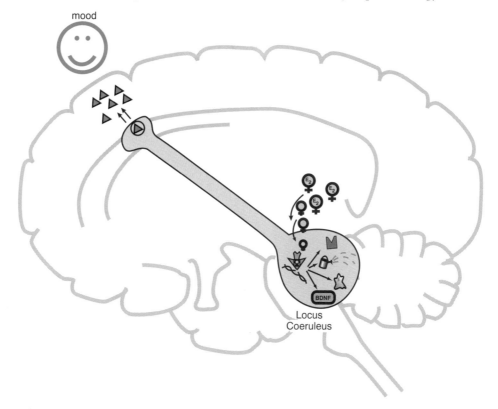

FIGURE 14–21. **Gene products** activated by estradiol interacting with **estrogen response elements** in the noradrenergic neurons of the brainstem locus coeruleus include not only **trophic factors** that nourish the growth and synapses of these neurons with nerve growth factor (NGF) and brain-derived neurotrophic factor (BDNF), but also the **enzymes and receptors** that facilitate **noradrenergic** neurotransmission. These receptors may also allow the neuron to have normal mood function and to be more responsive to antidepressant medications in case of a depressive episode.

skyrocket (Fig. 14–25). Estrogen levels then plummet precipitously immediately postpartum, and regular menstrual cycles begin again once the mother stops nursing (Fig. 14–25).

Although the median age of menopause, which is the time of complete cessation of menstruation, is 51, women do not begin menopause overnight. The transition period from regular menstrual cycles to complete cessation of menstruation, called perimenopause, can begin 5 to 7 years before menopause and is characterized on on-again off-again cycles and anovulatory cycles, prior to complete cessation of menstrual cycles (Fig. 14–25). Hormone levels can be chaotic and unpredictable during these years. This can be experienced both as a physiological and a psychological stressor. Menopause is the final stage of transition of estrogen in the female life cycle and can be associated with estrogen replacement therapy, which can restore estrogen to its physiological levels during the childbearing years.

There are potential links between these shifts in estrogen levels across the female life cycle and the observation that depression is much more common in women than in men during certain stages of the life cycle. In men, the incidence of depression

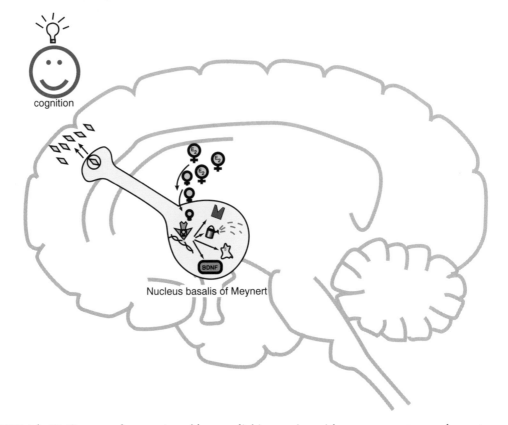

FIGURE 14–22. **Gene products** activated by estradiol interacting with **estrogen response elements** in the cholinergic neurons of the nucleus basalis of Meynert in the basal forebrain include not only **trophic factors** that nourish the growth and synapses of these neurons with nerve growth factor (NGF) and brain-derived neurotrophic factor (BDNF), but also the **enzymes and receptors** that facilitate **cholinergic** neurotransmission. These receptors may also allow the neuron to function optimally in memory formation, particularly verbal memory in aging women, and to be more responsive to cholinesterase inhibitors in the case of Alzheimer's disease.

rises in puberty and then is essentially constant throughout life, despite a slowly declining testosterone level from age 25 onward (Fig. 14–26). By contrast, in women the incidence of depression mirrors their changes in estrogen across the life cycle (Fig. 14–27). As estrogen levels rise during puberty, the incidence of depression skyrockets, falling again after menopause (Fig. 14–27). Thus, women have the same frequency of depression as men before puberty and after menopause. However, during their childbearing years when estrogen is high and cycling, the incidence of depression in women is two to three times as high as in men (Fig. 14–27).

Several other issues are of particular importance to women in terms of assessing their vulnerability to the onset and recurrence of mood disorders across their lifetimes. These are linked to shifts in reproductive hormone status, as outlined in Figure 14–28. *First episodes* of depression often begin in puberty or early adulthood, when estrogen is first rising; unfortunately these episodes are frequently unrecognized and untreated. Throughout the childbearing years of normal menstrual cycles,

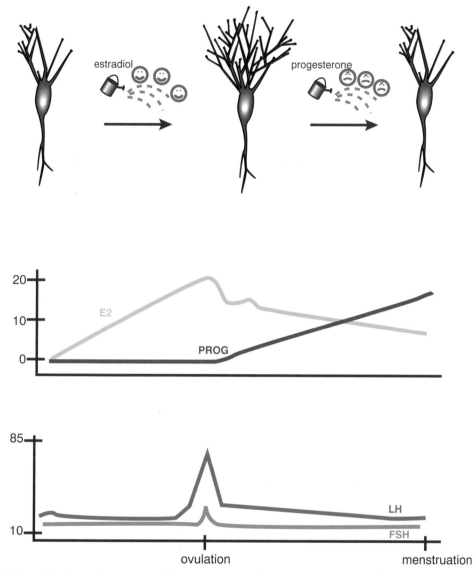

FIGURE 14–23. Dramatic evidence of **estrogen's trophic properties** can be observed in hypotha-lamic and hippocampal neurons in adult female experimental animals within days and **across a single menstrual (estrus) cycle**. During the early phase of the cycle, estradiol levels rise, and this trophic influence induces dendritic spine formation and synaptogenesis. Progesterone administration rapidly potentiates this, so spine formation is at its greatest when both estrogen and progesterone peak just after the first half of the cycle. However, once estrogen levels fall significantly and progesterone continues to rise, the presence of progesterone without estrogen triggers down regulation of these spines and removal of the synapses by the end of the estrus cycle.

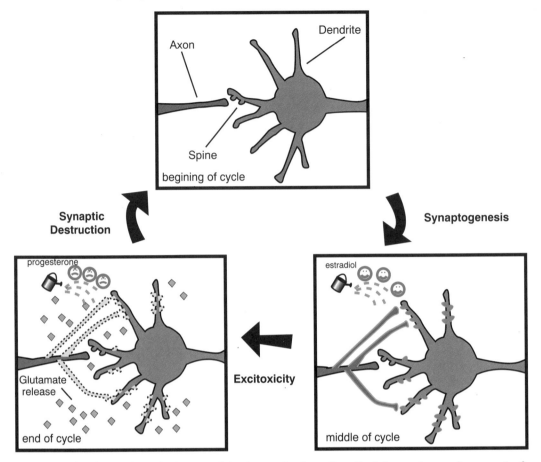

FIGURE 14–24. One hypothesis to explain the mechanism of **cyclical formation and removal of synapses** every menstrual (estrus) cycle in females is that estrogen may exert its trophic influence through low levels of glutamate activation, leading to spine formation and synaptogenesis. This, however, is followed by too much glutamate activation in the absence of estrogen, when progesterone alone leads to excitotoxicity and destruction of these same spines and synapses.

most women experience some irritability during the late luteal phase just prior to menstrual flow; however, if this is actually incapacitating, it may be a form of premenstrual syndrome (PMS), worthy of treatment with antidepressants or estrogen, sometimes just during the late luteal phase. In other patients, this end-of-the-cycle worsening is unmasking a mood disorder that is actually present during the whole cycle but is sufficiently worse at the end of the cycle that it becomes obvious in a phenomenon called *menstrual magnification*. This may be a harbinger of further worsening or may also represent a state of incomplete recovery from a previous episode of depression. Nevertheless, both PMS and menstrual magnification are important, not only for the symptoms they cause in the short run but for the risk they represent for a full recurrence in the future, signaling the potential need for both symptomatic and preventive treatment.

Figure 14–28 also indicates the two riskiest periods in a woman's life cycle for the onset of a first episode of depression or for the recurrence of a major depressive

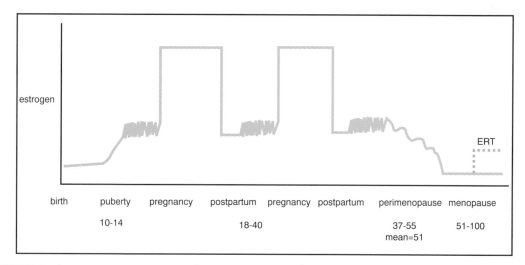

FIGURE 14–25. **Estrogen levels shift dramatically across the female life cycle,** all in relation to various types of reproductive events. Levels begin to rise and then cycle in puberty. Cycling persists during the childbearing years except in pregnancy, when a woman's estrogen level's skyrocket. Estrogen levels plummet precipitously immediately postpartum, and regular menstrual cycles begin again once nursing stops. Although the median age of menopause, when all menstruation stops, is 51, women do not stop menstruation overnight. The transition period from regular menstrual periods to complete cessation of menstruation is called perimenopause and can begin 5 to 7 years prior to menopause. The final transition phase is menopause, when estrogen replacement therapy (ERT) can restore estrogen levels to those of the childbearing years.

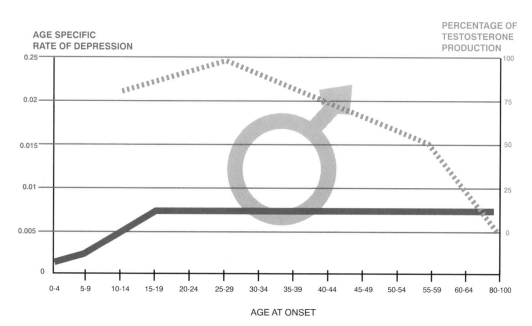

FIGURE 14–26. In **men,** the incidence of **depression** rises in puberty and then is essentially constant throughout life, despite a slowly declining testosterone level from age 25 on.

561

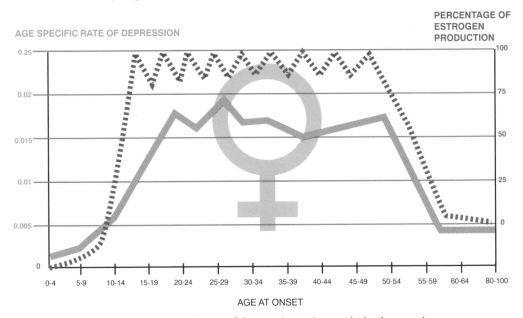

FIGURE 14–27. In **women, the incidence of depression mirrors their changes in estrogen across the life cycle.** As estrogen levels rise during puberty, the incidence of depression also rises, and it falls again during menopause, when estrogen levels fall. Thus, women have the same frequency of depression as men before puberty and after menopause. However, during their childbearing years when estrogen is high and cycling, the incidence of depression in women is two to three times as high as in men.

episode if she has already experienced one. Both are associated with major shifts in estrogen. The first is the *postpartum period*, when skyrocketing levels of estrogen plummet immediately after delivery of the child. The second occurs during *perimenopause*, when chaotic hormonal status characterizes the transition from regular menstrual cycles to menopause with no menstrual cycles.

There is an increasing risk that a woman will have a recurrence of a major depressive episode after any shift in her estrogen status across her lifetime, a phenomenon some experts have called "kindling." For example, a woman's risk of having a postpartum depression increases severalfold if she had a depressive episode after a previous pregnancy. A woman who has a depressive episode triggered by any endocrine shift is quite vulnerable to a recurrence of depression after another reproductive "event" later in her life cycle, such as those shown in Figure 14–28, which include puberty, miscarriage, postpartum, perimenopause, taking oral contraceptives, and taking hormone replacement therapy, especially progestins. The increasing chances of a recurrent episode of depression in women whose episodes are linked to reproductive events and shifts in estrogen status may be related to the phenomenon of recurrence in other psychiatric disorders, such as bipolar disorder and schizophrenia. Thus, it is possible that certain mental illnesses, including recurrent depression, are potentially damaging to the brain owing to excitotoxic brain damage (see Chapters 4 and 10). Perhaps life cycle shifts in estrogen status trigger excitotoxicity, just as they seem to do every menstrual cycle (see Figs. 14–23 and 14–24), but huge life cycle shifts in estrogen may trigger depressive episodes in some women that not

**Risk of Depression Across Female Life Cycle**

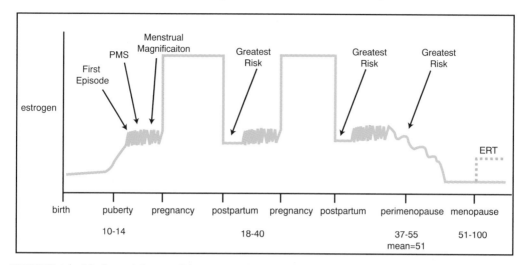

FIGURE 14–28. Several issues of importance in assessing **women's vulnerability** to the onset and recurrence of depression are illustrated here. These include first onset in puberty and young adulthood; premenstrual syndrome (PMS) and menstrual magnification as harbingers of future episodes or incomplete recovery states from prior episodes of depression; and two periods of especially high vulnerability for first episodes of depression or for recurrence if a woman has already experienced an episode, namely, the postpartum period and the perimenopausal period.

only cause suffering during the episode of depression itself, but also damage the brain, so that recovery is associated with an increased risk of subsequent episodes with diminishing the responsiveness to medication with each subsequent episode. This has also been hypothesized to explain the clinical course of schizophrenia as well, as discussed in Chapter 10 (Fig. 10–20). Whatever the cause of the high recurrence rate of depression in women across their life cycles and the associations with shifts in estrogen status, the importance of recognition and treatment of current episodes of depression in women, as well as use of medications to prevent future episodes, is extremely important since recurrence is so predictable, treatable, and potentially preventable.

Selecting treatments for the symptoms of mood disorders and their prevention must also take into account shifts in estrogen status and reproductive events across the life cycle of a woman. The potential impact of estrogen itself as a treatment, as well as antidepressants, must also be considered. Guidelines on how to use antidepressants and/or estrogen during these various phases of a woman's life cycle are only now being developed, and the issues to be considered are outlined in Figure 14–29.

First, a high index of suspicion for *first episodes of depression* should accompany the assessment of adolescent girls (Fig. 14–29), since this illness is frequently missed, and despite the lack of formal approval of antidepressants for use in anyone under the age of 18, the newer antidepressants are frequently used for this purpose, and their safety has been well established in children and adolescents for related conditions such as obsessive-compulsive disorder (see Chapter 5). Also, the use of *oral*

**Integrating Use of Estrogen and/or Antidepressants Across Female Life Cycle**

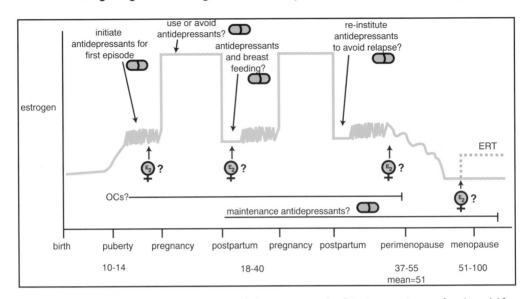

FIGURE 14–29. This figure illustrates some of the issues involved in integrating **endocrine shifts** and events related to a woman's life cycle with **treatment of a mood disorder** with antidepressants and/or estrogen. These include use of antidepressants prior to age 18 if necessary; understanding how to select oral contraceptives to minimize depression; calculating risks versus benefits of antidepressant maintenance during pregnancy and during breast-feeding; and deciding whether to include estrogens as adjunctive treatments for women with mood disorders. There are also various options and flexible and creative regimens for administering hormones with antidepressants to perimenopausal and post-menopausal women with mood disorders to optimize their treatments.

*contraceptives* can affect adolescents as well as all females of childbearing potential and must be taken into consideration (Fig. 14–29), because these agents may sometimes cause depression or worsen preexisting depression. Triggering of depression by oral contraceptives can be especially problematic in those with a previous episode of depression and with contraceptives containing progestins only. Switching to oral contraceptives containing low-dose progestins combined with estrogens can sometimes prevent mood problems in these patients.

A'nother key treatment issue to be managed in a disorder with such a high risk of recurrence is whether to treat with *maintenance antidepressants during pregnancy* (Fig. 14–29). This decision involves calculating a risk/benefit ratio for the individual patient in terms of risk to the mother of recurrence of her depression during pregnancy due to stopping antidepressant treatment versus risk to the developing fetus due to the mother taking antidepressant treatment. Since the greatest risk to the fetus is at the beginning of pregnancy (i.e., during the first 12-week trimester, when the brain and other critical tissues are being formed) and the greatest risk to the mother is postpartum, the tradeoff is often to wait until later in pregnancy, until the mother begins to have a recurrent episode, or after delivery.

However, this brings up another problem. What about *taking antidepressants during lactation and nursing* (Fig. 14–29), in terms of risk of exposure of the baby to antidepressants in the mother's breast milk? Again, a risk/benefit ratio must be calculated for each situation, with account taken of the risk of recurrence to the mother if she does not take antidepressants (given her own personal and family history of mood disorder), and the risk to the bonding between baby and mother if she does not breast-feed or to the baby if exposed to trace amounts of antidepressants in breast milk. Although the risk to the infant of exposure to small amounts of antidepressants is only now being clarified, it is quite clear that the risks to the mother with a prior postpartum depression who neglects to take antidepressants after a subsequent pregnancy has a 67% risk of recurrence if she does not take antidepressants and only one-tenth of that risk of recurrence if she does take antidepressants postpartum.

Another issue is whether to use *estrogens for the treatment of mood disorder* symptoms (Fig. 14–29). Estrogens can improve mood and a sense of well-being in normal women during perimenopause, especially if they are experiencing vasomotor symptoms such as "hot flashes." However, it is quite controversial whether estrogen has any antidepressant role for women with major depressive disorder. Antidepressants are still first-line treatments for major depressive disorder across the female life cycle, but when they fail, novel approaches that integrate the use of estrogen are now being investigated, including the use of estrogen by itself or in combination with antidepressants, particularly during specific life cycle–related mood disorders (Fig. 14–29). For example, some patients with PMS seem to benefit from antidepressants and others from late luteal phase supplementation with low doses of estrogens, particularly if delivered transdermally via a skin patch. Some patients with profound collapse into a postpartum depression will respond rapidly to antidepressants, others to electroconvulsive therapy, and still others to reinstitution of estrogen with a "softer landing" to physiological postpartum levels. There are no objective means to determine who will benefit from which approach, but those who receive estrogen tend to be those who fail other better accepted first-line treatment approaches.

Particularly in women with perimenopausal depressions and especially when these are recurrent and resistant to antidepressants, treatment with estrogen replacement therapies can be effective. This was discussed in Chapter 7 as one of the combination strategies to add to antidepressants when various treatment strategies fail and illustrated conceptually in Figure 7–34. There are no accepted guidelines for when to try this approach, but these are hopefully evolving. Treating postmenopausal depression may also benefit from a boost from estrogen replacement, as indicated in Figures 14–20 and 14–21, as a result of the beneficial effects that estrogen may have on critical monoaminergic systems involved in mood, such as norepinephrine and serotonin. In the absence of estrogen, these systems may not function adequately, resulting both in a mood disorder and in failure to respond to antidepressants. Restoring estrogen to monoaminergic neurons allows their estrogen receptors to "reawaken" estrogen response elements in these neurons and may either extinguish problems with mood or allow the patient to become responsive to antidepressants.

Another issue for postmenopausal women has to do with the roles of both progesterone and estrogen in managing their mood disorder. Since progesterone can act as an estrogen antagonist in some tissues, such as those in the uterus and in some brain areas (see Fig. 14–24), it should not be surprising that progesterone can counteract the positive effects that estrogen has on mood in some women. In these cases, administration of progesterone as a component of hormone replacement ther-

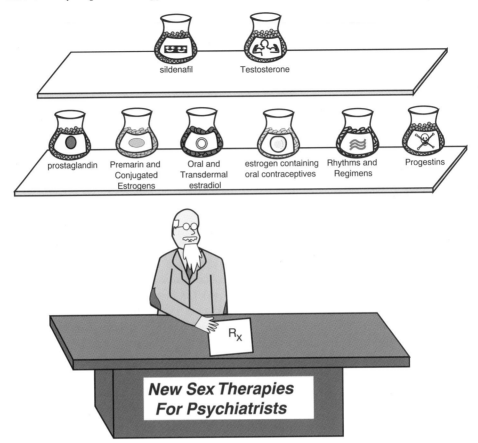

FIGURE 14–30. Psychopharmacology is beginning to identify new **therapies that are sex-specific** and related to **sexual functioning**. These include treatments for the human sexual response, especially for erectile dysfunction in men, as well as a better appreciation of the role of hormones in managing mood and cognitive disorders in women.

apy may precipitate depression, or cause a magnification reminiscent of menstrual magnification during normal menstruation (when endogenous progesterone was presumably causing the same thing). For postmenopausal women, progesterone is necessary to prevent uterine cancer when estrogen replacement is being given. Thus, in a woman who has had a hysterectomy, progesterone treatment can be avoided. In a woman with her uterus, it may be less disruptive to her mood to give estrogen and progestin daily rather than to give the progestin just at the end of the cycle.

These various hormone strategies to consider in the management of mood and cognition in the treatment of women across their life cycles are summarized in Figure 14–30, along with some therapies for erectile dysfunction in men. Components of this emerging pharmacy for managing issues specific to each sex and issues of sexual function in psychopharmacology include sildenafil and prostaglandins for erectile dysfunction and numerous reproductive hormones, including oral and transdermal skin patches for estrogens, progestins, and testosterone. Even the pattern of taking these hormones, such as daily, end of the menstrual cycle only, cyclically, counter-cyclically, etc. (i.e., rhythms and regimens) can make a big difference in a woman's response to them. It is also important to avoid some hormones (e.g., progestins) in some patients.

## Cognition, Alzheimer's Disease, and the Role of Estrogen in Sex Differences

Although there are no sex differences in full-scale IQ scores on standardized tests of general intelligence, some cognitive differences exist between men and women. The best established of these are that on average, men excel in spatial and quantitative abilities, whereas women excel in verbal abilities and in perceptual speed and accuracy. However, the magnitude of these differences is modest. Whatever differences exist may be due to prenatal influences of reproductive hormones on brain organization during fetal brain development. Interestingly, after menopause, there is a loss of verbal memory skills in women, which is restored with estrogen replacement therapy. This suggests that estrogen is necessary to maintain optimal verbal memory functioning in women (Fig. 14–22), that loss of estrogen may lead to lack of expression of critical genes necessary to maintain this function in cholinergic memory pathways, and that this process can be reversed and restored with reinstitution of estrogen signals to turn gene expression back on. These effects of estrogen on memory in normal postmenopausal women, like those differences between cognitive functions of men and women, are on the whole modest in magnitude.

Alzheimer's disease is also more common in women than in men. Memory disturbances in Alzheimer's disease are linked to disruption in cholinergic neurotransmission (see Chapter 12, Fig. 12–13). About one and one-half to three times as many women have Alzheimer's disease as men. Although women live longer than men on average and so are at greater risk for Alzheimer's disease (because more of them are alive at ages when this illness is most common), this does not account for their increased rates of Alzheimer's disease or for their longer survival as compared with men after the onset of Alzheimer symptoms. After statistical adjustments for these facts, there appears to be a sex-specific risk for Alzheimer's disease, which preliminary studies suggest may be reduced in those women who take estrogen replacement therapy. It is hypothesized that loss of estrogen after menopause may be responsible for this sex-specific increased risk of Alzheimer's disease, perhaps particularly because of loss of the normal trophic actions that estrogen has upon cholinergic neurons that mediate memory (Fig. 14–22), but also due to the general loss of estrogen's trophic influence throughout the brain (Figs. 14–17, 14–18, and 14–19). Thus, estrogen replacement therapy hypothetically allows critical estrogen response elements in cholinergic neurons (Fig. 14–22) and throughout the brain to turn back on and protect against the onset of Alzheimer's disease. In Chapter 12, we discussed how several studies are in progress to determine whether estrogen can protect against the development of Alzheimer's disease in randomized controlled trials. It has also been observed that once Alzheimer's disease is diagnosed, estrogen may boost the effectiveness of cholinesterase inhibitors (cholinesterase inhibitors for Alzheimer's disease were discussed in Chapter 12).

## Summary

In this chapter, issues in psychopharmacology related to sex and sexuality were discussed. This included an overview of the neurotransmitter mechanisms involved in the three psychopharmacological stages of the human sexual response, namely libido, arousal, and orgasm. Neurotransmitters that mediate each of these three stages were discussed, as well as drugs that facilitate and inhibit these stages. A specific introduction to the nitric oxide neurotransmitter system was outlined.

The clinical features and pathophysiology of and treatment approaches to erectile dysfunction in men was reviewed, including the new phosphodiesterase inhibitor sildenafil (Viagra). The role of estrogen across the female life cycle, including estrogen's profound behavioral and neurobiological properties, was also reviewed. The role of reproductive hormones, particularly estrogen, was outlined with a view to integrating it into psychopharmacology by taking account of a woman's stage in her life cycle (i.e., childhood, childbearing potential, pregnancy, and the postpartum, lactating/nursing, perimenopausal, and postmenopausal states) and whether she is taking estrogens when choosing a psychotropic drug for her in the treatment of either a mood disorder or a cognitive disorder.

# SUGGESTED READING

Alexander, S.P.H., and Peters, J.A. (1999) Receptor and ion channel nomenclature supplement. *Trends in Pharmacological Sciences*. Elsevier Press. Trends Journals, Cambridge, U.K.

Bloom, F.E., and Kupfer, D.J., (Eds.) (1995) *Psychopharmacology: the fourth generation of progress*. New York, Raven Press.

Bond, A.J., and Lader, M.H. (1996) *Understanding drug treatment in mental health care*. Chichester, John Wiley & Sons.

Broks, P., Preston, G.C., Traub, M., Poppleton, P., Ward, C., and Stahl, S.M. (1988) Modelling dementia: effects of scopolamine on memory and attention. *Neuropsychologia* 26, 685–700.

Carey, P.J., Alexander, B., and Liskow, B.I. (1997) *Psychotropic drug handbook*. Washington, DC, American Psychiatric Press, Inc.

Carrier, S., Brock, G., Weekour, N., and Lue, T.R. (1993) Pathophysiology of erectile dysfunction. *Urology* 42, 468–81.

Cooper, J.R., Bloom, F.E., and Roth, R.H. (1996) *The biochemical basis of neuropharmacology*, 7th edition, New York, Oxford University Press.

Crenshaw, T.L., and Goldberg, J.P. (1996) Sexual Pharmacology. New York, W.W. Norton.

*Depression in primary care, volume 1, detection and diagnosis*; clinical practice guideline, number 5, U.S. Department of Health and Human Services, AHCPR Publication No. 93-0551, Public Health Service, Agency for Health Care Policy and Research, Rockville, MD, April, 1993.

*Depression in primary care, volume 2, treatment of major depression*; clinical practice guideline, number 5, U.S. Department of Health and Human Services, AHCPR Publication No. 93-0551, Public Health Service, Agency for Health Care Policy and Research, Rockville, MD, April, 1993.

*Diagnostic and statistical manual of mental disorders, 4th edition (DSM-IV)*. (1994) Washington, DC, American Psychiatric Association.

Drummond, J.M. (1997) *Essential Guide to Psychiatric Drugs*, 3rd edition. New York, St. Martin's Press (Paperback).

Dubovsky, S.L. (1998) *Clinical Psychiatry*. Washington, DC, American Psychiatric Press, Inc.

Duman, R.F., Heninger, C.R., and Nestler, E.J. (1997) A molecular and cellular theory of depression. *Archives of General Psychiatry* 54, 597–606.

Feldman, R.S., Myer, J.S., and Quenzer, L.F. (1997) *The Principles of Psychopharmacology*. Sunderland, MA, Sinauer Associates Inc.

Foa, E.B., and Wilson, R. (1991). *Stop obsessing! How to overcome your obsessions and compulsions*. New York, Bantam Books.

Foster, M.C., and Cole, M. (1996) *Impotence*. London, Martin Dunitz Press.

Frank, E. (2000) *Gender and its effects on psychopathology*. Washington, DC, American Psychiatric Press, Inc.

Games, D., et al. (1995) Alzheimer-type neuropathology in transgenic mice overexpressing V717F beta-amyloid precursor protein. *Nature* 373, 523–7.

Gauthier, S. (1999) *Clinical diagnosis and management of Alzheimer's disease*, Second edition. London, Martin Dunitz Press.

Gelenberg, A.J., and Bassuk, E.L. (1997) *The practitioner's guide to psychoactive drugs*, 4th edition. New York, Plenum Medical Book Co.

Gitlin, M.J. (1990) *The Psychotherapist's guide to psychopharmacology*. New York, The Free Press; Toronto, Collier Macmillan Canada.

Goldstein, I., Lue, T.R., Padma, N.H., Rosen, A.C., Steers, W.D., and Wicker, P.A. (1998) Oral sildenafil in the treatment of erectile dysfunction. *New England Journal of Medicine* 338, 1397–404.

Guttmacher, L.B. (1994) *Psychopharmacology and electroconvulsive therapy*. Washington, DC, American Psychiatric Press, Inc.

Hardman, J.G., and Limbird, L.E. (1996) *Goodman and Gilman's The pharmacological basis of therapeutics*, 9th edition, New York, McGraw-Hill.

Hyman, S.E. (1999) Introduction to the complex genetics of mental disorders. *Biological Psychiatry* 45, 518–21.

Hyman, S.E., Arana, J.W., and Rosenbaum, J.F. (1995) *Handbook of psychiatric drug therapy*, 3rd edition, Boston, Little Brown and Company.

Hyman, S.E., and Nelson, E.J. (1996) Initiation and adaptation: a paradigm for undertaking psychotropic drug action. *American Journal of Psychiatry* 153, 151–62.

*International classification of diseases, 10th edition (ICD-10) classification of mental and behavioral disorders: clinical descriptions and diagnostic guidelines*. World Health Organization, Geneva, 1993.

Janicak, P.G. (1999) *Handbook of psychopharmacology*. Philadelphia, Lippincott Williams & Wilkins.

Janicak, P.G., Davis, J.M., Preskorn, S.H., and Ayd, F.J. (1997) *Principles and practice of psychotherapy*, 2nd edition. Baltimore, Williams & Wilkins.

Jenkins, S.C., and Hansen, M.R. (1995) *A pocket reference for psychiatrists*, Second edition. Washington, DC, American Psychiatric Press, Inc.

Jensvold, M.F., Halbreich, U., and Hamilton, J.A. (1996) *Psychopharmacology and women*. Washington, DC, American Psychiatric Press, Inc.

Joffe, R.T., and Calabrese, J.R. (1994) *Anticonvulsants and Mood, Disorders*. New York, Marcel Dekker, Inc.

Kandel, E.R. (1998) A new intellectual framework for psychiatry. *American Journal of Psychiatry* 155, 457–69.

Kaplan, H.I., Freedman, A.M., and Sadock, B.J. (1995) *Comprehensive textbook of psychiatry*, 6th edition. Baltimore, Williams & Wilkins.

Kaplan, H.I., and Sadock, B.J. (1993) *Pocket Handbook of Psychiatric Drug Treatment*. Baltimore, Williams & Wilkins.

Kaplan, H.I., Sadock, B.J., and Grebb, J.A. (1994) *Kaplan and Sadock's Synopsis of Psychiatry*. Baltimore, Williams & Wilkins.

Kramer, M.S., Cutler, N., Feighner, J., et al. (1998) Distinct mechanism for antidepressant activity by blockade of central substance P receptors. *Science* **281**, 640–5.

*Journal of the American Academy of Child and Adolescent Psychiatry*, **38**(5) May 1995: Special section: Current knowledge in unmet needs in pediatric psychopharmacology.

Leibenluft, E. (editor). (1999) Gender in mood and anxiety disorders. In *Bench to bedside*. Washington, DC, American Psychiatric Press, Inc.

Leonard, B.E. (1997) *Fundamentals of psychopharmacology*. Chichester, John Wiley & Sons, Ltd.

Martindale, W. (1996) *The extra pharmacopoeia*, 31st edition, London, Royal Pharmaceutical Society of Great Britain.

McClue, S.J., Brazell, C., and Stahl, S.M. (1989) Hallucinogenic drugs are partial agonists of the human platelet shape change response: a physiological model of the 5-HT$_2$ receptor. *Biological Psychiatry* **26**, 297–302.

McDowell, D.M., and Spitz, H.I. (1999) *Substance abuse: from principles to practice*. New York, Brunner/Mazel, Inc.

Meltzer, H.Y., and Stahl, S.M. (1976) The dopamine hypothesis of schizophrenia: a review. *Schizophrenia Bulletin* **2**(1), 19–76.

Nelson, J.C. (Ed.) (1998) *Geriatric psychopharmacology*. New York, Marcel Dekker, Inc.

Nemeroff, C.B., and Schatzberg, A.F. (1999) *Recognition and treatment of psychiatric disorders: A psychopharmacology handbook for primary care*, Washington, DC, American Psychiatric Press, Inc.

NIH Consensus Conferences (1993) Impotence. *Journal of the American Medical Association* **270**, 83–90.

*Physician's desk reference*, 54th edition. (2000) Oradell, N.J., Medical Economics Data Production Co.

Pies, R.W. (1998) *Handbook of essential psychopharmacology*. Washington, DC, American Psychiatric Press, Inc.

*Practice guidelines for major depressive disorder in adults.* American Psychiatric Association, Washington, DC, 1998.

Preskorn, S.H. (1999) *Outpatient management of depression*, 2nd edition. Caddo OK, Professional Communications, Inc.

Preston, G.C., Brazell, C., Ward, C., Broks, P., Traub, M., and Stahl, S.M. (1988) The scopolamine model of dementia: determination of central cholinomimetic effects of physostigmine on cognition and biochemical markers in man. *Journal of Psychopharmacology* **2**(2), 67–79.

Prien, R.F., and Robinson, D.S., (eds.) (1994) *Clinical evaluation of psychotropic drugs: principles and guidelines*. New York, Raven Press.

Quitkin, F.M., Adams, D.C., Bowden, C.L., Heyer, E.J., Rifkin, A., Sellers, E.M., Tandon, R., and Taylor, B.P. (1998) *Current psychotherapeutic drugs*, 2nd edition. Washington, DC, American Psychiatric Press, Inc.

Robins, L.N., and Regier, D.A. (1991) *Psychiatric disorders in America: the epidemiologic catchment area study*. New York, The Free Press (Macmillan, Inc.)

Sachs, O. (1983) Awakenings, New York, EP Dutton Press.

Sambunaris, A., Keppel Hesselink, J., Pinder, R., Panagides, J., and Stahl, S.M. (1997) Development of new antidepressants. *Journal of Clinical Psychiatry* **59**(Suppl. 6), 40–53.

Schatzburg, A.F., Cole, J.O., and Debattista, C. (1997) *Manual of clinical psychopharmacology*, 3rd edition. Washington, DC, American Psychiatric Press, Inc.

Schatzburg, A.F., and Nemeroff, B. (Eds.) (1998) *Textbook of psychopharmacology*, 2nd edition, Washington, DC, American Psychiatric Press, Inc.

Schuckit, M.A. (1995) *Drug and alcohol abuse: a clinical guide to diagnosis and treatment*, 4th edition, New York, Plenum Publishing Corp.

Shader, R.I. (1994) *Manual of psychiatric therapeutics*. Boston, Little, Brown & Co.

Siegel, G., Agranoff, B., Albers, R.W., and Molinoff, P. (1999) *Basic neurochemistry: molecular, cellular and medical aspects*, 6th edition. Philadelphia, Lippincott-Raven.

Sinha, S., and Lieberburg, I. (1992) Review article. Normal metabolism of the amyloid precursor protein (APP). *Neurodegeneration* 1, 169–75.

Stahl, S.M. (1994) Is serotonin receptor down regulation linked to the mechanism of action of antidepressant drugs? *Psychopharmacology Bulletin* 30(1), 39–43.

Stahl, S.M. (1997) Mixed depression and anxiety: serotonin 1A receptors as a common pharmacological link. *Journal of Clinical Psychiatry* 58(Suppl. 8), 20–6.

Stahl, S.M. (1997) *Psychopharmacology of antidepressants*, London, Dunitz Press.

Stahl, S.M. (1998) Basic psychopharmacology of antidepressants (part 1): antidepressants have seven distinct mechanisms of action. *Journal of Clinical Psychiatry* 59(Suppl. 4), 5–14.

Stahl, S.M. (1998) Basic psychopharmacology of antidepressants (part 2): estrogen as an adjunct to antidepressant treatment. *Journal of Clinical Psychiatry* 59(Suppl. 4), 15–24.

Stahl, S.M. (1998) Enhancing cholinergic neurotransmission with the new cholinesterase inhibitors: implications for Alzheimer's disease and cognitive disorders. *Hospital Practice* 33(11), 131–6.

Stahl, S.M. (1988) Selecting an antidepressant using mechanism of action to enhance efficacy and avoid side effects. *Journal of Clinical Psychiatry* 59(Suppl. 18), 23–9.

Stahl, S.M. (1998) Mechanism of action of serotonin selective reuptake inhibitors: serotonin receptors and pathways mediate therapeutic effects and side effects (mechanism of action of SSRIs). *Journal of Affective Disorders* 12:51(3), 215–35.

Stahl, S.M. (1999) *Psychopharmacology of antipsychotics*, London, Dunitz Press.

Stahl, S.M. (1999) Selecting an atypical antipsychotic by combining clinical experience with guidelines from clinical trials. *Journal of Clinical Psychiatry* 60(Suppl 10), 31–41.

Stahl, S.M., and Shayegan, D. (2000) New discoveries in the development of antipsychotics with novel mechanisms of action: beyond the atypical antipsychotics with serotonin dopamine antagonism. In *Atypical antipsychotics* (MDT), Ellenbroek, B.A. and Cools, A.R. (Eds.). Boston, Birkhauser.

Taylor, D. McConnell, H., McConnell, D., Abel, K., and Kerwin, R. (1999) *The Bethlem and Maudsley NSH Trust. Prescribing Guidelines*, 5th edition. London, Martin Dunitz.

Vanhatalo, S., and Soinila, S. (1998) The concept of chemical neurotransmission: variations on the theme. *Annals of Medicine* 30, 151–8.

Walsh, B.P. (1998) *Child psychopharmacology*. Washington, DC, American Psychiatric Press, Inc.

Zolle, M., Jansson, A., Sykova, E., Agnati, L.F., and Fuxe, K. (1999) Volume transmission in the CNS and its relevance for neuropsychopharmacology. *Trends in Pharmacological Sciences* 30, 142–50.

# Brainstorm Features 1997–2000

Stahl, S.M. (1997) Apoptosis: neuronal death by design. *Journal of Clinical Psychiatry* 58(5), 183–5.

Stahl, S.M. (1997) Excitotoxicity and neuroprotection. *Journal of Clinical Psychiatry* 58(6), 247–8.

Stahl, S.M. (1997) Mental illness may be damaging to your brain. *Journal of Clinical Psychiatry* 58(7):289–90.

Stahl, S.M. (1997) Are two antidepressant mechanisms better than one? *Journal of Clinical Psychiatry* 58(8), 339–41.

Stahl, S.M. (1997) Awakening from schizophrenia: intramolecular polypharmacy and the atypical antipsychotics. *Journal of Clinical Psychiatry* 58(9), 381–2.

Stahl, S.M. (1997) Estrogen makes the brain a sex organ. *Journal of Clinical Psychiatry* 58(10), 421–2.

Stahl, S.M. (1997) Sex therapy for psychiatrists has a new partner: reproductive hormones. *Journal of Clinical Psychiatry* 58(11), 468–9.

Stahl, S.M. (1997) Serotonin: it's possible to have too much of a good thing. *Journal of Clinical Psychiatry* 58(12), 520–1.

Stahl, S.M. (1998) Brain fumes: yes, we have NO brain gas. *Journal of Clinical Psychiatry* 59(1), 6–7.

Stahl, S.M. (1998) How psychiatrists can build new therapies for impotence. *Journal of Clinical Psychiatry* 59(2), 47–8.

Stahl, S.M. (1998) Nitric oxide physiology and pharmacology. *Journal of Clinical Psychiatry* 59(3), 101–2.

Stahl, S.M. (1998) Brain tonics for brain sprouts: how neurotrophic factors fertilize neurons. *Journal of Clinical Psychiatry* 59(4), 149–50.

Stahl, S.M. (1998) Recognition molecules are trailblazers for axon pathways. *Journal of Clinical Psychiatry* 59(5), 215–6.

Stahl, S.M. (1998) When neurotrophic factors get on your nerves: therapy for neurodegenerative disorders. *Journal of Clinical Psychiatry* 59(6), 343–4.

Stahl, S.M. (1998) No so selective serotonin reuptake inhibitors. *Journal of Clinical Psychiatry* 59(7), 343–4.

Stahl, S.M. (1998) What makes an antipsychotic atypical. *Journal of Clinical Psychiatry* 59(8), 403–4.

Stahl, S.M. (1998) Neuropharmacology of obesity: my receptors made me eat it. *Journal of Clinical Psychiatry* 59(9), 447–8.

Stahl, S.M. (1998) How to appease the appetite of psychotropic drugs. *Journal of Clinical Psychiatry* 59(10), 500–1.

Stahl, S.M. (1998) Getting stoned without inhaling: anandamide is the brain's natural marijuana. *Journal of Clinical Psychiatry* 59(11), 566–7.

Stahl, S.M. (1998) Using secondary binding properties to select a not so selective serotonin reuptake inhibitor. *Journal of Clinical Psychiatry* 59(12), 642–3.

Stahl, S.M. (1999) Peptides and psychiatry, part 1: How synthesis of neuropeptides differs from classical neurotransmitter synthesis. *Journal of Clinical Psychiatry* 60(1), 5–6.

Stahl, S.M. (1999) Substance P and the neurokinins, part 2: Novel peptide neurotransmitters in psychopharmacology. *Journal of Clinical Psychiatry* 60(2), 77–78.

Stahl, S.M. (1999) Peptides and psychiatry, part 3: Substance P and serendipity: novel psychotropics are a possibility. *Journal of Clinical Psychiatry* 60(3), 140–1.

Stahl, S.M. (1999) Why settle for silver, when you can go for gold? Response vs. recovery as the goal for antidepressant therapy. *Journal of Clinical Psychiatry* 69(4), 213–4.

Stahl, S.M. (1999) Mergers and acquisitions among psychotropics: antidepressant takeover of anxiety may now be complete. *Journal of Clinical Psychiatry* 60(5), 282–3.

Stahl, S.M. (1999) Antidepressants: the blue-chip psychotropic for the modern treatment of anxiety disorders. *Journal of Clinical Psychiatry* 60(6), 356–7.

Stahl, S.M. (1999) Antipsychotic polypharmacy, part 1: therapeutic option or dirty little secret. *Journal of Clinical Psychiatry* 60(7), 425–6.

Stahl, S.M. (1999) Antipsychotic polypharmacy, part 2: Tips on use and misuse. *Journal of Clinical Psychiatry* 60(8), 506–7.

Stahl, S.M. (1999) Molecular neurobiology for practicing psychiatrists, part 1: overview of gene activation by neurotransmitters. *Journal of Clinical Psychiatry* 60(9), 572–3.

Stahl, S.M. (1999) Molecular neurobiology for practicing psychiatrists, part 2: how neurotransmitters activate second messenger systems. *Journal of Clinical Psychiatry* 60(10), 647–8.

Stahl, S.M. (1999) Molecular neurobiology for practicing psychiatrists, part 3: how second messengers "turn on" genes by activating protein kinases and transcription factors. *Journal of Clinical Psychiatry* **60**(11), 731–2.

Stahl, S.M. (1999) Molecular neurobiology for practicing psychiatrists, part 4: transferring the message of chemical neurotransmission from presynaptic neurotransmitter to postsynaptic gene expression. *Journal of Clinical Psychiatry* **60**(12), 813–4.

Stahl, S.M. (2000) Molecular neurobiology for practicing psychiatrists, part 5: how a leucine zipper can turn on genes: immediate early genes activate late gene expression in the brain. *Journal of Clinical Psychiatry* **61**(1), 7–8.

# INDEX

Note: Page numbers of followed by f indicate illustrations; page numbers followed by t indicate tables.

Dementia (*Continued*)
  cognitive dysfunction in, 370, 371f, 446–447,
      447f
  memory disorders in, 478–479
  neuronal degeneration in, 117
  pathogenesis of, 114–115, 116f
  positive symptoms in, 369, 370f
  treatment of, 446–447, 447f
    quetiapine in, 435
    risperidone in, 434
    ziprasidone in, 436
Demethylation, of antidepressants, 208, 208f
Dendrites, 2, 2f, 3f, 30, 30f–32f
  destruction of, 127f
  spines on, 3f
    formation of, during menstrual cycle, 553–
        554, 559f, 560f
Dependence, drug, 500t, 501–502
  benzodiazepines, 526–527, 534f
  detoxification after, 502
  nicotine, 519, 525f
  opioids, 521
Dephosphophatases, in neurotransmission, 42f
Deprenyl, in Alzheimer's disease, 492
Depression
  in adolescents, treatment of, 154
  anxiety with, treatment of, 298–305, 300f, 304f
  in benzodiazepine withdrawal, 527
  biologic basis of, monoamine hypothesis in, *See*
      Monoamine hypothesis of depression
  in bipolar disorder, *See* Bipolar disorder
  in children
    estrogen levels and, 558
    treatment of, 153–154
  clinical features of, 136–139, 137t–141t
  vs. cocaine withdrawal, 509
  description of, 136
  diagnostic criteria for, 137, 138t, 139t
  double, 144, 147f
  epidemiology of, 137–139, 140t, 141t
  erectile dysfunction in, 546, 548f
  vs. estrogen levels during female life cycle, 557–
      558, 560, 561f–564f, 562–567, 566f
  first episode of, in adolescent girls, 563–564
  gender differences in, 557–558, 561f, 562f
  longitudinal course of, 153–154
  mania with, 136
  misconceptions about, 136–137, 137t
  natural history of, 137–139, 140t, 141t, 142,
      142f
  neurokinin hypothesis of, 188–196, 190f–197f
  neurotransmitter receptor hypothesis of, 185–
      186, 185f, 186f, 188f, 189f
  normal, vs. illness, 136
  partial remission in, 151, 151t
  patient education on, 140t
  postpartum, 561f, 562, 562f, 563f
  predisposition to, 111f
  pseudodementia in, 479
  as pseudomonoamine deficiency, 187–188, 188f,
      189f
  psychotic
    positive symptoms in, 368, 370f
    treatment of, 445

recovery from, 142, 142f, 143f
recurrence of, 142, 144f, 144t, 150, 150t
refractory, 152, 152t
  diagnosis of, 283
  treatment of, 293–294, *See also* Polypharmacy
relapse in, 142, 144f, 148, 149f
remission in, 142, 142f, 143f, 147–148, 148t,
    151–152, 151t
risk factors for, 140t
in schizophrenia, 372f, 373–374
somatization in, 136–137
suicide in, 139, 141t
as syndrome, 137, 139t
treatment of, *See also* Antidepressants
  in adolescents, 154
  antipsychotics in, 445–446
  bad news about, 150–153, 150t–152t
  in children, 153–154
  estrogen status considerations in, 563–567,
      564f, 566f
  five Rs of, 142–144, 142f–147f, 144t
  good news about, 147–148, 148t–150t, 149f,
      150
  long-term outcomes of, 142–144, 142f–147f,
      144t
  maintenance, 150, 150t
  "pooping out" in, 150–151
  refractory, 293–294, *See also* Polypharmacy
  response to, 142, 143f, 144–145, 147–148,
      147f–149f, 148t, 149t, 151–152
  vs. subtype, 144–147, 147f, 148f
  unipolar, 137
untreated, 137–139, 140t, 141t, 142, 142f
Depressive psychosis, 367–368, 444, 445f
Desferrioxamine, in Alzheimer's disease, 490–491
Designer drugs, 511, 513f
Desipramine
  in depression, 286, 287f, 290f, 293f
  in panic disorder, 353–354
Detoxification, 502
Development, of brain, *See* Neurodevelopment
Diabetes mellitus, erectile dysfunction in, 547
Diazepam
  as mood stabilizer, 271
  in panic disorder, 354–355
Diet, monoamine oxidase inhibitor interactions
    with, 214–215, 217, 219f–221f
Diethylpropion, in depression, 291f–293f
Dihydroxyphenylalanine, in dopamine synthesis,
    157, 158f
2,5-Dimethoxy-4-methylamphetamine, 511
Dimethyltryptamine, 511
Disorganization, conceptual, in psychosis, 367
Disorganized-excited psychosis, 367
Disorientation, in psychosis, 367
Dizziness
  antipsychotic-induced, 412f
  tricyclic antidepressant-induced, 226f
DMT (dimethyltryptamine), 511
DNA, *See also* Gene(s)
  in human genome, 21
  neurotransmitter effects on, 56, 57f
  in receptor down regulation, 66f
  in receptor up regulation, 67f

# REGISTRATION FORM FOR CME CREDIT

### Essential Psychopharmacology (2nd Edition)
### Stephen M. Stahl

Name of Registrant: _____

Address where CME certificate is to be sent:

_____

_____

_____

Number of category I CME credit hours claimed: _____
*(CME fee: $10 for each credit hour; $395 discounted fee for all 54 credits)*

Mail:
1. A check for the appropriate amount made payable to "UCSD, Department of Psychiatry" together with your answers and your evaluations

To:
    Stephen M. Stahl, M.D., Ph.D.
    Department of Psychiatry
    University of California, San Diego
    9500 Gilman Drive
    La Jolla, CA 92093-0603

# Essential Psychopharmacology Continuing Medical Education (CME) Post Test

## University of California San Diego Department of Psychiatry School of Medicine

### ACCME Accreditation

The University of California, San Diego School of Medicine is accredited by the Accreditation Council for Continuing Medical Education (ACCME) to sponsor continuing medical education (CME) programs for physicians. The University of California San Diego School of Medicine designates this continuing medical education activity for 54 hours of category I of the Physicians' Recognition Award of the American Psychiatric Association. Each physician should claim only those hours of credit he/she actually spent on the educational activity.

## European CME CNS Accreditation

The European Accreditation Committee for Continuing Medical Education designates this educational activity for up to 54 hours of CME CNS credit points. Partial credit is designated for each unit. Physicians should claim only those hours of credit that he/she actually spent on the educational activity. A 70% pass rate on unit tests is required for successful completion of this activity. Accreditation fee is waived for those physicians wishing to obtain European CNS credit.

## Instructions

This CME activity incorporates instructional design to enhance your retention of the didactic information and pharmacological concepts which are being presented. You are advised to go through this program unit by unit, in order, from beginning to end. You will first study the figures and read the figure legends for a single unit of instructional materials, and then go back and read the text that corresponds to that unit, reviewing the figures again as you go. After completing the text, you will then go back over the figures alone for another time. This will allow interaction with the materials, and also provide repeated exposure to the data and concepts presented both visually and in written explanations. Hopefully, this will be fun and interesting, and you will retain new information far more efficiently than you would after just reading the text or listening to a lecture on this topic.

Follow these directions to optimize your learning and retention of "Essential Psychopharmacology".

1. Go through each chapter unit one by one, from beginning to end and in order.
2. View each figure and read each figure legend.
3. Next, read the text while reviewing each figure as you go.
4. Complete the written post-test, using the answer sheet located at the end of the textbook.
5. Review the figures once again, checking any answers of which you are uncertain.
6. Photocopy and fill out the evaluation for the unit you just completed.
7. Fill out the CME registration form.
8. Pay $10 for each category I CME credit you are claiming, or a discounted fee of $395 if you are claiming all 54 credits (a $540 value, or 25% discount off the individual unit price).
9. Send the test answers, evaluations and check for the appropriate amount, payable to "UCSD Department of Psychiatry" to:

   Stephen M. Stahl, M.D., Ph.D.
   Department of Psychiatry
   University of California San Diego
   9500 Gilman Drive
   La Jolla, CA 93037

# OVERALL CONTINUING MEDICAL EDUCATION OBJECTIVES 14 INDIVIDUAL EDUCATIONAL UNITS IN TOTAL

*Up to 54 Hours of Category I Credits in Total*

Upon completing this educational program, the participant should be able to:

1. Understand the scientific basis of chemical neurotransmission.

2. Know how abnormalities in neurotransmission underlie major psychiatric disorders, including depression, anxiety disorders, psychosis, and cognitive disorders, including dementia, and drug and alcohol abuse.

3. Know that psychotropic drugs act by specific modifications of chemical neurotransmission.

4. Understand the major psychiatric disorders treated with psychotropic agents, including depression, anxiety disorders, psychosis, cognitive disorders including dementia and drug and alcohol abuse.

5. Be able to understand the unique psychopharmacological mechanisms of action of the major antidepressants, anxiolytics, antipsychotics, cognitive enhancing agents, and drugs of abuse.

6. Be knowledgeable of the mechanism of therapeutic action versus the side effects of the major members of each class of psychotropic agents.

Please see each individual unit for the specific objectives of each individual unit.


## UNIT 1: PRINCIPLES OF CHEMICAL NEUROTRANSMISSION

*Up to 3 Hours of Category I CME Credit*


## *Objectives*

1. To learn all three dimensions of neurotransmission: namely the spacial dimension, the dimension of time and the dimension of function.

2. To understand the spacial dimension as a chemically addressed vs. an anatomically addressed nervous system.

3. To understand the time dimension by knowing the difference between fast onset vs. slow onset chemical neurotransmission.

4. Understand the functional dimension of neurotransmission, gaining familiarity with excitation secretion coupling, receptor occupancy, and second messenger systems.

5. To gain an overview of molecular neurobiology as a basis for subsequent concepts developed later in this text, including how chemical neurotransmission results in the activation of neuronal genes.

6. To gain an overview of neuronal plasticity, as a basis for understanding the aging process, the development of the brain, and the action of growth factors.

## Self Assessment and Post Test

1. Please indicate which of the following is true for synaptic neurotransmission.
   a. An electrical impulse jumps from one nerve to another
   b. A chemical impulse jumps from one nerve to another
   c. An electrical impulse in one nerve is converted to a chemical impulse at the synaptic connection between two nerves which is then reconverted into an electrical impulse in the second nerve
   d. An electrical impulse in one nerve is converted to a chemical impulse at the synaptic connection between two nerves which is then converted into a chemical cascade reaching the post-synaptic genome
   e. c and d

2. The anatomically addressed nervous system is analogous to a complex wiring diagram. True or False.

3. The chemically addressed nervous system acts via a sophisticated chemical soup. True or False.

4. Some neurotransmitters act faster than others. True or False.

5. Glutamate is the universal excitatory neurotransmitter. True or False.

6. GABA is the universal excitatory neurotransmitter. True or False.

7. GABA and glutamate act by fast signals and not by slow signals. True or False.

8. Other neurotransmitters such as serotonin and norepinephrine act as slow neurotransmitters. True or False.

9. The headquarters or command center for the neuron is the DNA in its cell nucleus located in the cell body. True or False.

10. Receptor occupancy by neurotransmitters is specific to a single neurotransmitter and acts like a key fitting into a receptor lock. True or False.

11. Each neuron only contains one neurotransmitter. True or False.

12. Enzymes and receptors are both proteins synthesized in the cell body by the neuron's cell nucleus. True or False.

13. Alterations in the structure of an enzyme or a receptor can lead to a disease. True or False.

14. Once the brain is wired at the beginning of life, it stays that way forever and does not have the capability of changing once an individual reaches adulthood. True or False.

15. Although it has classically been held that neurons do not replicate after birth, recent evidence suggests that there may be replication of neurons in the mammalian brain, possibly even in humans. True or False.

16. The degree of branching of the dendritic tree of a neuron may imply how much functioning that neuron can perform. True or False.

17. Growth factors can promote synaptic connections. True or False.

18. The brain has a mechanism for revising synapses and even eliminating them throughout the lifetime of a neuron. True or False.

19. A second messenger is electrical, not chemical. True or False.

20. Some therapeutic drugs like Valium, Elavil and morphine as well as some drugs of abuse such as heroin and marijuana can act very similarly to naturally occurring neurotransmitters in the brain. True or False.

## Evaluation

|  | Strongly Agree | Somewhat in Agreement | Neutral | Somewhat Disagree | Strongly Disagree |
|---|---|---|---|---|---|
| 1. Overall this unit met my expectations to learn about principles of chemical neurotransmission. |  |  |  |  |  |
| 2. My general knowledge abut chemical neurotransmission was enhanced. |  |  |  |  |  |
| 3. The time spent reviewing chemical neurotransmission and brain function was just right. |  |  |  |  |  |
| 4. The time spent reviewing neurobiology and brain functioning was just right. |  |  |  |  |  |

| | Strongly Agree | Somewhat in Agreement | Neutral | Somewhat Disagree | Strongly Disagree |
|---|---|---|---|---|---|
| 5. The time spent reviewing three dimensions of chemical neurotransmission was just right. | | | | | |
| 6. What topics would you like to see deleted or condensed from this unit? | | | | | |
| 7. What topics would you like to see added or expanded in this unit? | | | | | |
| 8. What is your overall opinion of this unit? | | | | | |
| 9. What is your overall opinion of the usefulness of this training unit to your clinical practice? | | | | | |

## UNIT 2: RECEPTORS AND ENZYMES AS THE TARGETS OF DRUG ACTION

*Up to 3 Hours of Category I CME Credit*

## *Objectives*

1. To understand how receptors and enzymes are the targets of drug action.

2. To learn about the organization of receptor molecules, including the three parts of each receptor.

3. To gain familiarity with ion channels, transport carriers and active transport pumps.

4. To gain familiarity with second messenger systems.

5. To understand how drugs may modify chemical neurotransmission by interacting with receptors.

6. To understand how drugs may modify chemical neurotransmission by interacting with enzymes.

## Self Assessment and Post Test

1. Psychopharmacological agents act by:
   a. Inhibiting enzymes
   b. Antagonizing receptors
   c. Stimulating receptors
   d. All of the above

2. Which is not a property of the receptor super family of G protein linked receptors?
   a. Seven transmembrane regions
   b. Presence of a G protein
   c. Presence of an enzyme
   d. Presence of a second messenger
   e. Presence of an ion channel

3. A receptor is a chain of:
   a. Amino acids
   b. Fatty acids
   c. Sugars
   d. Fats

4. One of the most common organizations of a receptor in the central nervous system is for it to weave in and out of the cell membrane seven times thus creating seven transmembrane regions. True or False.

5. Transmembrane regions of receptors can be quite similar from one family of receptors to the next. True or False.

6. A neurotransmitter released from a neuron travels to a post synaptic neuron and:
   a. Interacts with a receptor in the membrane of the second neuron
   b. Gets inside the cell where it acts as a second messenger
   c. Travels straight to the nucleus of the second neuron
   d. None of the above

7. Receptors are theoretical sites of malfunctioning which could lead to nervous or mental disorders. True or False.

8. Neurotransmitters can serve as a gatekeepers to open or close a channel for an ion in a neuronal membrane. True or False.

9. Transport carriers act as a shuttle bus to allow molecules to get from the outside of the cell to the inside of the cell. True or False.

10. An active transport pump is a type of transport carrier which is linked to an energy utilizing system. True or False.

11. Neurotransmitter reuptake from the synapse is an example of molecular transport using an active transport pump. True or False.

12. In the neurotransmission process, the first event is the firing of the presynaptic neuron which releases neurotransmitter. True or False.

13. Once a neurotransmitter interacts with the receptor, it:
    a. Diffuses off the receptor
    b. Can be destroyed by enzyme
    c. Can be transported back into the presynaptic neuron
    d. All of the above

## Evaluation

| | Strongly Agree | Somewhat in Agreement | Neutral | Somewhat Disagree | Strongly Disagree |
|---|---|---|---|---|---|
| 1. Overall the unit met my expectations. | | | | | |
| 2. My general knowledge about receptors and enzymes was enhanced. | | | | | |
| 3. The time spent reviewing the pharmacology receptors was just right. | | | | | |
| 4. The time spent reviewing the pharmacology of enzymes was just right. | | | | | |
| 5. The explanation for how various chemicals work together in neurotransmission was explained well. | | | | | |
| 6. What topics would you like to see deleted or condensed from the unit? | | | | | |
| 7. What topics would you like to see added or expanded in the unit? | | | | | |
| 8. What is your overall opinion of this training unit? | | | | | |
| 9. What is your overall opinion of the usefulness of this training unit to your clinical practice? | | | | | |

# UNIT 3: SPECIAL PROPERTIES OF RECEPTORS

*Up to 2 Hours of Category I CME Credit*

## *Objectives*

1. To understand how receptors can have multiple subtypes.

2. To know the difference between an agonist and an antagonist.

3. To know the difference between an inverse agonist and an antagonist.

4. To understand both positive allosteric modulation and negative allosteric modulation.

## *Self Assessment and Post Test*

1. Allosteric modulation is:
   a. Two drugs competing for the same enzyme or receptor at the same site
   b. One drug helping or inhibiting another drug at the same receptor but at a different site on that receptor
   c. Unrelated to the presumed mechanism of action of any psychotropic drugs
   d. Presumed to be the cause of depression

2. There is only one type of receptor for each neurotransmitter. For example, there is only one serotonin receptor type. True or False.

3. Which is not a property of the super family of ligand gated ion channels?
   a. Neurotransmitter as gatekeeper ligand
   b. A G protein
   c. Allosteric modulating sites
   d. A column of receptors surrounding a central ion site

4. An agonist is the opposite of an antagonist. True or False.

5. An inverse agonist is the opposite of an agonist. True or False.

6. A partial agonist is in between a full agonist and an antagonist. True or False.

7. An antagonist can reverse both an agonist and an inverse agonist. True or False.

8. A partial agonist can be a net agonist when neurotransmitter is deficient but a net antagonist when a neurotransmitter is in excess. True or False.

9. Allosteric modulators help a neurotransmitter or hinder a neurotransmitter performing that neurotransmitter function. True or False.

10. There are two major super families of receptors including:
    a. Ligand gated ion channel
    b. Seven transmembrane G protein linked second messenger systems
    c. Allosteric modulators
    d. Both a and b

# Evaluation

| | Strongly Agree | Somewhat in Agreement | Neutral | Somewhat Disagree | Strongly Disagree |
|---|---|---|---|---|---|
| 1. Overall the unit met my expectations. | | | | | |
| 2. My general knowledge about special properties of receptors and enzymes was enhanced. | | | | | |
| 3. The time spent reviewing the pharmacology of agonists and antagonists was just right. | | | | | |
| 4. The time spent reviewing allosteric modulation was just right. | | | | | |
| 5. Time spent reviewing receptor super-families was just right. | | | | | |
| 6. What topics would you like to see deleted or condensed from the unit? | | | | | |
| 7. What topics would you like to see added or expanded in the unit? | | | | | |
| 8. What is your overall opinion of this training unit? | | | | | |
| 9. What is your overall opinion of the usefulness of this training unit to your clinical practice? | | | | | |

## UNIT 4: CHEMICAL NEUROTRANSMISSION AS THE MEDIATOR OF DISEASE ACTIONS

*Up to 2 Hours of Category I CME Credit*

## Objectives

1. To understand receptors and enzymes as targets of disease action in the central nervous system.

2. To understand the differences among three disciplines: neuroscience, biological psychiatry and psychopharmacology.

3. To understand various ways in which diseases modify synaptic neurotransmission, including molecular neurobiology and psychiatric disorders.

4. To understand how neuronal plasticity can impact psychiatric disorder.

5. To understand general principles of excitotoxicity.

6. To understand other mechanisms of disease action, including no neurotransmission, too much neurotransmission and ineffective wiring.

## Self Assessment and Post Test

1. Complex genetics suggests that psychiatric disorders are:
   a. Due to a single gene mutation
   b. Due to two gene mutations which cause all persons with such genetic abnormalities to manifest an illness
   c. The cause of psychiatric disorder is predominantly environmental
   d. Multiple lesions in the victim's DNA must be present in the right sequence and during the correct critical periods possibly with the need to have specific environmental inputs simultaneously in order to manifest the psychiatric illness

2. Neurobiology is the study of brain and neuronal functioning usually emphasizing normal brain functioning in experimental animals rather than man. True or False.

3. Biological psychiatry is the discipline evaluating abnormalities in brain biology associated with the causes or consequences of mental disorders. True or False.

4. Psychopharmacology is the discipline of discovering new drugs and understanding the actions of drugs upon the central nervous system. True or False.

5. Which of the following is not a key factor in the development of a psychiatric disorder:
   a. Genetic vulnerability to the expression of a disease
   b. Life event stressors
   c. The individual's personality, coping skills and social support
   d. Environmental influences
   e. All of the above are critical

6. For a neuron to develop properly, it must have adequate plasticity. True or False.

7. The neuron has a mechanism to destroy its synapses called excitotoxicity. True or False.

8. If excitotoxicity gets out of control, it could potentially destroy a dendrite or an entire neuron. True or False.

9. Drugs may at times be able to replace neurotransmitters which are absent from a synapse due to the death of a neuron. True or False.

10. Glutamate is the neurotransmitter which mediates excitatory neurotransmission as well as excitotoxicity. True or False.

11. Potassium is the ion which works with glutamate to mediate both excitation and excitotoxicity. True or False.

## *Evaluation*

| | Strongly Agree | Somewhat in Agreement | Neutral | Somewhat Disagree | Strongly Disagree |
|---|---|---|---|---|---|
| 1. Overall this unit met my expectations. | | | | | |
| 2. My general knowledge about how chemical neurotransmission is the target of disease action was enhanced. | | | | | |
| 3. The time spent reviewing the disciplines of neuroscience, biological and psycho-pharmacology was just right. | | | | | |
| 4. The time spent reviewing molecular neurobiology and neuroplasticity was about right. | | | | | |
| 5. The time spent reviewing excitotoxicity was just right. | | | | | |
| 6. What topics would you like to see deleted or condensed from the unit? | | | | | |
| 7. What topics would you like to see added or expanded in the unit? | | | | | |
| 8. What is your overall opinion of this unit? | | | | | |
| 9. What is your overall opinion of the usefulness of this unit to your clinical practice? | | | | | |

# UNIT 5: DEPRESSION AND BIPOLAR DISORDERS

*Up to 6 Hours of Category 1 CME Credit*

## Objectives

1. To review the diagnostic criteria for depression and bipolar disorders.

2. To review the definitions of response, remission and recovery.

3. To learn the epidemiology and natural history as well as longitudinal course of depression.

4. To understand the biological basis of depression, including the monoamine hypothesis, the neurotransmitter receptor hypothesis and the hypothesis of reduced activation of brain neurotrophic factors.

5. To understand the functioning of noradrenergic, dopaminergic and serotonergic neurons.

## Self Assessment and Post Test

1. The standard(s) usually targeted by studies seeking approval of most new antidepressants is (are):
   a. Response rates
   b. Remission rates
   c. Recovery rates
   d. Both a and b
   e. All of the above

2. Risk of relapse from depression is related to:
   a. The number of previous episodes
   b. Incomplete recovery
   c. Severity of index episode of depression
   d. Duration of index episode of depression
   e. All of the above

3. What is the best estimate for the risk of relapse into another episode of depression if an antidepressant is stopped within the first 6 to 12 months following a treatment response:
   a. Less than 5%
   b. At least 10%
   c. At least 33%
   d. At least 50%

4. What is the best estimate for the risk of relapse into another episode of depression while taking an antidepressant for the first six months following a treatment response:
   a. Less than 5%
   b. At least 10%
   c. At least 33%
   d. At least 50%

5. The chances of a depressed patient responding to any known antidepressant is one out of three.
   a. True
   b. False

6. The chances of a depressed patient responding to a placebo is one out of three.
   a. True
   b. False

7. Presynaptic alpha 2 receptors:
   a. Control norepinephrine release
   b. Control serotonin release
   c. Both
   d. Neither

8. Which serotonin receptor(s) is (are) most involved with regulating the release of serotonin?
   a. 5HT1A
   b. 5HT1D
   c. 5TH2A
   d. Both a and b
   e. All the above

9. The locus coerulus is the principal location of the cell bodies of serotonergic neurons.
   a. True
   b. False

10. The locus coeruleus in the brainstem is the principal location of the cell bodies of nonadrenergic neurons.
    a. True
    b. False

11. The monoamine hypothesis of depression suggests that depression is predominantly caused by deficiency of serotonin.
    a. True
    b. False

12. The monoamine receptor hypothesis of depression suggests that depression is caused predominantly by an absence of key monoamine receptors in the brain.
    a. True
    b. False

13. The monoamine receptor hypothesis of gene activation suggests that depression is caused by:
    a. A problem in monoamines activating critical neuronal genes
    b. An inherited genetic deficiency in a specific gene for monoamines
    c. Stress-induced reduction in the expression of genes for neurotrophic factors such as BDNF
    d. a and c
    e. All of the above

14. The neurokinin neurotransmitters include:
    a. Substance P
    b. Neurokinins A and B
    c. Tachykinins 1 and 2
    d. a and b

15. Neurokinin receptor antagonists:
    a. Are effective in reducing pain
    b. Are potential antidepressants
    c. Are effective in reducing neurogenic inflammation

## *Evaluation*

| | Strongly Agree | Somewhat in Agreement | Neutral | Somewhat Disagree | Strongly Disagree |
|---|---|---|---|---|---|
| 1. Overall the unit met my expectations. | | | | | |
| 2. My general knowledge of depression was enhanced. | | | | | |
| 3. The time spent reviewing the natural history and longitudinal course of depression was just right. | | | | | |
| 4. The time spent reviewing neurotransmitter pharmacology was just right. | | | | | |
| 5. The time spent reviewing biological theories of depression was just right. | | | | | |
| 6. What topics would you like to see deleted or condensed from this unit? | | | | | |
| 7. What topics would you like to see added or expanded in this unit? | | | | | |
| 8. What is your overall opinion of this unit? | | | | | |
| 9. What is your overall opinion of the usefulness of this unit to your clinical practice? | | | | | |

# UNIT 6: CLASSICAL ANTIDEPRESSANTS, SEROTONIN SELECTIVE REUPTAKE INHIBITORS AND NOREPINEPHRINE REUPTAKE INHIBITORS

*Up to 4 Hours of Category I CME Credit*

## Objectives

1. To review the monoamine receptor hypothesis of depression.

2. To review the two classical categories of antidepressants, namely MAO inhibitors and tricyclic antidepressants.

3. To review the mechanism of action of the five serotonin selective reuptake inhibitors.

4. To review adrenergic modulators such as dopamine and norepinephrine uptake inhibitors.

5. To review selective inhibitors of norepinephrine reuptake.

6. To understand how drug actions can explain not only therapeutic effects but also side effects for antidepressants.

7. To review pharmacokinetic interactions of antidepressants with other drugs.

## Self Assessment and Post Test

1. All antidepressants act by inhibiting the reuptake pump for serotonin, norepinephrine, or both.
   a. True
   b. False

2. When tricyclic antidepressants are given concomitantly with SSRIs such as fluoxetine or paroxetine:
   a. Plasma levels of the tricyclic antidepressants may rise
   b. Plasma levels of the tricyclic antidepressants may fall
   c. Plasma levels of fluoxetine or paroxetine may rise
   d. a and c

3. MAO inhibitors should not be administered concomitantly with:
   a. SSRIs (serotonin selective reuptake inhibitors)
   b. Meperidine
   c. Tyramine-containing foods
   d. All of the above

4. The mechanism of therapeutic action of SSRIs is:
   a. Stimulation of the serotonin transport pump
   b. Increasing the sensitivity of 5HT2A receptors
   c. Desensitizing somatodendritic 5HT1A autoreceptors
   d. None of the above

5. Side effects of the SSRIs such as anxiety, insomnia and sexual dysfunction may be mediated by stimulation of which serotonin receptor subtype?
   a. 5HT1A
   b. 5HT1D
   c. 5HT2A
   d. 5HT3

6. At high doses, which secondary property may apply to sertraline:
   a. 5HT2C agonist actions
   b. Blockade of dopamine transporters
   c. Blockade of muscarinic cholinegic receptors
   d. Blockade of cytochrome P450 1A2
   e. None of the above

7. At high doses, which secondary property may apply to fluoxetine:
   a. 5HT2C agonist actions
   b. Blockade of dopamine transporters
   c. Blockade of muscarinic cholinergic receptors
   d. Blockade of cytochrome P450 1A2
   e. None of the above

8. At high doses, which secondary property may apply to paroxetine:
   a. 5HT2C agonist actions
   b. Blockade of dopamine transporters
   c. Blockade of muscarinic cholinergic receptors
   d. Blockade of cytochrome P450 1A2
   e. None of the above

9. At high doses, which secondary property may apply to citalopram:
   a. 5HT2C agonist actions
   b. Blockade of dopamine transporters
   c. Blockade of muscarinic cholinergic receptors
   d. Blockade of cytochrome P450 1A2
   e. None of the above

10. The therapeutic action of bupropion is mediated in part via direct interactions with serotonergic neurotransmission.
    a. True
    b. False

11. The therapeutic action of reboxetine is mediated in part via direct interactions with serotonergic neurotransmission.
    a. True
    b. False

12. Increasing norepinephrine may cause:
    a. Antidepressant effects
    b. Improvement in attention
    c. Increase in motivation/reduction of apathy
    d. All of the above

## Evaluation

| | Strongly Agree | Somewhat in Agreement | Neutral | Somewhat Disagree | Strongly Disagree |
|---|---|---|---|---|---|
| 1. Overall the unit met my expectations. | | | | | |
| 2. My general knowledge about tricyclic antidepressants was enhanced. | | | | | |
| 3. The time spent reviewing the pharmacology of classical antidepressants, including tricyclic antidepressants and MAO inhibitors, was just right. | | | | | |
| 4. My general knowledge about serotonin selective reuptake inhibitors was enhanced. | | | | | |
| 5. The time spent reviewing serotonin selective reuptake inhibitors was just right. | | | | | |
| 6. What topics would you like to see added or expanded in this unit? | | | | | |
| 7. What is your overall opinion of this unit? | | | | | |
| 8. What is your overall opinion of the usefulness of this unit to your practice? | | | | | |

## UNIT 7: NEWER ANTIDEPRESSANTS AND MOOD STABILIZERS

*Up to 4 Hours of Category I CME Credit*

## Objectives

1. To review the mechanism of action of dual reuptake inhibitors such as venlafaxine as well as other dual action antidepressants such as mirtazapine, and serotonin 2A antagonists such as nefazodone.

2. To review the mechanism of action of lithium and five anticonvulsants used as mood stabilizers (valproic acid, carbamazepine, lamotrigine, gabapentin and topiramate).

3. To discuss the use of antidepressants in combination with other drugs and antidepressants for the treatment of patients nonresponsive to monotherapies for depression and bipolar disorders.

## Self Assessment and Post Test

1. Which of the following are serotonin 2A antagonists:
   a. Fluoxetine
   b. Nefazodone
   c. Paroxetine
   d. Mirtazapine
   e. b and d

2. Blocking a monoamine reuptake pump with an antidepressant can oppose the actions of drugs which block presynaptic alpha 2 receptors.
   a. True
   b. False

3. Dual neurotransmitter action at both serotonin and norepinephrine is possible only by combining two different psychopharmacological agents simultaneously.
   a. True
   b. False

4. Which of the following does not have selectivity for the noradrenaline transporter over the serotonin transporter:
   a. Desipramine
   b. Maprotiline
   c. Reboxetine
   d. Venlafaxine

5. Venlafaxine is a dual reuptake inhibitor of both serotonin and norepinephrine with equal potency for both transporters.
   a. True
   b. False

6. Lithium:
   a. Inhibits inositol monophosphatase
   b. Interacts with second messenger systems
   c. Blocks monoamine reuptake
   d. a and b
   e. All of the above

7. Which mood stabilizers are thought to act in part by interacting with ion channels:
   a. Carbamazepine
   b. Valproic acid
   c. Lithium

d. a and b

e. All of the above

8. Antidepressants can worsen depression in patients with bipolar disorders by inducing mania or rapid cycling.
    a. True
    b. False

9. Successful combinations of drugs for treating depressed patients resistant to monotherapies exploit pharmacologic synergies, where the total therapeutic effect may be greater than the sum of the parts.
    a. True
    b. False

10. The most accurate statement about psychotherapy for depression is that psychotherapy:
    a. Can be used instead of antidepressants for patients with marked to severe depression
    b. Has been proven to be useful for depression in all its different types, including psychodynamic, group, cognitive, behavioral and psychoanalytical psychotherapies
    c. Has been demonstrated to be synergistic with antidepressants for standardized cognitive behavioral psychotherapy
    d. All of the above

## Evaluation

| | Strongly Agree | Somewhat in Agreement | Neutral | Somewhat Disagree | Strongly Disagree |
|---|---|---|---|---|---|
| 1. Overall the unit met my expectations. | | | | | |
| 2. My general knowledge about dual action antidepressants was enhanced. | | | | | |
| 3. The time spent reviewing the pharmacology of venlafaxine, mirtazapine and nefazodone was just right. | | | | | |
| 4. The time spent reviewing mood stabilizers was just right. | | | | | |
| 5. The time spent reviewing antidepressant combinations was just right. | | | | | |

| | |
|---|---|
| 6. What topics would you like to see deleted or condensed from this unit? | |
| 7. What topics would you like to see added or expanded in this unit? | |
| 8. What is your overall opinion of this unit? | |
| 9. What is your overall opinion of the usefulness of this unit to your practice? | |

# UNIT 8: ANXIOLYTICS AND SEDATIVE HYPNOTICS

*Up to 4 Hours of Category I CME Credit*

## Objectives

1. To review a clinical description of generalized anxiety.

2. To gain an overview of the biological basis of anxiety emphasizing gamma aminobutyric acid (GABA) and benzodiazepines.

3. To gain an overview of the biological basis of anxiety with an emphasis on norepinephrine and the locus coeruleus.

4. To gain an overview of the biological basis of anxiety emphasizing the role of serotonin.

5. To discuss how the treatment of anxiety disorders is transitioning from anxiolytics such as benzodiazepines to various antidepressants.

6. To discuss and understand the mechanism of action of benzodiazepines in the treatment of anxiety.

7. To understand the role of serotonin 1A partial agonists in the treatment of anxiety.

8. To gain perspective on long term possibilities for future treatments of anxiety.

9. To review a clinical description of insomnia and sleep disorders.

10. To review the drug treatments for insomnia, including newer nonbenzodiazepine hypnotics as well as benzodiazepine and other hypnotics.

## Self Assessment and Post Test

1. Which of the following is an effective treatment for generalized anxiety disorder.
   a. Benzodiazepines
   b. Buspirone
   c. Venlafaxine
   d. a and b
   e. All the above

2. Generalized anxiety disorder is more likely to remit spontaneously or with treatment than is major depressive disorder.
   a. True
   b. False

3. If a full agonist benzodiazepine reduces anxiety, it would follow that an inverse agonist benzodiazepine would actually produce anxiety.
   a. True
   b. False

4. All of the following are true for benzodiazepines except:
   a. They are allosteric modulators of the GABA A receptor subtype
   b. They are cotransmitters with GABA itself for the GABA A receptor subtype
   c. They facilitate the influx of chloride to a cell
   d. They facilitate the inhibition of neural firing

5. The locus coerulus:
   a. Is the principle site of axon terminals for the noradrenergic system
   b. Can regulate serotonergic cell firing by its innervation of the raphe
   c. Theoretically malfunctions in obsessive compulsive disorder
   d. Regulates release of norepinephrine from its neurons through presynaptic alpha 1 receptors.

6. Buspirone's mechanism of action is:
   a. Like the benzodiazepines only on serotonin neurons
   b. Partial agonist actions on serotonin 2A receptors
   c. Partial agonist actions on serotonin 1A receptors
   d. Partial agonist actions on serotonin 1A and serotonin 2A receptors

7. Excessive activity of noradrenergic neurons can accompany some of the signs and symptoms of anxiety.
   a. True
   b. False

8. Generalized anxiety disorder (GAD) is distinct from major depressive disorder with anxiety in that it is unusual for a patient to have GAD at one point in time and major depressive disorder with anxiety at another time.
   a. True
   b. False

9. GAD is distinct from major depressive disorder with anxiety in that the drugs which are well documented to treat major depressive disorder with anxiety are not necessarily also well documented to treat GAD.
   a. True
   b. False

10. There is no major difference in outcome or risk factors for major depressive disorder with anxiety versus major depressive disorder without anxiety.
    a. True
    b. False

## Evaluation

|  | Strongly Agree | Somewhat in Agreement | Neutral | Somewhat Disagree | Strongly Disagree |
|---|---|---|---|---|---|
| 1. Overall the unit met my expectations. | | | | | |
| 2. My general knowledge about the clinical features and biological basis anxiety was enhanced. | | | | | |
| 3. The time spent reviewing the use of antidepressants and anxiolytics for the treatment of anxiety was just right. | | | | | |
| 4. The time spent reviewing insomnia and sleep disorders was just right. | | | | | |
| 5. The time spent reviewing sedative hypnotics for the treatment of insomnia was just right. | | | | | |
| 6. What topics would you like to see deleted or condensed from this unit? | | | | | |
| 7. What topics would you like to see added or expanded in this unit? | | | | | |
| 8. What is your overall opinion of this unit? | | | | | |
| 9. What is your overall opinion of the usefulness of this unit to your clinical practice? | | | | | |

# UNIT 9: DRUG TREATMENTS FOR OBSESSIVE COMPULSIVE DISORDER, PANIC DISORDER AND PHOBIC DISORDERS

*Up to 4 Hours of Category I CME Credit*

## Objectives

1. To review a clinical description of obsessive compulsive disorder.

2. To review the biological basis of obsessive compulsive disorder based upon serotonin and dopamine.

3. To review drug treatments of obsessive compulsive disorder, emphasizing serotonin reuptake inhibitors.

4. To review the clinical description of panic attacks and panic disorders.

5. To review the biological basis of panic attacks and panic disorder.

6. To review the drug treatments of panic disorder, including benzodiazepines, serotonin selective reuptake inhibitors, cognitive behavioral therapy and other treatments.

7. To review the clinical description and pharmacological treatments for phobic disorders, including social phobia.

8. To review the clinical description and pharmacological treatments for post traumatic stress disorder.

## Self Assessment and Post Test

1. The therapeutic efficacy and onset of action of an SSRI in obsessive compulsive disorder is very similar to that of an SSRI in major depressive disorder.
   a. True
   b. False

2. Only those SSRIs with FDA approved indications for different anxiety disorder subtypes actually are efficacious in such anxiety disorder subtypes.
   a. True
   b. False

3. It is best to start with a higher dose of an SSRI for the treatment of panic compared to the dose of an SSRI for the treatment of depression.
   a. True
   b. False

4. It is best to start with a higher dose of an SSRI for the treatment of bulimia compared to the dose of an SSRI for the treatment of depression.
   a. True
   b. False

5. The tricyclic antidepressant desipramine is effective in panic disorder and obsessive compulsive disorder.
   a. True
   b. False

6. A leading theory of panic disorders called the false suffocation alarm theory, postulates that false alarm is triggered by the brain during a panic attack.
   a. True
   b. False

7. SSRIs are the only antidepressants which have efficacy in the treatment of panic disorder.
   a. True
   b. False

8. Behavioral therapies and cognitive therapies are commonly less effective for the treatment of panic disorder and obsessive compulsive disorder than are the SSRIs.
   a. True
   b. False

9. If an SSRI is effective in an anxiety disorder, this implies that serotonin levels are deficient in that anxiety disorder.
   a. True
   b. False

10. If an SSRI is effective in an anxiety disorder, this implies that enhanced serotonergic neurotransmission is therapeutic for that anxiety disorder.
    a. True
    b. False

## Evaluation

|  | Strongly Agree | Somewhat in Agreement | Neutral | Somewhat Disagree | Strongly Disagree |
|---|---|---|---|---|---|
| 1. Overall the unit met my expectations. | | | | | |
| 2. My general knowledge about anxiety disorder subtypes including obsessive compulsive disorder and panic disorder was enhanced. | | | | | |
| 3. The time spent reviewing the pharmacology of treatments for OCD was just right | | | | | |

| | Strongly Agree | Somewhat in Agreement | Neutral | Somewhat Disagree | Strongly Disagree |
|---|---|---|---|---|---|
| 4. The time spent reviewing the pharmacology of the treatments of panic disorder was just right. | | | | | |
| 5. The time spent reviewing the pharmacology of phobic disorders, social phobia and post-traumatic stress disorder was just right. | | | | | |
| 6. What topics would you like to see deleted or condensed from the unit? | | | | | |
| 7. What topics would you like to see added or expanded in the unit? | | | | | |
| 8. What is your overall opinion of this unit? | | | | | |
| 9. What is your overall opinion of the usefulness of this unit to your practice? | | | | | |

## UNIT 10: PSYCHOSIS AND SCHIZOPHRENIA

*Up to 4 Hours of Category I CME Credit*

## *Objectives*

1. To review the clinical descriptions of psychosis.

2. To understand the difference between paranoid, disorganized and depressive psychosis.

3. To discuss the five dimensions of symptoms in schizophrenia, including positive, negative, cognitive, aggressive/hostile and anxious/depressed symptoms.

4. To review the biological basis of the positive psychotic symptoms.

5. To understand the different functions of the various dopamine pathways in the brain, including the mesolimbic dopamine pathway, the nigrostriatal dopamine pathway, the mesocortical dopamine pathway and the tuberoinfundibular dopamine pathway.

6. To review neurodevelopmental and neurodegenerative hypotheses of schizophrenia.

## Self Assessment and Post Test

1. A psychotic disorder is defined as one with delusions, hallucinations, and a thought disorder. True or False.

2. Schizophrenia and drug induced psychotic disorders require the presence of psychosis as a defining feature of the diagnosis. True or False.

3. Mania, depression, and cognitive disorders like Alzheimer's disease may or may not be associated with psychotic features. True or False.

4. Paranoid psychosis is characterized by severe retardation, apathy and anxious self-punishment and blame. True or False.

5. It is rare for a schizophrenic patient to commit suicide. True or False.

6. Schizophrenia is more common than depression. True or False.

7. The following are characteristic of the negative symptoms of schizophrenia except:
   a. Affective flattening
   b. Alogia
   c. Anhedonia
   d. Acalculia

8. The leading hypothesis for explaining the positive symptoms of psychosis is the overactivity of dopamine in the nigrostriatal dopamine pathway. True or False.

9. Movement disorders are mediated by abnormalities in the mesolimbic dopamine pathway. True or False.

10. The tuberoinfundibular dopamine pathway mediates the secretion of prolactin. True or False.

11. Prolonged blockade of dopamine receptors in the nigrostriatal pathway may lead to an increased sensitization of post-synaptic dopamine 2 receptors and a disorder called:
    a. Parkinsonism
    b. New symptoms of schizophrenia
    c. Tardive dyskinesia
    d. Galactorrhea

12. The severity of which dimension of symptoms in schizophrenia is best correlated with long term outcome:
    a. Positive symptoms
    b. Cognitive symptoms
    c. Affective symptoms
    d. a and b

13. Cognitive deficits in schizophrenia
    a. Include problems with sustaining and focusing attention, and prioritizing and modulating behaviors based upon social cues
    b. Include problems with verbal fluency and serial learning
    c. Resemble the short term memory deficits seen in Alzheimer's disease
    d. a and b
    e. All the above

14. A neurodevelopmental etiology for schizophrenia is suggested by all the following except:
    a. Increased incidence in those with obstetric complications in utero
    b. Premorbid and prodromal negative and cognitive symptoms in childhood and adolescence prior to onset of psychotic symptoms
    c. Increased incidence in first degree relatives
    d. Adult onset of psychotic symptoms with a downhill course during adulthood

15. A neurodegenerative etiology for schizophrenia is suggested by:
    a. Functional and structural abnormalities of brains in schizophrenic patients
    b. A downhill course after onset of psychosis
    c. Less responsiveness to antipsychotic medications the longer treatment is delayed and the more episodes of illness experienced
    d. a and c
    e. All the above

## Evaluation

| | Strongly Agree | Somewhat in Agreement | Neutral | Somewhat Disagree | Strongly Disagree |
|---|---|---|---|---|---|
| 1. Overall the unit met my expectations. | | | | | |
| 2. My general knowledge about psychosis was enhanced. | | | | | |
| 3. The time spent reviewing the five dimensions of clinical symptoms of schizophrenia was just right. | | | | | |
| 4. The time spent reviewing the dopamine pathways in the brain was just right. | | | | | |
| 5. The time spent reviewing neurodevelopmental and neurodegenerative theories of schizophrenia was just right. | | | | | |

| | |
|---|---|
| 6. What topics would you like to see deleted or condensed from the unit? | |
| 7. What topics would you like to see added or expanded in the unit? | |
| 8. What is your overall opinion of this unit? | |
| 9. What is your overall opinion of the usefulness of this unit to your practice? | |

# UNIT 11: ANTIPSYCHOTIC AGENTS

*Up to 6 Hours of Category I CME Credit*

## *Objectives*

1. To review the pharmacology of conventional antipsychotic treatments: the neuroleptics.

2. To contrast the older conventional antipsychotics with the newer atypical antipsychotics.

3. To review the importance of serotonin 2A antagonism to the atypical clinical properties of atypical antipsychotics.

4. To review the regulatory role of serotonin in each of the four major dopamine pathways.

5. To explain why atypical antipsychotics have fewer extrapyramidal side effects, less tardive dyskinesia, less prolactin elevation and better improvement of negative and cognitive symptoms of schizophrenia compared to conventional antipsychotics.

6. To review the unique pharmacological properties of several atypical antipsychotics, including olanzapine, risperidone, quetiapine, clozapine, ziprasidone and others.

7. To discuss the pharmacokinetics and drug interactions of atypical antipsychotics.

8. To discuss new drug discovery efforts in schizophrenia, including serotonin dopamine antagonists and other novel agents such as those based upon molecular and neurodevelopmental approaches to drug discovery.

## Self Assessment and Post Test

1. The first treatments for schizophrenia were based upon the knowledge that dopamine was hyperactive in the brain. True or False

2. Conventional antipsychotic drugs are also called neuroleptics. True or False.

3. Atypical antipsychotic drugs
   a. Can theoretically block mesolimbic dopamine 2 receptors preferentially, compared to nigrostriatal dopamine 2 receptors
   b. Have selective dopamine 2 antagonist properties whereas conventional antipsychotics have serotonin 2A antagonist properties as well as dopamine 2 antagonist properties.
   c. Have less EPS side effects but also less efficacy for positive symptoms than conventional antipsychotics
   d. None of the above

4. Clozapine is the atypical antipsychotic best documented to improve psychotic symptoms which are resistant to treatment with conventional antipsychotics. True or False.

5. Which of the following serotonin dopamine antagonists (SDAs) is not considered to be a first line atypical antipsychotic drug?
   a. Risperidone
   b. Quetiapine
   c. Loxapine
   d. Olanzapine

6. The pharmacological property which all atypical antipsychotics share is serotonin dopamine antagonism. True or False.

7. The new atypical antipsychotics including risperidone, olanzapine and quetiapine act by:
   a. Blocking dopamine-2 receptors
   b. Blocking serotonin-2 receptors
   c. Both of the above
   d. None of the above

8. The ratio between the blockade of serotonin receptors and dopamine receptors differs for various classes of antipsychotic drugs. True or False.

9. The interaction between dopamine and serotonin in the nigrostriatal dopamine pathway may explain why serotonin dopamine antagonists have propensity for reducing extrapyramidal reactions. True or False.

10. Which pharmacologic properties in addition to serotonin 2A/dopamine 2 antagonism characterize one or more atypical antipsychotics?
    a. Dopamine 1, 3, and 4 antagonism
    b. Serotonin 1D, 3, 6 and 7 antagonism
    c. Serotonin and norepinephrine reuptake blockade
    d. Alpha 1, alpha 2, muscarinic and histaminic receptor blockade
    e. All of the above

11. Which atypical antipsychotics are substrates for CYP450 1A2?
    a. Clozapine
    b. Olanzapine
    c. Risperidone
    d. a and b
    e. All the above

12. Which atypical antipsychotics are substrates for CYP450 2D6?
    a. Risperidone
    b. Clozapine
    c. Olanzapine
    d. All of the above

13. Smoking could lower clozapine and olanzapine plasma levels. True or False.

14. Molecular approaches to the treatment of schizophrenia attempt to identify an abnormal gene product in order to compensate for this abnormality. True or False.

15. Treatment of schizophrenia in the future may involve the combinations of various mechanisms of action simultaneously. True or False.

## Evaluation

|  | Strongly Agree | Somewhat in Agreement | Neutral | Somewhat Disagree | Strongly Disagree |
|---|---|---|---|---|---|
| 1. Overall the unit met my expectations. | | | | | |
| 2. My general knowledge about serotonin regulation of dopamine was enhanced. | | | | | |
| 3. The time spent reviewing conventional neuroleptic drugs was just right. | | | | | |
| 4. The time spent reviewing the class of atypical antipsychotics was just right. | | | | | |
| 5. The time spent reviewing individual atypical antipsychotic drugs was just right. | | | | | |
| 6. What topics would you like to see deleted or condensed from this unit? | | | | | |

| | |
|---|---|
| 7. What topics would you like to see added or expanded in this unit? | |
| 8. What is your overall opinion of this unit? | |
| 9. What is your overall opinion of the usefulness of this unit to your practice? | |

## UNIT 12: COGNITIVE ENHANCERS

*Up to 4 Hours of Category I CME Credit*

## *Objectives*

1. To review the clinical description of cognitive disorders, including both disorders of attention and disorders of memory.

2. To review the psychopharmacology of attention, including the roles of norepinephrine and dopamine.

3. To review the use of stimulants in disorders of attention, including attention deficit disorder in children and adults.

4. To discuss the role of acetylcholine pharmacology and cholinergic pathways in mediating memory functions.

5. To discuss how memory disorders, including Alzheimer's disease, impact cholinergic neurotransmission.

6. To discuss the new cholinesterase inhibitors and treatments for enhancing memory or slowing the pace of memory loss in Alzheimer's disease.

7. To compare and contrast the cholinesterase inhibitors tacrine, donepezil, metrifonate, rivastigmine, and others.

8. To review the neuropathology of Alzheimer's disease, and its relationship to the amyloid cascade hypothesis and the glutamate excitotoxic hypothesis of Alzheimer's disease.

9. To discuss future cognitive enhancers, including enhancement of attention and memory.

## *Self Assessment and Post Test*

1. Disorders of attention may be mediated via disruption of dopaminergic and/or noradrenergic neurotransmission in the cerebral cortex. True or False

2. The following are enhancers of attention in attention deficit disorder:
   a. Stimulants such as methylphenidate and d-amphetamine
   b. Alpha 2 agonists such as guanfacine and clonidine
   c. Stimulating antidepressants such as bupropion
   d. a and b
   e. All of the above

3. What is true about the pharmacology of d-amphetamine versus the pharmacology of d,l-amphetamine?
   a. d-Amphetamine acts at both norepinephrine and dopamine synapses whereas d,l-amphetamine acts predominantly at dopamine synapses
   b. d-Amphetamine acts predominantly at dopamine synapses whereas d,l-amphetamine acts at both dopamine and norepinephrine synapses
   c. d-Amphetamine acts predominantly at norepinephrine synapses
   d. d,l-Amphetamine acts predominantly at dopamine synapses

4. In attention deficit hyperactivity disorder
   a. Inattention and hyperactivity are both mediated by the nigrostriatal dopamine pathway
   b. Inattention and hyperactivity are both mediated by the mesocortical dopamine pathway
   c. Inattention is mediated by the mesocortical dopamine pathway but hyperactivity is mediated by the nigrostriatal dopamine pathway
   d. Inattention is mediated by the nigrostriatal dopamine pathway but hyperactivity is mediated by the nigrostriatal dopamine pathway.

5. Acetylcholine can be destroyed by:
   a. Acetylcholinesterase
   b. Butyrylcholinesterase
   c. Both
   d. Neither

6. The area of the brain where acetylcholine controls memory includes:
   a. Cholinergic pathways throughout the brain
   b. Cholinergic pathways in brainstem and striatum
   c. Cholinergic pathways arising from the nucleus basalis of Meynert
   d. a and c

7. Alzheimer's disease is a clinical diagnosis and not a pathological diagnosis. True or False.

8. Neuropathology of Alzheimer's disease includes:
   a. Neuritic plaques
   b. Amyloid deposition
   c. Neurofibrillary tangles
   d. All of the above

9. The amyloid cascade hypothesis of Alzheimer's disease states that:
   a. The DNA codes for an abnormal amyloid precursor protein
   b. The amyloid precursor protein initiates a lethal chemical cascade in neurons resulting in the formation of plaques and tangles

c. Plaques and tangles are linked to the formation of dementia symptoms in patients who develop these abnormalities in their neurons
   d. All of the above

10. Apo-E is:
   a. A binding protein which binds to beta amyloid and normally removes it
   b. The amyloid itself
   c. Only exists in an abnormal form
   d. Is unrelated to theories of Alzheimer's disease

11. The pharmacological benefits of cholinesterase inhibitors include:
   a. Functional improvement of central cholinergic neurotransmission at cholinergic synapses in the neocortex
   b. Stimulation of both muscarinic and nicotinic cholinergic receptors
   c. Possible protection against neuronal degeneration mediated through nicotinic receptor activation
   d. Possible modification of amyloid precursor protein processing, mediated through muscarinic receptor activation
   e. All of the above

12. Which of the following cholinesterase inhibitors is selective for acetylcholinesterase over butyrylcholinesterase:
   a. Donepezil
   b. Tacrine
   c. Rivastigmine
   d. Metrifonate
   e. a and c

13. There are two major subtypes of acetyl choline receptors called:
   a. Muscarinic and nicotinic
   b. M1 and M2
   c. Cholinergic and adrenergic

14. Current drugs approved for the treatment of Alzheimers disease in the United States have the common mechanism of action being:
   a. Blockade of cholinergic receptors
   b. Direct stimulation of cholinergic receptors
   c. Blockade of cholinesterase, destruction of acetyl choline
   d. Enhancing release of acetyl choline

15. Treatments of Alzheimer's disease in the future will likely involve multiple pharmacology approaches with mixing and matching different mechanisms of therapeutic action. True or False.

## Evaluation

| | Strongly Agree | Somewhat in Agreement | Neutral | Somewhat Disagree | Strongly Disagree |
|---|---|---|---|---|---|
| 1. Overall the unit met my expectations. | | | | | |
| 2. My general knowledge about disorders of attention was enhanced. | | | | | |
| 3. The time spent reviewing the pharmacology of stimulants for treating attention deficit was just right. | | | | | |
| 4. The time spent reviewing the pharmacology of cholinergic neurons and cholinesterase inhibitors was just right. | | | | | |
| 5. The time spent reviewing the pathophysiology of disorders of memory, including Alzheimer's disease, was just right. | | | | | |
| 6. What topics would you like to see deleted or condensed from this unit? | | | | | |
| 7. What topics would you like to see added or expanded in this unit? | | | | | |
| 8. What is your overall opinion of this unit? | | | | | |
| 9. What is your overall opinion of the usefulness of this unit to your practice? | | | | | |

# UNIT 13: PSYCHOPHARMACOLOGY OF REWARD AND DRUGS OF ABUSE

*Up to 4 Hours of Category I CME Credit*

## Objectives

1. To define various terms used in the study of drug abuse, including use, abuse, dependence, intoxication, withdrawal.

2. To review the psychopharmacology of reward, with special reference to the mesolimbic dopamine pathway use and abuse of benzodiazepines.

3. To review the pharmacology of marijuana and the endocannabinoids (i.e., the brain's own marijuana).

4. To review the pharmacology of stimulants, including cocaine and amphetamine and their actions on dopaminergic systems.

5. To review the hallucinogens and designer drugs and their actions on serotonin neurons.

6. To review the pharmacology of phencyclidine and its actions on glutamate neurons.

7. To review the pharmacology of nicotine.

8. To review the pharmacology of alcohol, and agents to reduce alcohol consumption including acamprosate and naltrexone.

9. To review the pharmacology of the opiates.

10. To review the psychopharmacology of obesity.

## Self Assessment and Post Test

1. DSM-IV has an accepted definition for addiction based upon a very severe form of drug abuse. True or False.

2. Benzodiazepines are rarely abused and are not known to create dependence or to produce withdrawal when discontinued. True or False.

3. There are three types of opiate receptors called alpha, beta and gamma. True or False.

4. Stimulants are thought to act predominantly upon the dopamine system. True or False.

5. Hallucinogens are thought to have important actions as partial agonists at serotonin-2A receptors. True or False.

6. Marijuana acts on:
   a. Norepinephrine receptors
   b. Serotonin receptors

c. Glutamate receptors

d. Endogenous cannabinoid receptors

7. Nicotine from smoking acts upon:
   a. Muscarinic cholinergic receptors
   b. Nicotinic cholinergic receptors
   c. Both a and b
   d. None of the above

8. A leading hypothesis for a final common pathway of drug abuse is the meso-limbic dopamine pathway and the psychopharmacology of pleasure. True or False.

9. Transdermal nicotine administration can assist in the withdrawal of:
   a. Alcohol
   b. Smoking cessation
   c. Benzodiazepine cessation

10. Pharmacology of alcohol is understood to be:
    a. Action as an enhancer of GABA neurotransmission
    b. Action as an inhibitor of glutamate neurotransmission
    c. Possible modulator of opioid systems
    d. Possible modulator of endogenous cannabinoid systems
    e. All of the above

11. Treatment of alcohol abuse and dependence can be facilitated by:
    a. Acamprosate which can reduce the withdrawal distress and craving when alcohol is withdrawn
    b. Naltrexone which blocks the euphoria of alcohol when alcohol is drunk
    c. 12 Step programs
    d. a and b
    e. All of the above

## Evaluation

| | Strongly Agree | Somewhat in Agreement | Neutral | Somewhat Disagree | Strongly Disagree |
|---|---|---|---|---|---|
| 1. Overall the unit met my expectations. | | | | | |
| 2. My general knowledge about drug abuse was enhanced. | | | | | |
| 3. The time spent reviewing the pharmacology of stimulants, hallucinogens and opiates was just right. | | | | | |

| | Strongly Agree | Somewhat in Agreement | Neutral | Somewhat Disagree | Strongly Disagree |
|---|---|---|---|---|---|
| 4. The time spent reviewing the pharmacology of marijuana, nicotine and alcohol was just right. | | | | | |
| 5. The time spent reviewing the psychopharmacology of pleasure was just right. | | | | | |
| 6. What topics would you like to see deleted or condensed from this unit? | | | | | |
| 7. What topics would you like to see added or expanded in this unit? | | | | | |
| 8. What is your overall opinion of this unit? | | | | | |
| 9. What is your overall opinion of the usefulness of this unit to your practice? | | | | | |

## UNIT 14: SEX-SPECIFIC AND SEXUAL FUNCTION–RELATED PSYCHOPHARMACOLOGY

*Up to 4 Hours of Category I CME Credit*

## Objectives

1. To explore the psychopharmacology of the human sexual response, including libido, arousal and orgasm.

2. To discuss the pathophysiology of erectile dysfunction (impotence) in men.

3. To review nitric oxide as a neurotransmitter system.

4. To review estrogen's function as a neurotrophic factor in the brain.

5. To clarify the role of estrogen and how it is linked to mood and mood disorders across the female life cycle.

6. To discuss the potential role of estrogen in cognitive function and cognitive disorders such as Alzheimer's disease.

## Self Assessment and Post Test

1. Which psychopharmacological mechanism(s) are most closely linked to libido (sexual desire):
   a. Dopamine
   b. Prolactin
   c. Nitric oxide
   d. Phosphodiesterase
   e. a and b

2. Which psychopharmacological mechanism(s) are most closely linked to sexual arousal (i.e., erections in men and lubrication and swelling in women)
   a. Nitric oxide
   b. Acetylcholine
   c. Phosphodiesterase
   d. All of the above

3. Which neurotransmitter can inhibit orgasm (and ejaculation in men)?
   a. Nitric oxide
   b. Serotonin
   c. Acetylcholine
   d. Norepinephrine

4. What percentage of men with severe depression experience erectile dysfunction?
   a. 15%
   b. 33%
   c. 60%
   d. 90%

5. What is false about nitric oxide?
   a. It is an anesthetic
   b. It is present in car exhaust fumes
   c. It is synthesized from arginine
   d. Its target of neurotransmission is iron in the enzyme guanylate cyclase

6. Seldenafil (Viagra) is
   a. An inhibitor of nitric oxide synthetase (NOS)
   b. An inhibitor of guanylate cyclase
   c. An inhibitor of phosphodiesterase V
   d. An inhibitor of adenylate cyclase

7. Estrogen receptors
   a. Can form transcription factors when they bind to estrogen that activate genes called estrogen response elements
   b. Are active in brain only during neurodevelopment and sexual differentiation
   c. Have neurotrophic actions on monoamine neurons through the lifetime of both men and women
   d. a and c
   e. All of the above

8. Which of the following is true about depression and reproductive hormones?
   a. Depression is linked to testosterone levels in men across their life cycles
   b. Depression is linked to estrogen levels, especially rapid shifts in estrogen levels, in women across their life cycles
   c. Depression is linked to reproductive events in women
   d. b and c
   e. All the above

9. Which are the greatest periods of vulnerability for depression across the female life cycle?
   a. Prepubescence
   b. Postpartum
   c. Postmenopausal
   d. Perimenopausal
   e. b and c

10. Which of the following is not true about estrogen?
   a. It is an antidepressant with comparable efficacy to SSRIs in the treatment of major depressive disorder
   b. Can improve mood in perimenopausal women with prominent vasomotor symptoms such as hot flushes and insomnia
   c. Can enhance the actions of antidepressants in some women
   d. Can reduce the chances of developing Alzheimer's disease
   e. All are true

## Evaluation

|  | Strongly Agree | Somewhat in Agreement | Neutral | Somewhat Disagree | Strongly Disagree |
|---|---|---|---|---|---|
| 1. Overall the unit met my expectations. | | | | | |
| 2. My general knowledge about the role of neurotransmitters in the human sexual response was enhanced. | | | | | |
| 3. The time spent reviewing the actions of psychotropic drugs upon libido, arousal and orgasm was just right. | | | | | |
| 4. The time spent reviewing nitric oxide pharmacology and neurotransmission were just right. | | | | | |

| | Strongly Agree | Somewhat in Agreement | Neutral | Somewhat Disagree | Strongly Disagree |
|---|---|---|---|---|---|
| 5. The time spent reviewing estrogen as a neurotrophic factor, and its links to mood and cognition across the female life cycle was just right. | | | | | |
| 6. What topics would you like to see deleted or condensed from this unit? | | | | | |
| 7. What topics would you like to see added or expanded in this unit? | | | | | |
| 8. What is your overall opinion of this unit? | | | | | |
| 9. What is your overall opinion of the usefulness of this unit to your practice? | | | | | |

# ANSWER SHEET

## UNIT 1: PRINCIPLES OF CHEMICAL NEUROTRANSMISSION

1. a b c d e
2. True False
3. True False
4. True False
5. True False
6. True False
7. True False
8. True False
9. True False
10. True False

11. True False
12. True False
13. True False
14. True False
15. True False
16. True False
17. True False
18. True False
19. True False
20. True False

## UNIT 2: RECEPTORS AND ENZYMES AS TARGETS OF DRUG ACTION

1. a b c d
2. a b c d e
3. a b c d
4. True False
5. True False
6. a b c d
7. True False

8. True False
9. True False
10. True False
11. True False
12. True False
13. a b c d

## UNIT 3: SPECIAL PROPERTIES OF RECEPTORS

1. a b c d
2. True False
3. a b c d
4. True False
5. True False

6. True False
7. True False
8. True False
9. True False
10. a b c d

## Unit 4: Chemical Neurotransmission as the Mediator of Disease Actions

1. a b c d
2. True False
3. True False
4. True False
5. a b c d e
6. True False
7. True False
8. True False
9. True False
10. True False
11. True False

## Unit 5: Depression and Bipolar Disorders

1. a b c d e
2. a b c d e
3. a b c d
4. a b c d
5. True False
6. True False
7. a b c d
8. a b c d e
9. True False
10. True False
11. True False
12. True False
13. a b c d e
14. a b c d
15. a b c

## Unit 6: Classical Antidepressants, Serotonin Selective Reuptake Inhibitors and Noradrenergic Reuptake Inhibitors

1. True False
2. a b c d
3. a b c d
4. a b c d
5. a b c d
6. a b c d e
7. a b c d e
8. a b c d e
9. a b c d e
10. True False
11. True False
12. a b c d

## Unit 7: Newer Antidepressants and Mood Stabilizers

1. a b c d e
2. True False
3. True False
4. a b c d
5. True False
6. a b c d e
7. a b c d e
8. True False
9. True False
10. a b c d

# UNIT 8: ANXIOLYTICS AND SEDATIVE HYPNOTICS

1. a b c d e
2. True False
3. True False
4. a b c d
5. a b c d

6. a b c d
7. True False
8. True False
9. True False
10. True False

# UNIT 9: DRUG TREATMENTS FOR OBSESSIVE COMPULSIVE DISORDER, PANIC DISORDERS AND PHOBIC DISORDERS

1. True False
2. True False
3. True False
4. True False
5. True False

6. True False
7. True False
8. True False
9. True False
10. True False

# UNIT 10: PSYCHOSIS AND SCHIZOPHRENIA

1. True False
2. True False
3. True False
4. True False
5. True False
6. True False
7. a b c d
8. True False

9. True False
10. True False
11. a b c d
12. a b c d
13. a b c d e
14. a b c d
15. a b c d e

# UNIT 11: ANTIPSYCHOTIC AGENTS

1. True False
2. True False
3. a b c d
4. True False
5. a b c d
6. True False
7. a b c d
8. True False

9. True False
10. a b c d e
11. a b c d e
12. a b c d
13. True False
14. True False
15. True False

## Unit 12: Cognitive Enhancers

1. True False
2. a b c d e
3. a b c d
4. a b c d
5. a b c d
6. a b c d
7. True False
8. a b c d

9. a b c d
10. a b c d
11. a b c d e
12. a b c d e
13. a b c
14. a b c d
15. True False

## Unit 13: Psychopharmacology of Reward and Drugs of Abuse

1. True False
2. True False
3. True False
4. True False
5. True False
6. a b c d

7. a b c d
8. True False
9. a b c
10. a b c d e
11. a b c d e

## Unit 14: Sex-Specific and Sexual-Function Related Psychopharmacology

1. a b c d e
2. a b c d
3. a b c d
4. a b c d
5. a b c d

6. a b c d
7. a b c d e
8. a b c d e
9. a b c d e
10. a b c d e